The Nurse Practitioner in Long-Term Care

Guidelines for Clinical Practice

Barbara White

DrPH, APRN, BC

Adult Gerontological Nurse Practitioner

Deborah Truax

MS, APRN, BC

Adult Gerontological Nurse Practitioner

JONES AND BARTLETT PUBLISHERS

Sudbury, Massachusetts

BOSTON   TORONTO   LONDON   SINGAPORE

World Headquarters
Jones and Bartlett Publishers
40 Tall Pine Drive
Sudbury, MA 01776
978-443-5000
info@jbpub.com
www.jbpub.com

Jones and Bartlett Publishers
Canada
6339 Ormindale Way
Mississauga, Ontario L5V 1J2
Canada

Jones and Bartlett Publishers
International
Barb House, Barb Mews
London W6 7PA
United Kingdom

Jones and Bartlett's books and products are available through most bookstores and online booksellers. To contact Jones and Bartlett Publishers directly, call 800-832-0034, fax 978-443-8000, or visit our website www.jbpub.com.

Substantial discounts on bulk quantities of Jones and Bartlett's publications are available to corporations, professional associations, and other qualified organizations. For details and specific discount information, contact the special sales department at Jones and Bartlett via the above contact information or send an email to specialsales@jbpub.com.

The authors, editor, and publisher have made every effort to provide accurate information. However, they are not responsible for errors, omissions, or for any outcomes related to the use of the contents of this book and take no responsibility for the use of the products and procedures described. Treatments and side effects described in this book may not be applicable to all people; likewise, some people may require a dose or experience a side effect that is not described herein. Drugs and medical devices are discussed that may have limited availability controlled by the Food and Drug Administration (FDA) for use only in a research study or clinical trial. Research, clinical practice, and government regulations often change the accepted standard in this field. When consideration is being given to use of any drug in the clinical setting, the health care provider or reader is responsible for determining FDA status of the drug, reading the package insert, and reviewing prescribing information for the most up-to-date recommendations on dose, precautions, and contraindications, and determining the appropriate usage for the product. This is especially important in the case of drugs that are new or seldom used.

Production Credits
Executive Editor: Kevin Sullivan
Acquisitions Editor: Emily Ekle
Associate Editor: Amy Sibley
Editorial Assistant: Patricia Donnelly
Production Director: Amy Rose
Production Editor: Carolyn F. Rogers
Senior Marketing Manager: Katrina Gosek

Cover Design: Kate Ternullo
Cover Image: © Photodisc
Composition: Pre-Press Company, Inc.
Printing and Binding: Malloy, Inc.
Cover Printing: Malloy, Inc.
Figures 7-1 and 7-3 through 7-40 are courtesy
of Dr. Habif.

Library of Congress Cataloging-in-Publication Data

The nurse practitioner in long-term care : guidelines for clinical practice / [edited by] Barbara White,
Deborah Truax.
    p. ; cm.
    Includes bibliographical references and index.
    ISBN-13: 978-0-7637-3429-9 (casebound : alk. paper)
    ISBN-10: 0-7637-3429-2 (casebound : alk. paper)
1. Geriatric nursing. 2. Nurse practitioners. 3. Long-term care of the sick. I. White, Barbara S. II. Truax, Deborah.
    [DNLM: 1. Long-Term Care. 2. Nurse Practitioners. WY 152 N9733 2007]
RC954.N87 2007
    618.97'0231—dc22

                                              2006022671

6048
Printed in the United States of America
10 09 08 07 06   10 9 8 7 6 5 4 3 2 1

~ *Dedication* ~

To my husband, Dick, who shows me daily the wisdom, strength, generosity, and spirit of successful aging.

Barbara White

To my parents, Ed and Gloria Hamwi; thank you for all your love, guidance, and support throughout my life. And to my husband, Steve; you're the best husband I could ask for.

Deborah Truax

Contents

SECTION III   Special Considerations

22 Pain Management   515
Pegi Black

Preface

As the population of the United States increases, so will the need for nursing home care. Approximately one-fifth of the United States population will be 65 or older by the year 2030. Even now, the fastest growing segment of the population is 85 years of age and older. Despite our efforts at health promotion and disease prevention, it is estimated that the nursing home population will more than double by the year 2030.

There is a growing trend in health care to use advanced practice nurses (APNs) to manage patients in nursing homes. Currently, advanced practice nurses provide patient care in about 20% of the nation's more than 16,000 nursing homes (Mezey et al., 2005). It is hoped that this trend will grow as the population ages. APNs serve as integral members of the healthcare team. APNs are ideal providers in this setting, as we bring expertise in direct patient care and patient advocacy. APNs also possess additional knowledge and skills, through master's education, in the diagnosis and management of acute and chronic illness within our scope of practice.

Several models of practice have developed to help the advanced practice nurse provide services in long-term care settings: (a) the private practice model, in which the nurse practitioner sees the patients in a nursing home for subacute care, rehabilitation, or as long-term residents; (b) the health maintenance organization model, in which nurse practitioners are assigned to nursing homes to manage subscribers' care on a daily basis with a collaborating physician; (c) nurse practitioners and other APNs employed by a facility to provide care to residents; (d) nurse practitioners working with organizations that contract to manage the nursing home patients for a practice; and (e) nurse practitioner-owned businesses that provide care for patients in a variety of residential settings. In each case, the nurse practitioner assumes responsibilities for the medical management of older adults with multi-system disease as part of an interdisciplinary team.

The goal of long-term care is to provide health related services in an efficient and cost effective manner, without compromising quality of care while preserving quality of life. Using advanced practice nurses as care providers in nursing homes has clearly demonstrated positive patient outcomes.

The types of services and care delivered in long-term care facilities have dramatically changed over the past two decades. The nursing home population is becoming more medically complex. Patients admitted directly from the acute care hospital require skilled care, such as administration of intravenous antibiotics, wound care, tube feeding, and rehabilitation. They present management challenges to the nurse practitioner because of their complex medical needs and psychosocial issues.

While many gerontological nurse practitioner programs include theoretical content and clinical experiences in long-term care settings, many nurse practitioners who elect to practice in these settings may not have had in-depth preparation in medical management of patients with multiple chronic and sub-acute diseases, in rehabilitation medicine, in coordination of care with several disciplines and agencies, in the multitude of government regulations that must be taken into account to maintain a legal practice in nursing homes, and in the interpersonal and end-of-life issues and decision making required of a care provider in these settings. Additionally, many nurse practitioners working in long-term care settings may have been educated as family or adult nurse practitioners and have had limited education in medical management of the geriatric patient or in the special needs of such clients in long-term care settings.

As the population ages, most APNs will have a caseload that includes a large number of older adults. Because the burden of illness continues to increase with advancing age, all nurse practitioners will face the management of patients with comorbidities and increasing frailty. It will be important for all APNs to have an understanding of the unique presentations of disease in the elderly and their unique responses to illnesses and medications.

The purpose of this book is to provide APNs, particularly nurse practitioners, with a collection of guidelines specific to the needs of frail elderly patients in nursing homes. It is also intended for use by nurse practitioners and other APN students to guide their clinical experiences in the nursing home setting. The guidelines will also be useful for any APN working with older adults in primary, sub-acute, or acute care settings. To date, few books in the field have focused specifically on the nursing home patient. This book is intended to fill this gap by addressing many of the issues unique to this setting.

The book is not intended to be a substitute for but rather an adjunct to the protocols required for legal practice as a nurse practitioner. The guidelines in this book are not tailored to any specific nurse practice act. The nurse practitioner using these guidelines must be familiar with the scope of practice where he or she resides. The American Nurses Association *Scope and Standard of Advanced Practice Registered Nurses* (ANA, 1996) concludes:

> The individual advanced practice registered nurse is responsible for identifying the scope of practice permitted by state and federal laws and regulations, the professional code of ethics, and professional practice standards. Furthermore, the nurse's competence is circumscribed by his or her experience, education, knowledge, and abilities.

The book is written in three sections. The first section deals with general principles of patient management in the nursing home, including specifics of the environment, general principles of patient management, and legal and ethical issues of care. Section II deals with selected diseases and conditions commonly encountered in nursing homes, arranged alphabetically by system. The third section discusses special considerations and situations encountered in the nursing home, including wound care, nutrition, podiatry, pain management, and end-of-life issues.

Discussions of specific diseases and conditions address epidemiology, assessment, diagnosis, and nonpharmacologic as well as pharmacologic management. Patient, family, and staff education as well as recommendations for consultation are also included. The authors have made every attempt to present material that is age-specific and that agrees with current clinical evidence. We recognize that the field of geriatrics is constantly evolving as new information regarding the treatment and management of our patients emerges. Available Internet resources and references or bibliographies are included to allow the reader to investigate topics in greater depth and to remain current in clinical practice issues.

Though the authors acknowledge that younger, disabled individuals currently reside in long-term care facilities, we have not addressed their care in this current edition.

REFERENCES

American Nurses Association (ANA). (1996). *Scope and standards of advanced practice registered nursing.* Washington, DC: Author.

Mezey, M., Burger, S. G., Bloom, H. G., Bonner, A., Bourbonniere, M., Rowers, B., et al. (2005). Experts recommend strategies for strengthening the use of advanced practice nurses in nursing homes. *Journal of the American Geriatrics Society, 53,* 1790–1797.

Acknowledgments

The authors gratefully acknowledge the generous gift of willing and enthusiastic contributors who shared their expertise in the development of this project. We also want to thank the reviewers who helped assure that our content is relevant and accurate. We would like to thank our editors, Kevin Sullivan, Amy Sibley, and Carolyn Rogers, for their vision, commitment, persistence, and patience during the writing and production of this manuscript. Finally, we would like to thank the hundreds of patients and residents in nursing homes and elsewhere with whom we have learned our practice and honed our skills. They have taught us that growing old is not for the weak but for the strong and persevering; and that the latter part of our lives is as precious as our youth.

Contributors and Reviewers

AUTHORS

Barbara S. White, DrPH, APRN, BC
California State University, Long Beach, CA

Deborah Truax, MS, APRN, BC
Kaiser Permanente, Southern California

CONTRIBUTORS

Doreen Bacon, NP, MSN
Kaiser Permanente, Southern California

Pegi Black, MSN, NP-BC
VA Long Beach Healthcare System

A. Christine Butler, CRNP
Palliative Care, Washington Adventist Hospital, Takoma Park, MD

Cathleen K. Case, MS, APRN, BC
Fallon Clinic, Dermatology, Worcester, MA

David F. Casey, MD
Kaiser Permanente, Southern California

Deborah Caswell, MS, APRN-C
Assistant Director, Gonda (Goldschmied) Vascular Center, UCLA

Yung-In Choi, MD
Joslin Diabetes Center at University of California, Irvine

Deborah Cox, MSN, CRNP-F
Caroline Nursing & Rehabilitation Center

Eileen Croke, EdD, APRN
California State University, Long Beach, CA

Guy D. Danon, DPM
Private Practice, Long Beach, CA

Julia A. Eggert, PhD, GNP-C, AOCN
Clemson University

Michelle Eslami, MD
Professor of Medicine, Division of Geriatrics, David Geffen School of Medicine, UCLA

Evonne Fowler, CNS, CWOCN
Kaiser Permanente Southern California

Mary Jacob, PhD, RD
California State University, Long Beach, CA

Bethsheba Johnson, MSN, CNS, GNP-BC
Southside Health Association/Luck Care Center Midwest AIDS Training & Education Center

Marianne C. McCarthy, PhD, APRN, BC
Arizona State University

Theodore Holmes O'Leary
Medical Defense Attorney, Los Angeles, CA

Debra Priest-Bakerjian, PhD, FNP
President, GeriHEALTHsolutions

Leslie Saltzstein Wooldridge, MSN, RNCS, GNP
Hackley Health at the Lakes Women's Center, Bladder Control Clinic, Muskegon, MI

Valisa Saunders, MN, APRN, GNP, BC
Kaiser Permanente Hawaii

Eileen Simpson, MS, PNP, AGNP
Kaiser Permanente Southern California

Aquilina T. Saw, MD
Clinical Professor, Department of Physical Medicine and Rehabilitation, University of California, Irvine

REVIEWERS

Janice T. Chussil, ANP

Jane Jeys, LVN, WCC

Patrice Leonard, MD

Jennifer Rogers, MS, FNP

Eileen Seibert, MD

James R. Sides, MD

David Snook, MD

SECTION I

General Principles

CHAPTER 1

The Nurse Practitioner in the Skilled Nursing Facility

Debra Priest-Barkejian

INTRODUCTION

Historically, long-term care facilities, and particularly nursing homes, were believed to be places where elderly, frail, and disabled people were placed to receive assistance in basic activities of daily living (ADLs). The typical image is the elderly woman with no family who had to go to the nursing home because she could no longer care for herself and, to some extent, this is still true. However, skilled nursing facilities are much more complex now, accepting patients from the hospital just a few days postoperatively or with recent acute illness. Nurse practitioners working in a skilled nursing facility must not underestimate the complexity of the patients who reside there long term or who are admitted for a short-term stay. This chapter will provide an overview of issues important to nurse practitioners who provide care to nursing home patients.

UNDERSTANDING THE OVERALL ENVIRONMENT

Long-term care encompasses a variety of healthcare services provided over a sustained period of time (weeks to years) to all ages of patients for a wide range of health conditions. Long-term care can be provided in institutional settings such as nursing homes and residential care facilities, or in community-based settings and private homes. Care requirements vary but include assistance with ADLs, acute posthospitalization rehabilitation, respite care, and total care for dependent patients with multiple chronic illnesses. Although nurse practitioners play an integral role in providing care in all settings, the focus here will be on issues that are specific to the nursing facility.

Long-term care facilities are a subset of the overall health delivery system in the United States that includes acute hospitals, long-term care inpatient facilities, outpatient clinics, and physician offices. In addition, there are a variety of specialized freestanding facilities that include clinics, pharmacies, physical therapy, radiology, dialysis centers, and other allied health offices. The key factor in determining whether a facility provides long-term care is whether the mission of the facility is to provide ongoing care versus acute care and how the facility is licensed in the state. This chapter will focus primarily on the skilled nursing facility with an occasional reference to other types of long-term care facilities.

Skilled nursing facilities must be licensed by the state for long-term, chronic care residents and/or for short-term hospital patients admitted for the purpose of rehabilitation prior to discharge home. Short-term stay patients typically are acutely ill and may have a higher acuity of care than the chronic long-term care residents. Medicare covers patients in skilled nursing facilities who have a 3-day qualifying stay in the acute care hospital for short-term rehabilitation. Medicare covers all of the facility charges under Medicare Part A as a hospital benefit. Nurse practitioners (and other clinicians) are paid through Medicare Part B for all Medicare patients in the nursing facility.

Skilled nursing facilities are organized in different ways. They may be privately or publicly owned, they may be for profit or not for profit, and they may have as few as 10 beds or up to thousands of beds. The average size facility in the United States is approximately 100 beds and is typically a for-profit facility. The facility may have a single owner or may be part of a chain of facilities. The facility characteristics are important for nurse practitioners to know so that they can understand how the facility operates and who is responsible for establishing the internal administrative processes and procedures. Before considering the internal environment of the nursing home, it is important that nurse practitioners understand the overall regulatory environment in which they must operate.

THE REGULATORY ENVIRONMENT

Nurse practitioners, as all other clinical providers, are subject to a variety of federal and state laws and regulations. Nursing practice is regulated by the State Nurse Practice Act; however, how a nurse may practice within the skilled nursing facility is subject to additional regulations. The regulations may differ depending on whether they are aimed at nursing practice or at how nurse practitioners are reimbursed. It is critical that nurse practitioners understand the regulations that guide both practice and reimbursement in order to be in compliance. Regulations may differ somewhat depending on whether a facility is licensed for Medicare, Medicaid, both, or neither.

In general, individual states are responsible for establishing the regulations for how skilled nursing facilities function. In addition, the federal government sets minimum standards of care for all facilities. Nurse practitioners must know how the regulations affect not only their individual practice, but also the nursing facility itself, the staff that is employed there, and the residents who are cared for in the facility.

QUALITY OF CARE IN THE SKILLED NURSING FACILITY

In a pivotal 1986 report, the Institute of Medicine (IOM) Committee on Nursing Home Regulations published recommendations to Congress to enact major reforms of the regulations later embedded in the Omnibus Reconciliation Act of 1987 (OBRA 87). OBRA 87 added several standardized requirements for all United States nursing homes such as a uniform Resident Assessment Instrument (RAI), a set of essential assessment items in the Minimum Data Set (MDS), more detailed Resident Assessment Protocols (RAP), and a standardized Online Survey Certification and Reporting (OSCAR) System (Hawes, et al., 1997). These changes substantively changed the nursing home industry and began to address the quality of care problems described in the report.

Subsequently, a follow-up study found that, while there was some improvement in the overall quality of nursing home care, there remained several serious problems such as pressure sores, malnutrition, urinary incontinence, and untreated pain that needed to be addressed (Wunderlich & Kohler, 2001). The committee made a number of recommendations to strengthen staffing, improve reimbursement, and ensure quality assurance through greater external oversight, all designed to improve the quality of nursing home care. Nurse practitioners need to be familiar with these facility requirements in order to understand their role in facility compliance issues.

The Center for Medicare and Medicaid Services (CMS) is responsible for establishing nursing home standards and monitoring compliance through the survey process. Following up on the 2001 IOM report, all US nursing facilities now have unannounced surveys conducted every 9–15 months to monitor compliance with CMS and state standards. States are responsible for conducting these surveys; however, they evaluate compliance with both state and federal regulations. In addition, all complaints regarding poor quality of care must be investigated by the state (Harrington & Carrillo, 1999).

Deficiencies in meeting the standards are rated by scope and severity. There are 12 categories of severity from *A* to *L*, with *L* being the most severe. Scope refers to the number of patients that are affected by a particular deficiency. Deficiencies below the level of *C* are considered to be "not in substantial compliance" and are subject to sanctions and even termination from the Medicare and Medicaid programs. The greater the scope, the more severe the sanctions are for the facility. State surveyors may be in the facility for a range of days, typically 2–7 days, depending on the size of the facility and the problems found in the survey. During the survey, the nursing home staff is required to address issues that are brought up and have an opportunity to correct some problems on the spot. Nurse practitioners can assist the staff during the survey process by responding to surveyors' questions when appropriate. The survey process is an important element in monitoring the quality of care in the skilled nursing facility, and nurse practitioners should be familiar with the areas of deficiencies given to the facility. Deficiencies must be addressed by the facility with a plan of correction. Nurse practitioners can play an important role in assisting in the development of correction plans by providing staff education or suggesting changes in policies, procedures, and processes.

Another important regulatory issue for nursing homes and nurse practitioners is the requirement of the MDS, a comprehensive patient assessment completed by the nursing staff for each patient admission to the facility. The MDS is standardized and required in all US nursing homes. It provides both administrative and clinical data about the patient. This data is transmitted to CMS and updated on a regular basis and provides a comprehensive profile of nursing home patients across the country. Nurse practitioners should not only be familiar with the MDS, but also have input into the changes that occur in the MDS on an ongoing basis. In fact, in order to bill for a comprehensive assessment visit, the MDS should reflect an annual history and physical update or a change in the patient's care plan. This requires coordination between the nurse practitioner and the staff and writing orders that are clear in terms of identifying and managing a new resident problem.

The MDS data are also the basis for individual quality indicators (QIs), which are specific elements that are designed to signal potential problems in care. These QIs are aggregated from individual scores to a facility-level total. Surveyors use the facility QIs to identify potential quality issues such as weight loss, pressure ulcers, incontinence, depression, bed fastness, and physical restraints. For example, if a facility has a large number (more than the state average) of residents with weight loss, that QI is triggered and surveyors will examine the charts of those individuals with weight loss to determine whether the facility is managing weight loss appropriately. It is important to remember though, that just because a QI is triggered, it does not mean that the facility is in the wrong. It is simply a mechanism for the surveyors to use to look to see if there is a pattern of poor quality care.

Nurse practitioners and physicians play an important role in managing these clinical problems as well as assisting the facility to improve quality by improving their care systems. Weight loss in residents is a prime example. By monitoring their resident's weights on a regular basis, nurse practitioners can intervene early to identify avoidable versus unavoidable weight loss. Interventions that address avoidable weight loss or documentation that weight loss is unavoidable is essential to ensure that quality of care standards are met. Many facilities have received deficiencies, not because they were necessarily doing anything wrong, but because the medical record lacked appropriate documentation to indicate the weight loss was unavoidable. Lastly, nurse practitioners may identify a systemic problem in a facility by highlighting issues that affect weight loss such as lack of a social dining environment or inadequate assistance with feeding residents. This is an excellent example of how, working with the other members of the clinical team (facility staff, dieticians, and medical directors), a nurse practitioner may affect positive outcomes in a facility's residents.

UNDERSTANDING THE INTERNAL NURSING HOME ENVIRONMENT

Nurse practitioners are an important part of the interdisciplinary team (IDT) in the nursing home. There are usually two levels of IDTs, patient level and facility level. The IDT that addresses individual patient problems typically consists of the facility director of nurses (DON) or designee, dietician (RD), social services director (SSD), physical or occupational therapy (PT/OT), and the activities director. These team members are responsible for quarterly meetings with the resident and/or their family to review and update the individual care plan. In addition, the primary care physician (PCP) and/or nurse practitioner, the medical director, facility administrator, pharmacy consultant, psychologist/psychiatrist, or geropsychiatric nurse practitioner collaborate depending upon the issues being discussed. The facility-level IDT is comprised of many of the members of the previous group plus the medical director, utilization review nurse, and the infection control nurse. This team is responsible for meeting quarterly to address facility wide issues.

To understand and be able to effectively function in the nursing home, nurse practitioners must be familiar with how nursing homes are staffed and how they function overall. Similar to acute care hospitals, nursing is the largest department in a nursing home. As opposed to the acute care hospital, however, certified nursing assistants (CNAs) comprise the largest group within nursing and provide the majority of direct patient care in a nursing home. Licensed nurses, including licensed vocational/practical nurses (LVNs, LPNs) and registered nurses (RNs), are a small percentage of the total "nursing staff" and most facilities have more LVNs/LPNs than RNs as nurses in charge of providing direct patient care.

The nurse to patient ratio varies between facilities and for each of the different shifts. However, the following ratios are the typical national average:

Day shift: 1 CNA to 8 residents
1 licensed nurse to 30 residents

Afternoon/
evening shift: 1 CNA to 10 residents
1 licensed nurse to 30 residents

Night shift: 1 CNA to 15 residents
1 licensed nurse to 60 residents

Nurse staffing ratios are a critical factor influencing the overall quality of care in a nursing home. Several studies have shown that higher ratios of nurses to patients, particularly registered nurses, improve the quality of care and quality of life of the residents (Harrington, et al., 2000; Kayser-Jones, et al., 2003; Kovner & Harrington, 2002). Whenever possible and appropriate, nurse practitioners should be sensitive to staffing levels and encourage hiring of a greater number of unlicensed and licensed staff, particularly RNs, to improve quality care.

Nursing Functions in Nursing Homes

Licensed nurses provide a variety of functions within the nursing home setting, including both direct and indirect care. Each facility differs in how they employ the nursing staff to provide different services, but the following are some examples found in most facilities.

Direct care functions include the following:

• Charge Nurse

The charge nurse passes medications, provides treatments, documents patient condition, and supervises CNA care for a group of residents

• Treatment Nurse

Some facilities use a separate treatment nurse who changes dressings, provides wound care, manages gastrostomy site care, and provides catheter care.

• Admission Coordinator

This nurse evaluates potential residents for admission, coordinates with hospital discharge planners to facilitate admissions from hospitals, and coordinates with families to admit patients directly from home or other nursing facilities.

• MDS Coordinator

This nurse is responsible for gathering and transmitting all of the facility MDS data to Medicare. The scope of this job varies among facilities. Some nursing homes require the MDS coordinator to actually perform each assessment and fill in the form; however, most facilities ask the MDS coordinator to work with the charge nurses and other staff to obtain the information and ensure that the document is filled out appropriately. MDS data is obtained upon admission and then updated quarterly and annually for all nursing home residents. Patients who are admitted from a hospital for rehabilitation under Medicare Part A require the initial assessment within 5 days and additional assessments at 14, 30, 60, and 90 days or until the patient is discharged.

• Infection Control Nurse

This nurse is responsible for identifying potential sources of infection and preventing the spread of infections within the facility. This is usually the nurse who organizes and coordinates vaccinations such as influenza and pneumococcal. In addition, this nurse is usually responsible for monitoring the tuberculosis (TB) program, making sure that residents get a tuberculin skin test, or chest X-ray if they are positive converters, upon admission and on a regular basis according to the facility policy. The infection control nurse often coordinates with the county or state on infection control issues such as infection control standards and procedures for organisms such as methicillin-resistant *Staphylococcus aureus* (MRSA). Nurse practitioners should be familiar with the infection control standards of care within their geographic area and work with the infection control nurse to maintain the safety of their residents.

- Utilization Review

This nurse is responsible for evaluating the status of each resident to determine the ongoing requirements of care. The utilization review (UR) nurse monitors whether the patient meets the requirement to stay in the facility in either a short-stay or long-stay status. The specific standards vary dependent upon who is paying for the services. For Medicare Part A, Medicaid, and most managed care organizations, patients must meet strict guidelines of needing skilled care and making progress in rehabilitation. In most instances, patients may pay privately to extend their stay beyond what third-party payers will allow. The UR nurse conducts regular meetings in conjunction with other members of the interdisciplinary team to evaluate that progress.

- Director of Staff Development

The director of staff development (DSD) nurse is responsible for the orientation and ongoing education of the unlicensed staff.

In some facilities this nurse also conducts programs to hire and train nursing assistants. There are strict federal guidelines on the continuing education requirements for CNAs, and each state establishes the number of hours CNAs must receive training. Some facilities require the DSD to maintain the CNA work schedule and act as their direct supervisor.

- Quality Assurance

All nursing homes must have a quality assurance (QA) or quality improvement program. In large nursing homes, one nurse may be assigned to this duty, but most often this position is combined with one of the others. The QA nurse is responsible for establishing a program and coordinating with the director of nurses and the medical director on a regular basis. The nurse practitioner can be an effective member of this team. Making contact with the QA nurse and offering assistance is a way to become involved in the quality improvement issues in the facility.

ALLIED NURSING HOME STAFF

State and federal regulations designate a number of services that must be available to nursing home residents. Each facility must provide social services, therapies, activities, and dietary services. The following services may either be in-house or be contracted, but they must be available as resident needs require.

- Social Service Staff

These individuals assist residents with a variety of issues such as finances, outside medical appointments, legal matters, discharge planning, and other social service issues. Nurse practitioners can work with the social service staff to obtain outside medical consultations and other social needs for their residents. Social service staff also are very effective in working with families and conservators to meet patients'/residents' needs. Social service staff document quarterly in the medical record.

- Activities Director

This staff member must develop an activity plan for each resident. The activities can be organized either in a group or one on one for residents who can't leave their rooms or who do not like group activities. The activity plan must be individualized and documented in the medical record. The activity director's documentation is often a source for nurse practitioners to understand the day-to-day life of their patients.

- Therapy Services

These services consist of physical therapy, occupational therapy, and speech-language therapy. Some facilities have in-house therapy departments that provide daily services. Others contract for services as needed by residents. Nurse practitioners should be familiar with how therapy can be ordered for residents. For Medicare Part A patients, therapy is often a required daily service. If the resident has Medicare Part B, therapy can be ordered on a less frequent basis, 2–3 times per week, and on discharge. The availability of acute therapy for Medicaid residents varies by state. Some states have generous programs, and others' programs provide extremely limited service, sometimes with no services available to the nursing home resident at all. This presents a challenge for the nurse practitioner to find appropriate services for residents who do not have Medicare or a private insurance. Familiarity with county or nonprofit programs can be helpful in identifying services such as pool therapy, transportation services, and other types of therapeutic treatments that might be available to

Medicaid-eligible residents. An excellent source for information on available Medicaid services is the local county hospital.

- Pharmacy Services

Facilities must contract with a consultant pharmacist to review each resident's medications on a monthly basis. The pharmacy consultant ensures that the resident's medications meet the regulatory guidelines as well as drug safety standards. Nurse practitioners should monitor the pharmacy recommendations for their residents and respond appropriately. These pharmacists can also provide consultation to the nurse practitioner on the therapeutic use of medications, drug-to-drug interactions, effective formulary substitution, and other practical issues on prescribing or furnishing.

- Registered Dietician

The registered dietician (RD) provides an individualized dietary plan for each resident. In addition, the dietician monitors nutritional needs on a regular basis and oversees the dietary department of the facility. Most nursing homes contract this service, which means the RD is not on site every day; however, the dietician must be available for admissions and for any nutritional problems that arise. Nurse practitioners should obtain dietary consultations for residents with nutrition-related problems such as anorexia, weight loss/weight reduction, or specialized dietary needs.

- Dental, Podiatry, Optometry, Audiometry, and Psychiatric Services

These services must also be available to residents and are typically contracted out to private clinicians. Nurse practitioners should ask who provides these services and how often the routine care is available. In most facilities, dental, podiatry, optometry, and audiometry services are regularly scheduled but can also be ordered for specific problems. Psychiatric consultations are typically requested on a case-by-case basis.

The nursing home is truly an interdisciplinary environment. As a primary care provider, the nurse practitioner is integral to facilitating the total care needs of their residents and must be familiar with what services are available and how they can be accessed in each facility.

NURSING HOME LEADERSHIP

The following sections detail the various positions most commonly found in the leadership structure of nursing homes.

Facility Administrator

This individual is responsible for the overall management of the facility, which includes hiring and supervising department managers, financial oversight, ensuring resident safety, providing leadership and guidance to the staff, and maintaining compliance with all local, state, and federal regulations. The administrator is the voice for the nursing facility owners and is responsible to the ownership, the staff, the residents and their families, and to the government agencies for the overall environment of the facility and the care that is provided. The administrator hires both the director of nursing and the medical director and works closely with these leaders on an ongoing basis. Nurse practitioners should introduce themselves to the facility administrator when first entering a facility to provide care.

Medical Director

All nursing homes must have a physician as the medical director who is responsible for ensuring that the standards of medical care are met within the facility. The medical director must participate in the oversight of resident medical care, infection control, and the quality improvement program. The medical director must provide direct patient care decisions when the primary care physician is unavailable. Some medical directors may also be primary care providers for several patients in the facility. Medical directors work closely with the director of nursing and other staff members to ensure that quality of care standards are met. Medical directors are responsible for making sure that medical staff is properly credentialed. It is in the nurse practitioner's best interest to find out the credentialing requirements of the facility and to provide a credentialing packet to the nursing home. In many facilities it is the administrator or the nursing director who actually maintains the packets. A typical credentialing packet in a nursing home includes copies of the following:

- Current licenses

- Professional certifications

- Drug Enforcement Agency (DEA) number

- National Provider Identifier (NPI)

- Malpractice insurance

- Standardized protocols, signed by both the nurse practitioner and the collaborating physician

Director of Nursing

All nursing homes must have a director of nursing (DON). This is the only position that is required to be a registered nurse by regulation. The scope of this position is dependent upon the size of the facility and the corporate climate of the ownership. Smaller facilities may have the DON actually providing direct patient care as a charge nurse in addition to fulfilling other nursing roles. Larger facilities usually have the DON in a management position, not providing direct patient care. The DON is responsible for all nursing services in the facility. The director usually reports to the facility administrator and works closely with the medical director as well. The DON plays a critical role in the nursing facility, particularly where there are no other registered nurses. The DON sets and maintains the quality standards of nursing care, is responsible for ensuring that systems of care are in place, hires and sustains the nursing workforce, and represents not only the nurses but also the patients and families in all facility-related activities. The DON is responsible for responding to patient and family complaints about care. The DON is responsible for overseeing the state survey as it relates to nursing care issues and for developing the plan of corrections for any patient care-related deficiencies. This is a critical position and one that requires extensive knowledge of the regulatory environment, nursing management, and patient care. Nurse practitioners should get to know the facility DON and maintain a working relationship, partnering with the DON in resident quality-of-care issues. As a team, the nurse practitioner and nursing director are a formidable force in improving the quality of care and quality of life for the nursing home residents.

THE ROLE OF THE NURSE PRACTITIONER IN NURSING HOMES

Nurse practitioners can play an integral role in the nursing home and can facilitate systematic improvements through their advanced practice role. Nurse practitioners have three overall roles in the nursing home, that of clinician, educator, and leader.

- The clinical role involves the provision of evidence-based direct patient care in collaboration with a physician.

- The educator role includes patient and family teaching as well as nursing facility staff instruction. Nurse practitioners have many opportunities to provide impromptu education during patient care rounds. An example might be when noticing improper positioning or an unusual rash. Calling for staff to come in to observe a problem and discussing a solution can be an effective means of education when framed in a positive manner. In addition, most nurse practitioners volunteer to conduct more formal classes for either the unlicensed or the licensed staff on such topics as falls, urinary incontinence, pressure ulcers, and weight loss.

- The leadership role includes setting exemplary professional standards for the entire nursing home staff in the role of nurse, educator, researcher, and patient advocate.

BECOMING A SKILLED NURSING FACILITY CLINICAL PROVIDER

Nurse practitioners may enter the nursing facility in a variety of ways. They may be employed directly by a facility, a physician or physician group, insurance company, or they may be self-employed, dependent upon state regulations.

Employment Models

Responsibilities within the nursing home may differ, depending upon employment status. Nurse practitioners may be employees or work as independent contractors for a group. In either case they may be paid a specific salary or work on a fee-for-service contract. Nurse practitioners should become knowledgeable about their state regulations and employment contracts prior to entering into any negotiations. In her book, *The Nurse Practitioner's Business Practice and Legal Guide*, Carolyn Buppert (2004) provides an excellent resource on employment contracts and other business and legal matters.

Nurse practitioners employed by a facility often are responsible for monitoring the day-to-day condition of all facility residents. They may be responsible for assessing acute changes, coordinating with the patient's physician, participating in meetings, working with families, as well as providing leadership and education to the nursing staff. Nurse practitioners employed or contracted by a physician or physician group usually work collaboratively with a physician to provide direct patient care to a specific set of residents. These nurse practitioners usually provide alternating routine visits after the physician has performed the initial admission visit. In addition, in this setting, nurse practitioners often provide many of the acute visits to the residents.

Some managed care organizations, such as Kaiser Permanente, have employed nurse practitioners to provide complementary care to the primary care physician for their insured. Another model is a subsidiary of United Healthcare, called Evercare, which started as a Medicare demonstration project using nurse practitioners to provide acute care and intensive subacute services in the nursing home to reduce hospitalization rates. This program continues to be an effective model for nurse practitioner practice. Another source of employment for nurse practitioners is the Veteran's Administration, which employs a large cadre of nurse practitioners to provide care for their long-term care residents. There are other, usually smaller, private for-profit businesses that either contract for or employ nurse practitioners in long-term care settings. Nurse practitioners interested in working for one of these companies can often gain information through a search on the Internet, attendance at conferences, or through the local telephone directory.

EDUCATIONAL PREPARATION OF NURSE PRACTITIONERS

Historically, nurse practitioners attended classes and received a certificate in a nurse practitioner specialty. Currently, however, most nurse practitioners are advance practice nurses with masters' degrees and are certified through a national certifying body such as the American Nurses Credentialing Center (ANCC) or the American College of Nurse Practitioners (ACNP). Nurse practitioners are independent practitioners who may work autonomously within the scope of their state's nurse practice act. For any procedures or processes that cross over into medical practice, nurse practitioners must work under standardized procedures or protocols that are created collaboratively with the physician with whom they work. This is particularly relevant when nurse practitioners diagnose illnesses or utilize their prescriptive authority. The scope of nurse practitioner practice varies by state. An excellent resource for understanding state to state differences is *The Pearson Report*, published annually in the *American Journal for Nurse Practitioners*.

Nurse practitioners who provide collaborative patient care should always ensure they are fully licensed and credentialed, have prescriptive authority as allowed by their state nurse practice act, and carry their own mal-practice insurance. Their collaborative role should be clearly stated within their standard-ized procedures and their contract with the employer. In addition, nurse practitioners in nursing homes must have National Provider Identifiers (NPIs) for both Medicare and Medicaid. Applications for Medicare NPIs can be downloaded from the Medicare Web site at www.cms.gov. The application is several pages long and must be filled out completely and correctly. Incorrect applications will be returned for corrections, which can substan-tially delay the process. It is in the nurse prac-titioner's best interest to read the instructions carefully. Medicaid provider applications differ by state, but most states have them available through their Department of Health Services Web sites. Some billing agencies can be help-ful in assisting nurse practitioners to obtain NPI numbers.

If billing for services, it is important that nurse practitioners ensure that the billing agency they hire will both bill secondary insurances and send out statements to patients who do not have a secondary insurance. Nurse practitioners who do not understand the billing process should look for a course that explains this process. Professional organi-zations such as the National Conference of Gerontological Nurse Practitioners (NCGNP) and the American Medical Directors Associa-tion (AMDA) present courses annually that focus on nursing home billing for practition-ers. In addition, nurse practitioners must be careful that the physician or physician group that employs them bill for their services cor-rectly. All nurse practitioners must have their own Medicare PIN and must bill under this PIN number even if their reimbursement is reassigned to their employer. Nurse practi-tioners are reimbursed at 85% of the physician allowed rate in most instances. The only exception is if the nurse practitioner is billing "incident to," which indicates the physician is

actually present onsite in an office setting. This is actually never allowable in a nursing facility unless the physician has a private office in the facility and the care provided occurred in that private office.

Nurse practitioners who are employees may either negotiate an hourly or monthly salary or they may negotiate a percentage of reimbursements.

DOCUMENTATION AND CHARTING IN LONG-TERM CARE

The long-accepted adage that if something has not been charted it has not been done has probably never been more true than it is in the nursing home setting. Nurse practitioners are held to the same standards and the same con-sequences as physicians when it comes to billing, coding, and documentation of their nursing home visits. Nurse practitioners should be cautious and not be lulled into a false sense of security because they are employed by a physician who does the med-ical billing. Medicare holds each practitioner responsible for their own billing, coding, and documentation.

Nursing home documentation standards are more rigorous than either office or hospi-tal standards. Nurse practitioners must become familiar with both the *Current Proce-dural Terminology* (CPT) *Manual*, which is pro-duced annually by the American Medical Association (AMA) and contains all medical procedure codes, and the *International Codes of Diagnosis* (ICD) *Manual*, which provides diag-nostic and procedure codes. Currently ICD version 9 is being used, however, ICD-10 will be implemented soon (Centers for Medicare and Medicaid Services, 2006). Both the CPT and ICD manuals are updated every year. It is the responsibility of the nurse practitioner to review the new codes each year, generally available in October.

Nurse practitioners must document accurately and appropriately to substantiate the billing code for each nursing home visit. Nursing home medical records are subject to frequent audits, and there are substantial fines associated with unsubstantiated codes. Failure to understand and comply with billing, coding, and documentation standards may result in charges of fraud that carry a $10,000 fine and loss of Medicare and Medicaid privileges. Accurate documentation does the following:

- Provides evidence of medical necessity of the visit, which is a CMS requirement for all nursing home visits

- Illustrates appropriateness of patient care

- Offers verification of Medicare compliance with codes used for billing

- Enhances communication between providers

- Substantiates the quality of care provided

- Facilitates utilization review

- Provides a method for other nursing home staff to understand the current condition and medical problems of the resident

- Aids in data collection for research and education

The Centers for Medicare and Medicaid Services has published extensive guidance for how clinicians must document nursing home care. This is based on a set of guidelines adopted by the AMA several years ago and revised several times. The revisions adopted in 1997 are currently being used for nursing home Evaluation and Management (E&M) services. According to these standards, the following is required:

- Medical records should be complete and legible.

- Patient encounter documentation should include the following:

  ○ The reason for the encounter

  ○ Any relevant history

  ○ Pertinent physical examination findings

  ○ Prior diagnostic test results

  ○ System specific assessment

  ○ Clinical impression or diagnosis

  ○ Plan of care

  ○ Date and legible identity of observer

- Rationale for ordering diagnostic and ancillary services should be easily inferred if not documented.

- Providers should have access to past and present diagnoses.

- Risk factors should be identified.

- There should be documentation of the patient's progress, response to treatment, changes in treatment, and revisions of diagnosis.

Documentation is an invaluable tool for long-term care providers and can be used for reasons other than proof of an action or evidence that a particular procedure has been performed. Inspections of provider documentation by Medicare officials, however, are a reality and appropriate charting is a necessity for Medicare reimbursement.

Documentation audits may be random or they may also be triggered by the nurse practitioner's practice pattern. This can occur when practice patterns fall outside an area standard. For example, nurse practitioners may get audited because they bill more frequently for comprehensive visits than the area average. This is usually easily explained because they spend more time with residents and families and perform more detailed examinations. In these cases the documentation will substantiate the codes. On the other hand, if the documentation does not substantiate the code, the visit will be down coded by the carrier. If a pattern develops, the nurse practitioner can be sanctioned or fined.

Appropriate documentation demands serious attention. Nurse practitioners must understand the elements of the exam, how to document properly, and then how to code to get the reimbursement they deserve for the time spent. It is poor policy to simply do minimal documentation and use the minimal code to avoid audits. Nurse practitioners who provide quality care should not be afraid to perform appropriate and necessary services and to bill for that service to the extent allowed by the guidelines.

Nursing Home Billing Codes

To document appropriately, nurse practitioners must understand the various billing codes that are used to describe the care provided. The CPT manual provides the entire list (hundreds) of these procedural billing codes (American Medical Association, 2006). Billing codes and document requirements are reevaluated annually by CMS, so clinical providers must be attentive to potential changes in the regulations. A list of references appears at the end of this chapter for current information on billing codes and appropriate documentation.

Fortunately, nursing home E&M codes are limited in number and are divided into three types of visits. Brief descriptions of the most typical reasons for these codes are listed below; however, to fully understand these codes, nurse practitioners are encouraged to read the E&M guidelines in detail. The E&M standards take into consideration the complexity of the problems, the extent of the examination required, the risk to the patient, and the level of medical decision making by the clinician.

Comprehensive Assessments

99304 Initial nursing facility care, per day, for the evaluation and management of a patient; requires the following three key components:

- A detailed or comprehensive history
- A detailed or comprehensive examination
- Medical decision making that is straightforward or of low complexity

Examples include the following:

- Nursing home admission for a dementia patient with no medical complications. Dementia has been documented and diagnosed previously to this admission.
- Readmission after brief hospitalization for acute illness with no changes to ongoing care.

99305 Initial nursing facility care, per day, for the evaluation and management of a patient; requires the following three key components:

- A comprehensive history

- A comprehensive examination

- Medical decision making of moderate complexity

Usually, the problem(s) requiring admission are of moderate severity. Examples include the following:

- Admission from home of stable patient with 1–2 chronic illnesses whose functional condition has deteriorated

- Readmission from acute hospital of patient with moderate problem such as pneumonia but no significant changes to baseline care. Requires management of acute illness and minor changes in chronic medications. May require straightforward therapy.

- Admission from hospital after surgery for routine rehabilitation with no medical complications

99306 Initial nursing facility care, per day, for the evaluation and management of a patient; requires the following three key components:

- A comprehensive history

- A comprehensive examination

- Medical decision making of high complexity.

Usually, the problem(s) requiring admission are of high severity. Examples include the following:

- New admission from acute care hospital or home with three or more chronic illnesses

or with complications of acute illness or surgical procedure that may cause unpredictable course

Subsequent Assessments

There are now four codes for subsequent nursing facility care, as outlined in the following sections.

99307 Subsequent nursing facility care, per day, for the evaluation and management of a patient, requires at least two of the following three key components:

- A problem-focused interval history

- A problem-focused examination

- Straightforward medical decision making

Usually, the patient is stable, recovering, or improving. Examples include the following:

- Straightforward conjunctivitis or otitis externa

- Recheck after an acute uncomplicated urinary tract infection

99308 Subsequent nursing facility care, per day, for the evaluation and management of a patient; requires at least two of the following three key components:

- An expanded problem-focused interval history

- An expanded problem-focused examination

- Medical decision making of low complexity

Usually, the patient is responding inadequately to therapy or has developed a minor complication. Examples include the following:

• Follow-up for patient with urinary tract infection requiring a change in antibiotic

• Otherwise stable patient with a simple upper respiratory infection

99309 Subsequent nursing facility care, per day, for the evaluation and management of a patient; requires at least two of the following three key components:

• A detailed interval history

• A detailed examination

• Medical decision making of moderate complexity

Usually, the patient has developed a significant complication or a significant new problem. Examples include the following:

• Diabetic patient with blood sugars out of control requiring a change of medication

• Hypertensive patient with lab results showing renal complications

99310 Subsequent nursing facility care, per day, for the evaluation and management of a patient; requires at least two of the following three key components:

• A comprehensive interval history

• A comprehensive examination

• Medical decision making of high complexity

The patient may be unstable or may have developed a significant new problem requiring immediate physician attention. Examples include the following:

• Patient with new onset of diabetes associated with hyperglycemia, dehydration, and/or infection

• Patient with peripheral vascular disease, hypertension, and congestive heart failure who has developed severe edema, significant weight gain, stasis ulcers, shortness of breath, and hypoxia

Discharge Codes

Discharge visits can be divided into two categories that are based on time only as described below. Discharge visits must be billed for the day of discharge.

• 99315—Nursing facility discharge day management; 30 minutes or less

• 99316—Nursing facility discharge day management; more than 30 minutes

Annual Assessment

There is one new annual assessment code:

• 99318—Evaluation and management of a patient involving an annual nursing facility assessment requires the following three key components:

  ○ A detailed interval history

  ○ A comprehensive examination

  ○ Medical decision making that is of low to moderate complexity

Miscellaneous Codes

In addition to the evaluation and management codes listed above, there are a variety of other procedures that are often performed by nurse practitioners. Some of the more common procedures are listed below as examples; however, there are many other procedures that can be performed by nurse practitioners depending upon their education and training and the collaborative agreement they have in place. The following procedures can only be billed when performed by the nurse practitioner:

- 43760—Change gastrostomy tube

- 43761—Reposition gastrostomy tube

- 51701—Straight bladder catheterization

- 51702—Insertion of Foley catheter

- 69210—Lavage of ears to remove cerumen impaction

- 90862—Psychiatric review of medications when performed at a separate visit

- 97597—Sharps wound debridement without anesthesia; less than 20 cm

- 97602—Wound debridement, no anesthesia; non-selective with assessment

Some of the codes listed above must be billed along with an E&M code; for example, Medicare will not reimburse the 97602 wound debridement code when submitted by itself.

Nursing Home Documentation

Documentation can be a reliable indication of Medicare compliance. Appropriate documentation must be used to substantiate the specific code used to describe the nursing home visit. Each of the comprehensive and subsequent billing codes require specific levels of documentation that describes the level of E&M services provided.

Evaluation and management (E&M) services are defined by the following seven components:

- *History*

- *Examination*

- *Medical decision making*

- Counseling

- Coordination of care

- Nature of presenting problem

- Time

The first three are key components, *history*, *examination*, and *medical decision making*, and are used to select the appropriate level of E&M services. In the event that the predominant components of a visit are counseling or coordination of care, time becomes the key factor. The total amount of time must be documented in writing on the medical record.

Diagnoses are submitted as International Classification of Diseases (ICD) codes, and these codes provide the reason for the billed visit. The use of ICD-9 codes can be complex. Nurse practitioners who do not have access to the ICD-9 code book should purchase one for their own personal use and become very familiar with how it works. The ICD manual establishes internationally recognized diagnostic codes that are used not only for billing, but also for budget planning, epidemiological studies, and other diagnostic-related research. Nurse practitioners may not have been educated in the use of this manual prior to establishing their practice, but it is essential that they learn to use this manual properly. Many bills are returned due to improper ICD diagnostic codes, which delay reimbursement and increase the cost of billing for everyone within the healthcare system. It is required that practitioners code to the most descriptive level in almost all cases. The ICD diagnostic codes are generally three digit numbers followed by a decimal point and two additional numbers. Each additional digit is more descriptive. For example, the diagnostic code for diabetes mellitus (DM), type 2 is 250.00, while patients with DM and renal complications are coded 250.85. In some instances, the bill will be rejected if the complete 5-digit code is not used. The ICD manual provides that information. Some clinicians either purchase or make themselves a quick-reference sheet of the most frequently used codes to assist in the proper diagnostic coding.

Documentation also serves as an invaluable means of communication from one provider to the next. Long-term care patients are frequently followed by multiple providers, including physicians, nurse practitioners, physician assistants, psychiatrists, psychologists, podiatrists, and dentists. The clearer the primary care provider documentation, the more easily subsequent providers will be able to assess for new problems and arrive at appropriate follow-up treatment. This is particularly true for nurse practitioners and physicians who provide alternating routine visits. The medical record provides subsequent long-term care providers with a knowledge base critical to assessing new or acute problems and to readdressing chronic problems. An accurate, chronological medical record facilitates the team of healthcare providers (including the staff nurses) in their efforts to evaluate and plan immediate treatment and to monitor a patient's health care over time.

Long-term care patients typically have multiple chronic medical diagnoses, some of which may be exacerbated by acute illness or a variety of psychosocial issues common to this population. Documentation by the long-term care provider should be organized in a manner that allows the problems of this population to be individually addressed in a clear and concise manner. Unambiguous documentation can enable the long-term care provider to sort through the many options of the differential diagnosis. With careful organization and charting of subjective and objective information, the provider can more easily reject inappropriate assessments and treatment options.

SOAP

SOAP charting is one method of effective diagnosis and documentation that satisfies Medicare requirements for the three key components of E&M services: history, examination, and medical decision making.

S—Subjective Data The recording of subjective data fulfills the E&M services requirement for the history key component.

- The chief complaint—Critical to establishing medical necessity for billing purposes. For routine mandatory visits, this may be to update the resident's condition or to monitor progress of rehabilitation.

- History of present illness—Recent medical history, including information from current hospital discharge summary or recent office visits or simply the onset of an acute condition

- Past medical history—Chronic illnesses, past hospitalizations, and surgeries

- Reports by nursing facility staff—Recent change in status, vital signs, intake and output, response to current treatment

- Reports by family and significant others— Prior level of activity, prior living arrangements, ability of family or significant others to care for patient, expectations regarding rehabilitation outcomes, discharge plan

- Recent laboratory and diagnostic findings

O—Objective Data *The recording of objective data fulfills the E&M services requirement for the examination key component.*

- Pertinent laboratory data reviewed

- Physical examination—Limited or detailed exam of affected body or organ system (subsequent nursing facility care visits, including the problem-focused visit), comprehensive exam of multiple organ systems, a single body area or organ system (comprehensive nursing facility assessments)

A—Assessment *The recording of an assessment fulfills the E&M services requirement for the medical decision making key component.*

- Diagnosis—The major differential diagnoses being considered should be either inferred or listed with the principle diagnosis being considered listed first.

- Status of condition—Resolution, improvement, exacerbation, deterioration, or additional problem

- Complicating factors such as dementia, behavioral issues, depression, compromised immune status, or other complications should be mentioned, as each of these raises the level of risk and makes decision making more complex.

P—Plan *The recording of a plan fulfills the requirements for the following E&M services key components: medical decision making, counseling and coordination of care.*

- Diagnostic and laboratory tests

- Treatments and medications

- Patient, family, and staff education— Describe the discussion and the amount of time required face to face and on the telephone with family

- Reevaluation of assessment and treatment plan based on results to tests or responses to previous treatments and medications

- Brief description of any new plan of care needed—The nursing staff can use this as a basis for the changes they make in the MDS and nursing care plan. This may include new monitoring of behavioral changes, vital signs, blood sugars, toileting program, fall prevention program, or other ongoing monitoring plans.

Alternative Documentation Methods

A number of clinicians are using alternative methods to handwritten SOAP charting notes. Some facilities have electronic medical records that provide quite comprehensive records of the visit. Some clinicians work with structured forms that typically provide a menu of choices to either circle or check off as appropriate, which shortens the handwritten note requirements. Structured notes must be personalized to each specific resident and meet all of the previously discussed components of care.

Table 1-1 contains a visual breakdown of the various component requirements for each type of E&M nursing home visit. This visual representation is helpful to aid in the overall

TABLE 1-1   Evaluation and Management (E&M) Brief Guide

INITIAL NURSING FACILITY ASSESSMENTS

99304	99305	99306
Detailed or comprehensive history	Comprehensive history	Comprehensive history
Detailed or comprehensive exam	Comprehensive examination	Comprehensive examination
Medical decision making that is straightforward or of low complexity	Medical decision making of moderate complexity	Medical decision making of high complexity

EXAMPLES

Admit for dementia w/o complicating illnesses	Admit from home with 2 or less chronic illnesses	Admit from home due to unstable condition, severe decline in functional status
Readmit after brief acute hospital w/o changes to ongoing care	Readmit from hospital with acute illness, little or no effect on functional status	Readmit from hospital with major decline or acute illness with severe effect on function

SUBSEQUENT NURSING FACILITY ASSESSMENTS

99307	99308	99309	99310
Problem-focused interval history	Expanded problem-focused interval history	Detailed interval history	Comprehensive interval history
Problem-focused examination	Expanded problem-focused examination	Detailed examination	Comprehensive examination
Straightforward medical decision making	Medical decision making of low complexity	Medical decision making of moderate complexity	Medical decision making of high complexity

EXAMPLES

Brief visit for UTI or cerumen impaction	Monthly visit for 2 or > straightforward problem	Monthly visit for 2 or > complex chronic conditions, may be declining	Monthly visit of patient with 3 or more complex conditions with instability
Recheck on acute illness that is stable, recovering, or improving	Recheck on acute problem that is not resolving or has minor complication	Recheck on acute problem w/significant complication OR significant new problem	Visit of unstable patient or significant new problem requiring immediate care

Annual H&P	Discharge—Simple	Discharge—Complex	
99318	99315	99316	
Detailed interval history	Nursing facility discharge day management; 30 minutes or less	NH discharge; more than 30 minutes	
Comprehensive examination			
Medical decision making that is of low to moderate complexity			
SHOULD COINCIDE WITH FACILITY MDS UPDATE			

understanding of what E&M components are required to bill each code and the level of documentation required to substantiate the visit.

CONFIDENTIALITY IN LONG-TERM CARE

Patient confidentiality is of critical importance. Under the Health Insurance Portability and Accountability Act of 1996 (HIPAA, Title II), the Department of Health and Human Services (HHS) established national standards for electronic healthcare transactions and national identifiers for providers, health plans, and employers. HIPAA also addresses the security and privacy of individual health data. Adopting these standards has improved the efficiency and effectiveness of the nation's healthcare system by encouraging the widespread use of electronic data interchange in health care.

Nurse practitioners must meet the same standards as all health professionals in protecting their patient's confidentiality. For the most part, common sense should guide nurse practitioners in how they address confidentiality. Specific concerns are in protecting all identifying information such as names, birth dates, and social security numbers, particularly when sending faxes or e-mail. Any information that can identify a resident must be kept confidential from all other persons; however, this does not include other health professionals involved or potentially involved in caring for this patient. Patient confidentiality is not compromised by giving identifying information to a consulting physician.

Confidential information can be inadvertently transmitted to persons who do not have the "need to know". The nurse practitioner must be sensitive to discussions about patients and residents carried out at the nurses' station, in other public areas of a facility, or in the presence of other patients, residents, or visitors. Reasonable care must be taken to preserve privacy in these situations.

In conclusion, nurse practitioners play a vital and influential role in the care of nursing home residents. To be fully effective, nurse practitioners must be familiar with both the external regulatory environment and the internal facility environment of the nursing home. It is essential to recognize the similarities and potential differences between nursing homes so that care can be tailored and residents can receive the quality of care they deserve.

Additionally, nurse practitioners need to be knowledgeable about how they can be employed in the nursing home. Whether they are salaried employees or self-employed nurse practitioners who bill independently, it is imperative that they bill appropriately for services and that legible, comprehensive medical records documenting care are kept. Nurse practitioners should be leaders within the interdisciplinary team, taking full advantage of working with their professional colleagues and setting the example for coordination of care. Nurse practitioners providing nursing home care not only need to be expert clinicians, educators, and leaders, they must also develop proficient business acumen to survive in the complex and highly regulated nursing home environment.

REFERENCES

Buppert, C. (2004). *The nurse practitioner's business practice and legal guide* (2nd ed.). Gaithersburg, MD: Jones & Bartlett.

American Medical Association. (2006). *Current procedural terminology* (4th ed.). Chicago: American Medical Association.

Centers for Medicare and Medicaid Services. (2006). *International classification of disease* (9th version). Baltimore: Centers for Medicare and Medicaid Services.

Harrington, C., Kovner, C., Mezey, M., Kayser-Jones, J., Burger, S., Moehler, M., et al. (2000). Experts recommend minimum nurse staffing standards for nursing facilities in the United States. *The Forum, 40*(1), 5–16.

Harrington, C., & Carrillo, H. (1999). The regulation and enforcement of federal nursing home standards, 1991–1997. *Medical Care Research and Review, 56,* 471–494.

Hawes, C., Mor, V., Phillips, C. D., Fries, B. E., Morris, J. N., Steele-Friedlob, E., et al. (1997). The OBRA-87 nursing home regulations and implementation of the Resident Assessment Instrument: Effects on process quality. *Journal of the American Geriatrics Society, 45,* 977–985.

Kayser-Jones, J., Schell, E., Lyons, W., Kris, A. E., Chan, J., & Beard, R. L. (2003). Factors that influence end-of-life care in nursing homes: The physical environment, inadequate staffing, and lack of supervision. *The Gerontologist, 43*(Spec No 2), 76–84.

Kovner, C., & Harrington, C. (2002). CMS study: Correlation between staffing and quality. *American Journal of Nursing, 102*(9), 65–66.

Wunderlich, G. S., & Kohler, P. O. (Eds.), (2001). *Improving the quality of long-term care.* Washington, DC: National Academy Press.

RESOURCES

Web Sites

- Medlearn Matters: Provides information on CMS regulations as they pertain to nurse practitioners and other clinicians. Nurse practitioners should become familiar with the site. In most instances anything that is important to the physician is important to nurse practitioners. Visit www.cms.hhs.gov/ MedlearnMattersArticles.

- The following URL provides specific guidance for documentation of the E&M visits: http://new.cms.hhs.gov/MedlearnProducts/ 20_DocGuide.asp

- Information on a variety of clinical and administrative issues can be found at www.medscape.com.

- Information on support services for nurse practitioners can be found at www.npcentral. net.

National Organizations

- American Academy of Nurse Practitioners (AANP)—www.aanp.org

- American College of Nurse Practitioners (ACNP)—www.nurse.org

- American Geriatrics Society (AGS)— www.americangeriatrics.org

- American Medical Directors Association (AMDA)—www.amda.com

- National Conference of Gerontological Nurse Practitioners (NCGNP)—www. ncgnp.org

Manuals

There are several publishers of both the CPT Manual and the ICD Manual. Nurse practitioners should choose one publisher for the manuals and sign up for annual upgrades.

Alternatively, the information can be accessed at the Medicare Web site. The following are publishers who provide a hard copy of the manuals:

- American Medical Association—www.amapress.com

- Ingenix (Medicode and St. Anthony's Publishing)—www.ingenixonline.com

- PMIC—www.medicalcodingbooks.com

CHAPTER 2

General Principles of Patient Management

Barbara White

Elderly patients present more diagnostic and management challenges than younger patients. The clinician must be able to distinguish among the physiological, functional, and psychosocial changes that can be attributed to the normal aging process and those that indicate acute or changing pathology. This is an especially challenging process in the nursing home setting where patients already have functional limitations, as well as chronic physical and/or mental disorders. To diagnose and manage these patients effectively the clinician must always take into consideration the following:

- The potential for altered disease presentations in the elderly

- The impact of multiple disease states that may interact with each other

- The potential for altered pharmacokinetics and pharmacodynamics in this population

- The challenges of accurate and swift diagnosis in patients with altered mental status

DIAGNOSTIC CHALLENGES OF DISEASE PRESENTATIONS IN THE ELDERLY

As an individual ages there are changes that influence the development of a disease or disability (Murray & White, 1999).

- A *decreased immune response* may increase susceptibility to infection, autoimmune disease, tissue rejection, and malignancy.

- *Altered homeostatic mechanisms* may prevent the expected response to physiologic stress. Absence of the expected tachycardic response to fever or circulatory compromise and/or slowed return of heart rate to baseline after stimulation may confound diagnosis. Similarly, there may be less temperature elevation in response to infection. Altered homeostasis is also indicated by slowed counterregulation resulting in orthostasis, idiosyncratic response to medications, decreased glucose tolerance, and increased thyroid dysfunction (e.g., sub-acute disease, euthyroid sick syndrome).

- *Altered drug absorption metabolism, elimination and utilization* result in increased incidences of adverse drug reactions.

- *Diminished functional reserves* challenge the ability to respond to adverse events. This may result in atypical signs and symptoms of disease, such as confusion and fatigue as the first signs of respiratory or urinary tract infection. The elderly may also decompensate more rapidly in the presence of physiological or psychological stressors. Conversely, recovery from illness may be slower than in the younger adult.

- The elderly patient may also *neglect to report symptoms or signs* of illness. This may be due to fear of consequences; misplaced expectations that the clinician will be able to discover them alone; attribution of symptoms to normal aging; or inability to communicate effectively due to aphasia, delirium, severe depression, psychiatric disorders, or dementia.

The high proportion of nursing home residents with dementia compounds the challenges of diagnosis and management. These residents may not be able to verbally express the nature of their discomforts or other symptoms. In these instances correct diagnosis and patient management must become a collaborative activity with the staff. Because of close daily contact with a resident, staff may better detect subtle changes in behavior that can signal a change in condition than the nurse practitioner who sees the patient less frequently.

The older adult usually has experienced social losses that can impact the response to an illness, the rate of recovery, and the will to recover. Nursing home residents may be affected by a new and unfamiliar environment, by temporary or permanent loss of independence, by role change, loss of personal possessions, and separation from or loss of family and friends.

The clinician must therefore expect that the older adult may present with the following

- Typical symptoms and signs

- Atypical symptoms and signs

- Subtle symptoms and signs

- No obvious symptoms or signs

■ PRINCIPLES FOR MANAGEMENT OF MULTIPLE DISEASE STATES

In 1999, according to the National Nursing Home Survey (National Center for Health Statistics, 2002), there were a total of 18,000 nursing homes in the United States with more than 1.6 million residents. This represented 4.3% of the U.S. population 65 years of age or older, 1.1% of persons aged 65–74 years, 4.3% of persons 75–84 years, and 8.25% of persons 85 years of age and older. Age distribution of residents in nursing homes included 9.8% under age 65 and 90.3% 65 and older. At the time of the survey 12% of residents were age 65–74 years, 31.8% were 75–84 years, and 46.8% were 85 years of age or older. The average length of stay was 2.4 years, and 75% of residents required assistance with three or more activities of daily living.

The nursing home offers a unique opportunity for the nurse practitioner, the primary care physician, and ancillary staff to provide close supervision and consistency of care to residents, most of whom suffer from multiple chronic diseases and disabilities. In this setting the nurse practitioner is able to apply the basic principles of chronic disease management. This includes (a) planned, regular evaluation and intervention; (b) functional assessment; and (c) prevention of exacerbations and complications.

The advance practice nurse is the ideal care manager in nursing home settings and can be instrumental in reducing costs and hospitalization rates for residents (Koppel, 2003). Chronic disease management presents a challenge in long-term care because of the frailty of many residents. With a change in condition, the nurse practitioner must evaluate whether the patient with multiple chronic conditions is experiencing any of the following:

• An exacerbation of an existing chronic condition

• Complications or extension of a chronic condition

• Development of a new condition unrelated to the known condition(s)

• An acute condition superimposed on chronic disease

This requires keen assessment skills, the ability to interpret information from a variety of sources, knowledge of pathophysiology and pharmacology, critical thinking skills, and close collaboration with other members of the interdisciplinary team and the primary physician. According to the American Geriatrics Society position statement on care management (2000), the care manager must address the medical, psychological, functional, and social domains of health care and must have a breadth of knowledge including knowledge and clinical experience in geriatrics and gerontology. To provide chronic disease management as a care manager the nurse practitioner must address the following:

• Geriatric syndromes

• Geriatric assessment

• Evidence-based management of chronic diseases

• Basics of rehabilitation

• Components of home and community-based care

• Cultural diversity

PRESCRIBING FOR THE ELDERLY NURSING HOME POPULATION

Geropharmacology is now recognized as a specialty area. The response of older adults to drugs is often unpredictable. Until recently, drug trials did not include women or adults over the age of 65. Because of normal changes with aging, effects of acute and chronic conditions on drug absorption and utilization, and the interaction of multiple drugs, adverse drug reactions are common in long-term care settings.

Pharmacokinetics

Pharmacokinetics is the process of drug absorption, distribution, metabolism, and elimination from the body. The properties of each drug, the interaction with other drugs, and the effects of chronic and acute conditions on pharmacokinetics can affect outcomes for nursing home patients.

Drug Absorption
In the elderly patient the predicted rate and amount of drug absorption from the gastrointestinal tract can be affected by altered gastric acidity. This may be due to decreased acid

secretion with aging, control of gastric acidity with antacid therapy, or altered function of mucosal cells. Other factors that may affect absorption include hyper- or hypomotility of the gastrointestinal tract and altered intestinal blood flow. Absorption of drugs by parenteral routes may be altered because of changes in muscle or subcutaneous tissue mass and peripheral blood flow. Likewise, intravenous administration and concentration may be altered because of changes in expected circulating fluid volume. Finally, topical absorption may be decreased because of changes in skin hydration, tissue keratinization, changes in surface lipids, and alterations in microcirculation and peripheral blood flow (Murray & White, 1999).

Drug Distribution

In the frail elderly, distribution of drugs to target sites may be adversely affected by altered levels of *serum albumin*, the principle plasma protein to which drugs are bound. Serum albumin levels can be affected by age, illness, and nutritional deficiencies. If there is insufficient serum albumin, drugs circulate in their active form and compete for binding sites. This increases the possibility of drug toxicity and adverse drug reactions.

Drug distribution can also be affected by *total body water*, which decreases as a normal change with aging. Coupled with dehydration, increased concentrations of water-soluble drugs decrease the volume of distribution. This may cause expected therapeutic response for a drug to occur at a lower than expected dose and produce toxicity or adverse drug reactions. Conversely, in the condition of fluid overload, there is an increased volume of distribution of water-soluble drugs, and therapeutic responses may require higher doses to be effective.

Increased *body fat* is a normal change with aging. Of particular concern is fat deposited abdominally. It occurs in both genders, but to a greater extent in females. The problem is exacerbated with obesity. In this state, fat-soluble drugs will accumulate, and drug action will be prolonged.

Drug Metabolism

Most drugs are metabolized by the liver. Blood flow to the liver may be compromised by conditions such as shock, congestive heart failure, and liver disease. Drug extraction and detoxification may be slowed, especially for those drugs that are ordinarily metabolized during the first pass, or oxidative phase, of metabolism. Cytochrome P450 isoenzymes are the major catalysts of these metabolic activities. Selected drugs may induce or inhibit the activities of these isoenzymes, thus affecting metabolic activities. Alteration in the process of metabolism may lead to drug toxicities and adverse drug reactions.

Drug Elimination

The kidney is the major organ for elimination of drugs from the body. With aging there is decreased blood flow to the kidneys, decreased glomerular filtration rate (GFR), and decreased tubular excretion or reabsorption. Additionally, conditions such as congestive heart failure, diabetes mellitus, dehydration, and nephrotic syndrome can further slow drug elimination. Creatinine levels may decrease in older adults because of loss of lean body mass. With reductions in GFR, however, creatinine levels may appear to be normal. An estimate of creatinine clearance can be calculated to measure GFR prior to prescribing drugs that are renally cleared. The Cockcroft–Gault formula calculates creatinine clearance based on age, weight, creatinine level, and gender:

$$\text{Creatine clearance (man)} = \frac{(140 - \text{age in years}) \times \text{body weight (in kg)}}{72 \times \text{serum creatinine (in mg/dL)}}$$

$$\text{Creatine clearance (woman)} = \text{Creatine clearance (man)} \times 0.85$$

Drug Half-Life

A final consideration in drug pharmacokinet-ics is drug half-life. This is the time it takes to eliminate one-half of the amount of drug remaining in the body. It usually takes about seven half-lives to completely eliminate a drug from the body and four to five half-lives to reach a steady state in which the amount of drug administered at an established dosing interval equals the amount eliminated. Half-life is directly affected by the volume of distri-bution and the rate of drug clearance. If half-life is prolonged because of altered distribution or clearance, toxicity will result.

Pharmacodynamics

Pharmacodynamics refers to the action of a drug at a target site. Drug actions can be affected by normal changes with aging or by pathological conditions that affect receptors in target organs. This may pro-duce any of the following idiosyncratic responses:

- Less reduction in cardiac output from beta-blockers

- Increased hypotensive effects of vasodila-tors and calcium channel blockers

TABLE 2-1   Beers Criteria (2002): Medications to Be Avoided in Older Adults, by Severity of Potential Adverse Outcomes

Severity	Drug Classification	Drugs
High severity	Amphetamines	Except anorexics and methylphenidate HCL (Ritalin)
	Analgesics/anti-inflammatories	Indomethacin (Indocin) plain and SR-long term, full dose; non-COX selective NSAIDs: naproxen (Naprosyn, Avaprox, Aleve), oxaprozin (Daypro), piroxicam (Feldene) Pentazocine (Talwin), oral meperidine (Demerol), ketoro-lac (Toradol)
	Antiarrhythmics	Disopyramide (Norpace, Norpace CR), amiodarone (Cor-darone), short-acting nifedipine (Adalat, Procardia)
	Anticholinergics/antihistamines	Chlorpheniramine (Chlor-Trimeton), diphenhydramine (Benadryl) *except for emergency treatment*, hydroxyzine (Vis-taril, Atarax), cyproheptadine (Periactin), promethazine (Phenergan), tripelennamine (PBZ), dexchlorpheniramine (Polaramine)
	Anticoagulants	Ticlopidine (Ticlid)
	Antidepressants	Amitriptyline (Elavil) and combinations (Limbitrol, Tri-avil), doxepin (Sinequan), daily fluoxetine (Prozac)
	Antiemetic	Trimethobenzamide (Tigan)
	Anti-infectives	Nitrofurantoin (Macrodantin)
	Antihypertensives/cardiac drugs	Methyldopa (Aldomet) and combinations (Aldoril); amio-darone (Cordarone), doxazosin (Cardura), guanethidine (Ismelin)
	Antipsychotics/neuroleptics	Thioridazine (Mellaril)

continues

TABLE 2-1   *(continued)*

Severity	Drug Classification	Drugs

	Anxiolytics	Meprobamate (Miltown, Equanil),
		Short-acting benzodiazepines in doses greater than:
		    3 mg lorazepam (Ativan)
		    60 mg oxazepam (Serax)
		    2 mg alprazolam (Xanax)
		    15 mg Temazepam (Restoril)
		    0.25 mg triazolam (Halcion)

		Long-acting benzodiazepines: chlordiazepoxide (Librium) and combinations (Limbitrol, Librax), diazepam (Valium), quazepam (Doral), halazepam (Paxipam), chlorazepate (Tranxene)
	Barbiturates	Avoid all (except Phenobarbital), *except for seizure control*
	Gastrointestinal antispasmodics	Dicyclomine (Bentyl), hyoscyamine (Levsin, Levsinex), propantheline (Pro-Banthine), belladonna alkaloids (e.g., Donnatal), clidinium-chlordiazepoxide (Librax)
	Hormones	Methyltestosterone (Android, Virilon, Testred)
		Desiccated thyroid
	Hypnotics	Flurazepam (Dalmane), diphenhydramine (Benadryl), all barbiturates (*except for seizure control*)
	Hypoglycemics	Chlorpropamide (Diabinese)
	Laxatives	Bisacodyl (Dulcolax), cascara sagrada, Neoloid (*except with opioid analgesia*), Mineral oil
	Muscle relaxants/ antispasmodics	Methocarbamol (Robaxin), carisoprodol (Soma), chlorzoxazone (Paraflex), metaxalone (Skelaxin), cyclobenzaprine (Flexeril), oxybutynin (Ditropan, and XL), orphenadrine (Norflex)
Low severity	Analgesics	Propoxyphene (Darvon) and combinations
	Antacid	Cimetidine (Tagamet)
	Antihypertensives/ cardiac	Clonidine (Catapres), digoxin greater than 0.125 mg (*unless used for atrial arrhythmia*), doxazosin (Cardura), reserpine greater than 0.25 mg., short-acting dipyridamole (Persantine)
	Diuretic	Ethacrynic acid (Edecrin)
	Hormones	Unopposed estrogens (oral)
	Minerals	Ferrous sulfate greater than 325 mg/dL
	Vasodilators	Ergot mesyloids (Hydergine), isoxsuprine (Vasodilan)

Source: Adapted from Fick, et al., 2003.

- Increased incidence of gastrointestinal bleeding with aspirin

- Decreased response to central nervous system stimulants

- Enhanced response to central nervous system depressants

- Stimulant response to central nervous system depressants (Murray & White, 1999, p. 47).

THE BEERS CRITERIA FOR PRESCRIBING DRUGS TO OLDER ADULTS

Based on the above considerations and the physical, psychosocial, and financial consequences of inappropriate medication prescribing for older adults, their families, healthcare providers and agencies, a consensus panel of experts developed and refined criteria for safe drug use for this population (Fick et al., 2003). The current Beers criteria identify 48 individual drugs or drug classes to avoid in older adults because of *potential* adverse outcomes. The Beers criteria are summarized in Table 2-1. The criteria also identify certain diseases or conditions and the specific drug classes that should generally be avoided in management plans for these disorders in an older adult population. These are summarized in Table 2-2. Potentially inappropriate medication management can be due to poor drug choices, excessive dose/duration, and drug-disease interactions (Beers, 1997).

The Beers criteria are not specific to the frail nursing home resident who may be at greater risk for adverse drug reactions than the general older adult population. In a study by Lau, Kasper, Potter, and Lyles (2004) using the Beers criteria and data from a 1996 nationally

TABLE 2-2	Beers Criteria (2002): Medications to Be Avoided in Older Adults, by Severity of Potential Adverse Outcomes for Patients with Specific Diagnoses/Conditions	
Severity	Disease/Condition	Drugs to Avoid
High severity	Anorexia/malnutrition	CNS stimulants with appetite suppressant effects: dextroamphetamine (Adderall), methylphenidate (Ritalin), methamphetamine (Desoxyn), pemoline (Cylert), fluoxetine (Prozac)
	Arrhythmias	Drugs with proarrhythmic and QT interval effects: tricyclic antidepressants (imipramine HCL, doxepin HCL, amitriptyline HCL)
	Bladder outflow obstruction	Drugs that promote urine retention: anticholinergics/antihistamines/decongestants, gastrointestinal antispasmodics, muscle relaxants, anticholinergic antidepressants, urinary antispasmodics (oxybutynin, flavoxate, tolterodine)
	Blood clotting disorders/anticoagulation	Aspirin, NSAIDs, dipyridamole (Persantine), ticlopidine (Ticlid), clopidogrel (Plavix)
	Cognitive impairment	Barbiturates, anticholinergics, antispasmodics, muscle relaxants, CNS stimulants
	COPD	Drugs that may cause respiratory depression such as long-acting benzodiazepines, beta-blockers

continues

TABLE 2-2   *(continued)*

Severity	Disease/Condition	Drugs to Avoid
	Depression	Long-term benzodiazepine therapy, sympatholytic agents such as methyldopa, reserpine, guanethidine
	Heart failure	Drugs with negative inotropic effects such as disopyramide (Norpace) and high-sodium content drugs (alginate bicarbonate, biphosphate, citrate, phosphate, salicylate, sulfate salts
	Hypertension	Drugs with strong sympathomimetic activity such as pseudoephedrine, diet pills, amphetamines
	Insomnia	Drugs with CNS stimulant effects such as decongestants, theophylline, methylphenidate (Ritalin, Concerta), monoamine oxidase inhibitors (MAOIs), amphetamines
	Parkinson's disease	Drugs with antidopaminergic/anticholinergic effects such as metoclopramide (Reglan), conventional antipsychotics, tacrine (Cognex)
	Peptic ulcer disease	NSAIDs (except coxibs), ASA over 325 mg
	Seizure disorder	Drugs that may lower seizure threshold such as bupropion (Wellbutrin), clozapine (Clozaril), chlorpromazine (Thorazine), thioridazine (Mellaril), thiothixene (Navane)
	Stress incontinence	Polyuric drugs such as alpha-blockers (Doxazosin, Prazosin, Terazosin), anticholinergics, tricyclic antidepressants, long-acting benzodiazepines
	Syncope/falls	Drugs that may produce ataxia, syncope, orthostasis such as short/intermediate acting benzodiazepines, tricyclic antidepressants, antihypertensives with orthostatic effects
Low severity	Chronic constipation	Calcium channel blockers, anticholinergics, tricyclic antidepressants
	Obesity	Appetite stimulants such as olanzapine (Zyprexa)
	SIADH/hyponatremia	SSRIs, including fluoxetine (Prozac), citalopram (Celexa), fluvoxamine (Luvox), paroxetine (Paxil), sertraline (Zoloft)

Source: Adapted from Fick, et al., 2003.

representative nursing home survey, resident characteristics associated with potentially inappropriate medication management in stays of 3 months to more than 1 year included the following:

- Residents with Medicaid health coverage were at 31% greater risk than with other coverage sources.

- Residents with mental disorders other than dementia were at 40% greater risk than those without such disorders.

- Younger residents (ages 65–74) were at greater risk than those 85 and older

- Residents taking less than five drugs were 75% less likely, and those taking 5–9 drugs were 50% less likely than those taking 9 or more drugs to risk drug problems

- Residents with communication problems were 30% less likely to have problems.

- More than one third of residents received a potentially inappropriate drug at least monthly during their stay.

Facility characteristics associated with potentially inappropriate medication management included the following:

- Facilities with the Joint Council on the Accreditation of Healthcare Organizations (JCAHO) accreditation were 30% less likely to have problems.

- Small facilities (less than 50 beds) were nearly 50% less likely to have problems than nursing homes with over 200 beds.

- Facilities with one registered nurse (RN) to every 20 residents were 40% more likely to have potentially inappropriate medication management than those with one RN to every 10 residents.

The American Medical Directors Association and the American Society of Consultant Pharmacists issued a joint position statement on the use of the Beers Criteria (Swagerty & Brickley, 2005). They cautioned that the Criteria were developed by a panel of experts rather than with the use of an evidence-based methodology. They suggested the Criteria be used only as guidelines in conjunction with individualized, patient-centered care rather than as regulations applicable to all older adults (Table 2-3).

CLINICAL PEARLS FOR SAFE DRUG PRESCRIBING IN LONG-TERM CARE

Considering the potential for harm related to the furnishing or prescribing of drugs for nursing home residents, the following clinical pearls are recommended:

TABLE 2-3   AMDA/ASCP Principles for Appropriate Medication Management in Older Adults

1. Prescribing decisions should be evidence based.

2. Make decisions based on the patient's medical and psychosocial condition, prognosis, quality of life, and the patient's, family's, and surrogate's wishes.

3. Recognize that overuse, underuse, and inappropriate use are equally important concerns.

4. Avoid use or disclosure of confidential medical information.

5. Identify and document the need for treatment or reasons not to treat.

6. Identify and document the objectives of drug treatment.

7. Consider and document benefits and risks of treatment.

8. Order appropriate precautions and instructions for monitoring effects and adverse reactions.

9. Assess and document the resident's status during or at the end of treatment.

Source: Swagerty & Brickley, 2005.

- Know the principle modes of action and major side effects and toxic effects of all drugs furnished.

- With few exceptions, start drug doses lower than that usually recommended for adults.

- Increase drug doses slowly.

- Introduce new drugs cautiously.

- Keep drug regimens as simple as possible.

- When introducing a new drug, regularly assess the patient for adverse drug reactions, with attention to potential affects of changes with aging and disease on drug pharmacokinetics and pharmacodynamics.

- Consider all changes in a patient's condition as possibly drug induced, and attempt to correlate with changes in drug regimens or condition.

- In collaboration with the physician and pharmacist, look for ways to discontinue drugs.

- With each patient visit, review the medication record to assess the frequency of use for "as needed" drugs, and discontinue those not used on a regular basis.

- Arrange for appropriate staff, patient, and family education about drug safety.

GOVERNMENT REGULATION OF MEDICATIONS PRESCRIBED IN NURSING HOMES

In addition to general considerations for safe drug prescribing for older adults, the healthcare provider in the nursing home setting is further restricted in medication selection by federal regulations established by the Nursing Home Reform Act within the Omnibus Budget Reconciliation Act of 1987 (OBRA 87) and its revisions. In response to past abuses, strict prescriptive guidelines have been established that regulate the use of certain drugs in nursing homes (Gurvich & Cunningham, 2000). The OBRA 87 regulations require that a resident's drug regimen be free of "unnecessary" drugs defined as the following:

- Excessive dose

- Excessive duration

- Inadequate monitoring

- Inadequate indication for use

- Causing adverse reactions

- Duplicate drugs

It further requires a monthly review of each resident's medication regimen by a consultant pharmacist.

Psychotropic Drugs

Of great concern is the use of psychotropic drugs in nursing homes. If these are used to control behavior when less aggressive methods are considered appropriate first-line treatment, they are termed *chemical restraints* and can only be used temporarily for a resident's immediate physical safety when no other means are effective.

When psychotropic drugs are prescribed, attempts to rule out medical or environmental causes, as well as psychosocial stressors, should be documented. The medical necessity for use must be clearly documented as well as attempts to withdraw the patient from the drug in a timely manner or at regular inter-

TABLE 2-4   Recommended Sleep Hygiene Strategies in Long-Term Care
• Discontinue caffeinated beverages in late afternoon and evening.
• Discourage daytime napping; encourage involvement in social activities.
• Encourage physical activity during the day, as appropriate, but not too close to bedtime.
• Encourage resident to stay out of the bedroom and the bed until ready for sleep, as feasible.
• Work with residents and staff to establish specific rituals immediately before bedtime (e.g., brushing teeth, washing face, combing hair).
• Toilet each resident before retiring.
• Order a backrub for residents with sleep problems.
• Try warm milk (melatonin) or a light snack at bedtime, if not contraindicated.
• Limit excessive fluid at bedtime.
• Order pain medication for chronic or acute pain at bedtime.
• Encourage bed checks by staff to be done quietly, using minimal light sources.
• Encourage staff to limit environmental noise and loud discussions at the nursing station.
• Offer ear plugs or ear muffs to the resident to block noise.
• Use white noise such as soft music to block environmental noises.

vals. Success, or lack thereof, must be documented in the medical record with descriptions of *specific* resultant patient behaviors.

Antipsychotic drugs are approved with a psychiatric diagnosis. In this instance such drugs may be prescribed without restrictions with periodic documented monitoring for drug side effects. When antipsychotic medications are used in residents with dementia, they may only be used for specified, persistent, risky, psychotic behaviors or for immediate patient safety. The practitioner must document evidence of attempts to wean at least twice per year and document side effect monitoring (e.g., tardive dyskinesia).

Agitated behaviors in the resident with dementia can be managed, if environmental measures fail, with a short-acting anxiolytic. Daily use should not exceed four months, and persistent symptoms should be documented along with attempts to wean at least twice per year. With treatment failure, a short-acting benzodiazepine may be tried using a similar regimen.

Insomnia is a common complaint in long-term care and requires evaluation for primary or secondary causes. Initial treatment should include nondrug sleep hygiene measures (Table 2-4). If these fail, a short acting sedative-hypnotic can be tried. Initial duration of the prescription should be no more than 10 days unless attempts to wean are unsuccessful. The healthcare provider should attempt to wean at least three times in six months and document results. With treatment failure, a short-acting benzodiazepine may be tried using a similar regimen.

Medicare D

Finally, the nurse practitioner in nursing facilities must now become familiar with new regulations affecting long-term care residents receiving Medicare Part D benefits. The following issues arise with this program:

- The need to establish relationships with multiple drug plans, formularies, and pharmacies

- Medicare responsibility for "dual-eligible" (Medicare, Medicaid) drug coverage

- Identification of residents using off-formulary drugs in order to make appropriate adjustments or accommodations

- Attention to coverage gaps as residents switch between Medicare Part A coverage and Medicare Part D coverage

- Drug classifications excluded from coverage (currently benzodiazepines, barbiturates, weight-control agents, and over-the-counter medications)

- Processes for exceptions and appeals

- Cooperation with the nursing homes in development of systems to inform resi-

dents of their drug plan choices and the financial impact of their drug plan selection on access to medications

Because nursing home residents may be disproportionately impacted by certain Medicare D drug plan formularies, the Centers for Medicare and Medicaid Services (CMS) allow nursing home residents to change drug plans on a monthly basis rather than a yearly one in order to assure adequate medication coverage.

■ MANAGING RESIDENT TRANSITIONS AND TRANSFERS

Movement to a nursing home for a short stay or as a permanent resident is usually a traumatic event for both the patient and caregivers. Likewise, transferring residents from the nursing home to an emergency department or acute care setting for medical necessity can be problematic for the resident, caregivers, and the healthcare providers.

Transition to Nursing Home Care

The transition from acute care to a skilled nursing facility for subacute care and/or rehabilitation is usually a short stay with a goal of return to a higher level of care or to independence within the community. Such transitions can be made easier if the patient and family are oriented to the nursing home by staff and the nurse practitioner. The practitioner should be aware of the admission procedures of the facility and encourage a patient orientation that includes an introduction to the environment, staff, services, legal rights, and opportunities to maintain and enhance quality of life. The clinician, in the course of the initial and subsequent visits should do the following:

- Confirm the patient's and the caregiver's understanding of the purpose of the transfer to skilled nursing care.

- Review the health history, physical examination, and physician's admission orders.

- Set mutual goals for the stay.

- Discuss patient's and the caregiver's concerns, fears, and preferences for care.

- Initiate discussion of discharge planning.

When the short-stay patient becomes a long-stay resident and when a person is admitted as a new resident of a nursing home, the transition may be more difficult because of the permanent loss of independence, accustomed lifestyle, and roles, as well as fear of the unknown. Similarly, family and caregivers may need support as they experience emotions such as relief, guilt, and fear. Ideally the new resident and caregivers will have the opportunity to visit the facility prior to admission to familiarize themselves with the surroundings, staff, residents, and activities. Including a current resident as a greeter or initiating support groups for residents and family caregivers may also be helpful in the transitioning process. Greeters will know the challenges of adjusting to a new and congregate setting (Hayden, 2005). The nurse practitioner can further support these efforts during initial and subsequent interviews by doing the following:

- Treating each resident as a responsible adult and not as a child

- Looking for ways to allow the resident a sense of control over aspects of his or her life and environment

- Providing the resident an opportunity to express concerns, dissatisfactions, and fears

- Collaborating with the resident and caregiver on goal setting

- Respecting a resident's ideas and recommendations

- Confirming the resident's Bill of Rights (Table 2-5)

Transfer To and From Acute Care Settings

Moving a patient between settings can be fraught with dangers for the patient, caregivers, and clinicians. Such transfers can threaten continuity and coordination of care. Poorly executed transitions increase the incidence of costly duplication of tests and services, risk medical errors and liabilities, and cause patient and family anxiety and frustration (Coleman & Fox, 2004a). Effective transitions can benefit all involved individuals and facilities. The administrative and advocacy roles of the nurse practitioner within any long-term care setting can facilitate continuity of care across healthcare organizations through working collaboratively with the facility's medical director and staff to accomplish the following:

- Develop policies and procedures for patient transfers between facilities.

- Identify core information required in each patient transition.

- Collaborate with agencies in the development of transition and transfer forms.

TABLE 2-5   The Residents' Bill of Rights

The Nursing Home Reform Act established the following rights for nursing home residents:

- The right to freedom from abuse, mistreatment, and neglect

- The right to freedom from physical restraints

- The right to privacy

- The right to accommodation of medical, physical, psychological, and social needs

- The right to participate in resident and family groups

- The right to be treated with dignity

- The right to exercise self-determination

- The right to communicate freely

- The right to participate in the review of one's care plan and to be fully informed in advance about any changes in care, treatment, or change of status in the facility

- The right to voice grievances without discrimination or reprisal

- Select transfer institutions and practitioners that uphold established standards of care continuity.

- Establish, monitor, and evaluate performance standards for transitions and transfers (Coleman & Fox, 2004a).

- Establish procedures for communication with the patient and caregivers about the transition or transfer process.

- Document all communications and outcomes involved in the transfer process, including the names of all healthcare providers involved.

- Require timely transfer orders and discharge summaries when receiving a patient from another facility or institution.

Emergency room nurses identified several pieces of information needed when receiving a patient from a nursing home setting (Davis, Brumfield, Smith, Tyler & Nitschman, 2005, p. 36). These included the following:

- Medical history

- A list of current medications

- Chief complaint that brought the resident to the emergency room

- Do-not-resuscitate status

- Name and contact information for the responsible family member or caregiver

- Telephone number of the transferring nursing home

- Specific changes from baseline for a patient with altered mental status

This information can be used to develop a resident transfer form (Figure 2-1) and provides a template for the development of similar forms for other transitions and transfers.

The Decision to Transfer to Acute Care

The nurse practitioner may need to weigh several options in making the decision to transfer a resident to the acute care setting. These include the following:

- Resident's wishes for aggressive treatment

- Existing advance directive

- Overall condition of the patient

- Anticipated outcomes of acute care

- Consequences of a transfer for patient comfort and quality of life

- Wishes and expectations of the family and/or responsible caregiver

- Availability of appropriate treatment at the nursing home

When possible, the nurse practitioner should make these decisions in consultation with the patient, the family or caregiver, the primary physician, and appropriate members of the interdisciplinary team. Discussion should include the benefits and risks of transfer. The nurse practitioner should clearly document the discussion and the final decision.

REFERENCES

American Geriatrics Society. (2000). *Care management position statement*. Retrieved June 14, 2006, from http://www.americangeriatrics.org/products/positionpapers/cmps.shtml

Beers, M. H. (1997). Explicit criteria for determining potentially inappropriate medication use in the elderly. An update. *Archives of Internal Medicine*, *157*, 1531–1536.

Coleman, E. R., & Fox, P. D. (2004a). One patient, many places: Managing health care transitions, part I: Introduction, accountability, information for patients in transition. *Annals of Long-Term Care*, *12*(9), 25–32.

Coleman, E. R., & Fox, P. D. (2004b). One patient, many places: Managing health care transitions, part II: Introduction, accountability, information for patients in transition. *Annals of Long-Term Care*, *12*(10), 34–39.

Coleman, E. R., & Fox, P. D. (2004c). One patient, many places: Managing health care transitions, part III: Financial incentives and getting started. *Annals of Long-Term Care*, *12*(11), 14–16.

Davis, M. N., Brumfield, V. C., Smith, S. T., Tyler, S., & Nitschman, J. (2005). A one-page nursing home to emergency room transfer form: What a difference it can make during an emergency! *Annals of Long-Term Care*, *13*(11), 34–38.

Fick, D. M., Cooper, J. W., Wade, W. E., Waller, J. L., Maclean, J. R., & Beers, M. H. (2003). Updating the Beers Criteria for potentially inappropriate medication use in older adults. *Archives of Internal Medicine*, *163*, 2716–2724.

Gurvich, T., & Cunningham, J. A. (2000). Appropriate use of psychotropic drugs in nursing homes. *American Family Physician*, *61*, 1437–1446.

Hayden, G. (2005). The move to a nursing home does not have to be a nightmare. *Long-Term Care Interface*, *6*(12), 24–28.

FIGURE 2-1   Resident Transfer Form—Nursing Home to Emergency Room

RESIDENT TRANSFER FORM

Name of Nursing Home_____

Address_____

Date of Transfer to the Emergency Room _____ / _____ / _____
Print only and answer each question (Please do not leave any blanks)
completed prior to the date of the emergency and updated as needed.

Resident's Last Name First Name MI	Sex ☐ M ☐ F	Date of Birth ___/___/___
Name of the unit/floor resident transferring from	Phone number of that unit/floor	Fax number of unit

Attending Physician	DNR orders ☐ Yes ☐ No	Advance Directive sent ☐ Yes ☐ No
Name Resident's Next of Kin/Health care power of attorney Phone number	Next of Kin notified ☐ Yes ☐ No	Religion

(Check if present)				Indep	Assist	Depend
Disabilities	Incontinence	Impairments	*Functional Status* Mental Status___A___O			
☐ Amputation	☐ Bladder	☐ Speech	Feeding	☐	☐	☐
☐ Paralysis	☐ Bowel	☐ Hearing	Bathing/Dressing	☐	☐	☐
☐ Contracture	☐ Saliva	☐ Vision	Transfer	☐	☐	☐
☐ Pressure Ulcer			Ambulation	☐	☐	☐

Behavior Issues

Copy of the MAR with current medication (within the last 24 hours) highlighted. ☐ Yes ☐ No *(If no, list current medications below)*	Allergies

Chief complaint(s) that bring(s) the patient to the Emergency Room (If altered mental status is the chief complaint, please describe behavior prior to the change). Date of onset/duration ___/___/___.	Diagnosis	Past Medical History

Lab or other Tests ordered prior to transfer or within 24 hours ☐ Yes (Send copy of results) ☐ No	Diet/Therapies

Resident uses	Sent with Resident
☐ Glasses ☐ Feeding tube ☐ Cane ☐ Other (explain)_____ ☐ Hearing aid ☐ Foley Catheter ☐ Crutches _____ ☐ Dentures ☐ Tracheostomy ☐ Walker ☐ Ostomy ☐ Dialysis Access (describe)_____	☐ Glasses ☐ Crutches ☐ Hearing aid ☐ Walker ☐ Dentures ☐ Other ____ ☐ Cane

Name of MD/NP/PA who made the decision to send patient Beeper Number	Physician's orders attached: ☐ Yes ☐ No
Vital signs at the time of transfer T_____, P, _____, R _____, B/P	Transport via ☐ Ambulance ☐ Other (explain)_____
Signature of the Transfer Nurse Print name	Date of transf. ___/___/___	Time of transf. ___/___/___

ER Dispatch FAX # — / — / — (Cover letter required.)
ER Dispatch # — / — / — (Phone notification of NH transfer to the ER. Call to be brief and to the point.
Give patient name, NH name, exact reason for patient transfer to the ER, & ETA. (Do not give a full report.)

Notes:
DNR, Do not resuscitate; MAR, medication administration record; NP, nurse practitioner;
PA, physician assistant; NH, nursing home; ER, emergency room; ETA, estimated time of arrival.

Source: Davis, Brumfield, Smith, Tyler, & Nitschman, 2005.

Koppel, P. D. (2003). The advance practice nurse: An ideal care manager. *Annals of Long-Term Care, 11*(4), 34–36.

Lau, D. T., Kasper, J. D., Potter, D. E. B., & Lyles, A. (2004). Potentially inappropriate medication prescription among elderly nursing home residents: Their scope and associated resident and facility characteristics. *Health Services Research, 39,* 1257–1276.

Malone, M. L., & Danto-Nocton, E. S. (2004). Improving the hospital care of nursing facility residents. *Annals of Long-Term Care, 12*(5), 42–49.

Murray, S. E., & White, B. S. (1999). *Critical care assessment handbook.* Philadelphia: Saunders.

National Center for Health Statistics. (2002). *The national nursing home survey: 1999 summary* (DHHS Publication No. 2002-1723). Washington DC: U.S. Government Printing Office.

Swagerty, D., & Brickley, R. (2005). American Medical Directors Association and American Society of Consultant Pharmacists joint position statement on the Beers list of potentially inappropriate medications in older adults. *Journal of the American Medical Directors Association, 6*(1), 80–86.

WEB SITES

- American Geriatrics Society information on Medicare Part D—www.americangeriatrics.org/news/medicarePart_D.shtml

- Centers for Medicare and Medicaid Services—www.cms.hhs.gov

CHAPTER 3

Health Promotion and Disease Prevention

Barbara White

Both short-stay patients and long-term residents in nursing homes deserve attention to traditional health promotion and disease prevention interventions appropriate to their age and circumstances. *Health promotion* includes those recommendations intended to optimize health status. *Disease prevention* includes screenings, chemoprophylaxis, and counseling to accomplish the following:

- Prevent the development of a disease (primary prevention)

- Detect a disease early in its course (secondary prevention)

- Treat an existing disease to deter or manage complications (tertiary prevention)

The focus of care for short-stay nursing home patients is subacute, rehabilitation, or palliative care. This may preclude the ordering of other age-specific screenings. In this case, counseling and postdischarge planning is appropriate for those returning to a lower level of care or to independent functioning in the community.

Long-term residents of nursing homes should have periodic reviews of their general health condition and at least annual screenings for conditions that do any of the following:

- Affect health and quality of life in this setting

- Have an acceptable cost-to-benefit ratio for treatment

- Respect the resident's wishes for diagnosis and treatment

- Have likelihood of successful outcomes with available treatments

HEALTH SCREENING

Several agencies recommend periodic health screening for early detection of disease. The following health screenings are appropriate for older adults in the nursing home *if treatment is feasible*. In making screening decisions the nurse practitioner must consider the patient's preferences, comorbid conditions, competing causes of death, estimated life expectancy (which should be greater than 5 years) (Walter & Covinsky, 2001), and the sensitivity and specificity of each test. Ordering screenings with low sensitivities and specificities may result in false positive and false negative results. False positive tests may require additional costly tests and anxiety, while the consequence of a false negative result is delayed diagnosis.

Screenings for Female Residents

The nurse practitioner should consider the following health screenings for the older adult female resident.

- Cervical cancer screening—Screening females with Pap testing may be discontinued at age 65 years (according to the United States Preventive Services Task Force [USPSTF]) or age 70 (according to the American Cancer Society).

- For women with an intact uterus who have been sexually active and for women who have not been previously screened or for whom no records are available, screening every 1–2 years should continue until there have been several consecutive normal screenings.

- Mammography and clinical breast examination (CBE)—Screening mammography should begin at age 40 years and be conducted every 1–2 years. There has been limited research on the effectiveness of screening for older women. The USPSTF suggests screening to age 70, the American College of Physicians to age 75, the American Geriatrics Society to age 85, and the American Cancer Society indefinitely. Risk of breast cancer increases with age, but available treatment options may not be appropriate or tolerated by some nursing home resi-

dents. There is no clinical evidence to recommend for or against clinical or self-examination of breasts for cancer screening.

Screening for Male Residents

The nurse practitioner should consider the following health screenings for the older adult male resident.

- Prostate cancer screening—Males with at least a 10-year life expectancy may be offered screening following discussion of risks and benefits. Consider screening males at greatest risk, including African-Americans and those with a family history of the disease in father or brothers. The effectiveness of the prostate-specific antigen (PSA) tests and digital rectal examination (DRE) remain controversial because of the high incidence of false positive results and the anxiety and advanced screening required to confirm a diagnosis. Treatment complications may also severely affect quality of life (impotence, incontinence) for a cancer that is often slow growing.

- Abdominal aortic aneurysm—The USPSTF recommends a one-time screening of males between the ages of 65–74 years with an abdominal computed tomography (CT) scan.

Screenings for All Residents

The nurse practitioner should consider the following health screenings for all older adult residents.

- Osteoporosis screening—If treatment will be considered, a dual-energy X-ray absorptiometry (DEXA) scan to measure bone mineral density should be ordered for the postmenopausal female at age 65 or older. It should be ordered at younger ages for those receiving chronic doses of corticosteroids, anticonvulsants, aluminum-containing antacids, cyclosporine (immunosuppressant), or those with a history of any post-menopausal fracture, including hip fracture. Males with similar risk factors or low testosterone levels should also be screened at advanced ages and considered for treatment.

- Colorectal cancer screening—Older adults for whom treatment is feasible should begin screening at age 50 (age 40 with family history of colorectal cancer or personal history of adenomatous polyps). Screening may generally be discontinued by age 80. Select from the following list the test best tolerated by the patient:

  ○ Annual fecal occult blood test (FOBT) or fecal immunochemical test (FIT)

  ○ Annual FOBT or FIT and flexible sigmoidoscopy every 5–10 years

  ○ Annual FOBT or FIT and double-contrast barium enema every 5 years

  ○ Colonoscopy every 10 years

- Depression and anxiety screening—The initial and quarterly resident assessments of nursing home residents using the Minimum Data Set (MDS) evaluate depressive symptoms and behaviors as perceived by nursing staff. Because symptoms of depression and anxiety may be subtle in older adults, it is advisable for the nurse practitioner to schedule evaluation of these conditions after several weeks in the facility and every 6–12 months thereafter. Screening should include those with dementia and patients who are terminally ill (Greenberg, Lantz, Likourezos, Burack, Chichin, & Carter, 2004). Several valid and reliable tools are available, including the Geriatric

Depression Scales (GDS 30, GDS 15, GDS 12, GDS 5), the Cornell Scale for Depression in Dementia, and the Zung Anxiety Self-Assessment Scale. Early recognition and treatment of depression and anxiety may improve quality of life, prevent increased morbidity, and improve palliative care efforts.

- Dementia screening—Although a large proportion of nursing home residents have an admitting diagnosis of dementia, others enter a facility with cognition intact, with benign senile forgetfulness, or with mild cognitive impairment, not yet appropriate for medication intervention. The nurse practitioner should continue periodic screening of patients for changes in cognitive function with use of the Folstein Mini Mental State Examination and clock drawing test. Early recognition and treatment may slow the progression of some dementias.

- Dental health—Evaluate teeth, gums, and dentures on admission and at least annually thereafter. Make referrals for dental care.

- Foot care—Evaluate feet and shoes on admission and at least annually thereafter. Lower extremities of diabetics should be examined at each visit. Make referrals for podiatry.

- Hearing—Because hearing loss can affect ability to function, safety, and social interaction, screen on admission and annually thereafter. In addition to reviewing data collected by nursing staff as part of a Minimum Data Set (MDS) evaluation, the nurse practitioner should ask each resident about any hearing problems and perform an otoscope examination for abnormalities and cerumen impaction.

- Vision—Because vision loss can affect ability to function, safety, and social interaction, it should be evaluated on admission and annually thereafter. In addition to reviewing data collected by nursing staff as part of the MDS evaluation, the nurse practitioner should ask each resident about vision problems. Handheld or wall vision screening charts may be used to collect objective data. Eye examination by an ophthalmologist or optometrist should be ordered annually beginning with the diagnosis of type 2 diabetes mellitus, and beginning 5 years after the diagnosis of type 1 diabetes mellitus. Screen for glaucoma in African-American residents or in residents with positive family history, severe myopia, or diabetes.

- Renal function—Because of the large number of drugs taken by nursing home residents, the majority of which are eliminated through the kidneys, it is advisable to evaluate renal function annually. Also, screen renal function annually beginning with the diagnosis of type 2 diabetes mellitus and beginning 5 years after the diagnosis of type 1 diabetes mellitus. Assess function by testing for microalbuminuria, and estimate glomerular filtration rate with blood creatinine levels.

- Peripheral neuropathy—Screen peripheral sensation annually beginning with the diagnosis of type 2 diabetes mellitus and beginning 5 years after the diagnosis of type 1 diabetes mellitus. Assess temperature sensation, vibratory sense (128 Hz tuning fork), and touch using a pinprick technique or a 10-g monofilament.

- Screen for hypertension on admission, review blood pressures with each visit, and evaluate blood pressures at least annually in the normotensive resident.

- Screen for weight on admission, and review monthly weight records for changes from appropriate baseline that may require interventions.

- Because of subtle or atypical disease presentations in the elderly, additional laboratory tests may be appropriate in annual screenings, including complete blood count, serum electrolytes, thyroid function, fasting blood glucose, and a lipid panel.

- Fall risk—Review fall risk and fall history on admission and periodically thereafter. If positive risk factors or history are present in the ambulatory resident, then review medications, evaluate gait and balance (Get Up and Go test), orthostasis, neuromuscular, and cardiovascular status.

CHEMOPROPHYLAXIS

Unless contraindicated by history of vaccine-associated allergy, anaphylaxis, or Guillain-Barre syndrome; severe acute illness, or patient refusal, the following immunizations and medications are recommended for all older adults. (Guidelines change frequently and the most current information can be found on the Web sites listed at the end of this chapter.)

- Annual influenza vaccination of residents *and staff*

- Access to adequate supplies of antiviral drugs for use in an influenza outbreak as treatment or prophylaxis, including the neuraminidase inhibitors, oseltamivir and zanamivir, which are currently effective again influenza A and B. Influenza A strains are becoming resistant to the adamantines (amantadine and rimantadine) and should not be used without verification of effectiveness each year (CDC, 2006).

- All residents should be screened for tuberculosis (TB) on admission. The American Geriatrics Association (2003) recommends two-step testing with purified protein derivative (PPD) given 1–3 weeks apart. Residents who react positively to either the first or second test (a phenomenon known as *boosting*) should be further evaluated with chest X-ray for active or latent disease. Residents who do not react to either step are susceptible to the development of disease on exposure or they may be anergic. Residents with negative results should be rescreened with single-step testing according to facility and state regulations. Screening should also occur during facility, local, or regional outbreaks. All residents should also be screened carefully for signs and symptoms of active disease. *All staff should also be screened for TB upon employment and annually thereafter.*

- Pneumococcal polysaccharide vaccine:

  ○ Administer at age 65 or later if original vaccination is uncertain.

  ○ Five years later revaccinate all persons at high risk for fatal infections or rapid antibody loss (e.g., renal disease).

  ○ Give a second dose if the first was received before the age of 65 and five or more years has elapsed (ACIP, 2005).

- Tetanus/diphtheria (Td) vaccine—Give a booster every 10 years following the primary series. For wound management, a booster dose may be needed in 5 years (ACIP, 2005).

- A Food and Drug Administration advisory panel in January 2006 recommended approval of a herpes zoster vaccine, Zostavax, for adults 60 years of age and older for the prevention of outbreaks and for the prevention or lessening of the severity of postherpetic neuralgia. Information on final approval and administration guidelines can be found on the Web sites listed at the end of this chapter.

- Chemoprophylaxis with aspirin (81–325 mg) daily for the primary prevention of cardiovascular events should also be considered, unless contraindicated by existing conditions.

- Vitamin and mineral supplements for health promotion and disease prevention should be ordered on an individual basis.

▬ HEALTH COUNSELING

In the nursing home setting, counseling for health promotion and disease prevention must include not only the patient, but also the staff. Patients should be assessed for readiness for behavior change and assisted to establish realistic goals. Counseling should include educational materials appropriate to the resident's age and condition, as well as ongoing support and monitoring as would be done in any primary care setting. The following are possibx home residents:

- Fall prevention strategies

- Weight management

- Physical activity and exercise

- Adherence to dietary requirements

- Smoking cessation

- Social interaction

- Development and review of an advance directive

Similarly, health promotion and disease prevention in nursing home settings requires staff cooperation to assure the health and safety of residents. Education and counseling for staff should include the following:

- Fall prevention strategies

- Infection control policies

- Drug safety

- Prevention and aggressive treatment of pressure ulcers

WEB SITES

- Agency for Healthcare Research and Quality guidelines (USPSTF)—www.ahrq.gov/clinic/uspstfix.htm

- American Academy of Family Physicians (AAFP)—www.aafp.org/exam.xml

- American Cancer Society—www.cancer.org

- American Medical Directors Association—www.amda.com

- American Geriatrics Society (AGS)—www.americangeriatrics.org/products/positionpapers

- Centers for Disease Control and Prevention, health information for older adults—www.cdc.gov/aging

- Advisory Committee on Immunization Practices (ACIP) at Immunization Action Coalition (IAC)—www.immunize.org/acip

- National Guideline Clearinghouse—http:www.ngc.gov

REFERENCES

American Geriatrics Society. (2003). *Two-step PPD testing for nursing home patients on admission.* Retrieved January 18, 2006, from http://www.americangeriatrics.org/products/positionpapers/PPD-test.shtml

Fields, S., & Nicastri, C. (2004). Health promotion/disease prevention in older adults—An evidence-based update. Part II: Counseling, chemoprophylaxis, and immunizations. *Clinical Geriatrics, 12*(12), 18–26.

McElhone, A. L., & Limb, Y. (2005). Health promotion/disease prevention in older adults—An evidence-based update Part III: Nursing home population. *Clinical Geriatrics, 13*(9), 24–31.

Nicastri, C., & Fields, S. (2004). Health promotion/disease prevention in older adults—An evidence-based update. Part I: Introduction and screening. *Clinical Geriatrics, 12*(11), 17–25.

Smith, R. A., Cokkinides, V., & Eyre, H. J. (2006). American Cancer Society Guidelines for the Early Detection of Cancer, 2006. [Electronic version] *CA: A Cancer Journal for Clinicians, 56,* 11–25.

Walter, L. C., & Covinsky, K. E. (2001). Cancer screening in elderly patients: A framework for individualized decision making. *Journal of the American Medical Association, 285,* 2750–2756.

CHAPTER 4

Ethical Issues in Long-Term Care

ELDER ABUSE

by Eileen Croke

Stanley, Blair, and Beare (2005) estimate that in the United States there are approximately 1.5 to 2 million elder, vulnerable adults abused annually. Vulnerable adults are defined by law as "persons with a mental or physical condition that significantly impairs their ability to care for themselves" (Guido, 2001, p. 417). The abuse may be intentional or unintentional. Intentional abuse requires a conscious and deliberate attempt to inflict harm or injury, whereas unintentional abuse occurs when an "inadvertent action" results in harm to the elder individual and usually results from caregiver ignorance, inexperience, lack of ability or desire to provide proper care (American Medical Association, 1992).

The Nursing Home Reform Act, as part of the Omnibus Budget Reconciliation Act of 1987 (OBRA 87), set national standards for care in nursing homes. All states have elder abuse (mistreatment) laws, though mandatory reporting laws vary from state to state. These laws are designed to protect the older, vulnerable adult from physical abuse, psychological abuse, fiduciary abuse, neglect, or abandonment. Reporting reasonably suspected or actual abuse is based upon "good faith" judgment. Most states grant immunity from civil or criminal prosecution for reporting, and some state laws prevent employment retaliation for reporting. Procedures for reporting and the agency to whom the report is made varies from state to state.

State agencies may include law enforcement, ombudsman's office, adult protective services, or a department of aging (Guido, 2001). Long-term care facilities are required by law to have a protocol in place for detection, assessment, and reporting of elder abuse. Federal laws require the ombudsman phone number be visibly posted within each long-term care facility. Nurse practitioners providing care in long-term care facilities must be aware of their facility's elder abuse protocol as well as their state laws regarding elder abuse.

Types of Elder Abuse

Physical abuse involves the intentional infliction of physical injury, impairment, or pain. Examples include slapping, hitting, shoving, shaking, kicking, pinching, burning, sexual assault, force-feeding, inappropriate use of medications, or physical restraints. Psychological abuse involves the infliction of mental anguish. Examples include verbal insults, threats, intimidation, harassment, humiliation, or purposeful social isolation.

Fiduciary abuse involves illegal or improper use of the elder's property, funds, or assets. Examples include fraud, misrepresentation, stealing the elder's possessions or money, and coercing the elder into changing a will.

Neglect involves failure to meet the vulnerable individual's basic or medical needs. Examples include withholding food, fluid, or medication; poor hygiene; malnutrition; or unattended pressure ulcers.

Abandonment involves the desertion or willful forsaking of care by any individual who has care or custody of an elderly person.

Detection of Elder Abuse

Detecting elder abuse may be difficult for the nurse practitioner as many signs and symptoms are often ascribed to the resident's medical conditions or are underreported. The resident may be unwilling or unable to discuss the abuse for fear of retribution or retaliation by the alleged abuser (caregiver). The resident may experience shame around the abuse, may have a desire to protect the abuser, or may not realize that they are being abused. Physical abuse, psychological abuse, and neglect are the most common types of elder abuse in long-term care facilities (Comer, 2005).

Nurse practitioners are well situated to play a role in the detection, management, and prevention of elder abuse in the long-term care facility. The nurse practitioner may be the only person outside of the long-term care facility or family who sees the elder individual on a regular basis. Nurse practitioners must be aware of any potential risk factors for elder abuse, its various signs and symptoms, and appropriate forms of intervention. Complete evaluation for elder abuse requires the nurse practitioner to obtain a detailed history from the resident, alleged abuser(s), and family members; conduct a thorough physical examination; order diagnostic tests as indicated; and report suspected or actual findings of elder abuse to the ombudsman and other agencies as required by agency protocol and state law. The nurse practitioner has cause to suspect elder abuse when the resident presents with unexplained injuries, the given explanation is not consistent with the physical examination findings, or when there are disparities in the explanations of the injuries provided by the resident and alleged abuser (caregiver).

Risk Factors for Elder Abuse

The various risk factors for elder abuse include the following (Comer, 2005):

- Presence of physical or cognitive impairment

- Functional impairment

- Prolonged caregiving with a heavy burden of care

- Psychiatric disorder

- Social isolation

Signs and Symptoms of Elder Abuse

The various signs and symptoms of elder abuse include the following:

- Bruising and skin lesions at various stages of healing, either unilateral or bilateral

- Rectal or vaginal bleeding, excoriation, or abrasions

- Depression, anxiety, withdrawal, suspiciousness, fear

- Unattended pressure sores

- Poor hygiene and grooming, urine- or feces-stained clothes or linens

- Recent or unreported evidence of past fractures

- Signs of malnutrition or dehydration

- Inappropriate use of medications or physical restraints

- Social isolation

Interventions for Elder Abuse

Subjective Data
The subjective data necessary before implementing an intervention includes the following:

- Interview resident and alleged abuser (caregiver) separately (assessing incongruence of histories).

- Evaluate the resident for current functional level for performing activities of daily living (ADLs).

- Check for alcoholism or substance abuse on the part of the resident or alleged abuser (caregiver).

- Check the resident's medical record for any past medical history indicative of similar signs and symptoms or complaints.

Objective Data

Perform and document results of a comprehensive physical examination including the following items (Kaiser Permanente, 1996):

- General appearance—Evaluate nutritional status (malnutrition and dehydration) unrelated to any preexisting medical conditions, evaluate resident and caregiver interactions, and evaluate resident's hygiene or other abnormalities.

- Mental status—Conduct a Folstein Mini Mental State Examination to assess for competency level, dementia, confusion, mental impairment, depression, delusions, changes in affect, or other abnormalities.

- Integumentary—Assess skin, hair, and nails (unilateral and bilateral) for signs of bruising (check for stages of bruising) or lesions that may indicate physical abuse. Photo documentation should be included.

- Musculoskeletal—Assess level of ambulation (with any recent changes noted) and for recent evidence of fractures, contractures, or other injuries.

- Genital and rectal—Assess for signs of recent sexual activity, lesions, trauma, or other abnormalities.

Assessment

Based on the initial assessment, the nurse practitioner has several courses of action (Kaiser Permanente, 1996):

- Positive for elder abuse—Reporting is mandatory to ombudsman and other state agencies as indicated by state laws and long-term care facility protocol.

- Highly suspicious of elder abuse—Reporting is mandatory to ombudsman and other state agencies as indicated by state laws and long-term care facility protocol.

- No evidence of abuse—Rule out cognitive, coagulopathy, functional, and metabolic imbalances.

Treatment Plan

Diagnosis is usually based upon history and the presence or absence of findings. Diagnostic workup may include the following as indicated:

- Radiology screening for fractures (chest, skull, long bones of arms and legs), aspiration, or presence of foreign body

- Computed tomography (CT) scan or abdominal ultrasound for abdominal trauma

- CT scan or magnetic resonance imaging (MRI) for imaging of head, if impaired neurological status or head trauma are noted

- Complete blood count (CBC) with differential and platelet count for bruising and to determine presence or absence of infection or anemia

- Prothrombin time (PT) and partial thromboplastin time (PTT) (coagulation studies) for bruising

- Albumin, prealbumin, and protein levels to determine nutritional status

- Metabolic screen to determine hydration and endocrine and electrolyte imbalances

- Urinalysis for hematuria with abdominal trauma

- Toxicology screen to determine evidence of medication misuse

- For suspected sexual abuse, take a specimen collection of vaginal secretions for DNA sampling and presence of STDs

If the resident is in danger, remove from current environment. Report actual or suspected elder abuse to the ombudsman and other state agencies as indicated by state laws and the long-term care facility protocol. Treat injuries and illnesses, as indicated, and inform resident and family members regarding reporting of abuse.

Consultation or Referral

- Contact physician and multidisciplinary team for therapeutic guidance on all actual or suspected elder abuse cases.

- Report suspected or actual findings of elder abuse to the ombudsman and other agencies as required by agency protocol and state law.

- Obtain consultation from other specialists, as indicated.

Follow-Up

- Determined by medical condition and status of investigation by state agencies

- Failure of prescribed treatment plan to remedy injuries or illness

- As needed to ensure the well-being of the resident

Education

- All long-term care facility staff need to be assessed (e.g., level of training and experience) and evaluated on their abilities to provide safe and competent care to residents at the facility. Monitor for staff burnout.

- All long-term care facilities need to have an elder abuse protocol in place, and each staff member needs to be made aware and educated about this protocol.

- All long-term care facility staff need to be educated on signs and symptoms of elder abuse and how to report this abuse.

- All long-term care facilities need to provide safe staffing levels and correct licensure staff mixture required by state law for providing safe and competent resident care.

- All long-term care facilities need to perform background checks on all employees to prevent hiring of individuals with known criminal or prior abuse histories.

ADVANCE DIRECTIVES

by Eileen Croke

In today's healthcare delivery system, attitudes toward end-of-life care have taken on new dimensions. Death and dying, once taboo subjects, have risen to a level of increased sensitivity and awareness for both the public and healthcare professionals alike. Health care providers often have feelings of discomfort and guilt when faced with patients who are dying, despite the healthcare provider's efforts for cure (Stanley, Blair, & Beare, 2005). Many healthcare professionals have not been educated in end-of-life care issues, yet are facing more exposure and challenges in how to deal with varying end-of-life care wishes of their patients, both orally and in writing— through advanced directives. Healthcare providers may be held liable for claims of medical battery based upon failure to implement (not following end-of-life care wishes of a patient) an advance directive.

In 1990, the US Congress introduced the Patient Self-Determination Act (PSDA), as part of the Omnibus Budget Reconciliation Act, and in 1991 this was enacted into federal law. The law does not "create any new rights for patients nor does it change state law" (Guido, 2001, p. 157). The PSDA requires all healthcare facilities receiving Medicare or Medicaid funding to implement the following regulations:

- Ask the patient on admission to the facility about the existence of an advance directive.

- Provide written information to all patients upon admission to the facility about their rights to accept or refuse medical or surgical treatment and procedures under state law.

- Patients must be given the opportunity to complete an advance directive, though the law does not mandate the patient execute an advance directive.

- Healthcare providers must document advance directives in each of the patient's records.

- Heath care providers and facilities must provide education to staff, caregivers, and patients on advance directives.

- Healthcare providers and facilities must not discriminate in care for or against patients with an advance directive.

- Every healthcare facility must have in place and communicate to staff, caregivers, and patients a policy about implementing advance directives (Painlaw, 2004).

In long-term care facilities, elders usually need two witnesses for their advance directive, one being a representative from the ombudsman's office who serves as the resident elder's advocate. When the resident wishes to make changes to an existing advance directive an ombudsman representative must be present. Healthcare professionals are not allowed to serve as a witness for their client's advance directives (Ebersole, Hess, & Luggen, 2004).

The Federal Health Care Privacy Law— Health Insurance Portability and Accountability Act (HIPAA) (2003) does not require any language changes in advance directives, and a person (a proxy, surrogate, or agent) authorized under his or her state's advance directive law to make healthcare decisions on behalf of a patient may still receive medical information on that patient. There are restrictions and limitations to personal representatives if a healthcare provider suspects domestic violence, abuse, neglect, or endangerment by the personal representative against the best interests of the patient (Partnership for Caring, 2004).

Types of Advance Directives

Formats of advance directives vary by state law. Advance directives inform healthcare providers what type of care the individual would like to have or not have if the individual becomes unable to make healthcare decisions. Two types of advance directives are the durable power of attorney for health care (DPAHC) and living wills. The DPAHC allows an individual (patient) to appoint someone (an agent, proxy, or surrogate) to make healthcare decisions for him or her. It becomes effective (active) when the patient becomes unconscious or loses the ability to make decisions or communicate his or her wishes. The healthcare agent is responsible for carrying out the patient's wishes as they are expressed in the advance directive or in discussions with the agent. The healthcare agent is not allowed to change the patient's wishes expressed in the DPAHC.

Living wills only come into effect when the patient is terminally ill, usually defined as less than six months to live. The living will provides specific instructions to healthcare providers about the specific types of treatment or procedures the patient would want or would not want to prolong life. Oral advance directives are allowed in some states if there is "clear and convincing" evidence of the patient's wishes. Advance directives can be revoked at any time by the patient—verbally or in writing. A physician's order in a patient's medical record is required to execute the end-of-life care issues expressed by the patient in the advance directive.

Laws pertaining to advance directives vary from state to state; therefore, nurse practitioners need to be cognizant of both federal and their state advanced directive laws as well as their long-term care facility's advance directive protocol to help decrease liability when dealing with end-of-life care issues. A list of the various state laws pertaining to advanced directives, as well as state-approved advance directive forms, are available upon request from the Partnership for Caring at pfc@partnershipforcaring.org.

▦ SEXUALITY IN LONG-TERM CARE

by Barbara White

Sexuality is a basic human need. It is the expression of intimacy, and includes physical, psychological, social, cultural, spiritual, and behavioral components. Surveys repeatedly indicate that 30–60% of older adults engage in sexual activities. Indeed, the generation of adults now entering, or soon to enter, long-term care were part of the sexual revolution and free love generation of the late 1960s and early 1970s. Conversely, the cohort of older adults currently residing in nursing homes comes from a more Victorian era in which sexuality was appreciated but not easily or openly discussed. The nurse practitioner must be sensitive to residents' past experiences and assist them to meet current needs for intimacy.

The aging process may change the way in which human sexuality is expressed. Hormonal changes, disease, and medications may affect sexual activities. Erections may be more difficult to achieve and repeat for the male. Clitoral stimulation may be diminished and vaginal dryness may cause dyspareunia for the older female. Physical disabilities may make coitus difficult or impossible. It is likely that coitus will occur less frequently, and signs of affection such as kissing, hugging, and touching may take its place.

Expressions of sexuality are an integral part of one's self-concept. With admission to a nursing home the resident's usual manner of expressing affection for a spouse or partner, or usual ways of attaining physical satisfaction, may be interrupted or curtailed.

Sources of disruption may include the following:

- Illness or injury affecting functional abilities

- Reliance on staff to assist in activities of daily living

- Medications that may affect sexual interest and performance

- Loss of stable relationships through death of a partner

- Healthcare provider discomfort with addressing issues of sexuality

- Family resistance and lack of understanding of a resident's sexual needs and desires

- Staff discomfort and/or insensitivity to resident needs and desires

- Lack of privacy: personal, visual, auditory

- A resident's altered mental status

Intimacy needs of residents can take any of the following several forms:

- Because of shared living arrangements and the encouragement of social interaction during meals and other group activities, nursing home residents may develop attractions and emotional bonds with other residents. This may, eventually develop into the desire for, and attempts at physical expressions of affection on the part of one or both parties to the relationship.

- Residents may have a spouse or significant other living in the community and desire intimate contact with the partner in the facility.

- Residents may desire to engage in self-stimulation for sexual satisfaction.

- Residents with cognitive impairment may have lost inhibitions for the expression of sexuality and seek expression of this need indiscriminately through inappropriate comments, actions, or disrobing.

In each of these circumstances the healthcare provider, in cooperation with the facility, must make decisions about the appropriate ways for the resident to express sexuality in the nursing home setting. Decisions will likely be made in consultation with the patient and family, as appropriate, by the physician and nurse practitioner, an interdisciplinary team, or an ethics committee.

The initial step in managing sexual activity in the nursing home is an assessment of the resident's need and desire for sexual expression. The PLISSIT model developed by Jack Annon in 1976 for assessment, education, and patient management of sexuality has been used with older adults (Wallace, 2003). It includes the following four levels of intervention:

- *P*—Request permission to discuss sexuality with the resident (e.g., "I'd like to talk about your sexual health with you. What concerns do you have about this area of your life, now that you are in the nursing home?").

- *LI*—Provide limited information about aging and sexuality (e.g., changes with aging, disease, injury, and medications that may affect sexual function; issues of safe sex).

- *SS*—Give specific suggestions to help the resident meet sexual needs (e.g., alternate methods of sexual expression, problem solving about family and privacy issues).

- *IT*—Refer for intensive therapy, as needed to deal with inhibition, issues of past abuse, and so on.

The expression of sexuality in the nursing home presents ethical implications and consequences for residents, family, and staff. It also presents legal challenges as the consequence of federal and state regulations that protect resident rights. Decisions about sexuality in long-term care settings include the following issues:

- Quality of life

- Preservation of dignity

- Competence to give informed consent

- Privacy issues

- Protection from physical and psychological harm, which may include the following:

  ○ Confidentiality and HIPAA regulations

  ○ Health considerations (e.g., sexually transmitted infections, HIV, hepatitis)

  ○ Medical concerns (e.g., cardiovascular conditions)

  ○ Safety issues (e.g., injury, falls, abuse)

Additionally, there are the following considerations related to staff and family or other surrogate decision makers' acceptance of residents' sexual activities:

- Allowing expressions of sexuality between adults who retain their decision-making capacity will likely involve educating staff and working with the facility to identify ways to provide privacy.

- Decisions involving consenting adults with mild cognitive impairment may involve the patient and family or surrogate decision makers in discussion about autonomy, decision-making capacity, and consistency of such activity with a resident's usual beliefs and values.

- Residents with moderate to severe cognitive impairment may elect to express sexuality in inappropriate places or ways. The healthcare provider should assist the staff to redirect a resident's attention and to set limits for acceptable behavior. In consultation with the physician, the nurse practitioner may consider appropriately documented pharmacologic management for rare instances of hypersexuality. This may include the use of antipsychotic medications, hormone manipulation, or the use of serotonergic drugs.

The nurse practitioner can play a pivotal role in facilitating appropriate sexual expression in the nursing home. This role should include the following activities:

- Evaluate personal values and biases

- Educate staff about the following:
  - Their personal values, biases, and fears
  - The importance of human sexuality and aging
  - The need to treat resident's sexual activities with respect and confidentiality
  - The importance of grooming and personal hygiene to sexual expression
  - The need to respect privacy of residents engaged in sexual activities

- Ways to set limits to inappropriate sexual expressions

- Work with the facility to identify methods to assure resident's privacy at times of intimacy.

- Educate and support families and surrogate caregivers in addressing the sexual needs of the resident.

- Protect the resident who is not able to give informed consent from situations in which he or she may be the victim or cause of sexual abuse in the setting.

- Advocate for the legitimate rights and needs of the client in all issues of sexual expression in the nursing home setting.

TABLE 4-1   Strategies to Meet the Sexual Needs of Residents with Cognitive Impairment
• Evaluate the resident with excessive or diminished interest in sexual activity for symptoms and signs of physical illness (e.g., urinary tract infection).
• Evaluate environmental reasons for inappropriate disrobing (e.g., room temperature, time of day, toileting needs).
• Consider alternate reasons for sexual displays (e.g., difficulty identifying one's partner, misinterpretation of a situation, boredom).
• Keep reactions to sexual displays neutral and matter of fact.
• Gently or firmly remind the resident when a behavior is inappropriate.
• Use distraction or redirection.
• Use touch to help the resident feel connected.
• Assist spouse and family caregivers to understand and accept changes in sexuality in the resident.

Source: Alzheimer's Association, 2004.

The Alzheimer's Association offers several suggestions about sexuality and the person with dementia that may be helpful for clinicians, staff, and caregivers in dealing with the sexual needs of residents with cognitive impairment. These are summarized in Table 4-1.

WEB SITES

- Alzheimer's Association: Sexuality and intimacy issues in Alzheimer's Disease— www.alz.org/Resources/Resources/ rtrlintim.asp

- National Center on Elder Abuse www. elderabusecenter.org

- American Bar Association: Facts about law and the elderly—www.abanet.org/media/ factbooks/eldtoc.html

- Clearinghouse on Abuse and Neglect of the Elderly—www.elderabusecenter.org/ default.cfm?p=cane.cfm

- National Academy of Elder Law Attorneys—www.naela.com

- National Eldercare Locator—www. eldercare.gov

REFERENCES

Alzheimer's Association. (2004). *Sexuality fact sheet.* Retrieved January 27, 2006, from http://www. alz.org/Resources/FactSheets/FSsexuality.pdf

American Medical Association. (1992). *Diagnostic and treatment guidelines on elder abuse and neglect.* Retrieved January 29, 2005, from http://www. ama-assn.org/ama/pub/category/3548.html

Comer, S. (2005). *Delmar's geriatric nursing care plans* (3rd ed.). Clifton Park, NY: Thompson Delmar Learning.

Ebersole, P., Hess, P., & Luggen, A. (2004). *Toward healthy aging: human needs and response* (6th ed.). St. Louis, MO: Mosby.

Gordon, M., & Sokolowski, M. (2004). Sexuality in long term care: Ethics and action. *Annals of Long-Term Care, 12*(9), 45–48.

Guido, G. (2001). *Legal and ethical issues in nursing* (3rd ed.). Upper Saddle River, NJ: Prentice Hall.

Kaiser Permanente. (1996). *Nurse practitioner, certified midwife, physician assistant protocols* (2nd ed.). Pasadena, CA: Southern California Permanente Medical Group.

Lantz, M. S. (2004). Consenting adults: Sexuality in the nursing home. *Clinical Geriatrics, 12*(6), 33–36.

Painlaw. (2004). *Failure to respect advance directives is medical battery.* Retrieved January 9, 2005, from http://www.painlaw.org/medicalbattery.html

Partnership for Caring. (2004). Caring connections. Retrieved January 5, 2005, from http://www. partnershipforcaring.org

Stanley, M., Blair, K., & Beare, P. (2005). *Gerontological nursing* (3rd ed.). Philadelphia: F.A. Davis.

Wallace, M. (2003). Sexuality and aging in long term care. *Annals of Long-Term Care, 11*(2), 53–59.

CHAPTER 5

Legal Considerations

Ted O'Leary

It has been reported that as many as 98,000 patients die each year as a result of medical errors (Marquis, 1999). The public is unhappy with and mistrustful of the medical professional as a result of managed health care, the loss of choice of one's providers (including, sometimes, being seen and/or treated by a nurse practitioner rather than a doctor), and the increase in bureaucratic delays and coverage restrictions. At the same time, people are more sophisticated about medicine and medical litigation (the population can now learn about medical/legal matters through a multitude of television programs, medical and legal reporters on news programs, online medical journals and Web sites, health sections of major newspapers, not to mention the abundance of lawyer advertising). Several factors have arguably affected the quantity of malpractice litigation, including recovery limitations (caps), the difficulty and expense of presenting a malpractice case, and an outcry by physicians. Despite this, elder abuse cases are of growing interest to plaintiff lawyers and are becoming more common.

The elderly population is rapidly increasing with the aging of the baby boomers. The elderly typically need more medical care and are at higher risk for chronic and/or severe disease states and postoperative complications. The higher the risk of serious complications, the higher is the risk of malpractice or elder abuse litigation arising out of those complications. Twenty years ago, when a 75-year-old died from surgical complications few lawyers would have been interested, but today, if that 75-year-old was in otherwise fair health and might have lived another 10 years, a lawyer is more inclined to take the case. More and more seniors find themselves in hospitals, nursing homes, and rehabilitation and skilled care facilities, thus affording greater opportunity for actual or claimed abuse by healthcare professionals. And because elder abuse laws actually encourage litigation by providing more lucrative remedies, which are either unavailable (multiplied damages, damages for pain and suffering of a decedent, and attorney fees) or exceedingly rare (punitive damages) in traditional medical malpractice actions, we are likely to see a continued growth in elder abuse litigation. To qualify for the "enhanced remedies" (those which go beyond indemnification) allowed under elder abuse and dependent adult laws, the patient need only be a statutorily prescribed age, in some states 60 years, but typically age 65 and older, or a dependent adult, which could be as young as age 18 (Elder Abuse and Dependent Adult Civil Protection Act [EADACPA], 1992d).[1]

For the nurse practitioner practicing in a long-term care facility, where the prognosis for the majority of patients is poor to begin with, discomfiting familiarity with malpractice and elder abuse litigation is all but inevitable. The purpose of this chapter is to educate the nurse practitioner in the basics of malpractice and elder abuse law and to provide a background for the practitioner's conduct and awareness in light of the risk of litigation. It is not intended to offer legal advice for any specific incident or case; if such advice is sought, the reader should consult an attorney familiar with the laws of his or her state. (Many of the references used in this chapter are to laws of California, where the author practices.)

LIABILITY OVERVIEW

Our system of justice is derived from the English common law. These are basic legal principles with which most people are familiar. For example, you may not trespass upon another's land and do harm to it, you must keep a promise to pay for another's product or work, and so forth. Most such laws have been either codified by statutes or established by judicial decisions interpreting, and many times expanding, the common law. Legal liability is a civil justice (noncriminal) concept in which a wrongdoer (tort-feasor) may be held accountable (liable) for monetary damages for any wrong (tort) that causes damage, harm, or injury to another. These actions may be

unintended, or, more typically, intended but with unintended consequences. Or they may be willful or done with reckless disregard for consequences that were either foreseeable or should have been foreseeable. The former is negligence, and, in the arena of the healthcare professional, more aptly termed *medical malpractice* (which includes the claim "lack of informed consent"). The latter, in the arena of the healthcare professional, might lead to a claim of battery (an unconsented-to harmful "touching," such as when a patient consents to the amputation of the left arm, but the right one is removed) or intentional infliction of emotional distress. *Elder abuse* is a hybrid term and may be based upon physical abuse, financial abuse, neglect, abandonment, isolation, or other treatment resulting in physical or mental harm to the patient. This harm is often claimed to be the result of fraud, malice, oppression, or the reckless disregard for the health and safety of the patient (EADACPA, 1992f; Book of Approved Jury Instructions, California [BAJI], 2002c). In either case, the person alleging harm—the plaintiff—sues the healthcare provider and alleged wrongdoer—the defendant.

Lawyers are almost always retained to represent both sides. The healthcare provider is usually, though not always, insured. The insurer provides a legal defense and indemnifies its insured against any verdict, judgment, or settlement.[2] The plaintiff files a complaint in a state or federal court.[3] The defendant files an answer in which the allegations of the complaint are (almost universally) denied. There is a discovery phase during which both sides may take depositions of witnesses,

---

[1] Note that in California, at least, the dependent adult must also have physical or mental limitations that restrict his or her ability to carry out his or her normal activities or protect his or her rights *and* be admitted as an inpatient to a 24-hour health care facility.

[2] In most states, public policy considerations prohibit insurance companies from insuring against and/or indemnifying policy holders for liability arising from acts of criminal conduct and for punitive damages.

[3] An action is filed in federal court when there is "diversity jurisdiction" or a "federal question." This is rare but not unheard of in medical malpractice and elder abuse actions.

exchange written responses to questions, produce documents, or sometimes require a physical or mental examination, usually of the injured party. During this phase, most if not all of the facts and theories of the case are developed or uncovered, and experts may be consulted and retained to express opinions at trial. Both sides evaluate the case fully, and if the case is not settled it proceeds to a trial or sometimes an arbitration (before one or several arbitrators rather than a jury). Either the jury, a judge, an arbitrator, or a panel of arbitrators renders a verdict or decision specifying whether the defendant is legally liable, and, if so, the amount of damages he, she, or it must pay to the plaintiff(s). This verdict or decision then becomes a judgment, and until paid or collected it remains outstanding and collectable, usually with interest accruing at a predetermined rate. Costs of the suit may be added to the verdict, for whichever side prevails, but these costs typically do not include attorney fees, unless the action is brought pursuant to a statute that allows for this exception (such as under many elder abuse laws) (EADACPA, 1992i).

From the filing of the complaint (suit) to the conclusion of a trial, anywhere from 6 months to several years may pass, depending upon the backlog of litigation in the particular jurisdiction. Generally, if the action is tried on its merits rather than disposed of by a technicality (such as the statute of limitations), a verdict *for the plaintiff* means that the defendant has been found legally liable for the damages incurred and must pay, or have his, her, or its insurer pay said damages; a verdict *for the defendant* means the plaintiff could not prove his or her case, and the defendant is not legally liable. A settlement, although resulting in some form of payment to the plaintiff, is not an admission of negligence, and most releases used to document the settlement terms specify that the settlement involves a compromise of a disputed claim and does not constitute an admission of liability. In some states, all

settlements must be reported to the applicable medical board; in others, only settlements above a certain dollar figure are reported (Ca. Bus. & Prof. Code, §§ 801, 801.1, 802, 803.2). Many states require that adverse verdicts or judgments be reported to the applicable state medical board. The applicable board may launch its own investigation into the case and may take action against the practitioner's license, such as suspension, revocation, or probation. The federal government requires that all settlements and adverse judgments be reported to the National Practitioners' Data Bank (Health Care Quality Improvement Act, 1986).

In the long-term care setting, a nurse practitioner is less likely to be sued alone; he or she is more likely to be sued together with the doctor or medical group employing him or her and perhaps the skilled nursing facility itself. Plaintiff attorneys prefer the *David v. Goliath* scenario of a patient or a patient's family up against a large and wealthy corporation (the skilled nursing facility) or at least a medical group; whereas, if only the nurse practitioner is sued, the jury may empathize as much with the nurse practitioner as with the patient or family. A jury may be concerned that a verdict for the plaintiff might cause the nurse practitioner to lose his or her job. Subconsciously, they may consider what might happen to them if they were found negligent at their own job or if they were hauled into court to pay damages. Employers (especially corporations), on the other hand, are notoriously unsympathetic—jurors may associate them with their own employers and expect them to be responsible for the conduct of their employees. Even a medical group receives less sympathy than an individual doctor or nurse practitioner. A jury may speculate that the nurse practitioner is uninsured and cannot afford to pay the money a plaintiff's attorney asks them to award, but they will typically assume the employer or corporate defendant is either wealthy, insured, or both (even though most states preclude any mention of insurance during the trial). Finally, suing the owner of a long-term care facility in an elder abuse case provides the basis for the enhanced remedies mentioned earlier, but suing only a nurse practitioner may not. It is the potential of the enhanced remedies that greatly increases the settlement value, and therein lies the attraction of such a case to a plaintiff's attorney.

The medical group employing the nurse practitioner, even if it has done nothing wrong itself, may be legally liable for the nurse practitioner's conduct under the vicarious liability doctrine of *respondeat superior* (BAJI, 2002e; California Civil Jury Instructions [CACI], 2005g).[4] This legal principle holds that the nurse practitioner, acting within the scope of his or her employment, does so for the benefit of the employer. The nurse practitioner is said to be the agent of his or her employer, who should, as a matter of public policy, be responsible for the nurse practitioner's acts in furtherance of that employment (Ca. Civ. Code, § 2295).[5]

With regard to the skilled nursing facility, however, the nurse practitioner will generally be considered an independent contractor just as a physician would be in relation to the hospital where he or she sees patients (*Malloy v. Fong*, 1951; *Hull v. Lopez*, 2002).[6, 7] This legal relationship typically does not create liability for the skilled nursing facility for the acts of the independent contractor nurse practitioner (*Welch v. Scheinfeld*, 2005; *Elam v. College Park Hospital*, 1982), and the plaintiff would be remiss for suing only the facility thinking that he or she could hold it liable for an act of the nurse practitioner alone.[8, 9] An exception to this rule may be found in recent case law holding that a facility may be held liable on a theory of "ostensible agency," in which it need only appear to, or be presumed by the patient that an emergency room physician is an employee, and the hospital takes no steps to inform the patient to the contrary. This concept could theoretically apply when the nurse practitioner sees a patient only in the skilled nursing facility, and the skilled nursing facility does nothing to inform the resident that the nurse practitioner is not its employee. This independent contractor status, therefore, is more likely to lead to the nurse practitioner being specifically named as a defendant in any lawsuit arising out of his or her actions. The nurse practitioner typically needs his or her own individual malpractice insurance.

When the nurse practitioner is employed by a medical group but is named in the complaint as a defendant along with the group, the nurse practitioner should consider, through his or her attorney, asking the plaintiff's attorney to dismiss the nurse practitioner in exchange for a "stipulation" on the record that the nurse

---

[4] The employer is liable in such cases of elder abuse only if it had advanced knowledge of the unfitness of the agent or employee and employed him or her with a conscious disregard of the rights and safety of others and authorized or ratified (confirmation and acceptance of a previous act) the conduct (BAJI No. 7.48).

[5] California defines *agent* as "one who represents another, called the principal, in dealings with third persons."

[6] The distinction between an independent contractor and an agent depends primarily upon whether the one for whom the work is done has the legal right to control the activities of the alleged agent. The existence of the right of control and supervision establishes the existence of an agency relationship.

[7] When the hospital actually employs the nurse practitioner, as with its nurses, then an agency relationship exists, which could make the hospital liable for the actions of its employed nurse practitioner.

[8] Whether a skilled nursing facility has any liability under a theory of corporate negligence for negligently screening the competency of its staff, including a nurse practitioner employed by an individual doctor or a medical group, is unclear and likely dependent on each state's law.

[9] In California, *Elam v. College Park Hospital* established such an action against hospitals under this theory, but the group-employed nurse practitioner may be one step too far removed.

practitioner was acting within the course and scope of his or her employment and that the group will be liable for any damages caused by any negligence attributed to the nurse practitioner by the trier of fact. In exchange for such a stipulation, there should be no need for the nurse practitioner to remain as an individual defendant, and the nurse practitioner may be dismissed. Should the nurse practitioner be uninsured, this will result in a significant reduction in anxiety related to the litigation. Even if the nurse practitioner is insured, either individually or as an "additional insured" under the group's insurance policy, a dismissal *could* (depending on the facts and the reporting requirements of each state) allow the nurse practitioner to avoid some of the reporting requirements and their consequences to the nurse practitioner's practice.

On the other hand, once the nurse practitioner is dismissed, there is uncertainty that the nurse practitioner's interests are fully protected in relation to the group or supervising physician, such as in how a settlement or judgment is reported to the appropriate board, unless the nurse practitioner stays involved with the litigation and in touch with the defense attorney. When the dismissal part of the stipulation is refused by the plaintiff, or when it has been strategically wiser not to offer it, the author has, in turn, conceded that a group is legally liable for any act of its nurse practitioner (which is generally true as a matter of law anyway) and then asked that the judge preclude any mention of the group as a party, either in describing the case to the jury, in questioning witnesses, or in the submission of jury instructions, thus leaving the jury to believe that the nurse practitioner is the sole defendant. This, then, removes the "deep pocket" consideration for the jury and invokes the aforementioned concern about the nurse practitioner individually, which may help the jury decide in favor of the nurse practitioner. Because the "vicarious" liability of the group has already been determined, unless there is a

specific claim that the group was negligent in its hiring or supervision of the nurse practitioner, there is no need to adjudicate anything as to the group. And, if the nurse practitioner wins, so too will the group. The judge's consideration in agreeing to this is that it will shorten the trial and reduce the legal issues to be decided by the jury, thus reducing the risk of error.

In a typical *medical malpractice* case, in which the error might be a misdiagnosis, prescribing or administering the wrong medication, a delay in treatment, failure to recognize a deterioration of symptoms, and so on, the focus is on whether the healthcare provider (nurse practitioner) made a mistake (not necessarily *why* the mistake was made) that amounted to a deviation from the standard of care and if so whether that mistake injured or harmed the patient, or, in the case of a wrongful death suit, whether it legally caused the death of the patient. If so, the practitioner becomes legally liable for the actual damages proved at trial. And, if it is proved that the practitioner was employed by or was otherwise an agent of a doctor or medical group, the doctor or group may also be held legally liable for the provider's malpractice. Damages consist of that amount of money that will compensate the plaintiff for the injury suffered and indemnify the plaintiff for any financial losses suffered as a consequence of the injury.

In an *elder abuse* case, however the focus is more typically on *why* the conduct that caused the alleged injury or death occurred. Did it result from inadequate staffing, training, or policies, or did it occur as a pattern of conduct by the employer or facility? (If so, the prospect of punitive damages being awarded increases substantially). The provider allegedly erred, not just because mistakes happen, but because he or she worked in an understaffed facility, doing tasks a more qualified provider should be doing, not knowing any better for lack of training or supervision, or struggling against unreasonable policies. The plaintiff's attorney will argue that the facility should be punished (punitive and/or multiplied damages, and so on) for providing a setting that puts more importance on profit than on the interests of its elderly patients and that in order to deter such practices, more than compensation and indemnification is required.

■ MEDICAL MALPRACTICE AND NEGLIGENCE

For a patient (or his heirs or family members) to prevail in an action against a nurse practitioner for medical malpractice, the patient must prove that the nurse practitioner had a duty to the patient under the law, that the nurse practitioner breached that duty, and that the breach of that duty (the malpractice) was a legal (sometimes referred to as *proximate*) cause of injury to the patient. *Duty* is first established by showing that the nurse practitioner was either directly caring for, was consulted on, or was supervising the care of the patient at the time of the error (even if the error did not *immediately* result in injury). The duty owed the patient is the duty to conform to a level or degree of conduct commonly referred to as the *standard of care* (*Planned Parenthood of Northwest Indiana, Inc. v. Vines*, 1989).[10]

The *standard of care* is typically broadly defined by the law, such as California's Civil Jury Instruction No. 501: "A [nurse practitioner] is negligent if he/she fails to exercise the level of skill, knowledge, and care in the diagnosis and treatment that other reasonably careful [nurse practitioners] would use in similar circumstances" (CACI, 2005c).[11] Note that the nurse practitioner may, under the law, make a mistake and yet not be negligent, so long as the mistake was reasonable and might have been made by any reasonably careful nurse practitioner. California's Civil Jury Instruction No. 505 reinforces this by stating: "A [nurse practitioner] is not *necessarily* negligent just because his or her efforts are unsuccessful or he or she makes an error that was reasonable under the circumstances" (CACI, 2005d).[12]

In reality, the standard of care is almost always more narrowly defined to fit the circumstances of the case by the testimony of an expert witness. Such a witness might testify, for example, that the standard of care requires a nurse practitioner to check a patient's chart for medication allergies before ordering an injection of penicillin, and that if the nurse practitioner orders penicillin without checking the chart, then he or she has fallen below the standard of care. (Note: Do not confuse *standard of care* with *standard care*—they are not the same.) The plaintiff's standard-of-care expert will almost always testify that the mistake or error was not reasonable under the circumstances. Also, if the nurse practitioner failed to follow or deviated from the standardized procedure approved by the supervising physician and the facility, the plaintiff attorney will argue this as further evidence the nurse practitioner was negligent in his or her duties to the patient. The defense standard-of-care expert often will testify that the nurse practitioner "exercised his or her best judgment under the circumstances" or that the standardized procedure does not set the standard of care, and based on this testimony, the defense

---

[10] Although most jurisdictions refer to the "standard of care in the community," unless the community is a small, rural area, the standard is similar in most medical centers and skilled nursing homes in America.

[11] Note the absence of the words "in the same or similar locality" (i.e., community), that had previously been included in BAJI No. 6.00.1 (2002).

[12] For example, the nurse practitioner's efforts would clearly be unsuccessful if, for instance, the patient died. But the law recognizes that healthcare providers cannot be a guarantor of success.

attorney will remind the jury that the law does not require perfection.

Injury is generally anything that a reasonable person might construe as physical or emotional harm and any financial consequence of same. The injury must be tied to the violation of the standard of care; if it is not, the plaintiff cannot prevail. If the injection in the above example caused even a small reaction, that injury was *caused by* the nurse practitioner failing to comply with the standard of care. But if the plaintiff sues for a malady not caused by allergic reaction to penicillin, there is no connection even though the nurse practitioner was technically negligent, and the plaintiff's case will fail likely before it ever reaches trial. Or, if a deviation from the standardized procedure or even the standard of care cannot be tied to the injury, then there is no causal connection between the deviation and the damages being claimed, and again, the claim will fail unless it is also predicated on other acts or omissions that are alleged to have been negligent.

The plaintiff must prove duty, breach, and injury by a "preponderance of the evidence" (BAJI, 2002a).[13] Plaintiff attorneys commonly explain this phrase to juries by referencing the scales held by Lady Justice—if one scale dips ever so slightly below the other, it is said that the weight of the evidence *preponderates* and thus, the plaintiff has proved his or her case. This burden is different from and less than the more familiar burden of proof in a criminal prosecution: "beyond a reasonable doubt." California no longer uses the term *preponderance*, electing instead to use the simpler language: "more likely true than not true" (CACI, 2005a). Thus, in California, it is the plaintiff's burden to prove it more likely than not that the nurse practitioner had a duty to the plaintiff, more likely than not that the nurse practitioner negligently breached that duty by failing to comply with the standard of care, more likely than not that the plaintiff was injured, and more likely than not that the negligence caused the injury. Similarly, the defense will try to attack one or more of these categories (negligence, causation, and damages); for if there is a defense to any one of them, the plaintiff's case cannot succeed.

The nurse practitioner has no burden of proving that he or she was *not* negligent, but would be foolish not to present convincing evidence nevertheless, for if the jury believes that the plaintiff's evidence causes the scale to dip even a little ("all you need is the weight of a feather" is a common argument), in reality the burden *is* now with the nurse practitioner to add weight to his or her side of the scales.

Unless the breach of duty was some simple act of negligence that is obvious to a lay person without the need of further education, an expert will be necessary to explain what the standard of care requires (*Landeros v. Flood*, 1976; CACI, 2005c).[14] Although in malpractice cases, an expert is almost always required, the plaintiff need not, in many instances, use another nurse practitioner to establish the standard of care. Indeed, in some jurisdictions, a physician with sufficient experience working with or supervising nurse practitioners may provide this testimony (*Cline v. Lund*, 1973; *Chaddock v. Cohn*, 1979).[15] It is even possible that a registered nurse may provide the expert testimony on the standard of care of a nurse practitioner if the conduct or action in question is also performed by registered

---

[13] The plaintiff has the burden of proving by a preponderance of the evidence all of the facts necessary to establish proof. Preponderance of the evidence means evidence that has a more convincing force than that opposed to it.

[14] When you are deciding whether the defendant was negligent, you must base your decision only on the testimony of the expert witnesses (including the defendant) who have testified in this case.

[15] Many other examples are cited in McDonald, G. (2005). *California medical malpractice, law and practice* (Rev. ed., Vol. 1, p. 382). Eagan, MN: West.

nurses (McDonald, 2005).[16] A plaintiff attorney may use such an expert, then argue to the jury that "even a registered nurse" should know not to do what the nurse practitioner did (however, a sharp plaintiff attorney would more likely have his doctor expert testify "even a registered nurse would know that"). Because nurse practitioners do not generally give expert testimony as often as do physicians, and because a physician's testimony may be perceived as carrying more weight than a nurse practitioner's, it is not unusual for either side to retain a doctor rather than a nurse practitioner to provide expert testimony. The plaintiff's attorney might argue that the standard of care required the nurse practitioner to consult with or call in a physician or physician-specialist to evaluate or treat the patient. Or the attorney might argue that the nurse practitioner defendant failed to possess a sufficient degree of skill and learning by, for example, not having a certification as a gerontologic nurse practitioner. If the nurse practitioner defendant did not make the aforementioned referral and the patient suffered adverse consequences through inaction, omission, or ineffective treatment, then the plaintiff attorney will ask the judge to instruct the jury that the nurse practitioner is held to the same standard of care as the physician or physician/nurse practitioner specialist. Such an instruction is found in California's Civil Jury Instructor No. 508: If a reasonably careful [nurse practitioner] in the same situation would have referred [the patient] to a [specialist], then the defendant was negligent if

he or she did not do so" (CACI, 2005e). For example, a suit may contend that the nurse practitioner should have consulted a surgeon for a patient's pressure ulcer or a psychiatrist for a patient's depression, and when she did not, she assumed the same (higher) standard of care as would be required of a surgeon or psychiatrist. Jurors are likely to believe that a surgeon, who determines if and when to surgically debride or otherwise treat a skin ulcer, or a psychiatrist, a specialist in mood disorders, would naturally provide more specialized if not better care than the nurse practitioner. The defense must then have a surgeon or psychiatrist testify that the nurse practitioner met the standard of a reasonable surgeon or psychiatrist *and* that the injury or event would have occurred even in the hands of such a specialist. The defense then must not only argue that the nurse practitioner should *not* be held to a higher standard but also that the nurse practitioner's conduct complied with that higher standard should the jury choose to apply it.

ELDER ABUSE LAW

Although outside the scope of this chapter, it should be noted that many states have enacted laws that make the willful causing or permitting of elder abuse a crime, punishable by either imprisonment, fine, or some combination of both (Ca. Penal Code, § 368; EADACPA, 1992h).[17]

A key distinction between elder abuse and malpractice cases, as pointed out earlier, is that

---

[16] This cites cases where a physician of a specialty other than the defendant was allowed to testify as to whether the defendant met the standard of care where the expert nevertheless demonstrated a professional knowledge and experience with the particular procedure or treatment. See also, 85 A.L.R. 2d 1022 (2005 West Group) for a comparison of various state decisions, most to the effect that if the proffered expert was not licensed in the school of medicine to which he or she was to testify, his or her testimony would not be found competent. Thus, if the conduct of a nurse practitioner doing a function a nurse might also perform, such as drawing blood or giving an injection, is at issue, then the nurse would usually qualify as an expert; if, however, the conduct was one not ordinarily performed by a nurse, or one the nurse had no experience with, though she may have studied it, the nurse would not usually qualify as an expert.

[17] This code sets various punishments such as fines not to exceed $6000, imprisonment in either county jail (not to exceed one year), or state prison (not to exceed 4 years; if great bodily harm is done, then 3–7 years).

elder abuse laws, such as California's Elder Abuse and Dependent Adult Civil Protection Act (EADACPA), provide for additional remedies (or financial recoveries), making such cases more attractive to plaintiff lawyers. These enhanced remedies were provided in order to *encourage* the filing of elder abuse lawsuits, which, the California legislature reasoned, would be less likely to be brought without them (EADACPA, 1992a). The California statute provides for the following:

- Recovery of the plaintiff attorney's fees should plaintiff prevail (EADACPA, 1992i; BAJI, 2002d).

- Recovery for any pain and suffering of the plaintiff, even if the patient dies before the action is brought (and whether or not the death occurred as a result of any alleged wrongdoing) (EADACPA, 1992i; BAJI, 2002d; CACI, 2005).[18]

- Recovery of punitive damages when the plaintiff can prove by "clear and convincing" evidence that the conduct in question was willful, malicious, or with reckless disregard for the rights and/or safety of the patient (EADACPA, 1992i).[19]

Both state and federal governments have set forth the goals of such legislation. The Code of Federal Regulations, for instance, states the following:

- The resident has a right to a *dignified existence.*

- A facility must protect and promote the *rights* of each resident.

- A facility must care for its residents in a manner and in an environment that promotes *maintenance or enhancement* of each resident's *quality of life* (Omnibus Budget Reconciliation Act, 1987b).

- Each resident must receive . . . the necessary care and services to attain or maintain the *highest practicable* physical, mental, and psychological well-being . . ." (Omnibus Budget Reconciliation Act, 1987c).

California law states that it was designed to "set forth *fundamental human rights* that all patients *shall be entitled to* in a skilled nursing or intermediate care facility . . ." (Ca. Health & Safety Code, Div. 2), and it underscores the federal language by setting forth that "each patient *shall be* treated with *dignity* and *respect* and shall not be subjected to verbal or physical abuse of any kind" (Ca. Admin. Code, Title 22). Such lofty goals and purposes are laudatory but also provide standards nearly impossible to meet (and give rise to indignation, if not litigation, where conduct falls short), in part because of the subjective nature of the language itself. Such language can, unfortunately, give rise to spurious or extortionist suits based upon complaints as simple as a patient disliking the food he or she is served (and, as a result, not eating), or being "talked down to." Also, note the language requiring that the resident's quality of life be "maintained or enhanced." This is a tall order when quality of life is, in large part, dependent on the progression of a disease, illness, or just plain aging that brought the resident to the nursing facility in the first place.

---

[18] Both BAJI and CACI instructions are based on the California Welfare and Institutions Code section cited and require that the physical abuse, neglect, or fiduciary abuse be the result of recklessness, oppression, fraud, or malice, with authorization, ratification, advanced knowledge of the unfitness of the employee, or where the employee was also an officer or managing agent of the skilled nursing facility/corporation, and proved by *clear and convincing evidence. Clear and convincing* is a higher standard of proof than *by a preponderance of evidence* but not as high as the criminal standard *beyond a reasonable doubt.*

[19] Reckless disregard is defined in the California case of *Delaney v. Baker* 20 Cal. 4th 23 (1999) as "deliberate disregard of the high probability an injury will occur."

Another key distinction is the emphasis on the concept of *neglect*, as opposed to *negligence*. Negligence is the focus in traditional malpractice actions, but lacks the requisite willfulness or reckless disregard for the welfare or safety of the patient to form the basis for the recovery of punitive damages. Neglect, on the other hand, as defined by California law includes "failure to assist in personal hygiene," "failure to provide medical care for physical and mental health needs," "failure to protect from health and safety hazards," and "failure to prevent malnutrition or dehydration" (EADACPA, 1992e); this implies both a more ongoing process and a more conscious evasion of one's duty than a mere mistake.

Whereas malpractice actions focus on a healthcare provider, elder abuse laws focus instead on a care custodian of the nursing home patient. Of course, a physician or nurse practitioner may be considered as much a care custodian as the nursing home administration or the certified nursing assistant (in California, this is true so long as the doctor or nurse practitioner is an "employee of a public or private facility or agency providing care or services for elders or dependent adults" or is a person providing such care whether or not so employed) (Ca. Penal Code § 368; EADACPA, 1992c). In addition, with elder abuse laws the person receiving care is not referred to as the *patient*, but as the *resident*, which tends to deemphasize the professional treatment aspect of the care and emphasize the custodial aspect of the relationship.

In a trial, the plaintiff attorney emphasizes the deterioration of the resident's condition and looks to mechanical issues, such as the number of times a resident is turned in bed in order to prevent bedsores, any staff-to-resident ratio deficiencies, the development of contractures, the resident's weight loss, the number of times the resident refused to eat, or told her family that he or she had to lay in a bed covered with urine or feces. The defense emphasizes the natural progression of disease and the physiological aspects of aging. The plaintiff attorney may show photos of decubitus ulcers, often those taken by the facility itself. The defense usually presents evidence of degenerative disease states, previous skin breakdown, and poor circulation. It is difficult at best to convince a jury of lay people, many of whom are either elderly or whose parents are, that a patient with a weeping decubitus ulcer, perhaps with rotting flesh, has maintained a decent "quality of life."

Many states mandate reporting to one or more controlling agencies of any acts or incidents of suspected abuse of the elderly or dependent-adult patient. In California, the law provides that failure to do so can result in fine or imprisonment (EADACPA, 1992g).[20] This provision makes it clear how important California lawmakers believe it is to prevent and deter elder abuse.

Many states also require written policies to ensure the rights of the elderly patient and that the patient be given copies of or be apprised of the existence of such policies. This is typically a matter for the nursing home administration. However, such laws also require comprehensive periodic written assessments and care plans of the patient and determination whether the care plan is being followed or requires updating. In cases when the nurse practitioner is also subject to state law requiring standardized procedures in order to exceed the usual scope of nursing practice, the care plan may be compared to the standardized procedures to determine if the nurse practitioner is authorized to carry out or update

---

[20] This law provides that any elder or dependent-adult care custodian or health practitioner . . . is a mandated reporter. But EADACPA § 15630(b)(2)(A)(iv) provides that reporting may be excused if "in the exercise of clinical judgment the physician, surgeon, registered nurse, or psychotherapist . . . reasonably believes the abuse did not occur."

the plan without supervision or direct assessment by a physician.

Most skilled nursing facilities have policy and procedure manuals covering a multitude of topics, including, in many instances, nursing and medical care. Some actually use the term *standard of care* in describing procedures they wish to see followed. This terminology should be avoided, because plaintiff attorneys almost always try to introduce the manuals into evidence to show that the care provided did not meet the procedural or policy standards set by the facility itself. When *standard of care* is used in the manuals, it provides free expert testimony to the shortcomings of the care given (or not given). In fact, such manuals should contain disclaimers that they do not purport to establish any standards of care.

Violation of any statutory language may be used as a tool against the defendant in elder abuse litigation. The doctrine of "negligence per se," in which negligence may be established without further proof by showing a violation of an elder abuse statute (BAJI, 2002b; Ca. Evidence Code § 669) can turn the burden of proof around, with the burden now placed on the provider to prove that, despite the violation of the statute, the conduct was not negligent or did not cause injury or harm. This burden, needless to say, can be very difficult to overcome.

"No win" or "catch-22" situations can be created when the law creates two potentially conflicting duties, such as the duty to prevent falls and the duty not to unreasonably restrain; the duty to prevent bedsores and the duty not to move the patient against his or her wishes; the duty not to over medicate thus preventing the patient from participating in his own care and the duty not to abuse the patient by being unresponsive to complaints of pain, and so on.

The nurse practitioner should know that while the majority of elder abuse cases are directed against the skilled nursing facility owners and administration, the nurse practitioner may be one of the key players. The plaintiff attorney, as part of his indictment of the facility and his characterization of "profit over patient rights," may contend that the use of nurse practitioners is part of the cost-cutting plan that results in unacceptable or deficient care. To do so, he must make the nurse practitioner look relatively uneducated and unskilled, not to mention uncaring. Thus, the nurse practitioner, as well as the certified nursing assistants and the licensed nurses may be subject to accusations and aggressive questioning. The attorney will look for "sound bites" during the nurse practitioner's deposition that he might use during trial to demonstrate the nurse practitioner's lack of skill or understanding. The plaintiff attorney will also look to use the nurse practitioner's testimony against the facility wherever possible. It must also be kept in mind that the nurse practitioner can still be sued for an individual act of malpractice or a pattern of conduct constituting neglect that could be significantly tied to the claim of overall neglect or abuse against the nursing facility.

In prosecuting the elder abuse claim, a plaintiff attorney may not necessarily need an expert, certainly not as is almost universally required in a malpractice action. The plaintiff attorney may point to statute violations or Department of Health and Human Services/Department of Social Services survey deficiencies (to prove knowledge of any preexisting inability to provide adequate care in order to establish reckless disregard) or argue that the facts speak for themselves and that the jury doesn't need to hear from an expert when the abuse or neglect is obvious.

CHARTING AND DOCUMENTATION ISSUES

"If it is not in the chart, it didn't happen." This phrase has become a mantra among medical malpractice and elder abuse plaintiff attorneys. Such attorneys exploit the deficient chart in this fashion, interrogating the nurse practitioner (or other healthcare provider) on the stand:

- "Isn't the purpose of charting to document pertinent complaints, vital signs, and conditions, and to document your reaction to same, such as treatment or diagnostic testing?"

- "And isn't one of the major reasons for doing this so the next doctor or nurse practitioner reading the chart will know what was done and how the patient reacted?"

- "Well then, show me where in the chart during your care of the patient that you recorded such information? Where did you note in this chart that you were aware of or considered the patient's weight (loss), vomiting, (de)hydration, elevated white count, incontinence, abdominal distention, pain level, and so forth?"

- "Isn't one of the reasons for charting to document the progression of symptoms?"

- "Well then, where do you chart the condition of Mr. Smith's skin ulcer from October 2nd to October 30th?"

- "You wouldn't know the patient's vital signs without seeing them on the chart, would you?"

- "Well then, what were Mr. Smith's vital signs at any time from October 2nd to October 30th?"

- "Where in the chart does it say that Mr. Smith was turned every two hours as ordered, or that you were or were not aware your order was being carried out?"

- "I don't see any mention in the chart that you consulted the patient's physician—that *is* required by the standard of care, isn't it?"

- "You saw Mr. Smith on six occasions in the fall of 2004, yet you only recorded vital signs on three of those occasions. Why was it important to record the vital signs on three occasions and not the other three times?"

Truth is, whether or not your chart ends up in court, it is good practice to document as much as possible. Make your entries readable to prevent mistakes (and embarrassment at trial when you are unable to read your own entry to the jury. Imagine being questioned by an attorney: "And how did you expect the nurse to follow *that* order/know what you wanted/what you were thinking?"). Look through one of your old charts on a patient you do not recall, and see if your charting tells a good "story" of what went on, what you thought, whether you considered and ruled out alternative diagnoses, what you ordered, and what the patient's response was. What kind of nurse practitioner do you appear to be from a review of the chart alone? Charting differential diagnoses is recommended, for one reason, because you could conceivably be sued a year or two later and asked whether you considered and ruled out the diagnosis you are now accused of missing. Better to have thought of it and mistakenly felt you had ruled it out than not to have thought of it at all, which is what it may look like if your chart is scant and includes only your ultimate diagnosis. Many practitioners use the *SOAP* (Subjective complaint, Objective findings, Assessment, and Plan) format for their entries. This is a well-recognized method and should serve you well so long as it is not used simply to shorten your note taking. It is not a good idea to repeatedly use the same cryptic entry, such as "patient doing well" because the entry is too vague and gives no specifics, and repetition of the phrase infers an overly casual approach to patient assessment. Remember that juries may associate your entries with your care. If your entries are short and cryptic, they may believe that your assessments were quick and not thorough. If your handwriting is more like scribbling, they may conclude, even subconsciously, that you must have been in a hurry during your assessment.

As you are going through the risk-benefit analysis of detailed charting versus spending time on something more enjoyable, consider that if this patient should sue you and your case comes to court two years later, if there is a "he said/she said" type of dispute, the opposing attorney will point out that you've seen hundreds of patients and residents in the interim, and he will infer there is no way you could actually recall that which wasn't important enough to chart, while this was the only time his client was hospitalized, injured, and treated for this condition, and his memory is therefore more trustworthy. The patient may have his or her spouse testify in support of his or her version of the facts. But if your chart contains specifics, is detailed, and is trustworthy, that document will have more credibility than either you *or* the patient.

Good charting may, in fact, ensure the plaintiff testifies honestly about what happened or at least doesn't dispute what is written there. In this vein, quoting the patient can be quite helpful. In one case, when a patient sued a physician for missing the diagnosis of amaurosis fugax (temporary loss of vision in one eye due to insufficient flow of blood—often a precursor to stroke), the doctor noted that the patient described seeing a "white curtain" coming down over one of his eyes. Although a "curtain" is commonly associated with amaurosis fugax, white is not the "default" color for blindness, but is more akin to a flash or symptom of a migraine. In deposition, the patient testified that the curtain was grey or black (the default color), which would have made the diagnosis almost certain. The quotation marks emphasized the fact that the description came straight from the patient, was more believable than the patient's testimony in pursuit of a lawsuit, and helped explain the errant diagnosis of migraine.

If you do get sued, review the chart in question. If you feel that it does not tell the whole story, you must resist the temptation (and panic) of "fixing" the chart. I have represented healthcare professionals for 23 years and have seen enough "doctoring" of charts to know that this is one of the worst mistakes one can make. Altering medical records that might be admitted into evidence in a court of law can be either a misdemeanor or a felony (Ca. Penal Code, §§ 132, 134, 135). If your attorney finds out about it, he cannot ethically put the records into evidence or ask you to testify as to their contents unless you first admit under oath that you had altered them (Ca. Bus. & Prof. Code, 6106; Ca. Rules of Prof. Conduct, §§ 5–200, 5–220). If you testify that the records are unaltered, and you are proven wrong (almost always by a copy of the chart obtained prior to the lawsuit, but in many other potential ways), you will have perjured yourself and the judge may throw out all of your testimony as a result, you will have lost any credibility you may have had with the jury and almost certainly will lose your case. Some states allow a cause of action for the spoliation of records—you can be sued separately just for altering or disposing of the records. In California, you may not be separately sued, but the judge is given the discretion of throwing out all or part of your defense (*Cedars-Sinai Med. Center v. Superior Court*, 1998), which could make it nearly impossible to defend the case. There have been many cases that but for the alteration of records could otherwise have been won by the healthcare professional, even with the unaltered chart, but that had to be settled *because of* the alteration. Although document alterations are not always caught, most of the time they are. In many, if not most cases, a copy of the chart is obtained by the patient, the patient's family, or attorney before the provider is even aware they are being sued. Another copy is obtained during the litigation and they are scrutinized for discrepancies. Attorneys are trained to review records for such alterations, and if they have any suspicions, there are trained document examiners who can confirm the "doctoring" in any number of ways. Don't do it. Period.

If, while treating a patient (not after you have been sued), you feel the need to add a line or two for the sake of completeness, be certain to put the words *late entry* and your initials next to the addition as evidence that you are being up front and honest about the timing of the addition. Do not, however, make a late addition of false information. Even if done *before* you are sued, it will look like you *knew* you would be sued (because you already knew you had done something wrong) and tried to protect yourself ahead of time.

At all times, keep your entries professional Avoid any finger-pointing or entries of blame. Such entries will come back to haunt you in litigation when the person you blamed in the chart is now pointing the finger back at you as his only means of defense, or the plaintiff attorney claims that you made the entry to place *your* blame elsewhere, making your alleged transgression even worse. In one case, there was finger-pointing between two doctors, residents at the same hospital, each claiming in multiple entries that the other one's negligence was the cause of a newborn's brain damage, when a subsequent MRI revealed the damage was congenital, and not caused by either doctor. Nevertheless, the entries were so damaging, the defense of the case was severely compromised.

Also, resist the temptation to blame or label the patient. Such charting might actually be used as evidence of your bias against and your lack of concern for the patient. Should the patient refuse recommended treatment or therapy, note it carefully, including what you said to convince him or her otherwise, without characterizing the patient as "stubborn." You may wish to consider the language you use in your charting, noting that you "encouraged" the patient or that you "reassured," "supported," or "comforted" the patient, rather than saying the patient was "convinced" or "accepted" your explanation. Consideration of such language might even lead to an improved bedside manner.

Sometimes even a well-intentioned entry can pose a problem. In a case that went to arbitration, the plaintiff who claimed elder abuse was a nasty, uncooperative, sarcastic, and angry woman who missed no opportunity to criticize her care and caretakers. In short, she was the "patient from hell." (Of course, during the arbitration, she was as sweet as apple pie). Although *her* abuse of her caretakers was well documented, even admitted, one entry in the chart noted that she "responded to TLC." The arbitrator cited this entry in his ruling that it was the facility's (and doctors') *lack* of TLC (and "poor bedside manners") on other occasions that caused the patient to be upset and angry. When you see such a patient, you should recognize that the patient or his or her family is probably more likely to sue than a patient with a different disposition. Your entries and the entries of those you supervise should reflect ongoing efforts to meet the patient's social and psychological needs as well as his or her medical needs. Note your interactions with the patient, where you "explain" options and procedures and obtain the patient's understanding and consent. If nothing else, your chart should reflect that you were attentive to your patient.

Employees of nursing facilities can be underpaid, overworked, asked to do menial and objectionable tasks, and as a result may be neither long-term employees nor particularly loyal. They may be angry with the administration or even with a doctor or nurse practitioner. These ex-employees are often tracked down by plaintiff attorneys and may be more than willing to testify to the shortcomings of the administration, doctor, or nurse practitioner in order to justify or excuse their own conduct. The more entries you make in the chart, the less likely you will be accused of being absent, abandoning the patient, or not responding to calls. If a nurse or certified nurse assistant does the charting, ideally they should note in the chart whenever you are at the patient's bedside. Similarly, the nurse practitioner should note in the chart whenever he or she consults with the physician.

Although it may be argued that inadequate charting is, either by itself or in specific instances, below the standard of care or is evidence of an omission or mistake, inadequate charting alone, when it causes no harm to the patient, cannot be the basis of a claim of malpractice. In a trial, caution should be exercised so that inadequate charting is not exploited where it has no connection to any damage suffered by the patient. A plaintiff attorney may attempt to use such charting to infer that you have a character trait for sloppiness or carelessness where this type of character evidence is otherwise usually inadmissible. Even when not specifically pointed out or exploited, you may find one of your short chart entries—in which your handwriting is indecipherable, you misspelled *patient*, and your order for a dose of 5 cc looks like it could also be 50 cc—enlarged and placed in front of a jury, and as we attorneys like to say, it may "speak for itself."

Of course, you cannot live your life or manage your career constantly worrying about being sued or what might happen if you are sued. But as you nurse practitioners like to say, "An ounce of prevention is worth a pound of cure."

REFERENCES

BAJI (Book of Approved Jury Instructions, California), 9th ed., No. 2.60 (2002a).

BAJI, 9th ed., No. 13.03 (2002e).

BAJI, 9th ed., No. 3.45 (2002b).

BAJI, 9th ed., No. 7.41, 7.46 (2002c).

BAJI, 9th ed., No. 7.46 (2002d).

Ca. Admin. Code, Title 22, Div. 5, Chapter 3: 22 CCR § 72315(b) or 22 CA. ADC § 72315(b).

Ca. Bus. & Prof. Code § 6106.

Ca. Bus. & Prof. Code §§ 801, 801.1, 802, 803.2.

Ca. Civ. Code § 2295; Restatement Second of Agency, § 220.

Ca. Evidence Code § 413.

Ca. Evidence Code § 669.

Ca. Health & Safety Code, Div. 2, Chapter 3.9, § 1599.

Ca. Penal Code § 368(i).

Ca. Penal Code § 368.

Ca. Penal Code §§ 132, 134, 135.

Ca. Rules of Prof. Conduct, Rules 5–200, 5–220.

CACI (California Civil Jury Instructions), No. 200 (2005a).

CACI, No. 204 (2005b).

CACI, No. 3104, 3105 (2005f).

CACI, No. 3703 (2005g).

CACI, No. 501 (2005c).

CACI, No. 505 (2005d).

CACI, No. 508 (2005e).

Cedars-Sinai Medical Center v. Superior Court, 18 Cal. 4th 1 (1998).

Chaddock v. Cohn, 96 Cal. App. 3d 205, 208 (1979).

Cline v. Lund, 31 Cal. App. 3d, 755,766 (1973).

EADACPA (Elder Abuse and Dependent Adult Civil Protection Act), Ca. Welfare and Institutions Code § 15600 (1992a).

EADACPA, Ca. Welfare and Institutions Code § 15600(j) (1992b).

EADACPA, Ca. Welfare and Institutions Code § 15610.17 (1992c).

EADACPA, Ca. Welfare and Institutions Code § 15610.27 (1992d). Ill. Ann. Stat., Ch. 23, para 6602(e); Mass. Gen. Laws, ch. 19A, § 14 (age 60); Ca. W & I Code § 15610.23; Ark. Stat. Ann. § 5–28–101 (1) (Supp 1989); Mn. Stat. Ann. § 626.557(2)(b) (West Supp 1990); California's Book of Approved Jury Instructions (BAJI) 9th Ed. (2002), Instr. No. 7.40; Judicial Council of California Civil Jury Instructions 2005 (CACI) Instr. No. 3112 (age 18).

EADACPA, Ca. Welfare and Institutions Code § 15610.57(a)(b) (1992e).

EADACPA, Ca. Welfare and Institutions Code § 15630(a), (h) (1992g).

EADACPA, Ca. Welfare and Institutions Code § 15656 (1992h).

EADACPA, Ca. Welfare and Institutions Code §§ 15610.57, 15657 (1992f).

EADACPA, Ca. Welfare and Institutions Code §§ 15657 (1992i).

Elam v. College Park Hospital, 132 Cal. App. 3d 332 (1982).

Health Care Quality Improvement Act, 45 C.F.R. § 60.1 et seq. (1986).

Hull v. Lopez, 2002 Ohio 6162 (2002).

Landeros v. Flood, 17 Cal. 3d 399, 410 (1976).

Malloy v. Fong, 37 Cal. 2d 356, 370 (1951).

Marquis, J. (1999, November 30). California and the West: Medical errors kill thousands, panel says. *The Los Angeles Times.*

McDonald, G. (2005). *California medical malpractice, law and practice* (Rev. ed., Vol. 1, pp. 382, 383). Eagan, MN: West.

Omnibus Budget Reconciliation Act, 42 C.F.R. § 483.10 (1987a).

Omnibus Budget Reconciliation Act, 42 C.F.R. § 483.15 (1987b).

Omnibus Budget Reconciliation Act, 42 C.F.R. § 483.25 (1987c).

Planned Parenthood of Northwest Indiana, Inc. v. Vines, 543 N. E. 2d 654, 660 (1989).

Welch v. Scheinfeld, 801 N.Y.S. 2d 277, 282 (2005).

SECTION II

Management Guidelines for Common Disorders

CHAPTER 6

Cardiac Disorders

Barbara White

ATRIAL FIBRILLATION

Definition

Atrial fibrillation (AF) is a cardiac dysrhythmia characterized by ineffective atrial contractions with an irregular and usually rapid ventricular response pattern. The condition can be paroxysmal or persistent and can produce emergent symptoms requiring immediate attention. Untreated, especially in the elderly, it can lead to altered cardiac output and the risk of clot formation and resultant cerebral thromboembolism. It may also alternate with atrial flutter, characterized by rapid atrial contractions (200–300 per minute) with a blocked and slower ventricular response that may also decrease cardiac output and produce similar symptoms to atrial fibrillation.

Epidemiology

Atrial fibrillation is the most common cardiac dysrhythmia. The incidence increases with age, and there is a higher incidence in men than in women. Prevalence of nonvalvular AF in nursing homes exceeds that in the community and is estimated at 7.5–17% (Crecelius & Levenson, 2004). In addition to age and gender,

other risk factors for the development of AF include the following:

- Hypertension
- Coronary artery disease, myocardial infarction, pericarditis, myocarditis, cardiomyopathies
- Heart failure
- Valve disease including rheumatic and, especially, mitral
- Other supraventricular tachyarrhythmias (e.g., atrial flutter)
- Pulmonary embolus, other pulmonary disorders
- Diabetes
- Clinical and subclinical hyperthyroidism
- Alcohol overuse, especially binge drinking
- Familial tendency
- Cardiac surgery

In some instances correcting the acute cause of the arrhythmia may cure it. Heart failure may be either a cause or an effect of atrial fibrillation and may be the first indication of the dysrhythmia. The exact mechanism that produces AF is unclear, but likely involves fibrosis, hypertrophy, and/or inflammation of atrial fibers causing disruption of the normal conduction pattern through the sinoatrial node (Fuster et al., 2001). Persistent atrial fibrillation likely produces cardiac remodeling known as tachycardic cardiomyopathy (Fuster et al.). Atrial fibrillation can disrupt normal hemodynamics producing stasis, endothelial dysfunction, and hypercoagulability (Virchow's triad). This promotes thromboembolization and increases the risk of stroke.

Patients with atrial fibrillation may have low, moderate, or high risk for stroke. A risk stratification tool developed for use in community settings (CHADS-2) has also been recommended for use in nursing homes because it was validated with a recently hospitalized sample of adults ages 65–95 years (Latif & Messinger-Rapport, 2004). Level of risk will suggest management options (Table 6-1).

Common Presenting Signs and Symptoms

Atrial fibrillation may be asymptomatic or symptomatic. The first manifestation of the dysrhythmia may be a transient ischemic attack (TIA), stroke, or heart failure. Upon admission to the nursing home the nurse practitioner should review the medical record for evidence of a history of atrial fibrillation or risk factors for its development. If a patient is admitted on anticoagulation therapy, every effort should be made to ascertain (a) the reason for the treatment, (b) the duration of the treatment, (c) previous attempts to investigate underlying causes of the disorder that may be reversible, (d) stroke risk, (e) bleeding risk, and (f) patient and family preferences for treatment (Crecelius & Levenson, 2004).

TABLE 6-1	Stroke Risk Stratification and Recommended Anticoagulant Therapy for Patients with Atrial Fibrillation	
RISK LEVEL	**CRITERIA[a] AND CHADS-2 SCORE[b]**	**RECOMMENDED TREATMENT**
Low	Age < 65 with no cardiovascular disease	Aspirin 325 mg/day
Moderate	Age 65–75 *Diabetes mellitus (1)* Coronary artery disease with normal LVEF	Adjusted-dose warfarin to maintain an INR 2.0–3.0 *or* Aspirin 325 mg/day
High	Age > 75 (1) *Prior stroke, TIA, or systemic embolus (2)* *Hypertension (1)* *Abnormal LVEF (1)* Mitral valve disease Bioprosthetic or prosthetic heart valve	Adjusted-dose warfarin to maintain an INR 2.0–3.0 (2.5–3.5 with prosthetic valve) *or* Aspirin 325 mg/day if warfarin is contraindicated or refused

LVEF, left ventricular ejection fraction; TIA, transient ischemic attack; INR, international normalized ratio.

[a] American College of Chest Physicians (2001) risk stratification scheme, Albers et al. (2001).

[b] CHADS-2 risk stratification scores for five specific items (*in italic*): 0–1 = low risk; 2–3 = moderate risk; 4–6 = high risk.

Patients may present with the following transient or persistent symptoms:

- Palpitations
- Chest pain
- Dyspnea
- Fatigue
- Lightheadedness, confusion, or syncope
- Polyuria, possibly associated with release of atrial natriuretic peptide (Fuster et al., 2001)
- Signs and symptoms of underlying disease (e.g., hypertension, heart failure)

Patients with atrial fibrillation may present with the following signs:

- Irregular heart rate and rhythm by palpation and auscultation.
- Heart rate is usually rapid, but in the elderly it may be within normal range.
- Atrial flutter usually presents with a regular rhythm.
- A mitral or aortic cardiac murmur may be present.
- Signs of cardiogenic shock.

Differential Diagnoses

- Atrial flutter
- Other supraventricular tachycardias
- Reversible causes of atrial fibrillation

Essential Diagnostic and Laboratory Tests

- ECG or rhythm strip—If AF is present, RR intervals are usually irregular. This helps to distinguish AF from other supraventricular arrhythmias.
- Coagulation studies—Prothrombin time and international normalized ratio (PT/INR), complete blood count (CBC).
- Other tests that may be considered include Holter monitor for paroxysmal AF

and echocardiogram to determine underlying heart disease.

- Refer to cardiology for more extensive workup, if necessary.

Management Plan

The goals for the management of atrial fibrillation are to correct reversible causes, prevent stroke, and relieve symptoms.

Nonpharmacologic

- Regularly check rate and rhythm at rest, with exertion, and with any changes in medication (Crecelius & Levenson, 2004).
- If possible, discontinue cardiac stimulant drugs (e.g., sympathomimetics, caffeine) that may exacerbate the condition.
- If on warfarin, monitor dosing with any change in physical condition, medications, or diet (Table 6-2).
- Consult with the dietician to maintain consistency in vitamin K-rich foods.

Pharmacologic

Historically, atrial fibrillation has been undertreated in long-term care (Crecelius & Levenson, 2004). Current guidelines recommend that medication management should be directed at controlling cardiac rate, and in certain circumstances rhythm, and for provision of anticoagulation. Management of atrial fibrillation in the nursing home should be done in collaboration with the primary physician. Specific interventions depend on the duration of the condition when it is discovered.

New Onset

- *Refer for emergency treatment with electrical cardioversion or intravenous drug administration if the patient is hemodynamically unstable.*
- Look for underlying causes of AF that may be reversible.

TABLE 6-2   Warfarin Drug Interactions

Increase Warfarin Effects

Antimicrobials	Azole antifungals—Miconazole (Monistat) oral, intravaginal, topical; ketoconazole (Nizoral), fluconazole (Diflucan), itraconazole (Sporanox)
	Cephalosporins (parenteral)—Cefoperazone, cefamandole, cefotetan, cefmetazole
	Fluoroquinolones—Ciprofloxacin (Cipro), levofloxacin (Levaquin), norfloxacin (Noroxin), ofloxacin (Floxin)
	Macrolides (all)—Especially erythromycin, clarithromycin
	Metronidazole (Flagyl)
	Penicillins (high parenteral doses)—Penicillin-G, piperacillin, ticarcillin
	Sulfonamides—Trimethoprim-sulfamethoxazole, sulfamethizole, sulfamethoxazole, sulfisoxazole
	Tetracyclines—Doxycycline, tetracycline
Cardiovascular Drugs	Amiodarone
	Propafenone
Anti-inflammatories and Analgesics	NSAIDs—Especially celecoxib
	Acetaminophen ≥ 9.1 g/week
	Aspirin > low dose once daily
Gastrointestinal Drugs	Cimetidine
Decrease Warfarin Effects	
Antimicrobials	Griseofulvin
	Penicillins—Dicloxacillin, nafcillin
CNS Agents	Barbiturates
	Carbamazepine
	Phenytoin

- If hemodynamically stable and duration of AF is less than 48 hours, consider initial anticoagulation with heparin and refer for cardioversion.

- If hemodynamically stable and duration of AF is more than 48 hours, consider initial anticoagulation with warfarin for 3 weeks followed by referral for cardioversion. Continue warfarin therapy for at least 4 weeks after the procedure. Premature cardioversion increases the risk of thromboembolic events.

Duration Unknown

- *Refer for emergency treatment with electrical cardioversion or intravenous drug administration if the patient is hemodynamically unstable.*

- Look for underlying causes of AF that may be reversible such as Wolff-Parkinson-White syndrome (WPW) or atrioventricular (AV) node reentrant tachycardias.

- Manage heart rate to 70–90 beats per minute. Less drug-related adverse effects occur with rate control than with rhythm management, especially in the elderly, and efficacy is equivalent.

  ○ Beta-blockers atenolol and metoprolol have demonstrated efficacy in rate control at rest and during exercise by slowing conduction through the AV node. These are recommended as first-line therapy. The choice may be driven by potential interactions with comorbidities.

○ Calcium channel blockers diltiazem and verapamil have demonstrated efficacy in rate control at rest and during exercise by slowing conduction through the AV node. These are recommended as alternative first-line therapy. The choice may be driven by potential interactions with comorbidities.

○ Digoxin is effective for rate control only at rest and should be considered a second-line therapy for active patients.

○ If single-agent therapy fails, consider the combination of digoxin with diltiazem, atenolol, or betaxolol, which has demonstrated efficacy at rest and during exercise.

• Begin or continue anticoagulation as appropriate for patient condition (Table 6-3). Anticoagulation significantly decreases cerebrovascular accident (CVA) morbidity and mortality. Current guidelines do not consider fall risk, alone, as a reason to defer anticoagulation.

○ For patients with low- or one moderate-risk factor consider aspirin 325 mg/day or warfarin (American Geriatrics Society [AGS], 2000).

○ For patients with more than one moderate- or any high-risk factor consider chronic warfarin therapy (AGS, 2000).

○ Anticoagulation benefit usually outweighs risk. Warfarin therapy is not recommended for patients with the following (Institute for Clinical Systems Improvement [ICSI], 2005a):

  ▪ Low cerebrovascular accident (CVA) risk

  ▪ High risk for intracranial or gastrointestinal hemorrhage

  ▪ Active bleeding, hematocrit < 30

  ▪ Known coagulation defects

  ▪ Thrombocytopenia (platelets < 50,000/mm³)

▪ Recent hemorrhagic stroke

▪ Excessive alcohol intake

▪ Uncontrolled hypertension (> 180/100 mmHg)

▪ Daily NSAID use

▪ Pending invasive procedure

○ Titrate dose to maintain the INR at 2.5 (range 2.0–3.0). Patients with mitral valve disease or mechanical prosthetic valves should be maintained at an INR of 3.0 (range 2.5–3.5).

○ Initiate rhythm control only if the patient is unable to tolerate the atrial fibrillation or flutter. Recommended drugs for rhythm control are amiodarone, disopyramide, propafenone, or sotalol (Snow et al., 2003).

Patient, Family, and Staff Education

• Nature and course of the disorder

• Bleeding precautions for patients on anticoagulants

• Symptoms to report

• Medications and foods to monitor while taking warfarin

• Medic alert bracelet at discharge to the community, if taking warfarin

• Need to notify health care providers, if taking warfarin

• Emergency treatment for dangerously elevated INR, persistent bleeding

Physician Consultation

• Refer to the cardiologist for cardioversion.

• Consult with the primary physician on antiarrhythmic and anticoagulation therapy.

TABLE 6-3   Guidelines for Managing Oral Anticoagulation in the Elderly

- Obtain a baseline international normalizing ratio (INR) and activated partial thromboplastin time (APTT) if using concurrent heparin therapy.

- Evaluate the medication regimen for possible drug interactions with warfarin.

- Consider an initial dose of 5 mg or less of warfarin in the elderly.

- Order warfarin dose to be taken at the same time of day, in late afternoon or evening.

- Do not switch between generics or between brand name and generic warfarin formulations during therapy.

- Monitor INR daily until stable for two measurements (2.0–3.0). Obese patients and the elderly may take longer to reach a steady state.

- Discontinue any heparin when the INR is in the therapeutic range for two measures.

- Continue to monitor INR 2–3 times/week for 1–2 weeks; weekly for 1 month and monthly thereafter.

- When adjusting a warfarin dose, spread the adjustment over the total weekly dose, if possible. A 15% adjustment of the weekly dose is recommended. This is likely to result in approximately a 1.0 INR change.

- Increase the INR monitoring schedule during changes in patient condition, medications, or diet.

- If bleeding occurs at a therapeutic INR look for an underlying cause.

- If INR exceeds 3.0 initiate the following protocols:

  ○ INR 3.0–5.0—If no bleeding, withhold 1 dose or lower dose; monitor INR, and resume therapy when normal.

  ○ INR 5.0–9.0—If no bleeding, withhold 1–2 doses; monitor INR, and resume therapy when normal. In addition, consider the following:

    ▪ Consider vitamin K_1 (1–2.5 mg orally) for bleeding risk.

    ▪ Give 2–4 mg orally if rapid correction is needed.

    ▪ Add an additional 1–2 mg for persistently elevated INR.

  ○ INR > 9.0—Withhold warfarin; monitor INR. Give vitamin K_1 3–5 mg orally and additional doses if INR remains elevated in 24–48 hours.

- Significant bleeding—Discontinue warfarin; give vitamin K_1 10 mg slow IV infusion and refer for treatment of blood loss.

TABLE 6-3   *(continued)*

- Prior to invasive procedures:
  - ○ Moderate-risk patient—Discontinue warfarin about 4 days prior to procedure to allow INR to normalize. In addition, do the following:
    - Give low-molecular weight heparin (LMWH) or low-dose unfractionated heparin (LDUH) 5000 IU subcutaneously 2 days prior to procedure and following it.
    - Resume warfarin postprocedure, and discontinue heparin when INR is in the therapeutic range for 2 days.
    - For minor surgery or dental procedures weigh the use of topical agents to reduce bleeding instead of discontinuing warfarin.
  - ○ High-risk patient: Discontinue warfarin about 4 days prior to procedure to allow INR to normalize. In addition, do the following:
    - Administer full dose heparin subcutaneously or IV and discontinue about 5 hours prior to procedure, *or* give LMWH until 12–24 hours before procedure.
    - Resume heparin or LMWH and warfarin after procedure and discontinue when INR is in the therapeutic range for 2 days.

Source: American Geriatrics Society, 2000; ICSI, 2005a.

CORONARY ARTERY DISEASE

Definition

Coronary artery disease (CAD) is the condition resulting from the narrowing or occlusion of the arterial blood vessels that supply oxygen to the heart. Diminished oxygen supply results in myocardial ischemia that produces the characteristic pain of angina pectoris. Progression of the ischemia can further damage cardiac muscle and result in what is now termed *acute coronary syndrome* (ACS), and includes the following:

- Unstable angina
- Non-ST elevation myocardial infarction (NSTEMI)
- ST elevation myocardial infarction (STEMI)

Angina pectoris is a syndrome that causes discomfort in the chest, jaw, shoulder, back, or arm (American College of Cardiology/ American Heart Association [ACC/AHA], 2002) as a result of coronary ischemia. The pain may occur with or without precipitating factors. Additional causes include valvular heart disease, hypertrophic cardiomyopathy, and uncontrolled hypertension (ACC/AHA). Anginal episodes are characterized as predictable and readily managed (stable coronary artery disease [SCAD]) or difficult to control and a precursor to acute myocardial infarction (unstable angina).

The major end point of cardiac ischemia is acute myocardial infarction (AMI) resulting from occlusion of an epicardial artery causing cardiac muscle necrosis. Without rapid medical or surgical revascularization death can occur.

NSTEMI was formerly called the *subendocardial* or *non-Q-wave* MI. Unstable angina and NSTEMI are similarly characterized by unstable coronary artery thrombi. Both present with characteristic chest pain, ST segment depression, and/or T-wave inversion on the standard ECG. In NSTEMI, however, laboratory results indicate cardiac necrosis. Unstable angina progresses to NSTEMI in about 15% of cases (Awtry & Loscalzo, 2004).

STEMI, formerly called the *transmural* or *Q-wave* MI, demonstrates ST elevations greater than 1 mm in two or more contiguous limb leads, or greater than or equal to 2 mm elevation in precordial leads (ACC/AHA, 2002). Peaked T waves may also be seen in selected precordial and limb leads on the standard ECG. This infarction results from complete occlusion of a coronary artery.

Epidemiology

Coronary artery disease is the major cause of morbidity and mortality for adults 65 years of age and older. Age, alone, is a major risk factor for its development. Coronary artery disease is usually the result of generalized atherosclerosis that likely begins to develop early in life and contributes to diseases including hypertension, peripheral arterial disease, carotid artery disease, transient ischemic attacks, and stroke. Atherosclerosis may also be secondary to other diseases found frequently in nursing homes including diabetes mellitus, hypothyroidism, nephrotic syndrome, chronic renal failure, and diseases of the liver or pancreas. Generalized atherosclerosis increases the severity of any cardiac event.

Atherosclerosis begins with injury to blood vessel endothelium caused by chemical, mechanical, and inflammatory processes secondary to hypercholesterolemia. Low-density lipoprotein cholesterol (LDL-C) deposits produce an inflammatory reaction in blood vessels. Oxidized LDL-C is attacked by macrophages resulting in a lipid core encased in smooth muscle and fibrous tissue that forms the atheromatous plaque. Small plaques with minimal inflammation and a thick fibrous cap produce stable, slowly progressing angina.

Plaque with inflammatory edges stimulates release of digestive enzymes that dissolve the cap and initiate plaque rupture. This produces acute coronary syndromes (Wenger, Helmy, Patel, & Lerakis, 2005). The patient with CAD may develop symptoms of angina or remain asymptomatic before experiencing an acute episode.

Prevention of coronary events often involves the aggressive management of other diseases, including the following:

- Hypertension and hypotension
- Dyslipidemia
- Heart failure
- Cardiac arrhythmias
- Diabetes
- Anemia
- Thyroid disorders
- Infection

Angina pectoris can be triggered by a variety of circumstances including emotional stress, temperature extremes, large meals, alcohol, physical exertion, and cigarette smoking. The following are the three main types of angina:

- Stable angina—Characterized by predictable patterns and intensities of pain over time, and a predictable response to rest or medication.
- Unstable angina—Variable in frequency, intensity, timing, and level of activity that triggers the pain. Response to treatment may be unpredictable or ineffective. Unstable angina should be treated as a medical emergency because a myocardial infarction may be imminent.
- Variant or Prinzmetal's angina—Results from vasospastic narrowing of an atherosclerotic artery, often near the site of a potential blockage. Pain usually occurs at rest, often at night, or at a predictable time of

day. Episodes usually end within minutes and respond to traditional medical management. Because this type of angina is usually associated with atherosclerotic plaque, a myocardial infarction remains a distinct possibility.

Common Presenting Signs and Symptoms

Upon admission to the nursing home, review the new patient's chart for the following:

- History of coronary heart disease, angina, and/or myocardial infarction.

- Risk factors for cardiac events that should be managed, including hypertension, heart failure, dyslipidemia, and diabetes mellitus.

- Lifestyle factors requiring modification, including obesity, diet, exercise level, and smoking.

- Other precipitating factors that may increase oxygen demand in susceptible individuals such as obstructive pulmonary disease, anemia, overt and subclinical hyperthyroidism, and infection.

- Advancing age of residents, alone, will necessitate all residents be evaluated periodically for development or extension of CAD.

Angina Pectoris

History The most common symptom of angina is chest pain. For clinical evaluation purposes, chest pain can be classified as the following (ACC/AHA, 2002):

- Typical angina:
  - Substernal chest discomfort, heaviness, tightness with characteristic quality and duration
  - Precipitated by physical exertion or emotional stress
  - Relieved by rest or medication

- Atypical—Meets two of the above criteria
- Noncardiac—Meets only one of the above criteria

Typically, ischemic chest pain is described as a heavy sensation in the chest that may radiate to the jaw, arm, or back. In the elderly, women, and diabetics with CAD, these characteristics may be absent, mild, or atypical, or they may go unreported secondary to the presence of other chronic pain, dementia, depression, or delirium. Other indicators of chest pain might include the following:

- Fatigue
- Change in usual level of activity
- Dyspnea with activity or at rest
- Diaphoresis
- Restlessness
- Change in mental status

Chest pain characteristics should be evaluated to assist in differential diagnoses, including the following:

- Quality—Usually dull or heavy and not affected by position or respiration
- Location—Usually substernal, with or without radiation
- Duration—And any changes from the usual pattern
- Factors that provoke the pain—Activity at time of pain
- Factors that relieve the pain—Including effectiveness of prescribed medications

The American College of Cardiology/ American Heart Association guidelines for the management of chronic stable angina (2002) use the Canadian Cardiovascular Society Classification System to measure the severity of angina pectoris based on the patient's ability to function with the condition. This classification can provide baseline data and also assist in the evaluation of therapeutic interventions, although modifications may be necessary for nursing home residents with baseline limitations in activity level.

- Class I—Ordinary physical activity does not cause symptoms. Anginal symptoms occur with strenuous, rapid, or prolonged exertion.

- Class II—Slight limitation of activity. Angina occurs with strenuous activity such as walking or climbing stairs rapidly, walking an incline, walking activities after meals or in cold or wind. Angina occurs with extended duration of usual walking and stair-climbing activity. It occurs when under emotional stress or early in the day.

- Class III—Marked limitation of ordinary activity. Angina occurs walking less than two blocks on level ground and climbing one flight of stairs at a normal pace under normal conditions.

- Class IV—Inability to engage in any physical activity without discomfort. Anginal symptoms may be present at rest.

Physical Examination *The physical examination of the patient with chest pain may be negative. During chest pain the focus is on cardiorespiratory assessment. A full assessment includes other systems to rule out other causes of chest pain. Standard evaluation should include the following:*

- Assessment during chest pain includes the following:
  - Vital signs
  - Mental status
  - Respiratory—Rate, rhythm, adventitious sounds, friction rub
  - Cardiac—Heaves, displaced apical impulse, rate, rhythm, paradoxically split second heart sound (S2), mitral regurgitant murmur, third (S3) or fourth (S4) heart sounds, friction rub

- Assessment for other causes of chest pain or to confirm atherosclerosis include the following:
  - Skin—Color, temperature, thyroid disease changes, lipid lesions (xanthomas)
  - Eye—Arcus senilis, retinal exudates
  - Thyroid evaluation
  - Abdomen—Obesity, tenderness, evaluation of liver, gallbladder, pancreatic signs
  - Peripheral vascular assessment—Bruits, peripheral vascular disease signs
  - Musculoskeletal pain assessment for chest wall, joint pathology

Unstable Angina
According to current guidelines (ACC/AHA, 2002), patients with unstable angina have the following risk profile for death or non-fatal AMI:

- High risk—At least one of the following:
  - Prolonged resting chest pain (longer than 20 minutes)
  - Pulmonary edema
  - Angina at rest with ST changes greater than or equal to 1 mm
  - Angina with new or worsening mitral regurgitant murmur
  - Angina with S-3 or new/worsening crackles (rales)
  - Angina with hypotension

- Intermediate risk—No high-risk signs, and at least one of the following:
  - History of prolonged resting chest pain (longer than 20 minutes) currently resolved, but with likelihood of CAD
  - Prolonged resting chest pain (longer than 20 minutes) relieved with nitroglycerin
  - Nocturnal angina
  - Angina with dynamic T-wave changes

○ New onset Class III or IV angina with likelihood of CAD

○ Q-wave or resting ST segment depression less than or equal to 1 mm in multiple lead groups (anterior, inferior, lateral)

○ Age greater than 65 years

• Low risk—No high or intermediate risks, but any of the following:

○ Increased angina frequency, severity, or duration

○ Angina provoked at a lower threshold

○ New onset angina within 2–8 weeks

○ Normal or unchanged ECG

Acute Coronary Syndrome

Between 22–68% of myocardial infarctions in older adults are silent and old, discovered during routine electrocardiogram. Acute myocardial infarction may present with acute chest pain. If present, it may be similar to that of angina, but unrelieved with rest or medications and may be accompanied by the following:

• Dyspnea

• Weakness

• Anxiety

• Diaphoresis

• Nausea

• Loss of consciousness

Differential Diagnoses

Coronary heart disease typically presents with chest pain and dyspnea. Other non-atherogenic causes of these symptoms include the following (ACC/AHA, 2002):

• Cardiac—Aortic stenosis, aortic dissection, pericarditis, heart failure

• Pulmonary—Pneumonia, embolus, pneumothorax, pleuritis

• Gastroesophageal reflux, esophagitis, biliary diseases

• Skeletal muscle or costochondral chest pain, fibrositis, rib fracture, arthritis, Herpes zoster prodrome

• Anxiety, depression, somatoform disorders

Essential Diagnostic and Laboratory Tests

Selection of diagnostic tests depends on whether the patient has known CAD or is being worked up for the disorder with or without current symptoms. Selection of diagnostic tests is also based on the patient's comorbidities and advance directive orders. Diagnostic tests to consider include the following:

• 12-lead electrocardiogram, resting or with chest pain

• Chest X-ray or computerized tomography (CT) to rule out noncardiac causes

• Echocardiogram to evaluate left ventricular function and valvular disease

• Routine tests for evaluation of risk factors (hypertension, dyslipidemia, diabetes mellitus, anemia, thyroid disease)

• Laboratory tests for markers of coronary heart disease. Newer markers for diagnosis include (Agruss & Garrett, 2005):

○ Highly sensitive C-reactive protein (hsCRP)—A marker of endothelial inflammation and predictor of adverse cardiovascular events. The degree of elevation indicates level of risk and should be correlated with other known risk factors. Persistent elevation indicates the need for pharmacological therapy (e.g., aspirin, statins). If treatment fails to improve blood levels, consider the presence of non-cardiovascular inflammation.

○ Leukocyte count—A marker of systemic inflammation and a possible predictor of cardiovascular events, especially in females 50–79 years of age.

- Homocysteine—An independent risk factor for future cardiovascular events. A sulphur-containing amino acid that rises in response to dietary deficiencies of folic acid and vitamins B_6 and B_{12}. Elevated levels are associated with damage to vascular smooth muscle and endothelium resulting in turbulent blood flow and increased blood clotting.
  - Type B brain natriuretic hormone (hBNP)—A marker of cardiovascular disease and heart failure (see section on heart failure).
  - Nontraditional lipids—See section on dyslipidemia for details.
- Stress testing, as appropriate
- Angiography, as appropriate

Management Plan

The goals for management of coronary artery disease are to control anginal symptoms, treat underlying causes, and prevent nonfatal and fatal myocardial infarction.

Limited data is available on the management of the components of coronary artery disease in the older adult population, as advanced age has often been an exclusionary criteria in large clinical trials. In the long-term care setting recommended evidence-based guidelines must take into consideration the older individual's functional status, comorbidities, and the risk/benefit ratio in selecting therapies (Wenger, Helmy, Patel, & Lerakis, 2005).

Nonpharmacologic

Stable Angina Pectoris Treat modifiable risk factors with the following lifestyle interventions, as appropriate to the patient's overall condition:

- Weight control
- Dietary management of dyslipidemia, hypertension, and/or diabetes mellitus

- Addition of omega-3 fatty acids in diet or through supplementation (1 gram daily) has demonstrated decreased sudden death and overall mortality (ICSI, 2005f).
- Exercise, as tolerated
- Smoking cessation, as necessary
- Stress reduction

Acute Coronary Syndrome Diagnosis of any acute coronary syndrome in the presence of an advance directive that elects aggressive treatment requires immediate referral to the acute care setting for stabilization and treatment. The nurse practitioner should assure that a protocol is established for transfer of the patient to the acute care setting. While awaiting emergency medical services the clinician should provide supportive therapy, including the following:

- Oxygen
- Nitroglycerin
- Anticoagulation with aspirin (chew and swallow), unless contraindicated
- Pain management according to protocol (morphine)

For patients with written do-not-resuscitate (DNR) orders, the nurse practitioner, in consultation with the primary physician or hospice program, provides supportive care including oxygen therapy and pain relief measures for end stage disease.

Pharmacologic

Stable Angina Pectoris Principles for the medical management of angina include the following (see Table 6-4):

- Medications for hypertension, dyslipidemia, and/or diabetes mellitus management—Because several drugs used to manage angina can also be used for comorbid conditions, attempt to simplify drug regimens by using medications that can satisfy multiple conditions.

TABLE 6-4   Options for Medication Management of Stable Angina Pectoris

DRUG USUAL DOSE RANGE	ADDITIONAL CONSIDERATIONS
General Therapies for Cardiovascular Disease	
Aspirin (ASA) *81–162 mg/day or* *325 mg every other day*	• First choice for primary and secondary prevention of atherosclerotic events • Contraindicated with aspirin allergy • Contraindicated with recent intracranial bleed • Enteric coating or giving with meals may decrease gastric upset. • Low dose may be safe with warfarin therapy. • Avoid concurrent routine use of NSAIDs.
Clopidogrel (Plavix) *75 mg/day*	• Use when ASA cannot be tolerated. • May be used with ASA for high-risk patients.
Omega-3 fatty acid (EPA/DPA) *1 g/day*	• Evidence indicates a reduction of overall mortality and sudden death in patients with stable chronic angina.
Folic acid *0.4–1 mg/day*	• May use to reduce elevated homocysteine levels (inflammation). • Check for B_{12} deficiency prior to initiating therapy if anemia is suspected.
Vitamin B_6 (Pyridoxine) *10–50 mg/day*	• May use as adjunctive therapy with folic acid.
Vitamin B_{12} (Cyanocobalamin) *300–1000 mcg/day*	• May use as adjunctive therapy with folic acid.
Angina-Specific Therapy	
Nitroglycerin—sublingual or spray *0.3–0.6 mg* *May repeat three times*	• Use as an immediate rescue for chest pain. • Give smaller dose initially for headache or hypotension side effects. • If symptoms are not relieved, treat as a medical emergency.
Beta Blockers (BBs) Atenolol (Tenormin) *50–200 mg/day* Metoprolol (Lopressor) *50–200 mg 2x/day* Propranolol (Inderal) *20–80 mg 2x/day* Others[a]	• First choice for daily therapy with SCAD. • Order for all post-MI patients without contraindications. • Target heart rate 55–60 • Avoid abrupt withdrawal. • Avoid drugs with intrinsic sympathomimetic activity. • Do not use for vasospastic (Prinzmetal's) angina. • Also useful for hypertension and atrial fibrillation (with or without digoxin). • Avoid with severe heart failure, heart block, or asthma. • May mask hypoglycemia in diabetics.
Long-Acting Nitrates Isosorbide dinitrate (Isordil) *5–80 mg 2–3x/day* Nitroglycerin Transdermal *0.2–0.8 mg/hour every 12 hours* Isosorbide mononitrate *Imdur 60–240 mg/day; Ismo 20 mg* *2x/day, 7 hours apart; Monoket 5–20 mg 2x/day*	• Alternative when beta-blockers cannot be used • Also recommended for vasospastic angina • Controls angina, but with no evidence of effect on mortality • Tolerance can develop—allow nitrate-free intervals every 24 hours versus around-the-clock dosing. • Do not use with phosphodiesterase-5 inhibitors such as sildenafil.

continued

TABLE 6-4 *(continued)*	
DRUG USUAL DOSE RANGE	**ADDITIONAL CONSIDERATIONS**

Calcium Channel Blockers (CCBs)
Nondihydropyridines
  Verapamil LA (Calan SR, Isoptin SR, Verelan)
    120–320 mg/day
  Diltiazem LA (Cardizem CD, Dilacor XR)
    30–180 mg/day
Dihydrpyridines
  Nifedipine LA[b] (Procardia XL, Adalat CC)
    5–10 mg/day
  Amlodipine (Norvasc)
    5–10 mg/day
  Felodipine (Plendil)
    2.5–10 mg/day
Other[a]
	• A third line drug class for SCAD
	• Use long acting formulations for angina
	• Controls angina, but no evidence of effect on mortality
	• Dihydropyridines may exacerbate angina if used as monotherapy (ICSI, 2005)
	• Avoid with decompensated heart failure, bradycardia, AV node heart block

• Angiotensin-converting enzyme inhibitors (ACEI)—Use as routine secondary prevention for patients with known CAD, especially diabetics (ACC/AHA, 2005).

• Lipid-lowering therapy has demonstrated effectiveness in primary and secondary prevention of nonfatal MI and death.

[a] Many other drugs are appropriate in this class.
[b] Avoid monotherapy with nifedipine as it can cause a reflex increase in heart rate (ICSI, 2005f).
SCAD, stable coronary artery disease.

○ Angiotensin-converting enzyme inhibitors (ACEIs) have demonstrated effectiveness in decreasing the relative risk of death, MI, and stroke in patients with CAD. Drugs most extensively studied to date are ramipril and perindopril.

○ Lipid-lowering agents have demonstrated effectiveness in decreasing the relative risk of death, MI, and stroke in patients with hypercholesterolemia and CAD. Drugs most extensively studied to date are simvastatin and pravastatin.

○ Statin therapy in the absence of dyslipidemia is also appropriate for patients at risk for CAD secondary to conditions such as diabetes mellitus, peripheral arterial disease, and hypertension.

○ Discontinue hormone replacement therapy (HRT) in female patients if it was prescribed principally for cardioprotection. Recent research indicates that it is ineffective for this purpose and increases the risk for breast cancer (combination therapy) and venous thromboembolism.

• Aspirin (ASA), plain or enteric coated, 81–162 mg/day unless contraindicated (allergy, gastrointestinal bleeding, recent intracranial bleed, bleeding disorder, use of other anticoagulants, uncontrolled hypertension). If ASA is not tolerated or sufficient, order clopidogrel (Plavix) 75 mg/day. Regular use of NSAIDs should be avoided.

• Sublingual short-acting nitrates as needed for mild angina. Begin with a low-dose tablet to decrease side effects of headache and hypotension.

• Consider folic acid supplementation to reduce elevated homocysteine levels. May also add vitamins B$_6$ and B$_{12}$. Folic acid supplementation may mask a B$_{12}$ deficiency but will not correct the neurological symptoms of the anemia. It may be advisable to check for vitamin B$_{12}$ deficiency prior to ordering folate in older adults.

- Use beta-blockers as a first-line maintenance treatment for relief of anginal symptoms, unless contraindicated. Target a heart rate of 55–60 beats per minute (ICSI, 2005b).
- Oral or topical (patch) long-acting nitrates can be used as maintenance treatment for relief of anginal symptoms. Provide nitrate-free intervals during each 24-hour period to decrease the risk of tolerance (e.g., oral drugs during waking hours only; remove patch at bedtime). Nitrates are effective for symptom management, but they have no demonstrated effect on survival.
- Oral calcium channel blockers can be used as maintenance treatment for relief of anginal symptoms, but they have no demonstrated effect on survival.
- Combination therapy should be used cautiously, if needed (ICSI, 2005b).
  - In general, increase the dose of one drug to its maximum before considering combination therapy. If the patient does not tolerate high dosing consider trying low doses of medications in more than one class.
  - Combinations increase the risk of side effects.
  - A beta-blocker and long-acting nitrate are recommended as the first choice for combination therapy.
  - A beta-blocker and nondihydropyridines (diltiazem, verapamil) may induce severe bradycardia and should be avoided with heart failure, sinus bradycardia, and conduction disturbances.
  - A beta-blocker and nifedipine (dihydropyridine) may be effective, especially with conduction system disturbances.
  - Dihydropyridines and long-acting nitrates may cause excess vasodilation.
- Patients with chronic angina and acute coronary syndrome may experience depressive symptoms that can impede progress in rehabilitation. Evaluate these patients and treat depression, as needed with nonpharmacologic as well as pharmacologic interventions.

Postmyocardial Infarction Management Medication management of the patient following a myocardial infarction usually includes the following:

- Management of risk factors and comorbid conditions
- ASA or clopidogrel
- ACEI to reduce all-cause mortality
- Beta-blocker without intrinsic sympathomimetic activity to reduce all-cause mortality (e.g., metoprolol, carvedilol, propranolol, timolol)

Patient, Family, and Staff Education
- Nature and course of the condition
- Importance for patient and family to report chest pain.
- Importance for staff to contact a clinician for complaints of chest pain (pressure) or breathlessness in a timely manner. This may necessitate an in-service program about coronary artery disease.
- Correct use of nitroglycerin
- Importance of the advance directive and selection of treatment options.

Consultation
- Consult with primary physician for management of unstable angina or myocardial infarction.
- Refer appropriate patients with risk factors or unstable CHD to the cardiologist for evaluation for a revascularization procedure.

- Refer post-ACS patients to physical therapy for evaluation for cardiac rehabilitation.
- Refer to hospice for end-of-life care.

▇▇ DYSLIPIDEMIA

Definition

Dyslipidemia is a complex of abnormalities principally associated with derangements in total cholesterol (TC), low-density lipoprotein cholesterol (LDL-C), high-density lipoprotein cholesterol (HDL-C), and triglycerides. Abnormalities of these lipids are recognized as independent risk factors for the development and extension of cardiovascular disease.

Certain lipid derangements are also components of the metabolic syndrome—a collection of conditions associated with obesity and insulin resistance that increase the risk of heart disease, diabetes, and stroke. It is defined by the presence of any *three* of the following abnormalities:

- Triglycerides > 150 mg/dL
- HDL-C < 40 mg/dL in males and < 50 mg/dL in females
- Large waist circumference (40 inches in males, 35 inches in females)
- Fasting blood glucose > 110 mg/dL
- Blood pressure > 130/85

An elevated LDL-C is considered the principal lipid to be managed for the prevention and treatment of coronary heart disease (CHD). Low HDL-C and elevated triglycerides (≥ 200 mg/dL) are also considered independent risk factors for coronary heart disease. Conversely, an HDL-C of ≥ 60 mg/dL is considered a negative risk factor for the development of cardiovascular disease.

Epidemiology

Dyslipidemia develops through a number of mechanisms including heredity, advancing age, a diet high in cholesterol and saturated fatty acids, insulin resistance, and obesity. Dyslipidemia also develops secondary to other common disorders found frequently in nursing home patients, including diabetes mellitus, hypothyroidism, nephrotic syndrome, chronic renal failure, and diseases of the liver or pancreas. Certain drugs may also increase lipid levels (Table 6-5).

Cholesterol and triglycerides are major contributors to atherosclerosis. Exogenous sources in the diet and endogenous synthesis of these substances are transported in the blood stream as part of lipoprotein particles (Katzel & Goldberg, 2003, p. 875). The major lipoproteins in order of density include chylomicrons, very low-density lipoproteins (VLDL), LDL, lipoprotein (a), and HDL.

- Chylomicrons are synthesized in the intestine and transport both dietary cholesterol

TABLE 6-5	Drugs Associated with Dyslipidemia
Elevated cholesterol	Thiazide diuretics
	Corticosteroids
	Anabolic steroids
	Progestins
	Cyclosporine
	Amiodarone
	Antipsychotics:[a]
	Clozapine (Clozaril)
	Olanzapine (Zyprexa)
	Risperdone (Risperdol)
	Quetiapine (Seroquel)
Elevated triglycerides	Thiazide diuretics
	Corticosteroids
	Beta-blockers
	Bile acid-binding resins
	Estrogen, tamoxifen
	Protease inhibitors
	Isotretinoin

[a] May also cause hyperglycemia
Source: American Diabetes Association, American Psychiatric Association, American Association of Clinical Endocrinologists, North American Association for the Study of Obesity, 2004.

to the liver and triacylglycerols (triglycerides) to adipose tissue and muscle.

- VLDL is synthesized in the liver and transports cholesterol and triacylglycerols from the liver to the periphery.
- LDL, derived from VLDL, has a high concentration of cholesterol and transports it from the liver to the periphery.
- HDL has a high ratio of protein to lipid and transports excess cholesterol from the periphery to the liver where it can be converted to other lipoproteins or eliminated by bile acids.

The major source of cholesterol is from animal sources in the diet. Cholesterol is also synthesized within cells through a complicated biochemical pathway catalyzed by the enzyme hydroxymethylglutaryl-CoA (HMG-CoA) reductase. Cholesterol is an essential component of cell membranes and a precursor of all steroid hormones and of bile acids that are essential for fat metabolism.

Triglycerides are the plasma forms of fats ingested in the diet or synthesized in the body from energy sources such as carbohydrates. Excess triglycerides are stored in fat cells and skeletal muscle. They are metabolized through hormone action (glucagon) that signals lipase to release fatty acids into the blood stream to meet the body's energy needs and produce glycogen for brain use. Decreased insulin and increased glucose levels potentiate the synthesis of triacylglycerol, ketone bodies, and cholesterol in the liver that is then transported in the blood stream as VLDL.

High plasma levels of cholesterol and triglycerides are the result of a diet rich in cholesterol, fats, or carbohydrates that form acetyl-CoA, a cholesterol precursor. A hereditary defect in the LDL receptor that allows storage of cholesterol within cells may also lead to an excess of circulating cholesterol. This excess cholesterol may deposit in the skin (xanthomas), eyes (arcus senilis), tendons (nodules), or arteries (atherosclerosis).

Age-associated changes in lipid levels must be taken into consideration in making diagnostic and treatment decisions in the nursing home setting. Cross-sectional studies suggest that LDL-C and triglycerides increase to the seventh or eighth decades of life in males and somewhat more in postmenopausal females. Conversely, a decline in LDL-C, HDL-C, and total cholesterol in older adults may be attributed to comorbidities, changes in body composition, and poor nutrition (Katzel & Goldberg, 2003).

Controversy exists about the diagnosis and treatment of dyslipidemia in the very old. The American College of Physicians (1996) does not recommend for or against screening adults 65–75 years of age. It recommends against screening for those 75 years of age or older. Decisions about screening or treatment should not, however, be based solely on age. Consideration must also be given to the extent and seriousness of comorbidities and the effects of recommended treatment guidelines on the patient's perceived quality of life.

Common Presenting Signs and Symptoms

- Many patients in long-term care settings have a diagnosis of dyslipidemia on admission.
- Patients at risk for dyslipidemia include those with hypertension, diabetes, peripheral vascular disease, and/or a history of TIA or stroke.
- Patients may be admitted with conditions capable of producing dyslipidemias secondary to another disease (see differential diagnoses).
- Many nursing home patients may also be taking one or more drugs that may have an effect on lipid levels (Table 6-5).
- Physical examination may indicate signs of lipid disease such as xanthomas, arcus senilis (also an expected change with

advanced age), tendon nodules, vascular bruits, or peripheral arterial signs (pale, cool extremities with nail thickening, hair loss, distal ulcerations).

The Framingham Heart Study has identified an estimate of 10-year risk for CHD outcomes (myocardial infarction and death) for adults without current heart disease or diabetes. It is based on calculations of age, HDL level, systolic blood pressure, smoking history by age, and total cholesterol by age. The calculation of risk stops at the eighth decade of life (ages 70–79). They recommend that the person with a calculated risk of 10% or greater be treated to decrease morbidity and mortality from CHD. The National Cholesterol Education Program (NCEP, 2001), based on results of the Framingham Study, has developed a calculator to estimate the risk of cardiovascular disease. Although it is not specific to those over age 79 or those in nursing home settings, it may be helpful for the nurse practitioner in decision making. Both online and personal data assistant (PDA) versions can be found at http://hin.nhlbi.nih.gov/atpiii/calculator.asp?usertype=prof or http://hin.nhlbi.nih.gov/atpiii/riskcalc.htm.

Differential Diagnoses

Secondary dyslipidemia may be caused by the following conditions:

* Diabetes
* Hypothyroidism
* Chronic renal failure
* Nephrotic syndrome
* Obstructive liver disease
* Genetic disorders
* Drugs that affect lipids (Table 6-5)

Elevated triglycerides may be due to the following factors (National Cholesterol Education Program, 2001):

* Overweight or obesity
* Physical inactivity

* Cigarette smoking
* Excessive alcohol use
* Diet with greater than 60% carbohydrate content
* Diseases such as type 2 diabetes mellitus, chronic renal failure, and nephrotic syndrome
* Drugs that affect triglycerides (Table 6-5)
* Genetic disorders

Essential Diagnostic and Laboratory Tests

* Order a fasting lipid panel in all patients with CAD, peripheral arterial disease, history of TIA/stroke, and diabetes to establish a baseline and/or as a guide for continuing blood lipid management. In a recent small study in an academic nursing home LDL-C was measured in only 36% of the CAD patients not treated with statins, and levels were found to be elevated in 64% of those persons (Ghosh, Ziesmer, & Aronow, 2002).

* Don't measure lipids if the patient has a fever or major infection, is 4 weeks post-MI/stroke, during acute alcohol intoxication, with diabetes out of control, or during rapid weight loss.

* If triglycerides are greater than 400 mg/dL, order a direct measure of LDL-C, as the traditionally estimated value calculated as (LDL − C = TC − [HDL-C + TG/5]) is inaccurate in such cases.

* Consider additional lipid tests for patients with CVD whose LDL and HDL are normal to assess for nontraditional lipid values that may require management. These may include the following:

  ○ Very low-density lipoprotein (VLDL)—This can be estimated as the triglyceride value/5.

  ○ Lipoprotein (a) [Lp(a)]—A highly atherogenic lipoprotein, instrumental in deposition of cholesterol in arterial walls.

May indicate the need to add an additional drug class (niacin, fibrate) to the statin regimen to attain lipid control.

○ LDL subclasses—Subclass B (LpB) is an independent marker of CAD.

○ Calculate the non-HDL-C (total cholesterol–HDL). The value should be less than 130 for high-risk patients.

• Consider measurement of C-reactive protein (CRP) and homocysteine as indicators of cardiovascular disease risk.

• Consider laboratory/diagnostic tests to rule out secondary dyslipidemia.

• Evaluate baseline renal function and liver function in preparation for ordering drug therapy or to evaluate the effects of treatment.

• Order a creatine kinase if considering statin therapy or if the patient is taking a statin, statin/fibrate, or statin/nicotinic acid combination and complains of muscle fatigue, weakness, or pain (myositis, rhabdomyolysis).

Management Plan

The goal for management of dyslipidemia is to prevent cardiovascular morbidity and mortality.

Secondary goals may include preservation of renal function in patients with diabetes mellitus.

Nonpharmacologic

Traditional nonpharmacologic treatments for the management of dyslipidemia include the following therapeutic lifestyle changes (TLC) that should be part of every management plan (NCEP, 2001), as appropriate to the patient's overall condition:

• Decrease dietary saturated fats with the TLC diet (see Table 6-6). Consider this option carefully, as a low-fat diet may be nonpalatable to the older adult and thus may risk malnutrition.

• Consider the possible increased risk of CHD associated with low cholesterol levels (160 mg/dL) in the frail elderly, and adjust the diet accordingly.

• Consider additional LDL reduction with the addition of plant stanol/sterol esters (1 g/day) and increased soluble fiber (10–25 g/day).

• Consider the addition of omega-3 fatty acid supplementation (1 g EPA/DPA per day). Impairment of clotting has been associated with high doses.

TABLE 6-6	Components of the TLC Diet
Fats:	Limit to 25–35% of total calories
	Saturated fat—Less than 7% of total calories (8–10%, initially)
	Limited trans fatty acids
	Polyunsaturated fat—Up to 10% of total calories
	Monounsaturated fat—Up to 20% of total calories
	Cholesterol—Less than 200 mg/day (300 mg initially)
Carbohydrates:	50–60% of total calories
	Mostly complex carbohydrates derived from:
	Whole grains
	Fruits
	Vegetables
Fiber:	20–30 grams/day
Protein:	Approximately 15% of total calories

- Consider folic acid supplementation (0.4 mg/day) to reduce elevated homocysteine levels. May also add B_6 (25–50 mg/day) and B_{12} (0.5 mg/day). Folic acid supplementation may mask a B_{12} deficiency, but it will not correct the neurological symptoms of the anemia. It may be advisable to check for Vitamin B_{12} deficiency prior to ordering folate in older adults.
- Vitamin E should not be used as it may lower HDL-C and has demonstrated no angiographic improvement in vascular disease (ICSI, 2005e).
- If the patient is taking statins, limit the intake of grapefruit products. They inhibit the 3A4 isoenzyme in the gut and may increase statin absorption and the risk of myositis.
- Weight reduction, as needed
- Increased physical activity, as feasible
- Smoking cessation, as needed
- Management of alcohol consumption if the patient has access to it

Pharmacologic

In a recent small study in an academic nursing home it was found that only 21% of 77 eligible residents with coronary artery disease (CAD) received lipid-lowering drugs (Ghosh, Ziesmer, & Aronow, 2003). There is controversy surrounding how aggressive drug therapy should be for older adults. Recent studies suggest that statin therapy has a positive effect on cardiovascular morbidity and mortality. The studies had limited numbers of subjects in their 80s and 90s or older adults with several comorbidities and polypharmacy. Age is also a risk factor for cardiovascular disease, and the 5–10 year risk of adverse events may become less meaningful as life expectancy decreases.

Pharmaceutical management of dyslipidemia in the nursing home is likely dictated by a resident's risk profile, life expectancy, quality-of-life issues, and end-of-life care. Several pharmacologic options are available,

depending on the nature of the dyslipidemia (Table 6-7).

If therapy is not ordered for abnormal values, clearly document reasons for the decision in the medical record. This should be preceded by a discussion with the patient and/or caregiver.

The National Cholesterol Education Program guidelines for the diagnosis and management of dyslipidemia recommend target levels for TC, LDL-C, HDL-C and TG (Table 6-8). General principles of pharmaceutical management of dyslipidemia to reach these goals include the following:

- HMG-CoA reductase inhibitors (statins) have demonstrated effectiveness in both primary and secondary prevention of cardiovascular disease in the elderly. They decrease LDL-C, increase HDL-C, decrease triglycerides, improve vasomotor reactivity, stabilize atherogenic plaque, and produce antiplatelet and antioxidant effects (Omnicare, 2004). They have a greater effect on LDL-C than other drug classes.
  - Recent studies support the efficacy of statin therapy in older, high-risk patients with and without cardiovascular disease (Grundy et al., 2004).
  - Begin all statin therapy with a low dose.
  - If one statin is not tolerated, the recommendation is to try others in the class before selecting another drug class.
  - Avoid macrolide antibiotics and systemic azole antifungals greater than 200 mg/day if possible for patients taking statins. Consider temporary discontinuance of statins or dose reduction when these drugs are necessary (ICSI, 2005e).
  - If a patient complains of muscle fatigue, weakness, or pain prior to or during statin therapy, order a creatine kinase. If value is less than five times the upper limit, repeat in one week. If value is more than

five times the upper limit, discontinue the statin (ICSI, 2005e).

- When triglycerides are ≥ 200 mg/dL, management of non-HDL-C should become a secondary target for therapy (NCEP, 2001).
  - Triglycerides may be elevated secondary to hyperglycemia in diabetics. Controlling blood glucose may reduce triglyceride levels.
  - Nicotinic acid and fibrates are more effective than statins in the management of hypertriglyceridemia.
  - Bile acid resins have no effect or a negative effect on elevated triglycerides.
- Use of drugs from several classes to reach therapeutic goals requires assessment for multiple adverse drug reactions.
  - Combination drugs should not be used as initial therapy, but may be appropriate once lipid levels have been stabilized in order to simplify a medication regimen. Combination drugs should not be used in patients with abnormal renal or liver function.
  - Patients taking both a statin and fibrate or statin and nicotinic acid may be at increased risk for myositis.
- Adjust drug therapies in no less than 4-week increments, preceded by measurement of lipid levels and liver function.
- Goals for HDL-C are not set, and the emphasis should be on managing LDL targets.
- Consider aspirin therapy as an adjunct for primary and secondary prevention of cardiovascular disease.
- Lowering LDL-C levels below 70 mg/dL or total cholesterol levels below 150 may have a negative effect on morbidity and mortality.

Patient, Family, and Staff Education

- Nature and course of the disorders
- Dietary management of dyslipidemia
- Risks associated with dyslipidemia
- Signs and symptoms of adverse drug reactions to report

Consultation

- Lipid levels not responding to routine treatment.
- Use of combination drug therapy
- Consultation with the psychiatrist for dyslipidemia, hyperglycemia associated with antipsychotic use.
- Physical/recreational therapy for physical activity/exercise program, as possible.
- Consultation with the registered dietician for cholesterol control with diet.

HEART FAILURE

Definition

Heart failure is a clinical syndrome caused by a variety of disorders and diseases that affect the ability of the heart to pump sufficient blood to meet energy demands or requires it to do so at excessively high diastolic pressures or volumes (Massey, 2004, p. 291). Heart failure is described as the following:

- *Systolic* characterized by reduced myocardial contractility resulting in *reduced left ventricular ejection fraction* (LVEF) and signs of right-sided heart failure.
- *Diastolic* characterized by decreased left ventricular filling due to altered relaxation of the myocardium or ventricular stiffness, usually with an elevated left ventricular end diastolic pressure (LVEDP), *normal left ventricular ejection fraction,* and signs of left-sided heart failure. Diastolic disease may be more prevalent in older adults, especially women with hypertension (Shamsham & Mitchell, 2000; Tresch, 1997).

The New York Heart Association (NYHA) has classified heart failure based on the severity

TABLE 6-7   Drug Options for the Management of Dyslipidemia in Older Adults and Effects on Lipid Components

DRUG CLASSIFICATION (BRAND NAME)	DOSAGE RANGE	AVERAGE EFFECT ON LDL-C (%↓)	AVERAGE EFFECT ON HDL-C (%↑)	AVERAGE EFFECT ON TRIGLYCERIDES (%↓)	CONTRAINDICATIONS, SIDE EFFECTS (SE), SPECIAL CONSIDERATIONS BY DRUG CLASS
HMG-CoA Reductase Inhibitors					
Atorvastatin (Lipitor)	10–80 mg/day	38–54%	3–12%	26–46%	*Contraindicated with liver disease* *Use cautiously with certain drugs*[a] Increased liver enzymes (SE) Myopathy, rhabdomyolysis (SE) Measure liver function (AST, ALT) at baseline, at 3 months, before dose changes, and every 6–12 months Measure CK at baseline and with muscle soreness Use lower doses with reduced renal function (except fluvastatin, atorvastatin) Order lovastatin (Mevacor) with meals, all others at bedtime
Fluvastatin (Lescol)	20–40 mg twice/day	17–33%	2–8%	2–11%	
Lovastatin (Mevacor)	20–80 mg/day	29–48%	6–10%	10–19%	
Lovastatin ER (Altocor)	10–60 mg/day	23–40%	9–11%	17–25%	
Pravastatin (Pravachol)	10–80 mg/day	19–40%	4–8%	11–25%	
Rosuvastatin (Crestor)	4–40 mg/day	43–62%	8–13%	10–35%	
Simvastatin (Zocor)	10–80 mg/day	28–48%	5–20%	1–46%	
Fibrates[b]					
Fenofibrate (Tricor)	54–160 mg/day	17–35%	1–34%	15–53%	*Contraindicated with severe liver or hepatic disease* Gall stones (SE) Myopathy, rhabdomyolysis, especially with statins (SE)
Gemfibrozil (Lopid)	600 mg twice/day	12–35%	3–23%	40–50%	
Niacins (Nicotinic Acids)[c]					
Immediate release (crystalline)	1.5–3 g/day in 2–3 divided doses; begin at 100–200 mg 2–3 times/day	6–25%	15–35%	20–40%	*Contraindicated with chronic liver disease, severe gout* *Use cautiously with diabetes, peptic ulcer disease, hyperuricemia* Flushing (SE) Hyperglycemia (SE) Hyperuricemia (SE) Hepatotoxicity (SE) *Measure LFTs at baseline, at 3 months before dose changes, and every 6–12 months*
Extended release (Niaspan)	1–2 g/day	9–17%	15–26%	11–35%	
Sustained release	1–2 g/day; begin with 500 mg	6–50%	5–15%	10–40%	

Bile Acid Sequestrants[d]				
Cholestyramine (Questran, Prevalite)	4–24 g/day	15–30%	3–+11%	0–10%	*Contraindicated with triglycerides > 400 mg/dL, dysbetalipoproteinemia*
Colestipol (Colestid)	5–30 g/day				*Use cautiously with TG > 200 mg/dL*
Colesevelam (Welchol)	2.6–4.4 g/day				Constipation (SE)
					GI upset (SE)
					Decreased absorption from GI tract (SE)
					Order other drugs to be taken 1 hour before or after dose
Selective Cholesterol Absorption Inhibitor[e]					
Ezetimibe (Zetia)	10 mg/day	13–20%	1–6%	6–14%	*Contraindicated with liver disease*
					Avoid with fibrates
					Cholecystitis (SE)
Combination Drugs					
ER niacin/lovastatin (Advicor)	500/20–1000/20 mg twice/day	*Use as maintenance, not as initial therapy* Additive effect	Additive effect	Additive effect	See individual agents
Ezetimibe/simvastatin (Vytorin)	10/10–10/80 mg/day	Additive effect	Additive effect	Additive effect	See individual agents

[a] Atorvastatin, lovastatin, simvastatin are metabolized by CYP3A4 enzyme system. May interact with drugs that inhibit the enzyme such as amiodarone, erythromycin, clarithromycin, ketoconazole, verapamil, diltiazem, nefazodone, fluvoxamine, cyclosporine, grapefruit juice, etc. Fluvastatin is metabolized by CYP2C9 and can increase levels of phenytoin. Rifampin can lower fluvastatin levels. Rosuvastatin increases INR; cyclosporine and gemfibrozil increase rosuvastatin levels; lower doses in Japanese/Asian ancestry

[b] Fibrates may potentiate warfarin effect; monitor INR closely.

[c] Niacin and fibrates require caution with cyclosporine, macrolide antibiotics, antifungals, and cytochrome P450 inhibitors.

[d] Bile acid sequestrants require caution in older adults; closely monitor INR if on warfarin therapy; take other medications 1 hour before or 4 hours after dose.

[e] For selective cholesterol absorption inhibitors, use cautiously with cyclosporine; take bile acid sequestrant 2 hours before or 4 hours after.

TABLE 6-8   National Cholesterol Education Program (NCEP) Guidelines for the Diagnosis and Management of Dyslipidemia

RISK FACTOR LEVEL	LIPID LEVEL	SEVERITY	LIFESTYLE MANAGEMENT	BEGIN DRUG MANAGEMENT
	Total Cholesterol			
	< 150 mg/dL			
	150–199 mg/dL	Desirable		
	200–239 mg/dL	Borderline high		
	> 240 mg/dL	High		
	LDL Cholesterol			
CHD or risk equivalent[a]	< 70 mg/dL	Optimal in very high risk		
	< 100 mg/dL	Optimal	≥ 100 mg/dL	≥ 130 mg/dL
≥ 2 risk factors	< 100 mg/dL	Optional goal		
	100–129 mg/dL	Desirable	≥ 130 mg/dL	≥ 130–160 mg/dL
1 risk factor	130–159 mg/dL	Borderline high	≥ 160 mg/dL	≥ 160–190 mg/dL
	160–189 mg/dL	High		
	> 190 mg/dL	Very high		
	HDL Cholesterol			
	< 40 mg/dL	Low		
	> 40 mg/dL, male	Desirable		
	> 50 mg/dL, female	Desirable		
	> 60 mg/dL	Protective		
	Triglycerides			
	< 150 mg/dL	Normal		
	150–199 mg/dL	Borderline high		
	200–499 mg/dL	High		
	> 500 mg/dL	Very high		

[a] CHD risk equivalents include diabetes mellitus, peripheral arterial disease, abdominal aortic aneurysm, and symptomatic carotid artery disease.

of symptoms and their effect on functional ability, as shown below:

- Class I—Patients exhibit symptoms only at exertion levels similar to those of relatively healthy individuals.
- Class II—Patients exhibit symptoms with ordinary exertion.
- Class III—Patients exhibit symptoms with minimal exertion.
- Class IV—Patients exhibit symptoms at rest.

The American College of Cardiology and the American Heart Association (ACC/AHA, 2005) developed a complimentary classification of heart failure with four stages based on presenting cardiac structure, function, and symptoms:

- Stage A—Patients present with risk factors for heart failure but without structural abnormalities, signs, or symptoms of heart failure.
- Stage B—Patients present with structural abnormalities but without signs or symptoms of heart failure.
- Stage C—Patients present with structural abnormalities and with current or past signs and symptoms of heart failure.

- Stage D—Patients present with refractory heart failure that may require mechanical, pharmaceutical, transplant or end-of-life support.

Epidemiology

There are currently about 5 million individuals diagnosed with heart failure in the United States, and 550,000 diagnosed annually. Approximately 80% of heart failure patients are more than 65 years of age. Heart failure is the most common Medicare reported diagnosis, and costs the most Medicare dollars for treatment. The incidence of the disease is expected to rise with the increase in the older adult population (ACC/AHA, 2005).

Common disorders that contribute to the development of *systolic* heart failure include the following:

- Ischemic disorders (myocardial ischemia/infarction or hypoperfusion).
- Persistent vascular pressure (hypertension, obstructive valvular disease).
- Chronic volume overload (regurgitant valves, intra- or extracardiac shunting).
- Cardiac myopathies (genetic, toxic, immunologic, infectious, metabolic, infiltrative, idiopathic).

Diastolic heart failure does not involve valve disease and does not affect left ventricular ejection fraction (LVEF). It may be caused by conditions causing myocardial hypertrophy, including the following:

- Hypertension (most common cause)
- Aging
- Cardiac ischemia
- Rapid heart rates and rhythms
- Restrictive cardiomyopathies (amyloidosis, sarcoidosis)
- Fibrotic disorders

Additionally, heart failure may be caused by the following:

- Mechanical abnormalities
- Arrhythmias
- Pulmonary heart diseases (cor pulmonale, pulmonary vascular diseases).
- High-output states such as thyrotoxicosis and chronic anemia (Massey, 2004, p. 292).
- Severe subclinical hypothyroidism (TSH ≥ 7.0 mIU/ml with normal T-3 and T-4) was recently associated with increased risk of heart failure in older adults (Rodondi et al., 2005).

The body attempts to compensate for heart failure through a variety of physiological mechanisms, which may include the following (Riggs, 2006):

- Release of epinephrine and norepinephrine by the sympathetic nervous system to increase heart rate and improve cardiac output.
- Activation of the renin-angiotensin-aldosterone system to increase fluid volume and blood pressure
- Release of vasopressin (antidiuretic hormone) to promote vasoconstriction and prevent diuresis
- Release of endothelin 1 to promote vasoconstriction and stimulate growth of cardiac myocytes
- Secretion of aldosterone by the adrenal gland to retain sodium and water.
- Release of human atrial natriuretic peptide (hANP) and human brain natriuretic peptide (hBNP)—Atrial peptides are released in the atrium, and brain peptides in the ventricles to promote sodium and water retention by the kidneys.

Early stages of systolic or diastolic dysfunction can occur without symptoms. When the body can no longer compensate, cardiac output is compromised resulting, eventually, in hypoperfusion and organ failure. In certain circumstances heart failure may be reversible; in most, the condition will become chronic. Over time, ventricular remodeling results in cardiomyopathy and/or hypertrophy. Systolic and diastolic dysfunction and failure can coexist.

Coronary heart disease and myocardial infarction are the major causes of heart failure. Managing systolic hypertension, dyslipidemia, and diabetes to prevent initial or recurrent myocardial infarction are the principal therapies to control the incidence of heart failure.

Common Presenting Signs and Symptoms

Patients entering the nursing home without a current diagnosis of heart failure should, nonetheless, be evaluated for it. Upon admission clinicians should evaluate transfer documents to assess for a history of heart failure and disease risk factors (hypertension, diabetes mellitus, coronary artery disease, family history of heart disease). Lifestyle factors should also be evaluated, including a history of smoking, use of illicit and cardiotoxic drugs and alcohol, as well as obesity and limited exercise. Residents with risk factors should be assessed on a regular basis for signs and symptoms of acute heart failure.

Recognition of heart failure in the older adult may be challenged by the presence of comorbidities such as chronic respiratory or peripheral vascular diseases, or by attribution of signs and symptoms to aging alone. Because of this, diagnosis may be delayed. Signs and symptoms alone cannot clearly differentiate systolic from diastolic heart failure. Common symptoms of heart failure may include the following:

- Changes in activity level, decreased functional status

- Fatigue
- Altered mental status—confusion, delirium
- Insomnia
- Dyspnea, orthopnea, paroxysmal nocturnal dyspnea
- Unexplained cough, especially at night
- Abdominal discomfort, nausea
- Decreased food intake

Common signs of heart failure may include the following:

- Unexplained increase in weight (2 lb in a day or 5 lb in a week) and/or waist circumference
- Hyper- or hypotension
- Lateral displacement of the apical impulse (point of maximal impulse, PMI) in systolic dysfunction
- Tachycardia
- Third heart sound (S3) in systolic dysfunction and/or fourth heart sound (S4) in diastolic dysfunction, or an S3/S4 gallop in combined disease
- Low SaO_2
- Crackles (rales) over bilateral lung fields
- New or increasing lower extremity edema, usually bilateral
- Sacral or other dependent edema in the bedridden
- Positive jugular venous distention
- Abdominal distention, ascites
- Hepatomegaly
- Positive abdominojugular reflux
- Generalized edema (anasarca) in severe cases

Certain signs and symptoms suggest the need for emergent care (ICSI, 2005c, p. 18).

- Evidence of hypoperfusion such as cyanosis, cold/clammy skin, delirium

- Rapidly worsening dyspnea, shortness of breath at rest, air hunger
- Dizziness or syncope
- Coughing pink, frothy sputum
- SaO_2 less than 90%
- Systolic blood pressure less than 80–90 mmHg with symptoms
- Chest pain

Differential Diagnoses

- Lung diseases—Obstructive lung disease, asthma, pulmonary embolus, obstructive sleep apnea, severe pneumonia
- Severe hyper- or hypotension
- Coronary ischemia, acute coronary syndrome, cardiac dysrhythmia, valvular heart disease
- Altered metabolic states such as anemia, thyroid disease, obesity
- Venous insufficiency
- Renal insufficiency
- Sepsis
- Medication-induced symptoms
- High salt intake

Essential Diagnostic and Laboratory Tests

The decision to pursue aggressive diagnosis of heart failure must take into consideration the patient's overall condition, whether or not diagnosis would change the management plan, and the patient's willingness to cooperate with any proposed treatment. Any decision to modify usual guidelines for diagnosis should be discussed with the interdisciplinary team and caregivers and carefully documented in the patient record (American Medical Directors Association, 2002). Diagnostic tests may include the following:

- Review available ECG, echocardiogram, chest X-ray, etc., to confirm a previously established diagnosis.

- ECG for the presence of arrhythmia, ischemia, left ventricular hypertrophy.
- Two-dimensional and Doppler echocardiogram to assess valvular function, left ventricular systolic and diastolic function and filling pressures, left ventricular ejection fraction, and pulmonary artery pressures. This is the most cost effective first step in diagnosis. An ejection fraction < 50 should be considered abnormal.
- Radionuclide scanning, as tolerated, for precise measurement of ejection fraction.
- Chest X-ray to evaluate vascular congestion and pulmonary infiltrates and effusions.
- Laboratory tests to rule out reversible causes of heart failure—CBC, electrolytes including calcium and magnesium, TSH, BUN, creatinine, glucose, lipid profile, liver function, urinalysis (ACC/AHA, 2005).
- B-type natriuretic peptide (hBNP)—This blood test is a prognostic marker of heart failure in patients with dyspnea of unknown etiology. It is an amino acid peptide secreted from the cardiac ventricles in response to increased volume, elevated cardiac pressures, and the decreased myocardial contractility of acute heart failure (Strimike, 2006, p. 28). Elevated values correlate with left ventricular end-diastolic pressure and volume. Females and the elderly may have higher normal levels than younger males. Related diseases may also present with elevated values (severe aortic stenosis, pulmonary embolus, pulmonary hypertension, acute myocardial infarction, and severe renal failure and dialysis). This test is only used, therefore, as an adjunct in diagnosis. It can also be used to guide medical management and evaluate the effectiveness of treatment (Strimike).

Management Plan

Goals for the management of heart failure are to correct reversible causes; manage systolic hypertension, dyslipidemia, and diabetes; prevent initial or recurrent myocardial infarction; limit or control signs and symptoms; improve function; and decrease hospitalizations. If heart failure is or is associated with a terminal condition, the goal is to provide palliative care.

Nonpharmacologic
Lifestyle modifications are often indicated. Diet, smoking, alcohol use, and exercise level should be managed as appropriate to the patient's overall condition.

- Order positioning for comfort including elevation of the head of the bed to enhance breathing and elevation of affected extremities for relief of peripheral edema, as tolerated.
- Oxygen therapy, as needed
- Order and evaluate daily weights: same time, same clothing, same scale, same staff, as feasible.
- Consult with the dietitian to manage dietary intake to control risk factors including hypertension, dyslipidemia, diabetes, and fluid overload.
- Manage fluid and electrolyte imbalances associated with heart failure and medications, with particular attention to sodium (2400 mg/day); potassium balance; calcium, magnesium, and thiamine deficiencies; and fluid intake (restrict to 1500–2000 with edema or hyponatremia).
- Maintain caloric and protein intake by changing content, number and timing of meals, or adding supplements, as needed, for fatigued or anorexic patients.
- Encourage smoking cessation, as necessary.
- Encourage annual influenza vaccine and pneumonia vaccine per protocol.
- Physical therapy evaluation for cardiopulmonary rehabilitation following an acute exacerbation of heart failure.

Pharmacologic
Systolic Heart Failure Older adults have been underrepresented in drug trials. General principles of pharmacologic management of systolic heart failure include the following (ICSI, 2005c, pp. 27–28):

- Angiotensin-converting enzyme inhibitors (ACEIs) should be prescribed for all patients with left ventricular systolic dysfunction, unless contraindicated.
- Angiotensin II receptor blockers (ARBs) should be used primarily for patients who do not tolerate ACEIs. The addition of ARBs to standard therapy may be helpful, but more research is needed to validate their use in this capacity.
- ACEIs are more effective in decreasing mortality than isosorbide dinitrate/hydralazine combinations.
- The beta-blockers carvedilol, metoprolol succinate (extended release), and bisoprolol have demonstrated reductions in mortality over others drugs in the class.
- Diuretics should not be used alone but in combination with vasoactive drugs to manage volume overload.
- Loop diuretics are more effective than thiazide diuretics during severe failure, and a combination of the two drug classes is appropriate for refractory cases.
- Digoxin can be used for persistent symptoms. Use cautiously, if at all, in females because of reported increased incidence of morbidity and mortality (Aronow, 2006).
- Monitor patients for hypokalemia (thiazide diuretics) and hyperkalemia (ACEIs), hypomagnesemia, prerenal azotemia, digitalis toxicity, and orthostatic hypotension.
- Aldosterone-blocking agents (spironolactone, eplerenone) have been shown to reduce mortality in patients with severe failure who are on stable doses of digoxin and ACEIs.

- Calcium channel blockers (CCBs) should be used cautiously in patients with heart failure.
- For all pharmaceutical interventions, start with the lowest dose, and titrate slowly to the maximum dose, as required to control symptoms.
- Keep medication regimens as simple as possible in terms of the number and frequency of drugs.
- Monitor patients with chronic heart failure for signs and symptoms of depression that, if left untreated, can negatively affect morbidity and mortality.
- Monitor patients for pain that may be associated with coronary ischemia, respiratory distress, implanted defibrillators, psychological distress, comorbidities such as arthritis, etc., and treat appropriately.

Following are *specific* recommendations for management of systolic heart failure characterized by decreased ejection fraction (Table 6-9).

- Stage A—Control risk factors for heart failure including hypertension, dyslipidemia, diabetes, thyroid disorders, cardiac dysrhythmias, and myocardial infarction using current guidelines:
  - Consider angiotensin-converting enzyme inhibitors (ACEIs), or angiotensin II receptor blockers (ARBs) for those patients intolerant to ACEIs to manage risk factors. Also consider combination hydralazine/isosorbide dinitrate for ACEI intolerance (ICSI, 2005c).
- Stage B—Add a beta-blocker for all patients with a history of MI.
- Stage C—Add a diuretic and salt restriction for symptomatic patients with fluid overload.
  - If possible, avoid drugs that may potentiate symptoms, e.g., NSAIDs and glucocorticosteroids (fluid retention).
  - Consider introduction of digitalis for patients with atrial fibrillation, S3 gallop,

left ventricular dilation, or high filling pressures (ICSI, 2005c).
  - Consider a combined hydralazine/nitrate for patients with persistent symptoms. (Use cautiously in the elderly per the Beer's criteria.)

Diastolic Heart Failure Medication management of diastolic heart failure may differ somewhat because of its pathophysiology and the preservation of LVEF in most patients. Few randomized controlled trials have been conducted to validate current recommendations in the literature. Treatment goals include control of blood pressure and decrease of diastolic filling pressures while preserving cardiac output. General principles of pharmacologic management of diastolic heart failure include the following:

- Treat blood pressure to a goal of less than 130/85 (Gutierrez & Blanchard, 2004).
- Treat atrial fibrillation to control rate or restore rhythm, if it is not tolerated.
- Manage coronary artery disease with vasodilators.
- Control signs and symptoms of heart failure with ACEIs, ARBs, diuretics, and digitalis, as required.

Patient, Family, and Staff Education

- Nature and course of the disease
- Symptoms to report
- Purpose and techniques for accurate daily/weekly weights
- Purpose, importance, and techniques for accurate evaluation of intake and output
- Comfort care/hospice for terminally ill

Physician Consultation

Consult with the primary physician and/or cardiologist for patient management of unstable disease and for possible hospitalization

TABLE 6-9   Oral Drugs Commonly Used to Manage Nonrefractory (Stages B, C; NYHA I–III) Systolic Heart Failure

DRUG CLASS	ACC STAGE B NYHA I STRUCTURAL DAMAGE, ASYMPTOMATIC HF	POST MI	ACC STAGE C NYHA II, III STRUCTURAL DAMAGE, WITH SYMPTOMS HF	POST MI	DOSE RANGE	COMMON ADVERSE REACTIONS
Angiotensin-Converting Enzyme Inhibitors (ACEIs)	*Cornerstone of HF therapy. Use for postmyocardial infarction management, as an antihypertensive, as renal protection in diabetes, and as a vasodilator to increase stoke volume.*					
Captopril (Capoten) ++		X	X		6.25–50 mg tid	Dry cough
Enalapril (Vasotec) +++	X		X		2.5–20 mg bid	Angioedema
Fosinopril (Monopril) +++			X		5–40 mg/day	Hyperkalemia
Lisinopril (Prinvil, Zestil) +++		X	X		2.5–40 mg/day	Hypotension Worsening renal function
Perindopril (Aceon)	X				2–16 mg/day	
Quinapril (Accupril) +++			X		5–20 mg bid	
Ramipril (Altace)		X		X	1.25–20 mg/day	
Trandolapril (Mavik) +++		X		X	0.5–4 mg/day	
Angiotensin II Receptor Blockers (ARBs)	*Use for patients with intolerance to ACE inhibitors.*					
Candesartan (Atacand)	X		X		4–32 mg/day	As above, except cough
Losartan (Cozaar)		CV risk	X		12.5–100 mg/day	
Valsartan (Diovan) ++		X	X	X	20–160 mg bid	
Hydralazine/ Isosorbide Dinitrate	*Use for patients with intolerance to ACEIs or ARBs.*				Hydralazine 25–50 mg qid Isosorbide 20–40 mg tid	Hypotension
Diuretics: Thiazid	*Use for fluid overload with a loop diuretic or as maintenance. Also used to manage hypertension.*					
Chlorothiazide (Diuril)			X		250–1000 mg/day	Dehydration
Chlorthalidone			X		12.5–100 mg/day	Hypotension
HCTZ (HydroDIURIL, Microzide)			X		12.5–100 mg/day	Hypokalemia Hyponatremia Hypomagnesemia
Indapamide (Lozol)			X		2.5–5 mg/day	Hyperglycemia
Metolazone (Zaroxolyn)			X		2.5–20 mg/day	Hypercalcemia Hyperuricemia Elevated LDL, triglycerides
Diuretic: Loop	*First choice for fluid overload in HF*					
Bumetanide (Bumex)			X		0.5–10 mg/day	As above, except hypercalcemia
Furosemide (Lasix)			X		20–400 mg/day	
Torsemide (Demadex)			X		10–200 mg/day	Metabolic alkalosis Ototoxicity
Diuretic: Potassium Sparing	*Use as adjunct for fluid overload*					
Amiloride (Midamor) ^			X		5–20 mg/day	Dehydration
Spironolactone (Aldactone) +++			X		12.5–25 mg/day	GI disturbance Hyperkalemia
Triamterene Dyrenium ^			X		50–100 mg bid	

TABLE 6-9   *(continued)*

DRUG CLASS	ACC STAGE B NYHA I STRUCTURAL DAMAGE, ASYMPTOMATIC		ACC STAGE C NYHA II, III STRUCTURAL DAMAGE, WITH SYMPTOMS		DOSE RANGE	COMMON ADVERSE REACTIONS
	HF	POST MI	HF	POST MI		
Beta-Blockers	*Use to treat concomitant coronary artery disease, for heart rate reduction, and for negative inotropic effects in stable HF.*					
Bisoprolol (Zebeta)	X		X		1.25–10 mg/day	Hypotension
Carvedilol (Coreg)	X	X	X	X	3.125–25 mg bid (up to 50 mg for patients > 85 kg)	Worsening HF Bradycardia Heart block
Metoprolol succinate, extended release (Toprol XL)	X		X		12.5–200 mg/day	Asthma exacerbation
Aldosterone Antagonists	*Use to promote diuresis and as an adjunct to suppress aldosterone with ACEIs, beta-blockers, other diuretics, and digoxin.*					
Eplerenone (Inspra)		X		X	25–50 mg qid	Hyperkalemia
Spironolactone (Aldactone)			X		12.5 mg/day to 25 mg bid	Dehydration GI disturbance Gynecomastia (Spironolactone)
Digoxin	*Use as adjunct for symptom control with ACEIs, diuretics*					
			X		0.0625–0.25 mg/day	Toxicity Anorexia, nausea

HTN, hypertension; DMN, diabetic neuropathy; HF, heart failure; CV, cardiovascular; MI, myocardial infarction; NYHA, New York Heart Association.
Geriatric Pharmaceutical Guidelines: + + + = preferred; + + = acceptable; ^ = unacceptable.
Source: ACC/AHA, 2005; Veterans Health Administration, 2003; Omnicare, 2004; ICSI, 2005.

of patients with the following conditions (ICSI, 2005c, p. 19):

- Evidence of acute myocardial ischemia or infarction
- Heart failure symptoms refractory to nursing home treatment
- Pulmonary edema, severe respiratory distress
- Thromboembolic events
- Complicating medical illnesses such as pneumonia or renal failure
- Cardiac arrhythmias that compromise hemodynamic status
- Anasarca (generalized edema)
- Inadequate staffing for safe patient management
- Unmanageable hypoperfusion
- Hyperkalemia

Refer to the cardiologist for valve replacement, revascularization, pacemaker placement, or other invasive procedures for appropriate patients with good risk/benefit ratios.

Refer to hospice those patients in Stage D heart failure in consultation with family/caregivers.

▬ HYPERTENSION

Definition

The definition of hypertension is periodically redefined. The Seventh Report of the Joint National Committee on Prevention, Detection, Evaluation, and Treatment of High Blood Pressure (Chobanian et al., 2004) defines hypertension as follows:

- Normal blood pressure—Less than 120 mmHg systolic and less than 80 mmHg diastolic
- Prehypertension—120–139 systolic *or* 80–89 diastolic
- Stage 1 hypertension—140–159 systolic *or* 90–99 diastolic
- Stage 2 hypertension—Greater than 160 systolic *or* ≥ 100 diastolic

Systolic hypertension is defined as pressure greater than 140 mmHg. In persons older than 50 years of age it is considered to be a greater risk factor for cardiovascular disease (CVD) than diastolic hypertension greater than 90. In the older adult population *isolated systolic hypertension* with normal diastolic values also represents a cardiac risk factor that should be treated.

Epidemiology

Hypertension occurs in over 67% of adults older than 65 (Chobanian et al., 2004). This is also the population with the lowest rates of blood pressure control. The National Nursing Home Survey of 1999 (Jones, 2002) estimated that nearly 482,000 residents had a diagnosis of hypertension. This data is likely higher because it did not reflect the newest parameters of the disorder. It is reported elsewhere that 32–44% of nursing home residents are hypertensive (Levenson & Crecelius, 2003).

Adequate blood pressure is required to maintain perfusion to vital organs. Primary regulation of blood pressure is accomplished through the renin-angiotensin-aldosterone system (RAAS) in which angiotensin II induces vasoconstriction, sodium and fluid retention, renin and aldosterone release, and activation of the sympathetic nervous system. Intrinsic factors in blood vessel endothelium that relax (nitric oxide) or constrict (endothelin) blood vessels also contribute to autoregulation of blood pressure. Mechanisms that cause disruption of the autoregulation of blood pressure are not clearly understood, but heredity, age, obesity, diet, smoking, excessive alcohol intake, sedentary lifestyle, anxiety, and medications are implicated. Persistent hypertension can lead to vascular remodeling, left ventricular hypertrophy, atherosclerosis, and glomerulosclerosis (Graham & Sansoni, 2002).

The Seventh Report of the Joint National Committee on Prevention, Detection, Evaluation, and Treatment of High Blood Pressure indicates the following:

- The risk of CVD begins with blood pressure at 115/75 mmHg and doubles with each increase of 20/10 mmHg.
- Data from the Framingham Heart Study suggest that individuals who are normotensive at age 55 have a 90% lifetime risk of becoming hypertensive.
- Blood pressure control can decrease the incidence of stroke by 35–40%, of myocardial infarction by 20–25%, and of heart failure by 50%.
- Management of blood pressure may slow the progression of cognitive impairment and dementia (Chobanian et al., 2004).

Hypertension is classified as primary or essential if there is no identified organic cause for blood pressure elevation. Blood pressure elevation may also occur secondary to other disease conditions including renovascular hypertension, chronic kidney disease, obstructive uropathy, adrenal disorders (e.g., Cushing's syndrome, chronic steroid use, primary aldosteronism, and other mineralocorticoid excess), thyroid or parathyroid disease, sleep apnea, and drug-related causes.

Untreated or inadequately controlled hypertension may result in target organ damage, including the following:

- Heart—Left ventricular hypertrophy, heart failure, angina, myocardial infarction
- Brain—Transient ischemic attacks and cerebrovascular accident
- Kidney—Chronic renal failure
- Peripheral arterial disease
- Retinopathy

Common Presenting Signs and Symptoms

History
Presenting symptoms will vary and may include the following:

- Symptoms may be absent.
- Early morning headache
- Symptoms associated with end organ damage (see above)
- Presence of drugs that may elevate blood pressure (e.g., gluco- and mineralocorticosteroids, NSAIDs, cyclosporine, tacrolimus, erythropoietin, sibutramine, clozapine, lithium, ergots, sympathomimetics, inappropriate drug combinations (clonidine/ beta-blocker) (Chobanian et al., 2004)

Physical Examination
The exam may indicate secondary causes of hypertension, risk factors, and end organ damage.

- Persistently elevated blood pressure; two or more readings at separate assessments
- Osler's sign—Radial pulse remains palpable with blood pressure cuff inflation
- Obesity—BMI ≥ 30 or waist circumference > 35 inches (female), 40 inches (male)

- Fundoscopy—Hypertensive retinopathy (optic disc edema, arteriolar narrowing, arteriovenous crossing defects, retinal exudates, and hemorrhages)
- Thyroid enlargement, altered TSH
- Cardiac—Laterally displaced apical impulse, precordial heaves, abnormal rate/ rhythm, S3, S4, murmurs
- Abdomen—Obesity, kidney mass, aortic pulsation, renal artery bruit
- Peripheral arterial disease, peripheral edema, arterial bruits
- Neurological deficits

Differential Diagnoses
- White coat hypertension
- Incorrect blood pressure measurement technique
- Secondary causes of hypertension (see above)

Essential Diagnostic and Laboratory Tests
Patients who enter the nursing home without a prior history of hypertension should receive an initial accurate assessment of blood pressure. Prior to assigning a diagnosis of hypertension, blood pressure should be monitored on at least three occasions and the average of the readings used to establish the diagnosis, unless initial readings suggest a hypertensive crisis. The technique for blood pressure monitoring should include the following:

- Proper size blood pressure cuff—Too small a cuff yields a high reading; too large a cuff yields a low reading.
- Readings taken no sooner than 30 minutes after caffeine, cigarettes
- Patient's legs not crossed
- Restrictive clothing loosened

- Sphygmomanometer periodically calibrated for accuracy
- Cuff positioned on bare arm, not over clothing
- Patient's arm not placed higher than the level of the heart
- Palpate radial pulse while inflating the cuff and inflate to 30 mmHg after pulse disappears to correct for pseudohypertension and an auscultatory gap.
- Allow the needle or mercury column to descend no faster than 2–3 mmHg per second.
- Take initial readings in both arms with patient seated, and in one arm with patient standing or after transfer to a chair (to evaluate orthostatic hypotension).
- Evaluate for orthostatic hypotension defined as a drop in systolic pressure of 20 mmHg or more, or a drop in diastolic value of 10 mmHg or more two minutes after a position change.
  - ○ If symptoms occur with any drop in blood pressure, orthostasis exists.
  - ○ Palpate a peripheral pulse prior to and after position change as another indication of orthostatic changes (increased pulse and lower blood pressure suggest orthostasis).
- Avoid blood pressure evaluation immediately after a meal (postprandial hypotension).
- Order blood pressures to be taken at the same time of day; position and arm used should be noted in the patient record.

Further workup for hypertension and evaluation of therapies should include the following

- Electrocardiogram
- Urinalysis
- Blood glucose and hematocrit
- Serum potassium, calcium
- Creatinine or estimate of glomerular filtration rate

- Fasting lipid panel
- Consider measuring urinary albumin excretion or albumin/creatinine ratio.
- Holter monitoring may be indicated if diagnosis is unclear with traditional cuff pressures.

Management Plan

The goal for management of hypertension is prevention of end organ damage.

Nonpharmacologic

Several lifestyle modifications have been shown to effectively reduce systolic blood pressure values. At minimum, lifestyle interventions should be initiated for all patients diagnosed with prehypertension. Some of these may be appropriate in long term-care settings.

- Weight reduction, as needed
- Dietary Approaches to Stop Hypertension (DASH) diet (Chobanian et al., 2004)
- Sodium restriction—This may not be necessary in the diet of a frail elder, unless there is concurrent heart failure (Levenson & Crecelius, 2003). Consideration must also be given to patients diagnosed with hypertension who also have protein-energy malnutrition, which is common in nursing homes. In such instances imposing further dietary restriction may be counterproductive.
- Physical activity/exercise should be encouraged, as possible.
- Smoking cessation, if applicable
- Moderation in alcohol consumption for those who have access to it.

Pharmacologic

- Younger old adults (60–80) with hypertension, including isolated systolic hypertension, should be treated similarly to younger individuals. The Systolic Hypertension in the Elderly Program (SHEP) has demonstrated reduced incidence of stroke and heart failure episodes with treatment of isolated systolic hypertension in those over age 60 (Kostis et al., 1997; Perry et al., 2000).

- In the nursing home, lowering blood pressure to the recommended levels may lead to hypotension and risk of falls in some older persons and should be attempted with caution. This is especially true when a resident is prescribed a vasodilator in addition to a diuretic for blood pressure control. Fall risk may be particularly high postprandially.

- Evidence to support treatment of residents older than 80–85 is limited (Levenson & Crecelius, 2003). It may also be possible to wean the very old from antihypertensive medications. Lower systolic blood pressure, body mass index, and less evidence of left ventricular hypertrophy may predict successful weaning (Froom & Trilling, 2000).

- If tolerated, the blood pressure goal for most individuals is 130/85 mmHg. For residents with diabetes, renal disease, heart failure, or coronary artery disease the recommended blood pressure goal is 130/80 mmHg.

- In the nursing home setting, starting drug doses may initially be lower than for younger adults, but control may require dose increases and the addition of drug classes in order to achieve blood pressure control (Table 6-10).

- Drug regimens should be kept as simple as possible and patients should be monitored for subtle as well as overt adverse drug reactions, since most residents have multiple comorbid conditions and are at increased risk for reactions related to the number of drugs prescribed.

- Careful monitoring is required to prevent excess lowering of blood pressure and orthostatic hypotension that may affect cerebral perfusion and increase fall risk.

- Avoid aggressive management of isolated blood pressure elevations (treating the numbers) without evaluation of a resident's overall condition, comorbidities, treatment goals, and the technique used by staff to measure blood pressure (Levenson & Crecelius, 2003).

- The nurse practitioner, in consultation with the physician, may elect to discontinue medication management of blood pressure in certain terminally ill patients at end of life. This requires discussion with the patient and/or caregivers and the interdisciplinary team and clear documentation of decisions in the medical record.

There is evidence of overuse of calcium channel blockers (CCB) and alpha-blockers and underuse of diuretics, beta-blockers, and angiotensin-converting enzyme inhibitors (ACEI) in some nursing homes (Ziesmer, Ghosh, & Aronow, 2003). Specific recommendations for the management of hypertension in older adults include the following:

- In most patients, begin therapy with a low dose thiazide diuretic. These are well tolerated and offer the additional benefit of slowing demineralization of bone in osteoporosis. Use cautiously with a history of gout or with hyponatremia. In the Antihypertensive and Lipid Lowering Treatment to Prevent Heart Attack Trial (ALLHAT) chlorthalidone was found to be effective in both blacks and non-blacks in management of hypertension compared to an ACEI (lisinopril) and CCB (amlodipine) (Wright et al., 2005).

- Consider a loop diuretic when creatinine is > 2.0 mg/dL or glomerular filtration rate (GFR) is less than 30 mL/min per 1.73 m^2 (ICSI, 2005d).

- If blood pressure goal is not reached treatment options include the following:
  ○ Increase the initial agent towards the maximum dose.

TABLE 6-10   Preferred Antihypertensive Agents for Older Adults

DRUG	DOSAGE RANGE (DAILY FREQUENCY)	COMMON SIDE EFFECTS	SPECIAL CONSIDERATIONS
Thiazide Diuretics	*First-line drugs for uncomplicated hypertension*		
Chlorothiazide (Diuril)	500–1000 mg/day (1)	Hypokalemia	Preferred initial treatment for
Chlorthalidone	12.5–100 mg/day (1)	Hyponatremia	uncomplicated hypertension
Hydrochlorothiazide (HydroDIURIL, Microzide)	12.5–50 mg/day (1)	Hypotension Orthostasis	Effective for African-Americans Effective for isolated systolic
Indapamide (Lozol)	1.25–5 mg/day (1)	Hyperuricemia	hypertension
Metolazone (Microx, Zaroxolyn)	2.5–5 mg/day (1)	Hyperglycemia Hypertriglyceridemia	Effective for mild heart failure Action blocked by NSAIDs
		Fatigue	Digoxin toxicity with hypokalemia
		Dry mouth	ACEIs lessen hypokalemia
		Constipation	Increases lithium blood levels
		Nausea	
Angiotensin-Converting Enzyme Inhibitors (ACEIs)	*Start with low dose if patient is also taking a diuretic*		
Benazepril (Lotensin)	5–40 mg/day (1–2)	Angioedema	Effective for renal protection
Captopril (Capoten)	12.5–450 mg/day (3)	Cough	in diabetes
Enalapril (Vasotec)	2.5–40 mg/day (1–2)	Hyperkalemia	Effective for nondiabetic renal
Lisinopril (Prinivil, Zestril)	2.5–40 mg/day (1)	Hypotension	disease with proteinuria
Moexipril (Univasc)	3.75–30 mg/day (1)	Elevated serum	Effective for heart failure
Trandolapril (Mavik)	0.5–4 mg/day (1)	creatinine	Suggested for patients with
Fosinopril (Monopril)	5–40 mg/day (1)	Tachycardia	previous MI and impaired
Quinapril (Accupril)	2.5–80 mg/day (1–2)	Fatigue	left ventricular function
Ramipril (Altace)	1.25–20 mg/day (1–2)	Nausea	Suggested for those at high
Perindopril (Aceon)	4–16 mg/day (1–2)	Diarrhea	risk for coronary events
			Less effective monotherapy in African-Americans, except with renal insufficiency (AASK)
			Action blocked by NSAIDs
			Do not use with potassium sparing diuretics
			Expect a slight decrease in GFR or creatinine levels
Angiotensin II Receptor Blockers (ARBs)	*Start with a low dose if patient is also taking a diuretic*		
Candesartan (Atacand)	8–32 mg/day (1–2)	Angioedema	As above
Eprosartan (Teveten)	400–800 mg/day (1–2)	Hyperkalemia	
Irbesartan (Avapro)	150–300 mg/day (1)	Hypotension	
Losartan (Cozaar)	25–100 mg/day (1–2)	Increased serum	
Olmesartan (Benicar)	20–40 mg/day (1)	creatinine	
Telmisartan (Micardis)	40–80 mg/day (1)	Tachycardia	
Valsartan (Diovan)	80–320 mg/day (1)	Fatigue	
Beta Adrenergic Blockers (BBs)			
Acebutolol (Sectral)	200–800 mg/day (1)	Bradycardia	Suggested for all patients
Atenolol (Tenormin)	25–100 mg/day (1)	Dyspnea	postmyocardial infarction or at
Bisoprolol (Zebeta)	2.5–20 mg/day (1)	Wheezing	high risk for coronary events
Metoprolol (Lopressor)	12.5–400 mg/day (1–2)	Fatigue	Effective in heart failure
Metoprolol succinate (Toprol XL)	25–400 mg/day (1)	Lightheadedness, dizziness	Used with angina pectoris, supraventricular arrhythmias,
Nadolol (Corgard)	30–320 mg/day (1)	Confusion	hypertrophic cardiomyopathy

TABLE 6-10   *(continued)*

DRUG	DOSAGE RANGE (DAILY FREQUENCY)	COMMON SIDE EFFECTS	SPECIAL CONSIDERATIONS
Pindolol (Visken)	5–60 mg/day (2)	Sleep disturbances Depression Diarrhea Cold extremities	Avoid with severe asthma, COPD Avoid with second- or third-degree heart block and bradycardia Avoid in insulin-dependent diabetics prone to hypoglycemia Use with verapamil may potentiate complete heart block, negative inotropic effect Increased warfarin activity if BB metabolized in the liver Cimetidine and nicotine reduce bioavailability if BB is metabolized in the liver
Calcium Channel Blockers (CCBs) **Dihydropyridines** Amlodipine (Norvasc) Felodipine (Plendil) Isradipine (DynaCirc CR) Nicardipine SR (Cardene SR) Nifedipine SR (Adalat CC) Nifedipine SR (Procardia XL) **Nondihydropyridines** Diltiazem ER (Cardizem CD, Dilacor XR, Tiazac) Diltiazem SR (Cardizem LA) Verapamil (Calan, Isoptin) Verapamil LA (Calan SR, Isoptin SR)	 2.5–10 mg/day (1) 2.5–10 mg/day (1) 2.5–10 mg/day (2) 60–120 mg/day (2) 30–90 mg/day (1) 30–120 mg/day (1) 120–480 mg/day ((1) 120–240 mg/day (1) 40–480 mg/day (3) 120–480 mg/day (1–2)	 Elevated liver enzymes Hypotension Dizziness Peripheral edema Headache Flushing Heart block (verapamil) Constipation (verapamil)	 Effective for African-Americans without renal insufficiency (ALLHAT) Effective for angina pectoris Effective in hypertrophic cardiomyopathy without obstruction (verapamil, diltiazem) Avoid with severe heart failure (verapamil) Avoid with second- or third-degree heart block, Wolf-Parkinson-White syndrome (verapamil) Avoid with sick sinus syndrome (verapamil, diltiazem) Avoid with previous MI and heart failure (diltiazem) Additive negative inotropic effect with beta-blockers (verapamil) Verapamil increases digoxin levels Cimetidine increases nifedipine blood levels
Central Alpha-2 Agonists and Other Centrally Acting Drugs	*Avoid in the geriatric population due to side effects*		
Clonidine (Catapres) Clonidine patch (Catapres-TTS) Methyldopa (Aldomet) Reserpine	0.1–12 mg/day (2) 0.1–0.3 mg/day 125–3000 mg/day (3–4) 0.05–0.5 mg/day (1)	Memory loss Sedation, drowsiness Depression Orthostatic hypotension Peripheral edema, hemolytic anemia (methyldopa)	Discontinue slowly to prevent rebound hypertension

continued

TABLE 6-10 *(continued)*

DRUG	DOSAGE RANGE (DAILY FREQUENCY)	COMMON SIDE EFFECTS	SPECIAL CONSIDERATIONS
Direct Vasodilators	*Avoid in the geriatric population due to side effects*		
Hydralazine (Apresoline) Minoxidil (Loniten)	10–300 mg/day (4)	Lupus-like syndrome (hydralazine) Hirsutism (minoxidil) Reflex tachycardia Peripheral edema	Use with a diuretic and beta-blocker to combat tachycardia and peripheral edema Start with low dose at bedtime
Alpha-1 Blockers	*Not first-line treatment; use with extreme caution in the elderly, if at all*		
Doxazosin (Cardura) Prazosin (Minipress) Terazosin (Hytrin)	1–16 mg/day (1) 1–20 mg/day (2–3) 1–20 mg/day (1–2)	Increased risk of heart failure Dizziness Fatigue, lack of energy Orthostatic hypotension Edema, dyspnea (doxazosin) Palpitations, nausea (prazosin) Nasal congestion (terazosin)	Syncope with first dose–administer at bedtime Effective for benign prostatic hyperplasia

AASK, African American Study of Kidney Disease and Hypertension; ALLHAT, Antihypertensive and Lipid Lowering Treatment to Prevent Heart Attack Trial; GFR, glomerular filtration rate.
Source: Adapted from Chobanian et al., 2003; ICSI, 2005d; Omnicare, 2004; *Prescribers Letter,* 2003.

- ○ Add another agent from a different drug class.
- ○ Substitute an agent from another class.
- In older adults a combination of drugs may lessen the risk of side effects by keeping dosages for each drug low.
- Patients with chronic kidney disease may require three or more drugs for blood pressure control.
- For diabetics add an angiotensin-converting enzyme inhibitor (ACEI) or angiotensin receptor blocker (ARB) for hypertension treatment or for nephropathy prevention/management.
- ACEIs can reduce the risk of recurrent MI and manage concurrent heart failure in patients with deceased left ventricular function.
- For hypertensive patients with angina and/or postmyocardial infarction (MI) consider a beta-blocker instead of a diuretic as initial therapy. This drug class has been shown to reduce the risk of sudden death after an MI. Beta-blockers are also useful in treating atrial tachyarrhythmias, migraine, thyrotoxicosis, essential tremor, or perioperative hypertension. Beta-blockers should be avoided with a history of asthma, reactive airway disease, or second- or third-degree heart block.
- With isolated systolic hypertension (ISH) add a calcium channel blocker if a diuretic is not effective alone. This drug class may also be effective in Raynaud's syndrome and certain cardiac arrhythmias. It has also been effective in management of hypertension in African-Americans.
- With prostatism consider an alpha- or alpha-beta-blocker. The FDA has approved doxazosin (Cardura), prazosin (Minipress), and terazosin (Hytrin) for hypertension control. Side effects of dizziness, postural

hypotension, weakness, and fatigue are frequent so these drugs may not be appropriate for most patients in the nursing home.

- Avoid or discontinue drugs such as NSAIDs and sympathomimetics for all hypertensives, if possible, because they may cause or exacerbate blood pressure elevation.

Patient, Family, and Staff Education

- Nature and course of the disease
- Correct blood pressure measurement techniques
- Importance of blood pressure control and consequences of hypertension
- Importance of nonpharmaceutical interventions
- Discussion of blood pressure control at end of life

Physician Consultation

- Suspected secondary hypertension
- Hypertension not responsive to initial therapies
- Persistently elevating blood pressure
- Blood pressure control at end of life

WEBSITES

- American College of Cardiology—www.acc.org/clinical/statements.htm
- American Heart Association—my.americanheart.org/portal/professional/guidelines
- Institute for Clinical Systems Improvement, healthcare guidelines—www.icsi.org/knowledge/browse_bydate.asp?catID=29
- Detection, evaluation, and treatment of high blood cholesterol in adults (adult treatment panel III)—www.nhlbi.nih.gov/guidelines/cholesterol/index.htm
- Clinical practice guidelines for managing dyslipidemias in chronic kidney disease—www.kidney.org/professionals/kdoqi/guidelines_lipids/index.htm
- Lipid management in adults—www.icsi.org/knowledge/detail.asp?catID=29&itemID=197
- National Guideline Clearinghouse—www.ngc.gov
- Institute for Clinical Systems Improvement—www.icsi.org
- American Medical Directors Association—www.amda.com/info/cpg/heartfailure.htm
- National Heart, Lung, and Blood Institute—www.nhlbi.nih.gov/guidelines/hypertension

REFERENCES

Albers, G. W., Dalen, J. E., Laupacis, A., Manning, W. J., Petersen, P., & Singer, D. E. (2001). Antithrombotic therapy in atrial fibrillation. *Chest, 119,* 194S–206S.

Agruss, J. C., & Garrett, K. (2005). New markers for CVD. *The Nurse Practitioner, 30*(11), 26–27, 29–31.

American College of Cardiology/American Heart Association Task Force on Practice Guidelines. (2002). *Guideline update for the management of patients with chronic stable angina*. Retrieved March 26, 2006 from http://www.aacc.org/clinical/statements.

American College of Cardiology/American Heart Association Task Force on Practice Guidelines. (2005). ACC/AHA 2005 guideline update for the diagnosis and management of chronic heart failure in the adult—Summary article. *Circulation, 112,* 1825–1852.

American College of Physicians. (1996). Clinical guidelines, Part 1: Guidelines for using serum cholesterol, high-density lipoprotein cholesterol, and triglycerides levels as screening tests for preventing coronary heart disease in adults. *Annals of Internal Medicine, 124,* 515–517.

American Diabetes Association, American Psychiatric Association, American Association of Clinical Endocrinologists, North American Association for the Study of Obesity. (2004). Consensus development conference on antipsychotic drugs and obesity and diabetes. *Diabetes Care,* 27(2), 596–601.

American Geriatrics Society. (2000). Current guidelines for practice oral anticoagulation for older adults modified from *Chest,* 1998: *114,* 439S–440S. Retrieved January 3, 2006, from http://www.americangeriatrics.org/staging/products/positionpapers/oralanti.shtml

American Medical Directors Association. (2002). *Heart failure.* Retrieved February 11, 2005, from http://ngc.gov/ summary/summary.aspx?doc_id=3303&nbr=002529&string=heart+AND+failure.

Aronow, W. S. (2006). ACC/AHA guidelines update: Treatment of heart failure with reduced left ventricular ejection fraction. *Geriatrics,* 61(3), 22–29.

Awtry, E. R., & Loscalzo, J. (2004). Coronary artery disease. In T. E. Andreoli, C. C. J. Carpenter, R. C. Griggs, & J. Loscalzo (Eds.), *Cecil essentials of medicine* (6th ed., pp. 87–108). Philadelphia: Saunders.

Characteristics of the various statins. (2003). *Prescribers Letter,* 10(8). Retrieved February 25, 2006 from http://prescribersletter.com/(xcofzs55y10t0d55qy4w5455)/pl/ArticleDD.aspx?s=PRL&cs=&st=1&li=1&dd=190801&pb=&pt=2&fpt=10.

Chobanian, A. V., Bakris, G. L., Black, H. R., Cushman, W. C., Green, L. A., Izzo, J. L., Jr., et al. (2003). The seventh report of the joint national committee on prevention, detection, evaluation, and treatment of high blood pressure: The JNC 7 report. *Journal of the American Medical Association,* 289, 2560–2571.

Crecelius, C. A., & Levenson, S. (2004). Atrial fibrillation: Assessment and treatment of the most common cardiac arrhythmia in the LTC setting. *Caring for the Ages,* 5(5), 22, 24–25.

Froom, J., & Trilling, J. (2000). Reducing antihypertensive medication use in nursing home patients. *Archives of Family Medicine,* 9, 378–383.

Fuster, V., Ryden, L. E., Asinger, R. W., Cannom, D. S., Crijns, H. J., Frye, R. L., et al. (2001). Guidelines for the management of patients with atrial fibrillation. *Journal of the American College of Cardiology,* 38, 1231–1265.

Ghosh, S., Ziesmer, V., & Aronow, W. S. (2002). Underutilization of aspirin, beta blockers, angiotensin-converting enzyme inhibitors, and lipid-lowering drugs and overutilization of calcium channel blockers in older persons with coronary artery disease in an academic nursing home. *The Journal of Gerontology Series A: Biological Sciences and Medical Sciences,* 57, M398–M400.

Graham, A., & Sansoni, S. (2002). *The stroke of time: Controlling blood pressure in the elderly.* Columbia, MD: Medicalliance Education Institute.

Grundy, S. M., Cleeman, J. K., Merz, C. N. B., Brewer, H. B., Clark, L. T., Hunninghake, D. B., et al. (2004). Implications of recent clinical trials for the National Cholesterol Education Program Adult Treatment panel III guidelines. *Circulation,* 110, 227–239.

Gutierrez, C., & Blanchard, D. G. (2004). Diastolic heart failure: Challenges of diagnosis and treatment. *American Family Physician,* 69, 2609–2616.

Institute for Clinical Systems Improvement. (2005a). *Health care guideline: Anticoagulant therapy supplement.* Retrieved February 25, 2006, from http://www.icsi.org/knowledge/detail.asp?catID=29&itemID=151

Institute for Clinical Systems Improvement. (2005b). *Health care guideline: Diagnosis and treatment of chest pain and acute coronary syndrome (ACS).* Retrieved March 26, 2006, from http://www.icsi.org

Institute for Clinical Systems Improvement. (2005c). *Health care guideline: Heart failure in adults.* Retrieved February 11, 2006, from http://www.icsi.org/knowledge/detail.asp?catID=29&itemID=161

Institute for Clinical Systems Improvement. (2005d). *Health care guideline: Hypertension diagnosis and treatment.* Retrieved March 11, 2006, from http://www.icsi.org/knowledge/detail.asp?catID=29&itemID=173

Institute for Clinical Systems Improvement. (2005e). *Health care guideline: Lipid management in adults.* Retrieved January 31, 2006, from http://www.icsi.org/knowledge/detail.asp?catID=29&itemID=197

Institute for Clinical Systems Improvement. (2005f). *Health care guideline: Stable coronary artery disease* (10th ed.). Retrieved March 26, 2006, from http://www.icsi.org/display_file.asp?fileID=1575

Jones, A. (2002). *The National Nursing Home Survey: 1999 Summary. National Center for Health Statistics,* 13(152). (DHHS Publication No. (PHS) 2002–1723). Hyattsville, MD.

Katzel, L., & Goldberg, A. F. (2003). Dyslipoproteinemia. In W. R. Hazzard, J. P. Blass, J. B. Halter, J. G. Ousland, & M. E. Tinetti (Eds.). *Principles of geriatric medicine & gerontology* (5th ed.). New York: McGraw-Hill.

Kostis, J. B., Davis, B. R., Cutler, J., Grimm, R. H., Jr., Berge, K. G., Cohen, J. D., et al. (1997). Prevention of heart failure by antihypertensive drug treatment in older persons with isolated systolic hypertension. SHEP Cooperative Research Group. *Journal of the American Medical Association, 278*, 212–216.

Latif, A. A., & Messinger-Rapport, B. J. (2004). Should nursing home residents with atrial fibrillation be anticoagulated? [Electronic version] *Cleveland Clinic Journal of Medicine, 71*, 40–44.

Levenson, S., & Crecelius, C. (2003). Identifying and managing hypertension in the elderly. *Caring for the Ages, 4*(5), 12, 14–16.

Massey, B. M. (2004). Heart failure: Pathophysiology and diagnosis. In L. Goldman, & D. Ausiello (Eds.), *Cecil essentials of medicine* (22nd ed.). Philadelphia: Saunders.

National Cholesterol Education Program. (2001). *Third report of the National Cholesterol Education Program (NCEP) expert panel on detection, evaluation, and treatment of high blood cholesterol in adults (Adult treatment panel III) executive summary* (NIH Publication No. 01–3670). Washington, DC: National Heart, Lung, and Blood Institute, National Institutes of Health.

Omnicare. (2004). *Geriatric pharmaceutical care guidelines*. Covington, KY: Omnicare.

Perry, H. M., Jr., Davis, B. R., Price, T. R., Applegate, W. B., Fields, W. S., Guralnik, J. M., et al. (2000). Effect of treating isolated systolic hypertension on the risk of developing various types and subtypes of stroke: The Systolic Hypertension in the Elderly Program (SHEP). *Journal of the American Medical Association, 284*, 465–471.

Riggs, J. (2006, January/February). Managing chronic heart failure. *Nursing Made Incredibly Easy*, 28–31, 33–34, 36–39.

Rodondi, N., Newman, A. B., Vittinghoff, E., de Rekeneire, N., Satterfield, S., Harris, T. B., et al. (2005). Subclinical hypothyroidism and the risk of heart failure, other cardiovascular events, and death. *Archives of Internal Medicine, 165*, 2460–2466.

Shamsham, F., & Mitchell, J. (2000). Essentials of the diagnosis of heart failure. *American Family Physician, 61*, 1319–1328.

Snow, V., Weiss, K. B., LeFevre, M., McNamara, R., Bass, E., Green, L. A., et al. (2003). Management of newly detected atrial fibrillation: A clinical practice guideline from the American Academy of Family Physicians and the American College of Physicians. *Archives of Internal Medicine, 139*, 1009–1017.

Strimike, C. L. (2006). B-type natriuretic peptide: An emerging cardiac risk marker. *American Journal for Nurse Practitioners, 10*(3), 27–34.

Tresch, D. D. (1997). The clinical diagnosis of heart failure in older patients. *Journal of the American Geriatrics Society, 45*, 1128–1133.

Veterans Health Administration. (2003). *The pharmacologic management of chronic heart failure*. Washington, DC: Veterans Health Administration. Retrieved February 11, 2006, from http://www.oqp.med.va.gov/cpg/CHF/CHF_Base.htm

Wenger, N. K., Helmy, T., Patel, A. D., & Lerakis, S. (2005). Evidence-based management of coronary artery disease in the elderly—Current perspectives. *Medscape General Medicine, 7*(2), 75.

Wright, J. T., Dunn, J. K., Cutler, J. A., Davis, B. R., Cushman, W. C., Ford, C. E., et al. (2005). Outcomes in hypertensive black and nonblack patients treated with chlorthalidone, amlodipine, and lisinopril. *Journal of the American Medical Association, 293*, 1595–1608.

BIBLIOGRAPHY

Angeja, B. G., & Grossman, W. (2003). Evaluation and management of diastolic heart failure. *Circulation, 107*, 659–663.

Beers, M. H., & Jones, T. V. (2006). *The Merck manual of geriatrics* (3rd ed., updated). Retrieved January 31, 2006, from http://www.merck.com/mrkshared/mmg/home.jsp

Croft, J. B., Giles, W. H., Pollard, R. A., Keenan, N. L., Casper, M. L., & Amda, R. F. (1999). Heart failure survival among older adults in the United States. *Archives of Internal Medicine, 159*, 505–510.

Flaherty, E., Fulmer, T., Mezey, M. (Eds.). (2003). *Geriatric nursing review syllabus: A core curriculum in advanced practice geriatric nursing.* New York: American Geriatrics Society.

Gage, B. F., Waterman, A. D., Shannon, W., Boechler, M., Rich, W., & Radford, M. J. (2001). Validation of clinical classification schemes for predicting stroke: Results from the National Registry of Atrial Fibrillation. *Journal of the American Medical Association, 285,* 2864–2870.

Hirsh, J., Fuster, V., Ansell, J., & Halperin, J. L. (2003). American Heart Association/American College of Cardiology Foundation guide to warfarin therapy. *Circulation, 107,* 1692–1711.

Prithwish, B., Clark, A. L., & Cleland, J. G. F. (2004). Diastolic heart failure: A difficult problem in the elderly. *American Journal of Geriatric Cardiology, 13,* 16–21.

Subrato, G., & Aronow, W. S. (2003). Utilization of lipid-lowering drugs in elderly persons with increased serum low-density lipoprotein cholesterol associated with coronary artery disease, symptomatic peripheral arterial disease, prior stroke, or diabetes mellitus before and after an educational program on dyslipidemia treatment. *Journal of Gerontology: Medical Sciences, 58A,* 432–435.

CHAPTER 7

Dermatology

Cathleen Case

INTRODUCTION: SKIN AND AGING

The geriatric population is generally defined as persons 65 years of age and older, but it is important to recognize aging as a continuous process with a wide spectrum of appearance. External skin condition correlates with physiologic age more than chronologic age, and pathologic aging is further deterioration that occurs from disease.

Cutaneous aging includes changes due to the passage of time as well as chronic sun exposure (Figure 7-1). Changes in skin attributable to sun exposure have major morphologic and physiologic manifestations that represent the "old skin" look (Yaar & Gilchrest, 2003). True aging is inevitable and is demonstrated by physiologic alterations and subtle consequences for healthy and diseased skin. The following are important functions of skin that *decline* with age (Gilchrest, 1993):

- Cell replacement
- Injury response
- Barrier function
- Sensory perception
- Chemical clearance

- Mechanical protection
- Immune and vascular responsiveness
- Thermoregulation
- Sweat and sebum production
- Vitamin D production

Histologic features of aging skin are numerous. In the epidermis there is flattening of the dermal-epidermal junction that results in smaller surface between the two compartments with less communication and nutrient transfer. This poor adhesion explains the propensity to torn skin, superficial abrasions,

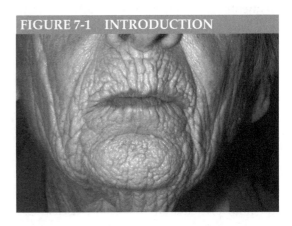

FIGURE 7-1 INTRODUCTION

TABLE 7-1	Primary Lesions	
PRIMARY LESION	DESCRIPTION	EXAMPLE
Macule	Circumscribed and flat, brown, blue, red, or hypopigmented	Freckle, lentigo, melasma, stasis dermatitis, vitiligo
Papule	Elevated solid lesion up to 0.5 cm, color varies, may coalesce and become plaques	BCC, dermal nevi, warts, hemangioma, seborrheic keratosis, eczema, psoriasis, scabies, melanoma
Plaque	Circumscribed, elevated, superficial, solid lesion more than 0.5 cm	Psoriasis, eczema, tinea corporis, Paget's disease, discoid lupus, seborrheic dermatitis
Nodule	Circumscribed, elevated, solid lesion more than 0.5 cm; large nodule is a tumor	BCC, SCC, melanoma, hemangioma
Pustule	Circumscribed collection of leukocytes and free fluid; varies in size	Acne, folliculitis, herpes simplex
Vesicle	Circumscribed collection of free fluid up to 0.5 cm	Acute eczema, herpes simplex or zoster, scabies
Bulla	Circumscribed collection of free fluid more than 0.5 cm	Bullous pemphigoid, fixed drug eruption
Wheal (hive)	Firm edematous plaque; dermis is infiltrated with fluid; transient and only last a few hours	Hives, urticaria, angioedema

and bulla formation in edematous sites. Dermal-epidermal separation may contribute to the increased prevalence of certain bullous dermatoses in the elderly. In the dermis there is atrophy with fewer mast cells, fibroblasts, and blood vessels, as well as abnormal nerve endings and shortened capillary loops. A rigid, unresponsive, and inelastic dermis does not repair well (Gilchrest, 1993).

The diseases and disorders in geriatric dermatology are numerous. The discussions in this section will focus on conditions most frequently seen in residents of skilled nursing facilities.

Dermatology Physical Exam

Dermatology is a morphologically oriented specialty, and the ability to describe what is seen is important. A full-body skin assessment is required because most skin diseases are dynamic and evolve through several stages. Identification of a primary lesion is the key to description of skin disease. Primary lesions are the most basic lesions identified during the initial presentation of the skin disease and

are the most prominent feature. Primary lesions are listed in Table 7-1.

It is important to use precise descriptive terminology for written and verbal documentation of a dermatologic condition. Note surface characteristics of lesions such as smooth, rough, pitted, or scaly, and whether the scale is fine, medium, heavy, thick, or silvery. Also describe precise color and uniformity, symmetry and shape, border regularity, distinctness, consistency, size, and distribution on the body. Secondary lesions such as scale, crust, fissures, or ulcers develop during the evolution of skin disease and are created by scratching or infection (Habif, 2004).

BULLOUS PEMPHIGOID

Definition

Blistering diseases in the elderly can be drug induced, autoimmune mediated, or caused by other systemic diseases. Diagnosis and treatment are important to avoid irreversible sequelae or death. Bullous pemphigoid (BP) is an autoimmune blistering disease of the

FIGURE 7-2   Primary Lesions

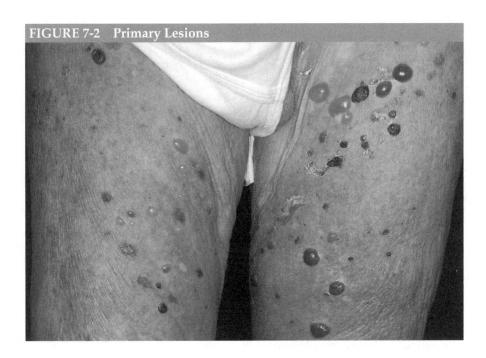

elderly and is also referred to as pemphigus of the elderly and senile pemphigoid (Lyon & Fitzpatrick, 1993). The disease is characterized by large tense bullae on flexor surfaces of the extremities, axilla, groin, and abdomen (Figure 7-2). It is mediated by IgG autoantibodies that bind to BP antigens. The resultant activity causes separation of the dermal-epidermal junction and the formation of a subepidermal blister.

Epidemiology

The mean age of onset for BP is 65 years, with 66% of patients older than 60. Estimated incidence is 6–7 cases per million per year, occurring in all races, and without gender predilection (Sami, Yeh, & Ahmed, 2004). There is little evidence of causal association of BP with internal malignancy (Habif, 2004); however, patients with BP have been reported with gastrointestinal, urinary tract, lymphoreticular, pancreas, genitalia, and breast malignancies.

There may also be an association with other autoimmune disorders such as diabetes, psoriasis, pernicious anemia, rheumatoid arthritis, and multiple sclerosis (Sami et al., 2004). Drugs such as furosemide and phenacetin are occasionally suspected as a cause (Habif, 2004).

Common Presenting Signs and Symptoms

1. Initial symptoms of pruritic, eczematous inflammation or urticarial plaques may be present for weeks or months in a preblistering stage. Itching is usually moderate to severe. This clinical picture can mimic a benign condition; if there is no response to initial treatment for pruritus, a biopsy needs to be done for appropriate diagnosis.

2. The bullae are tense, single or multiple, on erythematous or normal-appearing skin, about 0.5–7 cm in size, and the fluid is clear or hemorrhagic (Figure 7-3). The lesions

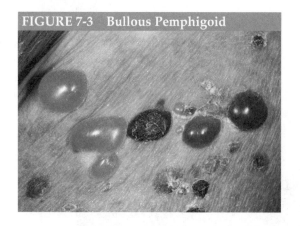

FIGURE 7-3   Bullous Pemphigoid

occur on flexor surfaces of the extremities, axilla, groin, and abdomen, but may also be a generalized distribution (Sami et al., 2004).

3. Once ruptured, the healing region is hyperpigmented as a result of inflammation.

Differential Diagnoses

- Pemphigus vulgaris
- Dermatitis herpetiformis
- Epidermolysis bullosa aquisita
- Erythema multiforme
- Cicatricial pemphigoid
- Porphyria cutanea tarda
- Bullous eruption of systemic lupus erythematosus
- Diabetic bullae

Essential Diagnostic and Laboratory Tests

- Dermatology referral for biopsies, including light microscopy and direct immunofluorescence, is essential for definitive diagnosis.
- The following may be present: peripheral blood eosinophilia, elevated serum IgE, and IgG antibodies revealed with serum indirect immunofluorescence (Habif, 2004).

Management Plan

The goal of therapy and management is to decrease blister formation, promote healing of all open erosions, and determine the minimal dose of medication required to control the disease process. Therapy must be individualized, and response must be closely monitored.

Nonpharmacologic

Domeboro soaks may be used 2 to 3 times a day to facilitate drying of blisters.

Pharmacologic

- Antihistamines, such as hydroxyzine HCL, for pruritus if tolerated without adverse effects.
- Systemic steroids.
- Topical corticosteroids, group I, have been effective combined with antibiotic therapy.
- Tetracycline, minocycline, doxycycline, and erythromycin have been used for localized or generalized BP; they increase cohesion at the basement membrane zone. Niacinamide may be used for synergistic effect.
- For patients with poor response, immunosuppressive therapy is considered with drugs such as azathioprine, methotrexate, or cyclosporine.

Patient, Family, and Staff Education

- The course of the disease is variable and depends on extent of involvement.
- Generalized BP in the older patient and individuals in poor general health have a poor prognosis.
- Localized BP may undergo spontaneous remission or become generalized.
- Meticulous skin care and monitoring for bacterial infection or ulcer formation is essential.
- Avoid physical trauma to skin surfaces.

CELLULITIS AND ERYSIPELAS

Definition

Cellulitis is an infection of the subcutaneous tissue with limited involvement of the dermis, usually caused by group A streptococcus and *Staphylococcus aureus* in adults. In patients with diabetes or immunosuppression the infection can be caused by gram-negative bacilli. Cellulitis typically occurs near areas of ulceration or a surgical site or in areas of venous or lymphatic compromise. Disruption of lymphatic circulation can occur after lymph node resection, radiation therapy, or previous cellulitis, leading to recurrent episodes (Habif, 2004). Predisposing factors for cellulitis in the geriatric patient include venous and/or arterial compromise, diabetes, trauma, xerosis with fissuring, and open areas created by chronic tinea infection on the foot (Lyon & Fitzpatrick, 1993).

Erysipelas is a superficial variant of cellulitis involving the dermis and superficial subcutaneous tissue with prominent lymphatic involvement. Lymphatic "streaks" may be present. Erysipelas is usually caused by group A streptococci. The area of involvement is well demarcated and raised above the surrounding skin. Most common sites include the face, ears (pinna), and lower legs. Recurrences may be spontaneous or secondary to trauma or obstruction of lymphatics (Habif, 2004).

Common Presenting Signs and Symptoms

Cellulitis

- Often a history of injury or ulcer followed by local erythema and tenderness
- Fever, malaise, chills, and pain
- Increased intensity of marked erythema, warmth, edema; not sharply defined or elevated (Figure 7-4)
- Proximal regional lymphadenopathy may be present.

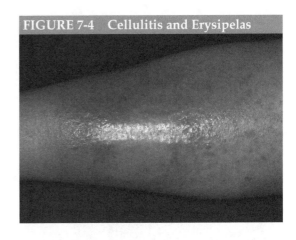

FIGURE 7-4   Cellulitis and Erysipelas

- Superficial vesicles or bullae may develop.
- Patients who have had saphenous venectomy may have recurrent cellulitis caused by non-group A beta-hemolytic streptococci. Tinea pedis in the web spaces has been observed on the affected leg, and the broken dermal barrier is thought to be a portal of entry for bacteria (Habif, 2004; Swartz & Weinberg, 1993).
- Dependent rubor may exaggerate the appearance of cellulitis in the lower leg; it is best to examine legs in the horizontal position each time for consistent evaluation.

Erysipelas

- May be more common in the lower leg with group B streptococci being the most common pathogen in adults over 50 (Habif, 2004). The facial infection involves the nose and one or both cheeks, or the pinna and same side cheek (Figure 7-5).
- Characteristic lesions are edematous, brawny, indurated, hot, shiny, red, well demarcated, and raised from the surrounding skin.
- Red, painful streaks lead toward regional nodes.

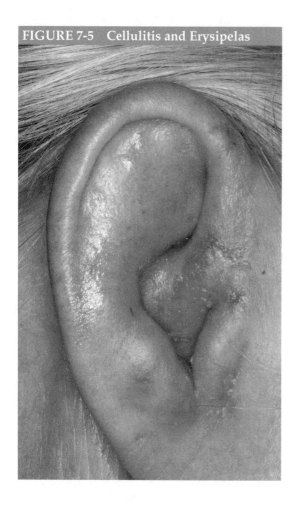

FIGURE 7-5   Cellulitis and Erysipelas

- Patients with chronic venous stasis and ulceration are prone to repeated attacks of erysipelas, which leads to lymphatic drainage impairment and permanent edema (Swartz & Weinberg, 1993).

Differential Diagnoses

Diagnosis is clinical for both conditions.

- Herpes zoster
- Osteomyelitis (facial or maxillary bones, and leg)
- Angioneurotic edema
- Contact dermatitis

Essential Diagnostic and Laboratory Tests

- Complete blood count, sedimentation rate, blood cultures
- It may be necessary to do a culture of a lesional biopsy specimen.

Management Plan

The goal of management is to clear infection with adequate and appropriate antibiotic coverage and aggressive monitoring for new infection.

Nonpharmacologic

- Burow's solution compresses or moist heat for pain
- Saline wet dressing to ulcers and necrotic lesions
- Leg elevation, rest, immobilization during acute phase
- Compression stockings for lower extremities following acute phase

Pharmacologic

- Empiric treatment for staphylococcal and streptococcal organisms is appropriate in adults. Dicloxacillin and first-generation cephalosporins are used most commonly. If response is poor, methicillin-resistant nosocomial or community acquired *S. aureus* needs to be considered. Severe infections, some elderly patients, and immunocompromised patients may require intravenous therapy.
- Vancomycin can also be used for penicillin allergy, and aminoglycoside agents should be considered if there is risk for gram-negative infection.
- Treatment of any existing tinea pedis according to fungal infection guidelines, along with treatment of the cellulitis, is important management and prophylaxis.

- For frequently recurrent cases, some suggest antibiotic prophylaxis with low doses of erythromycin, dicloxacillin, or cephalexin (Fitzpatrick, Johnson, Wolff, & Suurmond, 2001).
- Surgical intervention may be needed to drain an abscess or debride necrotic tissue.

Patient, Family and Staff Education
- General education about the care required, especially for chronic and recurrent cases of lower leg infections
- Adherence to treatment plans, especially compression stockings and leg elevation

Physician Consultation
- Consider referral to dermatology or surgery if biopsy is entertained for treatment failure or if diagnosis is uncertain.
- Infectious disease consult is helpful for antibiotic choice in difficult, resistant, or recurrent cases. Long-term prophylactic antibiotics are not commonly required and should only be implemented after consultation with an infectious disease expert.

CUTANEOUS MALIGNANCY

Definition

Nonmelanoma Skin Tumors
Basal cell carcinoma (BCC) and squamous cell carcinoma (SCC) are the two most common nonmelanoma skin cancers. Basal cell cancer is the most common malignant cutaneous neoplasm found in humans. Most BCCs occur on the head and neck region, 25% to 30% of these are on the nose. Squamous cell cancer has a stronger correlation with UV exposure than BCC (Habif, 2004).

Basal cell cancers arise in the basal layer of the epidermis and commonly present as a scab or bleeding lesion that persists, or heals and recurs. It grows by direct extension into normal surrounding tissue but rarely metastasizes to distant sites. It can, however, penetrate into subcutaneous tissue and bone, and if on the scalp, brain tissue can become invaded. Squamous cell cancer arises in the epithelium and is more common in the elderly population than younger ages. It has a definite risk of metastasis (Habif, 2004).

Malignant Melanoma
Malignant melanoma is a potentially lethal melanocytic neoplasm that can occur on the skin, eyes, ears, gastrointestinal tract, oral and genital mucus membranes, and leptomeninges (membranes surrounding the brain and spinal cord). Melanoma has the ability to metastasize to any organ. When detected early and properly treated, localized melanoma has a 5-year survival rate of 96% (Reyes-Ortiz, Goodwin, & Freeman, 2005). There are four proposed subtypes, although not all clinicians conform to the classifications. These include superficial spreading melanoma (SSM), lentigo maligna melanoma (LMM), nodular melanoma (NM), and acral lentiginous melanoma (ALM). Risk factors include prolonged exposure to UV radiation including the UVA of tanning booths, personal history of atypical moles, family history of melanoma, previous melanoma and nonmelanoma skin cancer history, more than 75–100 moles, immunosuppression, and giant congenital nevus > 20 cm (Habif, 2004).

Epidemiology

Nonmelanoma Skin Tumors
Basal cell carcinomas account for approximately 75–80% of all nonmelanoma skin cancers (Naylor, 2004). They occur at any age but mostly after the age of 40, and 85% are on the head and neck. One third of BCCs occur on skin that receives little or no UV radiation including sites of prior trauma. Squamous cell carcinoma is most common in areas of maximum solar radiation such as the head, back of the hands, top of the ear, and is more common in the older

population. Risk factors for SCC include sun exposure at a young age, sunburns, light color skin, hazel or blue eyes, blonde or red hair, freckling and telangiectasia on the face, living in southern regions, arsenic exposure, and human papilloma virus infection. Overall incidence of SCC increases with age and sun exposure (Habif, 2004).

Malignant Melanoma
The lifetime risk of malignant melanoma in Caucasians in 1987 was 1 in 123, and the estimate for the year 2010 is 1 in 50. The highest incidence is in New Zealand and Australia. Early recognition has been the goal of dermatologists monitoring for asymmetry, border irregularity, color variation, diameter enlargement, and local symptoms such as pain, itch, and tenderness (Habif, 2004).

Common Presenting Signs and Symptoms

Nonmelanoma Skin Tumors

- Nodular BCC is pearly white or pink, dome shaped with center depression or crust, and sometimes flat. Other features may include telangiectasia and specks of pigment floating within the lesions, irregular growth pattern, ulceration, crusting, and bleeding—and healing on occasion. Multinodular, ulcerative BCCs may extend deeply and peripherally (Figure 7-6).

- Superficial BCC is least aggressive. Found mostly on the trunk and extremities, the superficial BCC spreads peripherally; it is circumscribed, round or oval, and is a red scaling plaque containing an edge with a thin, raised, and pearly appearance. Figure 7-7 shows nodular BCC extending out of a superficial BCC.

- Actinic keratosis (AK) are precursor lesions to SCC and occur on sun-exposed skin (Figures 7-8 and 7-9). Characteristic AK papules are 2–6 mm thin/flat, pink, brown, and/or

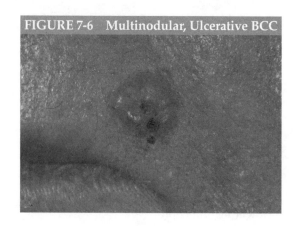
FIGURE 7-6   Multinodular, Ulcerative BCC

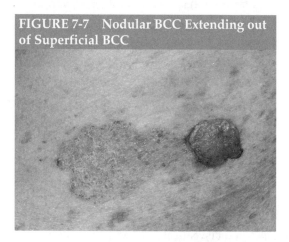
FIGURE 7-7   Nodular BCC Extending out of Superficial BCC

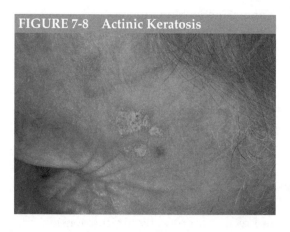
FIGURE 7-8   Actinic Keratosis

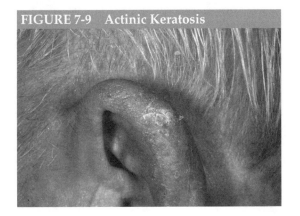

FIGURE 7-9   Actinic Keratosis

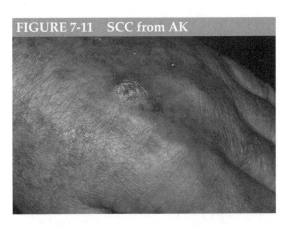

FIGURE 7-11   SCC from AK

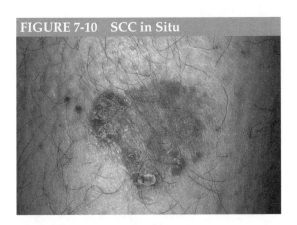

FIGURE 7-10   SCC in Situ

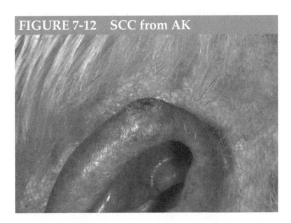

FIGURE 7-12   SCC from AK

rough; some lesions involute, others thicken, build up scale, and evolve to SCC.

- SCC in situ or Bowen's disease is found on sun-exposed areas, usually with sharp demarcation, erythema, and the papule or plaque can be smooth or scaly (Figure 7-10).

- SCC not from AK is usually a firm, movable, raised mass with sharp demarcation and little surface scale.

- SCC from AK is usually a thick papule or plaque with adherent scale, soft tumor, freely movable, red and with an inflamed base (Figures 7-11 and 7-12). Tumors on the

scalp, forehead, ears, nose, and lips are at higher risk for metastasis to regional lymph nodes. Tumors at sites of chronic inflammation, ulcers, scars, or previous radiation sites have higher rates of metastasis (Habif, 2004).

Malignant Melanoma

- Superficial spreading melanoma (SSM) is frequent on the back of both sexes and the legs of women. Hallmark presentation is often a haphazard combination of many colors including brown, black, and red. SSM begins in a nonspecific manner but changes shape by radial spread, can be flat

FIGURE 7-13   Superficial Spreading Melanoma

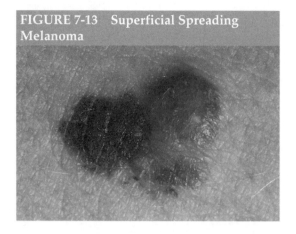

FIGURE 7-15   Lentigo Maligna Melanoma

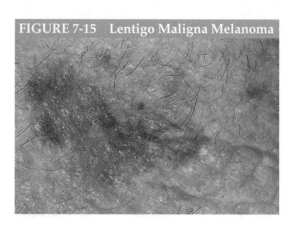

FIGURE 7-14   Nodular Melanoma

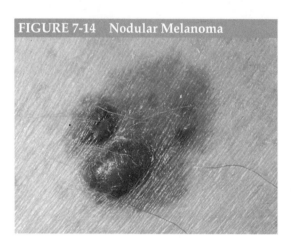

FIGURE 7-16   Acral Lentiginous Melanoma

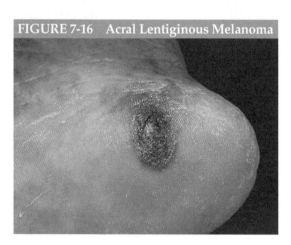

or elevated, any shape or size, irregular, and asymmetric (Figure 7-13). Of all melanomas, 70% are SSM.

- Nodular melanoma (NM) is more common in males than females. It can occur anywhere but is seen mostly on the trunk and legs; coloring can be dark brown, red brown, red black, or amelanotic (flesh color). NM can be dome shaped, polypoid, or pedunculated, and it can ulcerate and bleed. NM represents about 15–20% of melanomas (Figure 7-14).

- Lentigo maligna melanoma (LMM) is seen on the face, neck, arms, and legs, and represents

about 4–15% of melanomas. LMM is slow growing, starting as a lentigo maligna: a brown-black, irregular macule (Figure 7-15). Bluish black nodular tumors may develop within the macules after 10–15 years.

- Acral lentiginous melanoma (ALM) has clinical presentation similar to LMM. These occur on palms, soles (Figure 7-16), terminal phalanges, and mucus membranes. ALM is the most frequent form of melanoma in African-Americans, Asians, and Hispanics, and represents about 2–8% of melanomas in whites (Habif, 2004).

Differential Diagnoses

Nonmelanoma Skin Tumors

- Eczema
- Psoriasis
- Extramammary Paget's disease
- Wart
- Hypertrophic actinic keratosis
- Seborrheic keratosis
- Actinic keratosis

Malignant Melanoma

- Benign nevus
- Dermatofibroma
- Seborrheic keratosis
- Angioma

Essential Diagnostic and Laboratory Tests

- Any suspicious lesion should be evaluated, a biopsy performed, and a treatment plan established by a dermatology provider.
- After a melanoma's thickness is measured histologically, the need for further testing is determined. This often includes CXR, LDH, AST, ALT, and alkaline phosphatase.

Management Plan

The goals for treatment of skin cancer are to remove all of the cancer, preserve healthy skin tissue, minimize scarring after surgery, monitor for recurrence, and reduce the chance of recurrence with sun protection.

- Dermatology referral
- Options to treat BCCs include electrodesiccation and curettage, excision, and Mohs micrographic surgery. Radiation may be useful for the elderly patient who cannot tolerate a minor surgical procedure. Imiquimod 5% cream (Aldara), an immune response modifier, may be used on superficial BCCs.

- Actinic keratosis are treated with cryotherapy (liquid nitrogen), topical 5-fluorouracil, or imiquimod.
- SCC requires complete excision and occasionally radiation therapy and/or chemotherapy.
- Malignant melanoma requires complete excision, staging, and sentinel lymph node biopsy may be done for tumors thicker than 1.0 mm. Depending on the stage of disease, the patient is referred to oncology for consideration of chemotherapy, chemoimmunotherapy, vaccine therapy, and/or radiation.

Patient, Family, and Staff Education

- Understanding the different types of skin cancer and explaining the prognostic features of each is helpful. BCCs rarely metastasize and have a high cure rate with complete excision. Persons with multiple SCCs are at risk for metastasis and need monitoring for new lesions, recurrence, and lymphadenopathy at least every 6 months.
- Prognosis for malignant melanoma is dependent on the thickness and characteristics of the lesion, lymph node involvement, and presence of metastasis.
- Patients, family, and staff should perform meticulous skin assessment and alert the nurse practitioner and/or physician to suspicious lesions.

DRUG REACTIONS

Definition

Any dermatologic condition that begins within 2 weeks of starting a new drug should be considered for a drug reaction. Rashes are the most common adverse reaction to drugs, and they can mimic any dermatoses. The most common types of rashes are exanthematous or maculopapular eruptions, urticaria, and fixed drug eruption. Drug eruptions are caused by immunologic or nonimmunologic mechanisms and are provoked by administration of the drug. Some proposed immunologic mechanisms include immune complex dependency, T-cell mediation, and mast cell deregulation (Habif, 2004). Nonimmunologic mechanisms include accumulation of the drug, overdose, photosensitivity, irritancy, toxicity, idiosyncrasy, or other unknown processes (Fitzpatrick et al., 2001; Habif, 2004).

Epidemiology

Adverse cutaneous drug reactions are common in hospitalized and ambulatory patients. It has been reported that the most common adverse event for hospitalized patients is a complication of drug therapy (Fitzpatrick et al., 2001).

Adverse drug reactions are common in the elderly as they generally take more drugs and can be more difficult to assess secondary to a variable or atypical clinical presentation. The elderly are more likely to elicit an autoimmune disorder as an adverse reaction to medication such as pemphigus, bullous pemphigoid, or a lupus erythematosus-like rash. These are reversible when the drug is discontinued; however, resolution of an eruption in the older patient can be quite prolonged (Lyon & Fitzpatrick, 1993).

Common Presenting Signs and Symptoms

- Exanthems or maculopapular eruptions are the most common of cutaneous drug eruptions (Figure 7-17). Bright red macules and papules coalesce into a symmetric, widely distributed eruption often sparing the face and mucus membranes; palms and soles may be involved. It is generally pruritic. Usually starts 7–10 days after starting the drug. Scaling or desquamation may occur with healing. Life threatening, generalized exfoliative dermatitis may develop if drug is not discontinued. The reaction may take

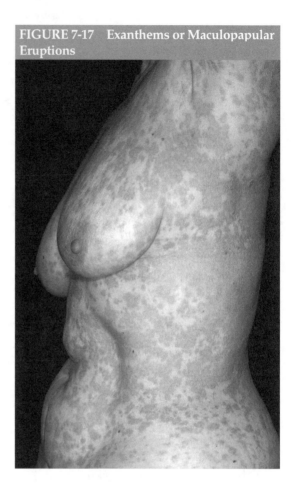

FIGURE 7-17   Exanthems or Maculopapular Eruptions

longer than 2 weeks to clear after the drug is stopped. This is the classic ampicillin and amoxicillin drug rash (Habif, 2004). Other culprits include other antibiotics, captopril, carbamazepine, chlorpromazine, gold, naproxen, phenytoin, and piroxicam (Litt, 2001).

- Urticaria, or hives, is a vascular reaction of the skin with itchy, red, edematous papules or plaques (wheals), usually symmetric and generalized (Figure 7-18). There is no scaling or vesicle formation. Aspirin, penicillin, and blood products are the most frequent causes of urticaria; however, any drug can induce the reaction. Hives fade in about 24 hours but recur in another body location.

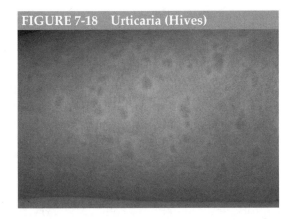

FIGURE 7-18   Urticaria (Hives)

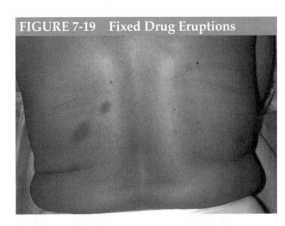

FIGURE 7-19   Fixed Drug Eruptions

Angioedema is urticarial swelling of subcutaneous tissue and the dermis and can include the mucus membranes. This may be a life-threatening reaction (Habif, 2004). Common causes of drug-induced urticaria include penicillin, captopril, quinine, rifampin, sulfonamides, NSAIDs, and vancomycin (Litt, 2001).

- Fixed drug eruptions (Figure 7-19) recur at the same cutaneous site each time the drug is ingested. The single or multiple, round, well-demarcated, red, dusky plaques are preceded or accompanied by itching and burning. The area may blister, erode, desquamate or crust, and then be brownish while healing. Sometimes the itching and burning presents by itself in an old patch; the glans penis is a common site. Length of time from reexposure to drug and onset of symptoms can be 30 minutes to about 8 hours (Habif, 2004). Some offending drugs include aspirin, barbiturates, sulfonamides, tetracyclines, phenytoin, and trimethoprim-sulfamethoxazole (Litt, 2001).

Differential Diagnoses

- Viral exanthema
- Lichen planus
- Psoriasis
- Cutaneous T-cell lymphoma

Essential Diagnostic and Laboratory Tests

Clinical identification of drug eruptions is mostly subjective, but estimating the probability that a given drug has a role in the adverse reaction is also possible. Below are six elements that can be used in the evaluation and management of the patient with a suspected cutaneous drug eruption (Blacker, Stern, & Wintroub, 1993).

- Previous experience—Investigate the frequency or rate of reactions to the drug in the general population. Evaluating the morphologic pattern (urticaria, maculopapular, or fixed eruption) can help determine the likelihood that a given drug is responsible.
- Alternative etiology—Is the eruption an unrelated dermatologic disease or an exacerbation of a preexisting disease? Skin biopsy may be necessary to categorize an eruption or identify other possible diseases.
- Timing of events—Most adverse drug reactions occur 1–2 weeks after starting the drug. Make a list of when the reaction started, all drugs, doses, duration, and any interruptions in ingestion.
- Drug levels—Some reactions are dose dependent or related to cumulative toxicity. Reactions to gold occur more in higher

doses. Drug levels may be helpful for co-matose or noncommunicative patients.

- Dechallenge—Most reactions improve with discontinuation of the offending drug. If the reaction improves without discontinua-tion, or if a patient fails to improve after dechallenge and therapy, the reaction may not be drug related. However, in the elderly the resolution may be prolonged.

- Rechallenge—This is the most definitive way to affirm a drug as the offending agent, but it is also the most difficult because of patient safety. A reaction that fails to recur with rechallenge of a drug is unlikely to be the cause.

Management Plan

The goals of management include identifying the offending agent and clearing the eruption with a focus on monitoring for escalating symptoms of urticaria, angioedema, or anaphylaxis.

Nonpharmacologic

Order the application of local moisturizing skin care when indicated. Patience is required waiting for improvement once the offending agent is discontinued.

Pharmacologic

Symptomatic relief is provided with antihista-mines, such as diphenhydramine or hydrox-yzine, and topical group V steroids (Table 7-2).

Patient, Family, and Staff Education

The importance of reporting any new erup-tion on the skin should be emphasized to fam-ily and staff.

Physician Consultation

Dermatology consult is warranted when the diagnosis is uncertain, the eruption has not responded to stopping a suspected agent, or

there is an atypical presentation such as dif-fuse purpura, bulla, desquamation, or sus-pected vasculitis.

ECZEMATOUS DISEASES

Definition

Eczema is a disease of the dermis and the epidermis. The etiology is thought to involve a cascade of events connected to inappropri-ate activation of T cells, histamine IgE re-ceptors, and Langerhans' cells (Dewberry & Norman, 2004). Dermatitis means inflamma-tion of skin but is not always synonymous with the eczematous process. Eczematous disorders are characterized by erythema, vesicles, and scale, as well as changes that occur secondary to scratching, irritation, and infection (Figure 7-20).

In acute eczematous inflammation the epi-dermis forms vesicles with intense redness; subacute eczema has redness, scaling, fissur-ing, and a scalded appearance; chronic eczema has excoriations and thickened skin with ac-centuated skin lines called *lichenification* (Habif, 2004). The geriatric population is particularly vulnerable to chronic forms of eczematous in-flammation because of the natural functional decline of the skin and comorbidities such as dementia, diabetes, and peripheral vascular disease. The sensation of pruritus leads to esca-lation of the condition because of the automatic response to scratch and rub. All of this leads to a decreased ability to combat and resolve the condition (Dewberry, Norman, & Bock, 2004).

Epidemiology

Eczematous conditions are among the most frequent dermatologic complaints (Moschella, 2001), and eczematous inflammation is the most common inflammatory skin disease (Habif, 2004). Not surprisingly, a frequent chief com-

TABLE 7-2   Topical Steroid Potency Ranking

GROUP	BRAND NAME	%	GENERIC NAME
I	Temovate cream	0.05	Clobetasol propionate
	Temovate ointment		
	Temovate gel		
	Ultravate cream	0.05	Halobetasol propionate
	Ultravate ointment		
	Diprolene lotion	0.05	Augmented betamethasone dipropionate
	Diprolene ointment		
	Diprolene gel		
	Psorcon ointment	0.05	Diflorasone diacetate
II	Cyclocort ointment	0.1	Amcinonide
	Diprolene AF cream	0.05	Augmented betamethasone dipropionate
	Diprosone ointment		Betamethasone dipropionate
	Elocon ointment	0.1	Mometasone furoate
	Halog cream	0.1	Halcinonide
	Halog ointment		
	Halog E cream		
	Halog solution		
	Lidex cream	0.05	Fluocinonide
	Lidex ointment		
	Lidex solution		
	Psorcon E cream	0.05	Diflorasone diacetate
	Psorcon E ointment		
	Topicort cream	0.25	Desoximetasone
	Topicort gel	0.05	
	Topicort ointment	0.25	
III	Aristocort A cream	0.5	Triamcinolone acetonide
	Cyclocort lotion	0.1	Amcinonide
	Cyclocort cream		
	Diprosone cream	0.05	Betamethasone dipropionate
	Diprosone lotion		
IV	Aristocort A ointment	0.1	Triamcinolone acetonide
	Elocon cream	0.1	Mometasone furoate
	Elocon lotion		
	Kenalog ointment	0.1	Triamcinolone acetonide
	Westcort ointment	0.2	Hydrocortisone
V	DesOwen ointment	0.05	Desonide
	Kenalog cream	0.1	Triamcinolone acetonide
	Kenalog lotion		
	Synalar cream	0.025	Fluocinolone acetonide
	Westcort cream	0.2	Hydrocortisone valerate
VI	Aclovate cream	0.05	Alclometasone dipropionate
	Aclovate ointment		
	Derma-Smoothe	0.01	Fluocinolone acetonide
	DesOwen cream	0.05	Desonide
	DesOwen lotion		
	Synalar solution	0.01	Fluocinolone acetonide
VII	Hytone cream	2.5	Hydrocortisone
	Hytone lotion		
	Hytone ointment		

plaint of the geriatric patient population is that of a pruritic rash or eruption representing an eczematous inflammation (Dewberry et al., 2004).

The prevalence of eczema in the private insurance population is about 2.4% as compared to about 2.6–4.1% of the Medicaid population.

Atopic eczema occurs in about 7–17% of the pediatric population, and of those individuals about 60% have persistent atopic eczema as adults (Ellis et al., 2002).

There are numerous clinical syndromes of eczema. The following list is not inclusive but

FIGURE 7-20   Eczematous Disease

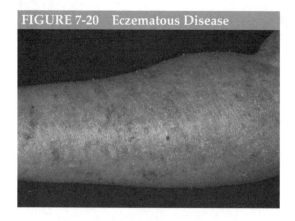

FIGURE 7-21   Asteatotic Eczema

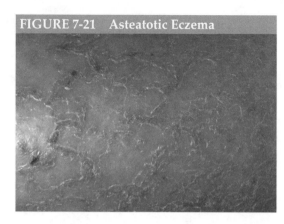

is representative of common clinical scenarios in the skilled nursing facility:

- Atopic eczema
- Asteatotic eczema (Figure 7-21)
- Nummular eczema (Figure 7-22)
- Lichen simplex chronicus (Figure 7-23)
- Contact dermatitis (Figure 7-24)
- Seborrheic dermatitis

FIGURE 7-22   Nummular Eczema

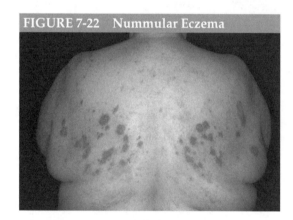

Common Presenting Signs and Symptoms

Atopic Eczema

- Diagnostic features—Pruritus, flexural involvement, cataracts, cheilitis, recurrent conjunctivitis, facial erythema, hand dermatitis, nipple dermatitis, orbital darkening, palmar hyperlinearity, wool intolerance, and xerosis (Habif, 2004)
- Itching is the primary symptom. Atopic and dry skin is sensitive, easily irritated, and itchy. Itching is what provides the basis for the development of the eczematous rash. It is called "the itch that rashes." Once the itch-scratch cycle is established there is no conscious control of scratching (Habif, 2004).
- Acute inflammation is characterized by erythematous papules and erythema; subacute

eczema has erythematous, excoriated, and scaling papules; chronic inflammation is thickened with accentuated skin markings (lichenification) and fibrotic papules.

- Involved areas include hands, flexor surfaces, eyelids, anogenital regions, and anywhere the hands can reach to scratch.
- Triggering factors include temperature change and sweating; decreased humidity; excessive washing; contact with irritating substances such as cosmetics, wool, cleaning chemicals or detergents; aeroallergens such as dust mites or pollen; *Staphylococcus aureus* overgrowth; food; or emotional stress (Habif, 2004).

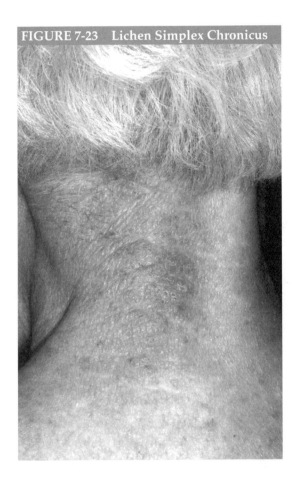

FIGURE 7-23   Lichen Simplex Chronicus

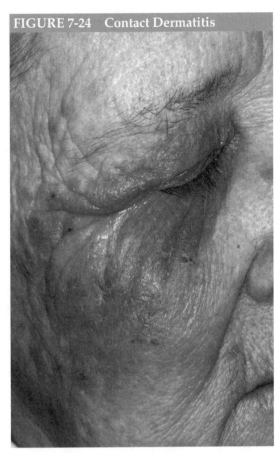

FIGURE 7-24   Contact Dermatitis

Asteatotic Eczema

- Excessively dry skin, especially in winter months and in the elderly. Most common on the anterolateral aspects of the lower legs but can occur in any location. Papules or plaque are usually the primary lesions.

- Red plaque, scaly accentuation of skin lines (xerosis), long and irregular fissuring, cracked porcelain appearance (eczema craquele)

- Seen in patients with atopic eczema, chronic renal or liver failure, myxedema, malabsorption, and in patients on diuretics (Dewberry et al., 2004)

Nummular Eczema

- Occurs mostly in middle aged and elderly

- Primary lesions are coin-shaped red plaques ranging in size from 1–5 cm, pruritic, and with thin scale that is sparse.

- Involved areas include the dorsum of the hands, extensor aspect of the forearms, and lower legs, flanks, and hips (Habif, 2004).

Lichen Simplex Chronicus

- Usually affects individuals with an obsessive component to their personality. Reasons for psychogenic disorders in the elderly are numerous: chronic disease, socioeconomics, anxiety, depression, and dementia (Moschella, 2001).

- Well-circumscribed eczematous eruption that is usually localized and created by habitual scratching. The condition is chronic.
- Primary lesion is usually a red papule that coalesces to form a red, scaly, thick plaque with lichenification.
- Moist scale, serum, crusts, and pustules are signs of infection.
- Most commonly affected areas are the outer portion of lower legs, scrotum, vulva, anal area, pubis, wrists and ankles, upper eyelids, back and side of neck, orifice of ear, extensor forearm near elbow, fold behind the ear, and scalp (pickers nodules) (Habif, 2004).

Contact Dermatitis

- Contact dermatitis is eczematous inflammation caused by exposure to substances that act as irritants or allergens. It can cause acute, subacute, or chronic eczematous inflammation.
- Everyone is at risk for irritant contact dermatitis; it is a nonimmunologic response, a physical and chemical alteration of the epidermis. Usually gradual onset. A few too many exposures to organic solvents or soaps are required for eruption of rash; borders of rash are usually indistinct.
- Allergic contact dermatitis is genetically predisposed; it is a delayed hypersensitivity response; one or several exposures are needed to cause sensitization. Once sensitized the onset may be rapid; eruption may correspond directly to contact.
- Patients with leg ulcers, venous insufficiency, and lower leg edema are more prone to contact dermatitis of the lower legs because of an altered sensitivity to chemicals such as lanolin, fragrance, wool, alcohols, parabens, neomycin, and bacitracin (Habif, 2004).

Differential Diagnoses

- Atopic dermatitis
- Asteatotic eczema
- Scabies
- Seborrheic dermatitis
- Tinea corporis
- Folliculitis
- Drug reaction
- Lichen simplex chronicus
- Neoplastic lesions
- Nummular eczema
- Dyshidrotic eczema
- Herpes zoster
- Neurodermatitis
- Stasis dermatitis
- Impetiginous dermatitis
- Contact dermatitis
- Psoriasis
- Mycosis fungoides

Essential Diagnostic and Laboratory Tests

- Personal, family, and clinical history
- The diagnosis is clinical. Recognizing a rash as eczematous and describing the quality and characteristics of the components of eczematous inflammation (erythema, scale, and vesicles) is fundamental to diagnosis. It is important to identify the primary lesion (Habif, 2004).
- Patch testing for allergic contact dermatitis and skin biopsy to rule out cutaneous malignancy is available with dermatology referral.

Management Plan

Treating eczematous conditions is easier than diagnosing them. Most of the diseases are treated the same. It is the stage of the condition that determines what is necessary. The goal of treatment is acute symptom relief, management of chronic eczema without skin atrophy or adrenal suppression, and long-term maintenance of skin integrity.

Nonpharmacologic
- Emollient creams and lotions restore water and lipids to the epidermis. Urea and lactic acid are especially effective but can cause irritation in some individuals. Phenol and menthol help control pruritus. Lubrication of the eczematous skin is essential. Soaking skin in the bath or shower and then sealing in the moisture immediately afterward while the skin is still wet is a good technique. Some examples include the following:
  - AmLactin, Lac-Hydrin, LactiCare, or Lactinol lotion (lactic acid)
  - Aquaphor, DML Forte, Eucerin, Moisturel (petroleum)
  - Cetaphil lotion or cream, Lubriderm lotion
- Superfatted soaps or cleansers are mild and nonirritating. These include the following:
  - Alpha-Keri
  - Basis
  - Cetaphil
  - Dove
  - Neutrogena dry skin formula
  - Oilatum
  - Purpose
- Antipruritic creams and lotions can be especially useful in patients who cannot receive oral steroids or antihistamines. Ingredients include menthol, camphor, pramoxine, and hydrocortisone. Some examples include the following:
  - Eucerin itch relief
  - Neutrogena anti-itch moisturizer
  - Sarna or Sarna with pramoxine

  - Aveeno anti-itch with menthol or 1% hydrocortisone
- Tar and tar combination lotions and shampoos can also provide relief for chronically eczematous and itchy skin. A few are listed here:
  - Denorex gel or lotion
  - Neutrogena T/gel or T/gel extra strength
  - Pentrax tar
  - Tegrin medicated cream or lotion
- Encourage adequate water intake along with review of patient's medications, which may frequently include a diuretic.
- Review the diet for adequate amounts of animal and fish oils and vitamin E.
- Environment humidity can be supplemented with ambient humidifiers, especially important in winter months (Dewberry et al., 2004).
- Avoidance of allergic contact substances, protection, and reduced exposure to irritants.

Pharmacologic
Acute Eczematous Inflammation
- Cool wet compresses with or without Burrow's powder macerates the vesicles and promotes evaporative cooling, vasoconstriction, and decreased serum production. Wet compresses should be changed after 30 minutes and treatment should be done for at least 1 hour, 2–3 times a day.
- Oral corticosteroids such as prednisone are useful for widespread inflammation and may be started at 30–60 mg a day for at least 3 to 5 days. It may take 3 weeks of slow taper for adequate control. Steroid dose packs provide treatment for too short a period to be effective.
- Antihistamines such as diphenhydramine, hydroxyzine, cyproheptadine, and clemastine may be useful for pruritus; patients

need to be monitored for adverse effects such as dizziness, confusion, and urinary retention. Providing itch relief helps with patient comfort and prevents worsening of the inflammation.

- High-potency corticosteroid (group II or III) ointments may be of benefit if prednisone cannot be used and/or if the surface area of involvement is small. See Table 7-2 for grouping of topical steroids.

- Oral antibiotics may hasten clearing if superficial secondary staphylococcus infection is suspected. Cephalexin and dicloxacillin are usually effective, but the incidence of nosocomial or community acquired methicillin-resistant *Staphylococcus aureus* (MRSA) is on the rise.

Subacute and Chronic Eczema

- Wet dressings must be discontinued when the acute inflammation is subdued because excess drying may cause cracking and fissures leading to infection.

- Topical corticosteroids are the treatment of choice. The anti-inflammatory action of the topical steroids occurs in the upper dermis. They are grouped based on strength, group I being the strongest, and VII the weakest (Table 7-2). The vehicle or base in which the active ingredient is dispersed determines the rate of absorption in the skin.

  - Creams are generally a mix of oils and water, versatile and cosmetically acceptable, slightly drying, and useful for the intertriginous areas.

  - Ointments are mostly greases, provide more lubrication and greater penetration of medicine than creams; are more potent and too occlusive for the intertriginous areas.

  - Gels are greaseless; some have alcohol and usually a clear base useful for exudative inflammation.

  - Solutions and lotions have water and alcohol and are most useful for the scalp.

- Suggested initial use of groups I–II topical steroids—Severe hand eczema, severe poison ivy, lichen simplex chronicus, chapped feet, severe nummular eczema, severe atopic dermatitis

- Suggested initial use of group III–IV topical steroids—Atopic dermatitis, nummular eczema, asteatotic eczema, stasis dermatitis, seborrheic dermatitis, postscabetic eczema, severe intertrigo, severe anal inflammation

- Suggested initial use of group VI–VII topical steroids—Eyelid and face dermatitis, mild anal inflammation, mild intertrigo. Eyelid use should be restricted to 2–3 weeks.

- Group I steroids can be used once or twice a day for 2 weeks followed by one week rest. No more than 50 grams of cream or ointment should be used in one week. This pulse dosing can continue until inflammation is controlled. Intermittent dosing with the group I or a weaker steroid can be used once or twice a week for maintenance.

- Groups II–V steroid use should be limited to about 3 weeks followed by a rest. Weaker steroids should be used for maintenance.

- Groups VI–VII can be used on gentle areas such as the face, groin, axilla, and under the breasts. Reevaluation is needed if the condition does not respond within 28 days.

- Potential adverse effects of topical steroid use include the following:

  - Steroid acne

  - Skin atrophy with telangiectasia, purpura, striae

  - Ocular hypertension, glaucoma, cataracts

  - Allergic contact dermatitis

  - Systemic absorption

  - Burning, itching, irritation, dryness caused by vehicle

○ Skin blanching

○ Hypopigmentation

- The nonsteroidal topical calcineurin inhibitors tacrolimus ointment (Protopic) and pimecrolimus cream (Elidel) are used for mild to moderate eczema, frequently face and neck eczema, or when topical corticosteroids have failed.

- Antihistamine use is generally effective to reduce pruritus, which will greatly reduce the production of new lesions or progression to chronic lesions secondary to scratching (Habif, 2004).

Patient, Family, and Staff Education

- Explain the need for meticulous care of skin and adherence to specified treatments for maintenance of good skin condition. The skin of the geriatric patient has decreased sebaceous (oil) production and stores a smaller amount of water.

- The patients with dementia or confusion have difficult management issues surrounding picking, scratching, and rubbing at the skin.

- Measures to be sure that the patient sleeps well at night decrease nighttime itching and scratching.

- Explain the difficulty in finding an exact cause for eczema.

Physician Consultation

- Any eczematous inflammation that does not respond to first-line therapy within 2–3 weeks in the skilled nursing facility should be referred to a dermatology specialist.

- Where feasible and available, teledermatology consultations offer minimal disruption to the functionally challenged nursing home patient.

▓ SUPERFICIAL FUNGAL INFECTIONS

Definition

Fungal infections are superficial mycoses that primarily affect the top layer of skin (stratum corneum or keratin layer), the hair, and the nails (Habif, 2004). The dermatophytes include a group of fungi (ringworm) that can infect and survive only on dead keratin. They cannot thrive on mucosal surfaces such as the mouth or vagina where keratin does not form. Dermatophytes are responsible for most skin, nail, and hair fungal infections. The yeastlike fungus *Candida albicans* and a few other *Candida* species live within the normal flora of the mouth, vagina, and gastrointestinal tract. Any depression of cell-mediated immunity may allow the yeast to become pathogenic.

Epidemiology

Infections caused by yeasts, dermatophytes, and nondermatophyte molds are one of the most prevalent skin conditions in the elderly (Loo, 2004). Although many species of dermatophytes have been identified and exist in nature, only a small number are responsible for development of disease in humans. The three genera responsible for dermatophyte infections in humans are *Trichophyton*, *Microsporum*, and *Epidermophyton*. Of these, *Trichophyton* species are responsible for most dermatophyte infections in the elderly (Glick, Zaiac, Rebell, & Zaias, 2001). Tinea infections are classified by body regions and produce a variety of disease patterns that vary with location and the species. The epidemiology of dermatophyte infections is dependent on many host and geographic factors, as well as the virulence of the infecting organism (Martin & Kobayashi, 1993). In the skilled nursing facility patient with immune suppression, dermatophyte infections are likely to be severe and resistant to treatment (Glick et al., 2001).

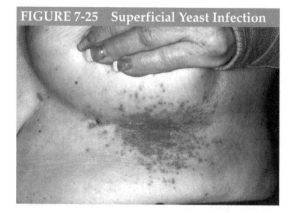

FIGURE 7-25   Superficial Yeast Infection

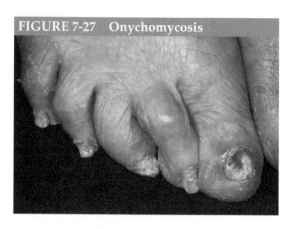

FIGURE 7-27   Onychomycosis

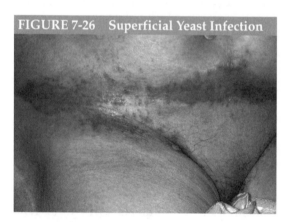

FIGURE 7-26   Superficial Yeast Infection

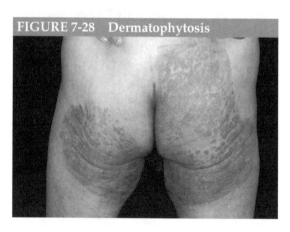

FIGURE 7-28   Dermatophytosis

C. albicans is a normal inhabitant of the intestinal flora but not a natural part of the normal skin flora. The organism opportunistically colonizes on skin that has become environmentally susceptible with conditions such as increased heat, moisture, occlusion, and compression of previously inflamed skin. Intertriginous skin folds under the breasts, between abdominal folds, in the axilla, and in the groin and rectal area can accommodate significant amounts of moisture and provide a setting that leaves the host susceptible to superficial yeast infections (Habif, 2004). See Figures 7-25 and 7-26.

- Onychomycosis (Figure 7-27) refers to fungal infection of the nail plate and the nail bed. Most onychomycosis is caused by dermatophytes (Tinea unguium). Other infections are caused by *Candida* and nondermatophyte molds (Loo, 2004).

Common Presenting Signs and Symptoms

Dermatophytosis

Dermatophytosis includes tinea corporis (body and face), tinea cruris (groin), tinea pedis and manus (foot and hand), and tinea unguium (nails).

- Primary lesion is usually a pink and scaling papule or plaque (Figure 7-28).
- Annular (ringlike) or arciform plaque with scale may be primary or secondary lesions. The annular plaques may be grouped together (polycyclic).
- Often found with an active border or leading edge of infection that is red, raised, and scaly with central clearing.
- Vesicles may appear at the active border with intense inflammation.
- Pruritus may be present.
- Tinea pedis can present as one of several variants: maceration, fissuring, and scaling in the web spaces; superficial white scales in a moccasin-type distribution with arciform pattern of scale; or small vesicles or vesicopustules near the instep (Martin & Kobayashi, 1993).
- Hands may be involved with "one hand, two feet" presentation.
- Tinea cruris (Figure 7-29) involves the proximal medial thighs and the crural (inguinal) folds. Primary lesion is red, pink or brownish, erythematous and/or macerated with fissures in the crural folds; usually with a scaling, annular, and well-demarcated border that can extend to the perianal region and buttocks.

- Onychomycotic nails are most commonly yellow and thick with hyperkeratosis under the nail, and separation of the nail from the nail bed (onycholysis) that is distal and/or lateral. The nail plate may look white and chalky on the dorsal surface, or there may be white discoloration of the proximal nail fold (Loo, 2004).
- *Candida* onychomycosis is seen in patients with chronic mucocutaneous candidiasis. The nail plate may be yellow, have dark brown streaks at the distal end growing proximally, and/or onycholysis (Habif, 2004).

Candida intertrigo

- Pustules on an erythematous base are the primary lesion, but they become eroded and confluent under opposing skin folds and form red papules with rings or fringe of scale.
- There may be red, shiny, moist, and well-demarcated plaque with fissuring in the skin creases, a wavy edge, and fringe of scale; satellite papules or pustules may be present outside of the intertriginous region (Habif, 2004).
- Angular cheilitis or perleche (Figure 7-30) occurs when saliva collects at the corners of the mouth. This environment is conducive for *Candida* to grow causing erythema, maceration, fissuring, and crusting (Loo, 2004).

FIGURE 7-29   Tinea cruris

FIGURE 7-30   Angular Cheilitis or Perleche

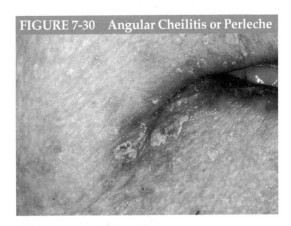

Differential Diagnoses

- Tinea corporis—Pityriasis rosea, psoriasis, subacute lupus erythematosus, nummular eczema. Examination of the feet, groin, scalp and hands may reveal the primary source of fungal infection.

- Tinea cruris—Erythrasma, *Candida* intertrigo, inverse psoriasis, and seborrheic dermatitis.

- Interdigital tinea pedis—Erythrasma or gram-negative infection.

- Tinea unguium—Psoriasis, lichen planus, pincer nail deformity, onychogryphosis, and crusted scabies. *Only about half of all patients with nail dystrophy have onychomycosis* (Loo, 2004).

- *Candida* intertrigo—Contact or irritant dermatitis, inverse psoriasis, tinea corporis or cruris, erythrasma, and frictional intertrigo.

Essential Diagnostic and Laboratory Tests

- Potassium hydroxide (KOH) wet mount preparation is the most important test for the diagnosis of dermatophyte infection when branching hyphae are directly visualized under the microscope. Tools for this test are not commonly found in the long-term care setting.

- Culture media for tinea include Dermatophyte Test Medium (DTM) and Sabouraud's agar. Sabouraud's agar allows for growth of most fungi including nondermatophytes, which is useful for nail infections. Acu-Nickerson is a medium used for isolation of *Candida* species.

  ○ A sterile cotton swab moistened with sterile water can be vigorously rubbed over the lesion and then over the surface of the agar.

  ○ Subungual debris should be collected from under the distal edge of the nail. The nail should be trimmed if possible

and the debris can be scraped into the medium with a curet or a #15 scalpel blade (Habif, 2004).

- Biopsy of skin tissue, nail clipping, or subungual debris for examination by routine histology and periodic acid-Schiff (PAS) staining may be necessary for accurate diagnosis.

Management Plan

The goal for management of superficial cutaneous fungal infections is symptom relief and complete therapy to prevent recurrence, secondary bacterial infection, or a rare fungemia. The goal for management of tinea unguium is to relieve pain symptoms and improve nail appearance.

Nonpharmacologic

Complete examination of the hands, feet, groin, and scalp in patients with tinea corporis may reveal a chronic fungal infection that is a primary source of infection. Tinea cruris is most often an autoinoculation from tinea manuum, tinea pedis, or tinea unguium (Loo, 2004).

Pharmacologic

- For tinea in any location, first-line therapy is any of the Azole topical creams (clotrimazole, econazole, ketoconazole) or terbinafine cream, twice a day for 2–4 weeks. Recommend using any topical cream for one week beyond clearing of the rash.

- Tinea pedis with interdigital maceration or vesicles requires compresses of Burow's solution to the area for 20–30 minutes twice or three times a day until the area is dry. Econazole nitrate and ciclopirox olamine creams have activity against bacteria that cause interdigital maceration and should be applied twice a day for 2–4 weeks.

- Recalcitrant tinea pedis or manus can be treated with terbinafine 250 mg every day for 2 weeks. Liver cytochrome P-450 enzymes metabolize terbinafine.

- Terbinafine inhibits the cytochrome P-450 enzyme CYP2D6. CYP2D6 is involved in the metabolism of antidepressants and psychotropic drugs.

- Terbinafine may decrease beta-blocker clearance, decrease cyclosporine levels, or increase theophylline levels.

- Cimetidine decreases terbinafine clearance, and rifampin may increase terbinafine clearance.

- Terbinafine is contraindicated in patients with chronic liver disease or active hepatitis. Adverse effects may include taste disturbance, dyspepsia, diarrhea, abdominal pain, and neutropenia. The manufacturer recommends obtaining baseline transaminases before treatment (Loo, 2004).

- Terbinafine is *not* active against *Candida* species.

- Feet should be dried completely after washing and antifungal powder or spray can be used in shoes once or twice a week. Application of antifungal cream to feet and toes once or twice a week, long term, can be effective for preventing reinfection.

- Extensive tinea corporis can be treated with terbinafine 250 mg every day for 2–6 weeks.

- *Candida* intertrigo requires Burow's solution, water or saline compresses, 20–30 minutes, 2 or 3 times a day for drying the skin. Any of the topical Azoles, miconazole nitrate (Monistat Derm lotion), or ciclopirox olamine (Loprox) should be applied twice a day for 2–4 weeks.

- *Candida* intertrigo is rarely cured but recurrent maceration can be prevented with drying the skin well and daily application of nystatin powder or miconazole (Zea-Sorb AF) powder.

- Angular cheilitis should be treated for inflammation, bacteria, and yeast. This includes iodoquinol/hydrocortisone 1% (Vytone) cream twice a day, any antifungal cream with a group V steroid twice a day, or mupirocin 2% (Bactroban) ointment or cream 3–4 times a day.

- Tinea unguium is treated with oral or topical medication. Not all patients need to be treated if they are asymptomatic; however, in diabetic patients onychomycosis can lead to bacterial infections, foot ulcers, and gangrene. In addition, patients with immunosuppression or immunodeficiency are likely to fail therapy. Terbinafine is the drug of choice for dermatophyte infection, 250 mg/day for 6 weeks for fingernails and 12 weeks for toenails. During a 12-week course a complete blood count (CBC) and aspartate transaminase (AST) should be checked at the 6-week interval.

Patient, Family, and Staff Education

- Explain the need for precise diagnosis for determining appropriate treatment.

- Review the risks and benefits of topical and oral therapy; topical therapy may need to be long term and intermittent to prevent recurrence of symptomatic rash, and many older patients on multiple medications may not be appropriate for oral therapy.

- Tinea pedis and tinea unguium are typically chronic, and symptom relief is an achievable goal.

- Total body skin evaluation is necessary to monitor for improvement, worsening, or recurrence. Chronic tinea pedis may contribute to recurrent tinea cruris, so long-term management of the foot fungus is a priority.

Physician Consultation

- Dermatology referral may be necessary for uncertain diagnosis if culture, scraping, or biopsy cannot be obtained in the nursing facility.

- Any persistent rash that does not respond to treatment should be referred to dermatology.

PSORIASIS AND SEBORRHEIC DERMATITIS

Papulosquamous diseases have similar primary lesion characteristics: scaly papules and plaques. Psoriasis and seborrheic dermatitis are among several conditions in this category and are quite common in the geriatric population. Pruritus will also be included in this section as it is most often associated with dry, rough, and scaly skin.

Definition

Psoriasis is a chronic and relapsing disease with a variable array of clinical features. Psoriasis is an immune system disorder driven by overactive white blood cells called T cells. T cells abnormally trigger other immune responses that lead to inflammation and rapid turnover of skin cells creating raised patches on the outer surface of the skin. The lesions are classified as erythrosquamous. The erythema is caused by increased vasculature, and there is increased scale formation in the epidermis (Christophers & Sterry, 1993). Drugs that can precipitate or exacerbate psoriasis include lithium, beta-blocking agents, nonsteroidal anti-inflammatory drugs, ACE inhibitors, and systemic steroids (Yaar & Gilchrest, 2003). Clinical presentations of psoriasis are numerous. This section will include chronic plaque (Figures 7-31 and 7-32), scalp psoriasis (Figure 7-33), and psoriasis inversus (flexural surface). See Figure 7-34 for intertriginous psoriasis.

Seborrheic dermatitis is a common, chronic, inflammatory condition of the scalp, face and trunk (Figure 7-35). The yeast *Pityrosporum ovale* may be a causative factor (Habif, 2004). The skin looks oily with an increase in sebum production (seborrhea) of the scalp and the follicle-rich areas of the face and trunk (Plewig, 1993). The papules and plaques are pink and edematous with yellowish brown scale and crust (Figure 7-36).

Pruritus is the sensation that leads to a desire to scratch. The scratching response is a

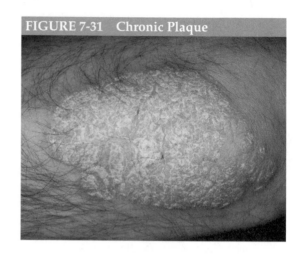

FIGURE 7-31   Chronic Plaque

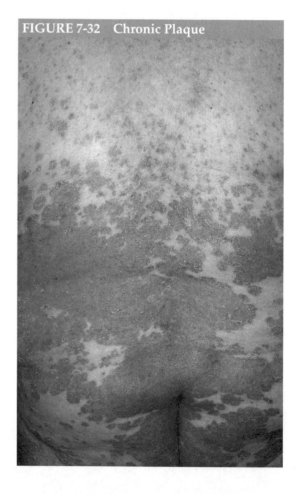

FIGURE 7-32   Chronic Plaque

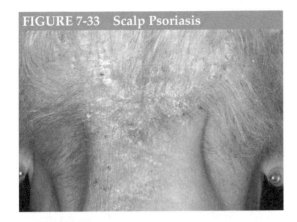

FIGURE 7-33   Scalp Psoriasis

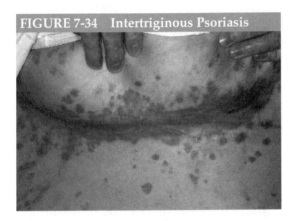

FIGURE 7-34   Intertriginous Psoriasis

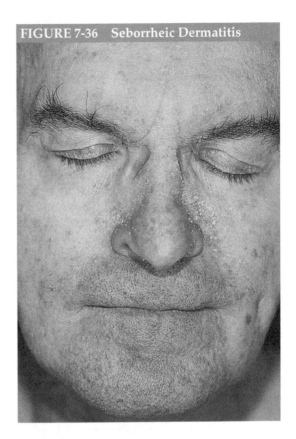

FIGURE 7-36   Seborrheic Dermatitis

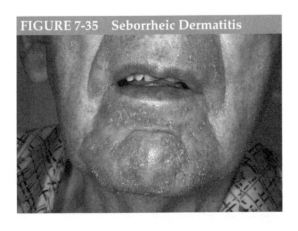

FIGURE 7-35   Seborrheic Dermatitis

spinal reflex. Excessive drying of the skin following bathing or low humidity leads to itchy skin especially in the elderly. Pruritus is the most common skin-related complaint of the elderly (Yaar & Gilchrest, 2003).

Epidemiology

Psoriasis has an unknown origin, is transmitted genetically, and affects about 1–3% of the population (Habif, 2004). With increasing age of onset there is a decrease in familial association. There are reports of psoriasis beginning from birth to 108 years. Most patients with psoriasis will present around the third decade; there is another peak of occurrence after 55 years. The elderly present with atypical eruptions; inflammatory reactions are muted with age because fewer vessels reduce the inflammatory cascade. Presentation of plaque-type psoriasis typically decreases with age, and flexural psoriasis is more common in patients over 60 years (Lyon & Fitzpatrick, 1993). Occurrence of the disease is universal, but the worldwide incidence varies considerably secondary to race, geography, and environment (Christophers & Sterry, 1993).

The cause of seborrheic dermatitis is not known, but it affects about 2–5% of the population. It occurs more often in males and has peaks of development in infancy and again in the fourth to seventh decades. Senescence may have a significant role in the natural history of this inflammatory condition, but there is also a neurophysiologic role suggested by the incidence in individuals with mental retardation and parkinsonism (Plewig, 1993). Low temperatures and humidity worsen seborrheic dermatitis.

Pruritus is the most common disorder in elderly skin particularly those over 85 years of age; about 50% of individuals over 75 have the complaint. Most pruritus stems from xerosis and is worse in winter with decreased humidity and increased indoor temperatures (Greaves, 1993). Severe pruritus that does not respond to conservative therapy should be evaluated for underlying systemic disorders that can cause this most annoying condition.

Common Presenting Signs and Symptoms

Psoriasis

- In chronic plaque psoriasis, the primary lesions are red scaling papules that coalesce to larger round or oval plaques. The scale is adherent and silvery white and bleeds when removed. Any cutaneous surface can be affected; however, the most common sites are extensor regions of elbows and knees, scalp (especially retroauricular), the lumbar area, umbilicus, and nails. Pruritus is variable.

- Psoriasis inversus involves major skin folds, the intergluteal fold being most common.

The axilla, groin, submammary folds, and the glans of the uncircumcised penis can be affected. In flexural areas the plaque is sharply demarcated, red, and smooth because the scale is macerated and dispersed.

- The scalp is a common site and may be the only area affected. A dense, tight, silvery scale that is anchored by the hair can cover the entire scalp. The psoriasis can extend down to the forehead with similar papules and plaques of the chronic plaque type.

- Factors that may provoke psoriasis include physical trauma, infections, stress, and drugs. There is systemic association of psoriasis with arthritis, inflammatory bowel disease, and clusive vascular disease (Christophers & Sterry, 1993).

Seborrheic Dermatitis

- A fine, white or yellow scale occurs on an erythematous base in seborrheic areas: scalp, scalp margins, posterior auricle, eyelid margins, eyebrows, nasolabial folds, external ear canals, and presternal region.

- Scaling can occur when a beard is grown and clear when shaved.

- Older patients who are bedridden and those with Parkinson's disease may have more extensive seborrheic dermatitis (Habif, 2004).

Pruritus

- Dry, scaling, cracked skin, or no clinical signs at all

- In most cases pruritus is attributable only to xerosis; however, there may be other causes that need to be pursued through appropriate laboratory evaluation.

Differential Diagnoses

Psoriasis

- Eczema
- Pityriasis rosea
- Seborrheic dermatitis
- Candidiasis

- Drug eruption
- Tinea
- Syphilis
- Cutaneous T-cell lymphoma
- Squamous cell carcinoma in situ
- Paget's disease

Seborrheic Dermatitis
- Psoriasis
- Tinea capitis
- Atopic dermatitis
- Impetigo
- Contact dermatitis
- Rosacea
- Pityriasis versicolor
- Pityriasis rosea

Pruritus
- Renal disease
- Biliary obstruction
- Polycythemia vera
- Lymphoma or leukemia
- Thyrotoxicosis
- Hypothyroidism
- Aquagenic pruritus
- Eczema
- Scabies
- Prebullous pemphigoid
- Pruritus of aged skin
- Psychoneurosis
- Diabetes

Essential Diagnostic and Laboratory Tests

- Clinical examination of all skin surfaces is imperative. Psoriasis and seborrheic dermatitis are diagnosed clinically. Typical psoriatic lesions are usually characteristic enough to make the diagnosis. The distribution of seborrheic dermatitis is a helpful clue. It may be difficult to distinguish seborrhea from psoriasis on the scalp. Skin biopsy may be necessary to confirm diagnosis in patients with atypical presentation.
- Workup for systemic pruritus includes the following:
  - Complete blood count
  - Thyroid, renal, and hepatic function tests including bilirubin and alkaline phosphatase
  - Fasting glucose
  - Stool for parasites if suspicion is high or the patient has eosinophilia
  - Chest X-ray

Management Plan

The primary goal of treatment is relief of pruritic symptoms without adverse effects from anticholinergic medications. In addition to managing pruritus, the goals for management of psoriasis and seborrheic dermatitis include clearing or improving skin lesions without skin atrophy or adrenal suppression from corticosteroid application, or adverse effects from systemic therapy.

Nonpharmacologic
Psoriasis and Seborrheic Dermatitis
- Control of psychologic stress factors can have a positive effect on the management of psoriasis (Habif, 2004).
- Management of skin itch and general dryness is as important in treatment of psoriasis as it is in eczema treatment. Some patients with heavy psoriatic scale find the application of Crisco helpful.
- Localized chronic plaques may respond to an occlusive dressing applied and changed every week (Habif, 2004). DuoDerm can be used with or without a group V through VII topical steroid.
- The scale of scalp psoriasis and seborrheic dermatitis needs to be thinned or removed for the topical medication to be effective.

Shampoos with tar (T-Gel) and salicylic acid (T-Sal) are most effective.

- Bakers' P & S liquid (phenol, sodium chloride, and liquid paraffin) is helpful in removing moderate scale and is well tolerated. It is applied at bedtime and washed out in the morning.

- Treatment of seborrheic dermatitis requires frequent washing of all affected areas with antiseborrheic preparations to suppress activity and then to maintain control. This includes zinc soaps (ZNP bar soap, Head & Shoulders shampoo), selenium sulfide (Selsun Blue, Head & Shoulders Intensive Treatment), tar (T-Gel, Pentrax, Denorex), salicylic acid (Neutrogena T-Sal, DHS Sal, Sebulex, P & S), and Nizoral shampoo (ketoconazole). It may be useful to alternate two or three different products for maintenance.

Pruritus

Anti-itch lotions are useful especially in patients who cannot tolerate sedating antihistamines. Sarna and Aveeno anti-itch cream are examples. These can be applied frequently day or night.

Pharmacologic

Psoriasis

- Topical steroids give fast relief, are useful for reducing inflammation and itching, but the relief is usually temporary.
  - Group I through V steroids applied twice a day in a cream or ointment base give best results.
  - Group V topical steroids can be used in the intertriginous areas and on the face.

- Calcipotriene (Dovonex) 0.005% ointment and cream is effective and safe for short- and long-term therapy. It is a vitamin D_3 analog that inhibits epidermal cell proliferation. Used in combination with a group I steroid such as diflorasone diacetate ointment, it is superior to either preparation alone. Suggested regimen includes the following:
  - Calcipotriene applied in the morning and a group I steroid in the evening for two weeks
  - Maintenance therapy—Topical steroid twice a day on weekends and calcipotriene twice a day during the week. This allows for less steroid use and limited side effects. Calcipotriene can cause an irritant contact dermatitis on the face and intertriginous areas and should be avoided in these areas. Less than 100 grams should be used in one week to avoid altered calcium parameters (Habif, 2004).

- Dermatology consult needed for phototherapy and systemic therapies such as acitretin (Soriatane), isotretinoin, cyclosporin, methotrexate, and the biologic agents (e.g., etanercept, alefacept, efalizumab).

- The scale in scalp psoriasis must be removed first so medication can penetrate. Derma-Smoothe FS oil (fluocinolone acetonide 0.01%) applied to a wet scalp and occluded with a shower cap overnight can be used nightly for 1–3 weeks. The oil loosens scale, and the steroid controls erythema.

- Groups I and II steroid solutions and gels are used for erythema and mild scale.

- Calcipotriene solution can be valuable for long-term therapy of scalp psoriasis either alone or in conjunction with steroid solution.

Seborrheic Dermatitis

- Derma-Smoothe FS oil treatment as above is helpful to remove scale.

- Lidex solution for the scalp and group V through VII topical steroid creams can be used for clearing scale and erythema. Antiseborrheic cleansers and shampoo should be used for remission maintenance.

- Ketoconazole (Nizoral) cream or ciclopirox olamine (Loprox cream or gel) applied twice a day to affected areas is effective. In addition, a group V through VII topical steroid may be required for control.

- Selenium sulfide lotion 2.5% can be applied daily for 10 minutes for 7 days, then used once or twice a week for maintenance.

Pruritus

- Treatment depends on identification of underlying cause.
- Topical steroids should only be used for active eruption.
- Antihistamines such as hydroxyzine (Atarax) or diphenhydramine, especially at bedtime, since most complain that itching is worse at night.

Patient, Family, and Staff Education

- There is no cure for psoriasis or seborrheic dermatitis, and occasionally puritis can only be partially controlled.
- Trigger factors for exacerbation or worsening of psoriasis include physical trauma, infections, stress, and drugs and alcohol ingestion. New lesions can be induced on clear skin by scratching and rubbing.
- Treatment goals need to be individualized.

Physician Consultation

- Patients with psoriasis that is resistant to topical treatment should have a dermatology referral to confirm the diagnosis and design an appropriate, individualized treatment plan.
- Dermatology referral for worsening conditions not responsive to usual therapies

SCABIES INFESTATION

Definition

Scabies is a pruritic and highly contagious infestation of the skin caused by the *Sarcoptes* *scabiei* mite. It is one of the earliest infectious diseases in history with a known cause (Stone, 2003).

Epidemiology

There are more than 300 million cases of scabies yearly, worldwide (Huynh & Norman, 2004). Scabies recognizes all social and socioeconomic levels and is not related to poor hygiene. There must be skin-to-skin contact for transmission of the mite; the prevalence is high within households, neighborhoods, schools, and in nursing homes. There is increased frequency with intimate personal contact, sharing inanimate objects, and healthcare workers providing care. Mites can live more than 2 days on clothing or in bedding; therefore, fomite transmission is a major factor in household and nosocomial passage of scabies (Habif, 2004).

The elderly population in assisted living facilities or skilled nursing facilities are at risk, especially debilitated and immobile patients. In the skilled nursing facility risk factors include the age of the institution (> 30 years), the size (> 120 beds), and ratio of beds to healthcare workers (< 10:1) (Fitzpatrick et al., 2001).

The adult mite is about 0.3–0.4 mm and has an oval shape with eight legs. Both males and females have a 30-day life cycle. As soon as the female mite is deposited on the skin she burrows into the stratum corneum and lays 2–3 eggs a day. She advances slowly in the burrow, not much more than 1 cm in her lifetime, and deposits the eggs and fecal pellets (scybala). The larvae hatch and mature in 14–17 days. The egg casings remain in the burrow. Adult mites copulate and repeat the cycle. After 3–5 weeks there are still only a few mites present, and only a few symptoms as well. When about 20 mites have matured and spread by migration and scratching, the initial minor itch becomes an intense generalized pruritus (Habif, 2004).

In scabies there is a type IV hypersensitivity reaction to the mites, eggs, saliva, and scybala

2–6 weeks after the infestation. This delayed inflammatory reaction causes the pruritus, which is the true hallmark of the disease. The pruritus is worse at night (Habif, 2004).

Common Presenting Signs and Symptoms

- The primary lesion is usually a burrow or vesicle and this is usually where the mites are found (Figure 7-37). Burrows are linear, curved or serpiginous, thin, 2–15 mm long, pink-white, and slightly elevated. Scratching destroys the burrows so they may not be visible. The lesions are usually in the finger webs (Figure 7-38), wrists, sides of hands and feet, penis, buttocks, scrotum,

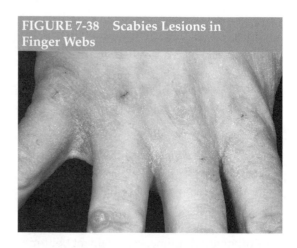

FIGURE 7-38   Scabies Lesions in Finger Webs

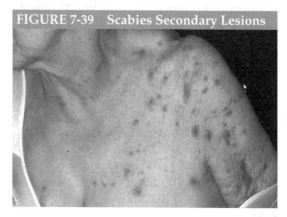

FIGURE 7-39   Scabies Secondary Lesions

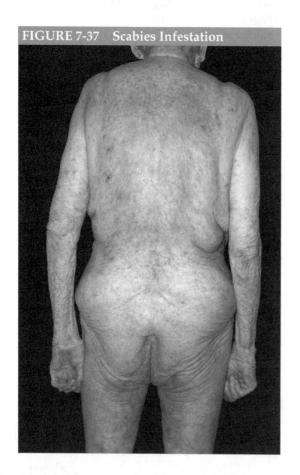

FIGURE 7-37   Scabies Infestation

nipples, waistline, and axillary folds. The face is usually spared. Vesicles are pinpoint, filled with serous fluid, discrete, and usually in the finger web spaces.

- Secondary lesions result from scratching (pinpoint erosion) or infection (pustules). Scaling, erythema, and all the characteristics of eczematous inflammation may be present as a result of the excoriation. Nodules occur in areas that are typically covered: buttocks, groin, scrotum, penis, axilla (Figure 7-39). Nodules may persist for months secondary to persistent antigens from the mite parts (Habif, 2004).

- The type of lesions and extent of involvement varies; the pruritus varies from periods of

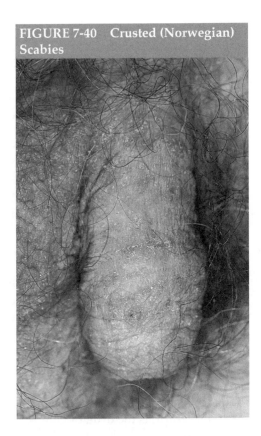

FIGURE 7-40   Crusted (Norwegian) Scabies

nocturnal itching to constant and frantic scratching.

- The elderly usually have severe pruritus but also an atypical presentation. They may have nothing other than dry skin, a few excoriations and scaling, and the lesions may be on the back and buttocks rather than the web spaces and axilla.
- Crusted (Norwegian) scabies is associated with hyperkeratotic and crusty lesions involving the hands and feet, trunk and extremities and occasionally the scalp. In regular scabies the host has about 10–15 mites, in crusted scabies there may be thousands or millions (Huynh & Norman, 2004). This condition has been associated with advanced age, debility, developmental disability, dementia, nutritional disorders, infectious diseases, and immunosuppression (Figure 7-40).

There can be facial desquamation, hair shedding, and itching may be absent or severe (Habif, 2004).

Differential Diagnoses

- Atopic dermatitis
- Dyshidrotic eczema
- Urticaria
- Pityriasis rosea
- Dermatitis herpetiformis
- Pediculosis
- Delusions of parasitosis
- Metabolic pruritus
- Impetigo
- Darier's disease
- Prurigo nodularis
- Seborrheic dermatitis
- Contact dermatitis
- Papular urticaria
- Adverse drug reaction
- Lichen planus
- Syphilis (Huynh & Norman, 2004)

Essential Diagnostic and Laboratory Tests

Microscopic identification of mites, eggs, or fecal pellets (scybala) is needed for definitive diagnosis. The burrows are often difficult to find, samples need to be taken from multiple sites: wrists, hands, finger webs, and waistline. Mineral oil is applied directly to the suspicious area and then shaved or scraped with a #15 scalpel blade. The samples and oil are placed on a glass slide, covered with a coverslip and examined under the microscope. Finding eggs, mites, or scybala confirms the diagnosis, but a negative scraping does not rule it out.

Overdiagnosis and underdiagnosis are common (Stone, 2001); early diagnosis is important especially when considering the potential for an epidemic outbreak in a skilled nursing facility.

Management Plan

The goal of treatment is complete clearing of infestation for the patient, family, and staff, and prevention of an outbreak in the facility.

Nonpharmacologic
- General environmental management requires all intimate contacts and household members be treated. Live mites have been found in dust samples, chairs, linens, and other inanimate objects for up to 96 hours after being removed from the host (Habif, 2004).
- All clothing, towels, and linens that have been in contact with the infected individual within the last 3 days should be washed in a hot washing machine cycle. General household cleaning is important, especially the rooms of those confined in single rooms of the skilled nursing facility.
- Hot water washing for at least 10 minutes, hot air tumble drying, dry cleaning, and hot ironing are effective for killing adult mites and their eggs (Stone, 2001).

Pharmacologic
- Permethrin 5% cream, a synthetic pyrethrin, is the drug of choice. One 60-gram tube is generally enough for two applications including the entire body from the neck down, including the underside of well-trimmed fingernails. Scalp and face should be included for those with recurrent or relapsing scabies and for the elderly. Nix is permethrin 1% cream rinse that can be used on scalp and face. The medication should be left on overnight, at least 10–12 hours, washed off, and treatment should be repeated one week later. Permethrin is reportedly more effective than Lindane (Habif, 2004).
- Ivermectin is an antiparasitic agent approved for the treatment and prevention of onchocerciasis ("river blindness") and other nematode intestinal parasites. Authors report an ivermectin dose of 200 mcg/kg body weight, given in divided doses one week apart, is an effective treatment to eradicate the scabietic nymph (Stone, 2003; Habif, 2004). Side effects of ivermectin may include transient tachycardia, flushing, and nausea. The medication is available in 3 mg and 6 mg tablets.
- Patients with crusted scabies may require combination treatment with topical permethrin and oral ivermectin.
- Postscabietic pruritus may persist for weeks after appropriate treatment and is usually attributed to the hypersensitivity response to dead mites and their body parts. Topical steroids, oral antihistamines, and occasionally systemic corticosteroids may be warranted.
- In the skilled nursing facility, early diagnosis is imperative. All infested patients should be treated within the same time period. Permethrin is the drug of choice, two applications one week apart. Residents with dementia and severe functional impairment may be resistant to treatment and require oral ivermectin. Permethrin and ivermectin used at the same time will increase cure rates (Habif, 2004).

Patient, Family, and Staff Education

Management of a scabies epidemic in a skilled nursing facility requires the following (Habif, 2004):

- Education about scabies, the spread, and the need for full cooperation with treatment for all patients, family, staff, and frequent visitors.
- Topical scabicide treatment for all patients, staff, contact staff, frequent visitors, and symptomatic family members of staff and visitors.

- All bedding and clothes worn in the last 48 hours need to be laundered in hot water or dry cleaned.
- Beds and floors should be cleaned just before scabicide is removed. Routine cleaning agents are appropriate.
- Treatments should be repeated in one week. Examine for treatment failures at 1 and 4 weeks.
- Treated healthcare workers should be considered noninfectious after one overnight application of permethrin and should be able to return to work the next day (Stone, 2001).

Physician Consultation

Early definitive diagnosis is imperative to avoid an epidemic in the skilled nursing facility.

WEB SITES

- DermNet NZ, Bullous Pemphigoid—www.dermnetnz.info/immune/pemphigoid.html
- Emedicine, Bullous Pemphigoid—www.emedicine.com/derm/topic64.htm
- DermNet NZ, Bacterial cellulitis—www.dermnetnz.org/bacterial/cellulitis.html
- SkinCancerNet—www.skincarephysicians.com/skincancernet/index.html
- CancerSociety.com, Treatment for Skin Cancer—www.cancersociety.com/skin_tp.cfm
- PDR (Physicians' Desk Reference)—www.pdr.net
- Litt's Drug Eruption Global Database—www.drugeruptiondata.com
- Indiana University School of Medicine, Drug Interactions—www.drug-interactions.com
- DermNet NZ, Eczema, Dermatitis, and Allergies—www.dermnetnz.info/dermatitis
- The National Eczema Society—www.eczema.org
- DermNet NZ, Fungal Skin Infections—www.dermnetnz.info/fungal
- National Psoriasis Foundation—www.psoriasis.org
- Psoriasis Net—www.skincarephysicians.com/psoriasisnet
- Center for Disease Control, Division of Parasitic Diseases, Scabies—www.cdc.gov/ncidod/dpd/parasites/scabies/factsht_scabies.htm
- DermNet NZ, Scabies—www.dermnetnz.info/rthropods/scabies.html

REFERENCES

Blacker, K. L., Stern, R. S., & Wintroub, B. U. (1993). Cutaneous reactions to drugs. In T. B. Fitzpatrick, A. Z. Eisen, K. Wolf, I. M. Freedberg, & K. F. Austen (Eds.), *Dermatology in general medicine* (5th ed., pp. 1783–1794). New York: McGraw-Hill.

Christophers, E., & Sterry, W. (1993). Psoriasis. In T. B. Fitzpatrick, A. Z. Eisen, K. Wolff, I. M. Freedburg, & K. F. Austen (Eds.), *Dermatology in general medicine* (4th ed., pp. 489–514). New York: McGraw-Hill

Dewberry, C., & Norman, R. A. (2004). Skin cancer in elderly patients. *Dermatology Clinics of North America, 22,* 93–96.

Dewberry, C., Norman, R. A., & Bock, M. (2004). Eczematous diseases of the geriatric population. *Dermatology Clinics of North America, 22,* 1–5.

Ellis, C. N., Drake, L. A., Prendergast, M. M., Abramouits, W., Boguniewicz, M., Daniel, C. R., et al. (2002). Cost of atopic dermatitis and eczema in the United States. *Journal of the American Academy of Dermatology, 46,* 361–370.

Fitzpatrick, T. B., Johnson, R. A., Wolff, K., & Suurmond, D. (2001). *Color atlas and synopsis of clinical dermatology: Common and serious diseases* (4th ed.). New York: McGraw-Hill.

Gilchrest, B. A. (1993). Aging of skin. In T. B. Fitzpatrick, A. Z. Eisen, K. Wolff, I. M. Freedburg, & K. F. Austen (Eds.), *Dermatology in general medicine* (4th ed., pp. 150–157). New York: McGraw-Hill.

Glick, B. P., Zaiac, M., Rebell, G., & Zaias, N. (2001). Superficial mycoses in the elderly. In R. A. Norman (Ed.), *Geriatric dermatology* (pp. 83–94). New York: Parthenon Publishing Group.

Greaves, M. W. (1993). Pathophysiology and clinical aspects of pruritus. In T. B. Fitzpatrick, A. Z. Eisen, K. Wolff, I. M. Freedburg, & K. F. Austen (Eds.), *Dermatology in general medicine* (4th ed., pp. 2297–2309). New York: McGraw-Hill.

Habif, T. B. (2004). *Clinical dermatology: A color guide to diagnosis and therapy* (4th ed.). Philadelphia: Mosby.

Huynh, T. H., & Norman, R. A. (2004). Scabies and pediculosis. *Dermatology Clinics of North America, 22*, 7–11.

Litt, J. Z. (2001). Adverse drug reactions on the skin. In R. A. Norman (Ed.), *Geriatric dermatology* (pp. 119–128). New York: Parthenon Publishing Group.

Loo, D. S. (2004). Cutaneous fungal infections in the elderly. *Dermatology Clinics of North America, 22*, 33–50.

Lyon, N. B., & Fitzpatrick, T. B. (1993). Geriatric dermatology. In T. B. Fitzpatrick, A. Z. Eisen, K. Wolff, I. M. Freedburg, & K. F. Austen (Eds.), *Dermatology in general medicine* (4th ed., pp. 2961–2972). New York: McGraw -Hill.

Martin, A. G., & Kobayashi, G. S. (1993). Superficial fungal infection: dermatophytosis, tinea, nigra, piedra. In T. B. Fitzpatrick, A. Z. Eisen, K. Wolff, I. M. Freedburg, & K. F. Austen (Eds.), *Dermatology in general medicine* (4th ed., pp. 2421–2451). New York: McGraw-Hill.

Moschella, S. L. (2001). Skin diseases of the elderly. In R. A. Norman (Ed.), *Geriatric dermatology* (pp. 17–34). New York: Parthenon Publishing Company.

Naylor, M. (2004). *The epidemic of nonmelanoma skin cancer: Prevention, diagnosis, and treatment.*

Retrieved May 2, 2005, from http://www.medscape.com/viewprogram/3129_pnt

Plewig, G. (1993). Seborrheic dermatitis. In T. B. Fitzpatrick, A. Z. Eisen, K. Wolff, I. M. Freedburg, & K. F. Austen (Eds.), *Dermatology in general medicine* (4th ed., pp. 1569–1574). New York: McGraw-Hill.

Reyes-Ortiz, C. A., Goodwin, J. S., & Freeman, J. L. (2005). *The effect of socioeconomic factors on incidence, stage at diagnosis, and survival of cutaneous melanoma.* Retrieved July 14, 2005, from http://www.medSciMonit.com/pub/vol_11/no_5/6929.pdf

Sami, N., Yeh, S. W., & Ahmed, A. R. (2004). Blistering diseases in the elderly: Diagnosis and treatment. *Dermatology Clinics of North America, 22*, 73–86.

Stone, S. P. (2001). Scabies and pediculosis. In R. A. Norman (Ed.), *Geriatric dermatology* (pp. 95–104). New York: Parthenon Publishing Group.

Stone, S. P. (2003). Scabies and pediculosis. In I. M. Freedman, A. Z. Eisen, K. Wolff, L. A. Goldsmith, S. I. Katz (Eds.), *Fitzpatrick's dermatology in general medicine* (6th ed., pp. 2283–2296). New York: McGraw-Hill.

Swartz, M. N., & Weinberg, A. N. (1993). Miscellaneous bacterial infections with cutaneous manifestations. In T. B. Fitzpatrick, A. Z. Eisen, K. Wolff, I. M. Freedburg, & K. F. Austen (Eds.), *Dermatology in general medicine* (4th ed., pp. 2354–2370). New York: McGraw-Hill.

Yaar, M., & Gilchrest, B. A. (2003). Aging of skin. In I. M. Freedman, A. Z. Eisen, K. Wolff, L. A. Goldsmith, S. I. Katz (Eds.), *Fitzpatrick's dermatology in general medicine* (6th ed., pp. 1386–1398). New York: McGraw-Hill.

CHAPTER 8

Endocrine Disorders

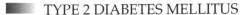 **TYPE 2 DIABETES MELLITUS**

by Doreen Bacon and Yung-In Choi

Definition

Diabetes mellitus is a group of diseases, each characterized by sustained hyperglycemia. Hyperglycemia can be attributed to insulin deficiency or resistance to insulin action in liver, adipose, and muscle tissue. A combination of insulin deficiency and resistance may also serve as the etiology of sustained hyperglycemia.

The three main types of diabetes mellitus are type 1 diabetes mellitus (T1DM), type 2 diabetes mellitus (T2DM), and gestational diabetes mellitus (GDM). T1DM, formerly known as insulin-dependent or juvenile-onset diabetes mellitus, is an autoimmune disease manifested by the immune destruction of pancreatic beta cells with loss of insulin secretion. GDM develops during the late stages of pregnancy and is caused by a combination of the hormones of pregnancy with a relative insulin secretory defect.

T2DM, the most common type of diabetes mellitus, is seen frequently in the frail elderly population in long-term care. Formerly known as non-insulin-dependent or adult-onset diabetes mellitus, T2DM is characterized by insulin resistance and a relative insulin secretory defect. The etiology of the insulin resistance and decreased insulin secretion is multifactorial and includes the following:

- Obesity—The majority of patients with T2DM are obese.
- Decreased physical activity
- Family history
- Side effects of certain medications
- Comorbid conditions such as cardiovascular disease
- An age-related decrease in beta cell mass

T2DM poses the following unique challenges for long-term care providers:

- A population with a frequently long history of sustained hyperglycemia
- Questionable efficacy of prior pharmacologic management
- Decreased activity
- Possibility of poor compliance or poor nutrition
- Increased frequency of significant comorbid conditions
  - Progressive dementia
  - Cardiovascular, peripheral vascular, cerebrovascular, renal, and respiratory diseases

Preterminal illnesses may significantly impact the life expectancy of the older diabetic. Some of these comorbid conditions may result in the contraindication of oral diabetic medications. Others may require treatment with medications that can exacerbate the illness through a drug-induced hyperglycemia.

Uncontrolled hyperglycemia in the elderly may potentiate or exacerbate urinary incontinence, urinary tract or skin infection, blurred vision, declining cognitive function, depression, chronic pain, recurrent falls, and organ damage. However, tight glycemic control, in the attempt to prevent chronic complications, may not be appropriate because of the increased risk of hypoglycemia, particularly if there is a potential for poor nutritional intake or medication noncompliance.

Epidemiology

Among adults 65 to 74, 18.5% have diabetes, and 20% have impaired glucose tolerance (Harris, Flegal, & Cowie, 1998). By 2000, diabetes was the sixth leading cause of death listed on U.S. death certificates. In 2005, 7% of the U.S. population, or 20.8 million people, had diabetes; 14.6 million diagnosed and 6.2 million undiagnosed. For those people 60 years and older, 10.3 million people in all, 20.9% of them had diabetes. Approximately 1.5 million new cases of diabetes were diagnosed in people aged 20 years or older in 2005. In the same year, 600,000 new cases of diabetes were diagnosed in patients over 60 years (National Diabetes Information Clearinghouse, 2005).

The cost of diabetes is increasing. For 2002, the total cost of diabetes in the United States was estimated at $132 billion, with $92 billion going to direct medical costs and $40 billion going to indirect costs. Worldwide, the total number of diabetics is projected to rise from 171 million in 2000 to 366 million in 2030 (Wild, Roglie, & Green, 2004), bringing the cost of diabetes to a phenomenal high.

Adults with diabetes have increased rates of hypertension as well as heart disease and death rates that are two to four times higher than nondiabetic adults. Diabetic adults are two to four times more likely to suffer a stroke. Diabetes is the leading cause of new-onset blindness and end-stage kidney disease in adults. Approximately 60% to 70% of people with diabetes have evidence of neuropathy, a major underlying cause of lower limb amputation (National Diabetes Information Clearinghouse, 2005).

Of the 20% of nursing home residents with diabetes, 90% have evidence of associated illnesses such as coronary artery disease, stroke, and/or peripheral vascular disease. Diabetic nursing home residents tend to have more diagnoses than their nondiabetic counterparts, with an average of 6.4 major diagnoses, compared to 2.4 major diagnoses in nondiabetic residents (Resnick, 2005).

Common Presenting Signs and Symptoms

- Most patients are asymptomatic
- Mild hyperglycemia detected through laboratory tests done for reasons other than detection of diabetes
- Polyuria
- Nocturia
- Dry mouth
- Excessive thirst
- Increased appetite
- Polydipsia
- Weight loss
- Anorexia
- Gastric upset
- Weakness
- Blurred vision
- Superficial fungal infections
- Impaired cognition, confusion
- Lower extremity pain or numbness
- Recurrent falls

Differential Diagnoses

- Systemic infection
- Side effect of diuretics
- Dehydration
- Dementia
- Malnutrition
- Medication-induced T2DM
- Secondary causes of T2DM:
  - Cushing's disease
  - Hyperthyroidism
  - Acromegaly
  - Pheochromocytoma
  - Hemochromatosis

Essential Diagnostic and Laboratory Tests

- Random plasma glucose = or > 200 mg/dL with symptoms of diabetes, *or*
- Fasting plasma glucose = or > 126 mg/dL confirmed by repeat testing on another day, *or*
- Plasma glucose = or > 200 mg/dL at 2 hours after 75 gm oral glucose, confirmed by repeat testing on another day
- Fasting plasma glucose in the morning is the preferred test for diagnosis.
- HbA1c, a tool for monitoring glycemic control, is not recommended for diagnostic screening.
- Fasting lipid panel
- Urinalysis
- Spot urine for microalbumin
- Serum creatinine
- History and physical
  - Height and weight
  - Blood pressure
  - Oral exam
  - Ophthalmoscopic exam
  - Thyroid exam
  - Cardiac exam
  - Neurologic exam
  - Skin exam
  - Foot exam
- Electrocardiogram
- Medication review—Evaluate for medications that may promote hyperglycemia.
  - Glucocorticoids
  - Thiazides
  - Dilantin
  - Alpha-adrenergic agonists
  - Nicotinic acid
  - Atypical antipsychotic drugs
    - Risperdal
    - Seroquel
    - Zyprexa
- Test everyone 45 years of age and older, due to the frequent lack of symptoms.
- Test everyone under the age of 45 with one of the following risk factors:
  - Overweight or obese (BMI > 25 or > 30)
  - Family history of diabetes in a parent or sibling
  - Latino, Black, American Indian, Asian, or Pacific Islander
  - Personal history of GDM or giving birth to a baby weighing > 9 lbs
  - Consistent blood pressure 140/90 or higher
  - HDL 35 or less
  - Triglyceride level 250 or higher
  - Inactivity—Exercising fewer than three times a week

Management Plan
Goals
- *Glycemic control, including symptomatic hyperglycemia, and avoidance of hypoglycemia:*
  - *HbA1c, < 7.0%*
  - *Preprandial plasma glucose 90–130 mg/dL*
  - *Postprandial plasma glucose < 180 mg/dL*

- *Maintain blood pressure to less than 130/80*
- *Maintain lipid level:*
  - *LDL < 100 mg/dL*
  - *Triglycerides < 150 mg/dL*
  - *HDL > 40 mg/dL (American Diabetic Association [ADA], 2005)*

Additional Management Goals
- *Prevention and treatment of acute and chronic complications*
- *Dietary compliance*
- *Weight management*
- *Safest and most effective pharmacological management*
- *Patient and family/caregiver education*
- *Long-term care staff education*

Nonpharmacologic
- Dietary recommendations of the American Diabetes Association (ADA, 2005)
  - Protein: 10–20%
  - Fat: Less than 30% total fat, less than 10% saturated
  - Carbohydrates: 50–55%
- Dietary therapy for elderly diabetic long-term care residents
  - Monitoring by a registered dietician
  - Small, frequent meals are associated with less glucose excursion, reduced free fatty acid levels, and lower insulin levels than larger, less frequent meals.
  - Diet consistent with the nursing home resident's likes, dislikes, lifestyle and any swallowing restrictions.
  - More soluble fibers
  - No fat restriction in the underweight elderly diabetic
  - Carbohydrates of low glycemic indices
  - Diet designed to correct dyslipidemias

- Meals with consistent calories, based on weight, comorbid illness, and physical activity
- Weight maintenance rather than weight reduction in the elderly
  - Elderly diabetics in long-term care settings tend to be underweight.
  - Comorbid conditions such as dementia can result in poor nutrition.
  - To prevent malnourishment, avoid food restrictions in the elderly nursing home resident.
  - Meals served at consistent times
  - Between meal snacks
  - Feeding assistance as needed
  - Monitoring of weight, protein levels
  - Include "bedtime snack" (HS) to avoid nocturnal hypoglycemia
- Exercise
  - Improves insulin sensitivity and glycemic control
  - Reduces fat mass
  - Lowers blood pressure
  - Improves lipid profiles
  - Enhances fitness and sense of well-being
  - Medical evaluation necessary before any exercise program
  - Potential risks are to insensate lower extremities and precipitation of cardiovascular complications.

Pharmacologic
- Nonpharmacologic management is usually attempted first.
- Pharmacologic management, in addition to dietary therapy, weight maintenance and exercise, is often necessary to achieve adequate glycemic control.
- Aspirin therapy
  - For cardiovascular prophylaxis

- Increased risk of gastrointestinal (GI) bleed in the geriatric population.
  - Add GI prophylactic therapy.
  - Monitor for anemia.
  - Monitor for signs of bleeding.
- Ace inhibitors
  - For cardiovascular and renal prophylaxis.
  - Increased risk of hyperkalemia, especially in renal insufficiency.
  - Monitor potassium level.
  - Monitor for side effect of cough.
- Statins
  - For cardiovascular prophylaxis
  - Monitor liver function
- Oral antidiabetic agents are usually the first pharmaceutical choice for hyperglycemia.
- For treatment of severe hyperglycemia (postprandial [PG] > 300 mg/dL), insulin should be used initially.
- Oral antihyperglycemics increase risk of hypoglycemia in the elderly, when combined with other risk factors.
  - Impaired liver or renal function
  - Hypoglycemia unawareness—no warning symptoms
    - Sweating
    - Palpitations
    - Hunger
  - Use of multiple antihyperglycemics
  - Nocturnal use of insulin without HS snack
  - Inadequate nutrition

Oral Antidiabetic Agents
- Dose of oral agent should be upgraded every 2–4 weeks until glycemic goal is reached.
- If single-agent therapy fails, add a second oral agent from another class.
- If two-agent therapy fails, add a third oral agent from a different class, or add, or switch, to insulin.
- Insulin secretagogues (glyburide, glipizide, glimepiride, repaglinide, nateglinide)
  - Often the first-line oral agents for non-obese or mildly obese patients
  - Avoid long-acting drugs in elderly patients who are at increased risk of prolonged hypoglycemia, especially in the setting of impaired renal function, such as glyburide and glimepiride.
- Biguanides (metformin—Glucophage, Glucophage XR)
  - A first-line agent for obese patients—promotes weight loss
  - Favorably affects lipid profile
  - Lactic acidosis
    - Rare, but potentially fatal adverse reaction
    - Usually in patients with severe kidney or liver disease, or congestive heart failure (CHF)
  - Contraindicated:
    - In patients over 80
    - Patients with kidney disease or dysfunction (serum creatinine >1.5 mg/dL in males and > 1.4 mg/dL in females; in elderly with creatinine clearance of < 60 mL/min)
    - In patients with CHF
    - In patients with respiratory insufficiency
    - In patients with liver disease
- Thiazolidinediones (pioglitazone, rosiglitazone)
  - Used in patients with significant insulin resistance or signs of metabolic syndrome
  - Can cause marked weight gain, especially when used with insulin

TABLE 8-1   Medications Used in Treating Diabetes

DRUG TYPE	DRUG ACTION	ADVANTAGES OF USE	SIDE EFFECTS
Insulin secretagogues	Pancreas is stimulated to increase insulin production	Improved control of blood sugar	Severe hypoglycemia, weight gain
Biguanides	Liver is stimulated to decrease release of glucose	Weight loss, improved lipid profile	Abdominal discomfort, flatulence, diarrhea; rarely, lactic acidosis
Thiazolidinediones	Adipocytes are shifted from peritoneum to subcutaneous space	Insulin resistance, metabolic syndrome	Edema, weight gain
Alpha-glucosidase inhibitors	Intestinal digestion of complex carbohydrate is slowed	Affects postprandial blood sugar; adjunct to other agents	Abdominal discomfort, flatulence, diarrhea

- Contraindicated:
  - In patients with alanine aminotransferase (ALT) > 2.5 times upper limit of reference range
  - In patients with CHF
  - In patients with significant lower extremity edema
- Alpha-glucosidase inhibitors (acarbose, miglitol)
  - Less potent than other classes of oral agents
  - Delay absorption of glucose
  - Used to control postprandial hyperglycemia
  - Used as an adjunct to other agents
  - Contraindicated:
    - In patients with irritable bowel syndrome
    - In patients with serum creatinine > 2.0 mg/dL
    - In patients with liver disease
- First-generation sulfonylureas (chlorpropamide, tolbutamide, and tolazamide)
  - Not widely used
  - Chlorpropamide (Diabinese)
    - Long half-life
    - Syndrome of inappropriate antidiuretic hormone secretion (SIADH)
  - Increased risk of hypoglycemia
  - Increased risk of weight gain

- The FDA recently approved sitagliptin (Januvia), a new class of drugs known as gliptins, for T2DM either as monotherapy or in combination with metformin or a thiazolidinedione.
- Combination drugs
  - Metformin/rosiglitazone (Avandament)
  - Glyburide/metformin (Glucovance)
  - Glipizide/metformin (Metaglip)
  - Generic glyburide/metformin
  - Use caution with elderly patients because of increased potential for hypoglycemia and other adverse reactions.

See Table 8-1 for more information.

Insulin Therapy
- Types of insulin
  - Human insulin
  - Insulin analogues
  - Prandial insulins
    - Lispro
      - Onset: 10–15 minutes
      - Peak: 1–1.5 hours
      - Duration: 4–5 hours
      - Target glucose: postprandial
    - Aspart
      - Onset: 10–15 minutes
      - Peak: 1–2 hours
      - Duration: 4–6 hours
      - Target glucose: postprandial

- Inhaled insulin (Exubera)
  - FDA approval in January 2006
  - Onset of action is significantly faster than regular insulin.
  - Duration of action between that of insulin Lispro and regular insulin
  - Target glucose: postprandial
  - Do not use in persons with the following:
    - Poorly controlled asthma
    - Chronic obstructive pulmonary disease
    - Other significant lung disease
    - Current smoker
- Regular insulin
  - Onset: 10–60 minutes
  - Peak: 2–4 hours
  - Duration: 5–8 hours
  - Target glucose: postprandial
  - It may be advisable to avoid bedtime use of regular insulin in the elderly to avoid potential for unobserved nocturnal hypoglycemia and to consider a conservative dose of peakless insulin such as insulin glargine at dinnertime instead.
- Basal insulins
  - NPH
    - Onset: 2.5–3 hours
    - Peak: 5–7 hours
    - Duration: 13–16 hours
    - Target glucose: midafternoon or next morning
  - Lente
    - Onset: 2.5–3 hours
    - Peak: 7–12 hours
    - Duration: 18 hours
    - Target glucose: midafternoon or next morning

- Glargine
  - Onset: 2–3 hours
  - Peak: no peak
  - Duration: 30 hours
  - Target glucose: premeal
  - May cause less nocturnal hypoglycemia than NPH or Lente
- Ultralente
  - Onset: 3–4 hours
  - Peak: 8–10 hours
  - Duration: 20 hours
  - Target glucose: midafternoon or next morning
- Detemir
  - Onset: 2–3 hours
  - Peak: no peak
  - Duration: 24 hours
  - Target glucose: premeal
- Initiation of therapy
  - Discontinue insulin secretagogues—glipizide, glyburide, and glimepiride—to avoid risk of prolonged hypoglycemia.
  - Continue metformin with insulin therapy.
  - Insulin combined with thiazolidinedione therapy may cause significant weight gain.
  - Addition of pioglitazone or rosiglitazone to insulin may result in improved glycemic control and significant reduction of insulin requirement.
  - For NPH, 10 units at bedtime is a reasonable starting dose.
  - Usual daily insulin requirement is 0.4–1.0 units/kg/day
- Indications
  - Patients who have failed to achieve glycemic control by diet, exercise, and oral agents
  - Uncontrolled T2DM patients unable or unwilling to take oral agents

○ For the short term in T2DM patients undergoing serious injury, infection, or other major stress

- Most T2DM patients require insulin after 15–20 years with the disease.
- Insulin is less expensive than the oral agents.
- Insulin reduces the risk of adverse effects of oral agents.
- Initiation of frequent blood sugar monitoring with a basal insulin and a short-acting prandial insulin (Aspart, Lispro, or regular) supplement (a regular insulin sliding scale) for plasma glucose (PG) > 300 mg/dL may be the safest way to control blood sugar in the elderly diabetic with inconsistent or poor intake.

Patient, Family, and Staff Education

- Diabetes is a chronic disease with multisystem involvement requiring a multidisciplinary approach.
- Signs and symptoms of hyperglycemia and hypoglycemia, with appropriate initial management of each.
- Blood glucose monitoring is an integral part of diabetes care.
- Glycemic parameters for notifying provider or initiating immediate management
- Familiarity with the basic aspects of diabetic nutrition, including the relationship of carbohydrate and blood glucose
- Ability to perform frequent skin and foot checks
- Understanding the importance of avoiding injury
- Knowing how to seek appropriate treatment for wounds and infections
- References and further education
  ○ Health care organizations, hospitals, and clinics provide diabetes education
  ○ Patients, families, and caregivers are encouraged to attend classes.

Nursing Facility Staff Education

- Familiarity and adeptness using blood sugar-monitoring equipment
- Understanding the need for frequent blood sugar monitoring
- Basic understanding of insulin onset, peak, and duration
- Assessment skills leading to early recognition of both hyperglycemia and hypoglycemia
- Recognizing subtle complications of hyperglycemia in the elderly
  ○ Dehydration
  ○ Infection
  ○ Decreased renal function
  ○ Wounds
- Recognizing subtle signs of infection in the elderly
  ○ Confusion
  ○ Lethargy
  ○ Hypotension
  ○ Anorexia
  ○ Chills
- Recognizing need to adjust insulin administration in the tube-fed patient
- Importance of diet and exercise for glycemic control
- Importance of maintaining nutritional status
- Specific guidelines and parameters for when to call provider
- Acute management of hypoglycemia, with parameters on when to initiate management
- Need for accurate documentation of glycemic levels and signs and symptoms
- Effective infection control measures

Physician Consultation

- Newly diagnosed diabetes mellitus
- Disease unresponsive to treatment
- Unexplained deterioration of renal function

- Exacerbation of comorbid diseases
- Annual ophthalmologic evaluation
- Vascular wounds unresponsive to treatment
- Podiatry referral

HYPERTHYROIDISM

by Doreen Bacon

Definition

Hyperthyroidism refers to the sustained increase in biosynthesis and secretion of thyroid hormones by the thyroid gland, such as occurs in Grave's disease. Thyrotoxicosis refers to the clinical syndrome of hypermetabolism that results when the serum concentrations of free T-4, free T-3, or both are increased, whether from endogenous or exogenous causes (White, 2004). Usually both hyperthyroidism and thyrotoxicosis are referred to as hyperthyroidism. Hyperthyroidism can be overt with symptoms, or subclinical without symptoms.

Etiology of Hyperthyroidism

- Grave's disease
- Toxic multinodular goiter (more frequent cause in the elderly)
- Excessive thyroid hormone ingestion
- Thyroiditis
- Single toxic adenoma
- Ingestion of iodine-containing compounds such as amiodarone (Woeber, 2005)

Hyperthyroidism in the elderly has been called apathetic hyperthyroidism (Lahey, 1931). Apathetic hyperthyroidism refers to the paucity of symptoms other than marked weakness seen in elderly patients. Hyperthyroidism can cause heart failure in the elderly (Felicetta, 2002), and should be considered as an etiology for heart failure in this age group.

The American Thyroid Association recommends screening all adults for thyroid disease at age 35, and every 5 years after that (Ladenson et al., 2000). It is important to screen older adults for subclinical hyperthyroidism because of the increased prevalence of the disorder in the older population.

Epidemiology

Hyperthyroidism was found in 1.3% (0.5% clinical and 0.7% subclinical) of the U.S. population in National Health and Nutrition Examination Survey III (NHANES III) (Hollowell et al., 2002). The prevalence of decreased thyroid-stimulating hormone (TSH) was 2.2% in the Colorado Thyroid Prevalence Study in 2000 (Canaris, Manowitz, Mayor, & Ridgeway, 2000).

In another study, elderly patients presented less frequently with the symptoms commonly seen in younger hyperthyroid patients, such as weight loss, increased appetite, nervousness, and palpitations (Davis & Davis, 1974). Women and men over 60 showed a 1.5% and 1% occurrence of subclinical hyperthyroidism, respectively, in a study of hyperthyroidism in older individuals (Helfand & Redfern, 1998).

Common Presenting Signs and Symptoms

- Enlarged thyroid
- Tremor
- Muscle weakness
- Moist skin
- Lid lag
- Lid tremor
- Stare
- Hyperreflexia
- Systolic hypertension
- Tachycardia
- Atrial fibrillation
- Congestive heart failure
- Angina
- Nervousness
- Anxiety
- Insomnia

- Weight loss
- Increased appetite
- Diarrhea
- Fatigue
- Weakness
- Heat intolerance
- Palpitations
- Grave's disease only:
  - Exophthalmos
  - Acropachy
  - Pretibial myxedema
- History
  - Family history of thyroid disease
  - History of cardiac disease
  - History of autoimmune diseases
  - Presence of symptoms
- Physical
  - Height and weight
  - Blood pressure
  - Thyroid exam
  - Goiter
  - Cognitive evaluation
  - Cardiac exam
  - Neurologic exam
- Medication review
  - Medications that increase T-4 or T-3

The following signs and symptoms are more commonly found in the elderly:

- Cardiac tachy-dysrhythmias (such as atrial fibrillation)
- Shortness of breath
- Edema
- Change in mental status
- Apathy
- Lethargy
- Depression
- Congestive heart failure

Differential Diagnoses

- Laboratory error
- AIDS (increased thyroid-binding globulin)
- Depression
- Acute psychiatric
- Atrial fibrillation
- Congestive heart failure
- High estrogen states
  - Tamoxifen
- Effects of high-dose glucocorticoids
- Acute illness
- Cushing's syndrome
- Other drugs such as the following:
  - Amiodarone
  - Amphetamines
  - Clofibrate
  - Heparin (dialysis method)
  - Methadone Perphenazine (Fitzgerald, 2005)

Essential Diagnostic and Laboratory Tests

- Thyroid-stimulating hormone (TSH) sensitive
  - The single most sensitive test for hyperthyroidism
  - Less than 0.1 microunits/mL in overt hyperthyroidism
  - Below reference range in subclinical hyperthyroidism
  - Not suppressed in the rare TSH-producing pituitary adenoma
- Free thyroxine (F-T-4)
  - Above normal in overt hyperthyroidism
  - Within reference range in subclinical hyperthyroidism
- Tri-iodothyronine (T-3) or free tri-iodothyronine (F-T-3)
  - Above normal in overt hyperthyroidism

○ Within reference range in subclinical hyperthyroidism

- Antithyroid peroxidase antibodies (TPO Ab)
  ○ Can be found in Grave's disease (Davies, 2000)
  ○ Measurement of radioactive iodine (RAI) uptake
    - Demonstrates thyroid gland function
    - High radioiodine uptake
      ♦ Graves' disease
      ♦ Toxic nodule
      ♦ Toxic multinodular goiter
    - Low radioiodine uptake
      ♦ Thyroiditis
      ♦ Factitious hyperthyroidism
    - Iodine-induced hyperthyroidism

- Imaging studies
  ○ Referral to endocrinologist
  ○ Thyroid scan
    - Gland structure and volume
    - Thyroid tissue location
    - Can differentiate between thyroiditis, Grave's disease, and multinodular goiter
    - Identifies nodules as hot or cold
  ○ Ultrasound
    - Confirms presence of nodules

- Fine-needle aspiration and biopsy
  ○ Referral to endocrinologist
  ○ Confirms diagnosis
  ○ Rules out malignancy

Management Plan
Goal
- *Alleviation of signs and symptoms*
- *Correction of TSH suppression*

Additional Management Goals
- *Correct resulting hypothyroidism after treatment*

Nonpharmacologic
- Treatment (nonpharmacologic or pharmacologic) is advised in symptomatic hyperthyroidism and asymptomatic patients with atrial fibrillation or severe osteoporosis.
- Asymptomatic subclinical hyperthyroidism
  ○ Treatment not indicated
  ○ Monitor T-4 and T-3 every six months.
- RAI ablation therapy
  ○ Treatment of choice for most patients
  ○ Safe
  ○ Not recommended in pregnant patients
  ○ Hypothyroidism can develop within 3 months
  ○ Monitor TSH every 4 to 6 weeks
- Thyroidectomy
  ○ Uncommon
  ○ Used for large nodular goiters
  ○ Used after failure of antithyroid therapy
  ○ Complications
    - Hypoparathyroidism
    - Vocal cord paralysis

Pharmacologic
- Beta-blocker (such as Atenolol)
  ○ All patients with overt hyperthyroidism
  ○ Patients with transient hyperthyroidism due to subacute or silent thyroiditis
  ○ Unless contraindicated by severe asthma
  ○ Can alleviate symptoms
    - Tachycardias
    - Nervousness
- PTU
  ○ Decreases thyroid hormone secretion
  ○ Inhibits conversion of T-4 to T-3
  ○ Used as pretreatment before RAI ablation in the elderly and those with cardiac disease

- ○ Usual dose: 100 to 150 mg three times a day
- ○ Monitor complete blood count (CBC) for agranulocytosis and neutropenia.
- ○ Monitor for hepatitis and vasculitis.
- Methimazole
  - ○ Decreases thyroid hormone secretion
  - ○ Used as pretreatment before RAI ablation in the elderly and those with cardiac disease
  - ○ Advantage of once-a-day dosing
  - ○ Usual dose: 10 to 15 mg daily
  - ○ Monitor CBC for agranulocytosis.

Patient, Family, and Staff Education

- Hyperthyroidism can cause or exacerbate cardiac disease.
- Hyperthyroid patients on antithyroid drug therapy need periodic thyroid function tests and follow-up by a physician.
- Radioiodine treated patients need periodic thyroid function tests for early detection of postablative hypothyroidism.
- It may be necessary to take thyroid replacement for a lifetime after treatment of hyperthyroidism.
- Appropriate dosing schedule for thyroid replacement
- References and further education
  - ○ Health care organizations
  - ○ Hospitals
  - ○ Clinics
- Monitor carefully for cardiac arrhythmias.
- Be aware of increased risk of fracture due to osteoporosis.
- Skin rash, itching, and unexplained fever can be adverse effects of antithyroid medications.
- Signs and symptoms of hypothyroidism in patients treated with radioiodine need thyroid function tests and evaluation.

Physician Consultation

- Newly diagnosed hyperthyroidism
- When the diagnosis is uncertain
- New-onset angina pectoris or cardiac arrhythmias
- Exacerbation of comorbid diseases

▬ HYPOTHYROIDISM

by Doreen Bacon

Definition

Hypothyroidism is a disease that results from decreased thyroid hormone levels. The three categories of hypothyroidism are primary, central or secondary, and subclinical hypothyroidism.

Primary Hypothyroidism

- Low thyroid hormone levels result from intrinsic disease of the thyroid gland itself.
- Hashimoto's thyroiditis
  - ○ Most common cause of primary hypothyroidism in the United States and other relatively iodine-sufficient areas of the world
    - ▪ Goitrous
    - ▪ Atrophic
- Other causes of primary hypothyroidism
  - ○ Prior thyroidectomy
    - ▪ Benign disease
    - ▪ Cancer
  - ○ Prior radioiodine ablation therapy
    - ▪ Hyperthyroidism
    - ▪ Thyroid cancer
  - ○ External radiation therapy to the head and neck
  - ○ Iodine load in the form of contrast dye
  - ○ Medications that may cause hypothyroidism in susceptible individuals
    - ▪ Interferon-α
    - ▪ Interleukin-2
    - ▪ Lithium

o Iodine insufficiency
  - Rare in iodine-sufficient areas such as the United States

Central or Secondary Hypothyroidism
- Caused by a decrease in the thyroid hormone level due to defective thyroid-stimulating hormone (TSH)
  o Pituitary disease
  o Hypothalamic disease

Subclinical Hypothyroidism
- Mild hypothyroidism with the laboratory finding of elevated TSH associated with normal thyroid hormone levels (free T-4 and T-3)
  o Symptoms may be mild or even absent.
  o Untreated, this form of hypothyroidism can progress to the overt form.

Epidemiology
A study of thyroid disease prevalence among 25,862 people attending a state fair showed that 9.5% had TSH values of over 5.01 mL/liter (Canaris et al., 2000). Evidence suggests an increase in hypothyroidism that is associated with sex, age, and ethnic origin. High TSH levels have been found in 7.5% of women overall, and 2.8% of men overall (Felicetta, 2002). The National Health and Nutrition Examination Survey (NHANES III) revealed that 10% of women and 4% of men over age 60 had elevated TSH, and that thyroid peroxidase (TPO) antibody was positive in 12% of men and 28% of women over age 60. NHANES III further showed that the TSH levels and the prevalence of TPO antibody are greater in women, increase with age, and are higher in Caucasians and Latinos than in African-Americans (Hollowell et al., 2002).

Common Presenting Signs and Symptoms
Nonspecific
- Signs and symptoms in the elderly
  o May be the same as in younger patients
  o May be subtle or absent

- Fatigue
- Lethargy
- Slowed cognition
- Constipation
- Fecal impaction
- Depression
- Mild psychiatric disturbances
- Heavy menstrual flow
- Arthralgias
- Myalgias
- Fluid retention
- Weight gain
- Syncope
- Cerebellar dysfunction
- Macrocytic anemia
- Increased cholesterol level
- Increased triglyceride level

More Specific
- Cold intolerance
- Dry skin
- Slow pulse rate
- Reduced deep tendon reflexes
- Slow, delayed relaxation phase of deep tendon reflexes
- Nonpitting edema (myxedema)
- Loss of scalp hair
- Periorbital puffiness

Severe Hypothyroidism
- Pleural effusion
- Pericardial effusion
- Sleep apnea
- Carpal tunnel syndrome
- Hyperprolactinemia
- Galactorrhea

Rarely
- Hypertrophic cardiomyopathy
- Heart failure

Differential Diagnoses

- Depression
- Acute psychiatric illness
- Disease-associated fatigue or malaise
- Unexplained congestive heart failure
- Pernicious anemia
- Adrenal insufficiency
- Recovery from non-thyroid-induced illness
- Myalgias
- Presence of heterophile bodies interfering with TSH assay
- TSH-secreting pituitary adenoma with hyperthyroidism
- TSH levels drawn at night, consistent with TSH surge

Essential Diagnostic and Laboratory Tests

- Thyroid-stimulating hormone (TSH)
  - The single most sensitive test for primary hypothyroidism
  - Consistently elevated
    - With a low free thyroxine (free T-4)
    - Confirms overt hypothyroidism
  - Consistently elevated
    - With a normal free T-4
    - Suggests subclinical or mild hypothyroidism
- Tri-iodothyronine (T-3)
  - Often remains normal
  - Cannot be considered diagnostic for the disease
- Antithyroid peroxidase antibodies (TPO Ab)
  - Positive in almost all patients with Hashimoto's thyroiditis
  - Positive in a majority of patients with postpartum thyroiditis and painless thyroiditis
- History
  - Family history of thyroid disease
  - History of thyroidectomy
  - History of thyroid cancer
  - Prior radioiodine ablation therapy
  - History of external radiation therapy to head and neck
- Physical
  - Height and weight
  - Observe for thyroidectomy scar
  - Thyroid exam
  - Goiter
- Medication review
  - Assess for medications that reduce L-T-4 absorption.
    - Ferrous sulfate
    - Aluminum hydroxide
    - Sucralfate
    - Cholestyramine
    - Colestipol
    - Raloxifene
    - Soy
    - Calcium salt
  - Assess for medications that enhance L-T-4 metabolism.
    - Dilantin
    - Tegretol
    - Phenobarbital
    - Rifampin
    - Amiodarone
    - Zoloft

Management Plan

Goal

- *Keep TSH within normal range.*
- *Keep free T-4 within normal range.*

Additional Management Goals

- *Avoid doses of thyroid replacement that can cause suppression of TSH, resulting in chemical hyperthyroidism.*
- *Avoid exacerbation of osteoporosis:*

○ *More than usual loss of bone mineral density can occur with a suppressed TSH level over an extended period.*

○ *Especially in elderly women (Felicetta, 2002)*

Pharmacologic

- Levothyroxine (L-T-4) replacement is the treatment for hypothyroidism.
  ○ Administer L-T-4 on an empty stomach to maximize absorption.
  ○ Usual starting dose is 50 mcg.
  ○ Increase dose to normalize TSH.
    ▪ Increase at monthly intervals.
    ▪ Usual dosage increase is 25 mcg.
- T-3 replacement is not needed.
  ○ L-T-4 acts as a prohormone.
  ○ L-T-4 is deiodinated into T-3 at the target tissue level.
- All cases of overt, or symptomatic, hypothyroidism should be treated.
- Some patients with subclinical hypothyroidism should be treated.
  ○ Especially in case of hyperlipidemia
  ○ Patients with even mild symptoms may feel better with pharmaceutical treatment.
- Elderly patients
  ○ Start with low dose and increase slowly to normalize TSH.
  ○ Starting dose: 12.5 or 25 mcg
  ○ Increase at 6-week intervals.
  ○ Monitor every 6 weeks for stabilization of TSH.
  ○ Avoid TSH suppression.
- Elderly patients with severe coronary artery disease
  ○ Even low dose of L-T-4 may cause the following:
    ▪ Severe angina
    ▪ Cardiac arrhythmias
  ○ Partially treated hypothyroidism (low dose of L-T-4):

- ▪ May cause hyperlipidemia
- ▪ May result in exacerbation of heart disease

Patient, Family, and Staff Education

- Hypothyroidism is a chronic disease.
- It is necessary to take thyroid replacement for a lifetime.
- Appropriate dosing schedule for thyroid replacement
- Signs and symptoms of hypothyroidism
- References and further education
  ○ Health care organizations
  ○ Hospitals
  ○ Clinics
- Assessment skills leading to early recognition of hypothyroidism
- Signs and symptoms in the elderly may be easily misinterpreted as the following:
  ○ The aging process
  ○ Comorbid diseases
  ○ The side effects of medications
- L-T-4
  ○ Long half-life
  ○ Give first thing in the morning on an empty stomach.
  ○ Without other medications
- Adherence to the optimal dosing schedule of L-T-4
  ○ Can help avoid underdosing
  ○ Can avoid overdosing
- Thyroid replacement must be taken for a lifetime.
- Thyroid function (TSH and free T-4) should be checked 6 weeks after each dosage adjustment.
- Assessment skills leading to early recognition of hyperthyroidism due to excessive doses of L-T-4

○ Angina

○ Arrhythmias

○ Myocardial infarction

○ Compression fractures secondary to osteoporosis

Physician Consultation

• Newly diagnosed hypothyroidism

• TSH cannot be kept in normal range despite adjustment of L-T-4 dosage.

• New-onset angina pectoris or cardiac arrhythmias

• If patient is on L-T-4 for postsurgical hypothyroidism

• Exacerbation of comorbid diseases

▧ THYROID NODULES

by Doreen Bacon and Yung-In Choi

Definition

Thyroid nodules are masses attached to the thyroid gland. Although most thyroid nodules are benign, infrequently they are malignant. Thyroid nodules with signs of hyperthyroidism point to a hot nodule or toxic multinodular goiter. Hot nodules are usually benign. A firm, irregular thyroid with signs of hypothyroidism suggests goitrous Hashimoto's thyroiditis. Cold nodules are hypofunctioning, and have a somewhat increased risk of malignancy.

Radiation therapy, widely used from the 1920s to the 1950s for treatment of benign diseases such as enlarged thymus, tonsils, and adenoids, as well as acne, increases risk of both thyroid nodules and thyroid cancer.

Thyroid nodules come to the attention of the medical provider through the following:

• Discovery by the patient

• An incidental finding during the following:

○ Routine physical examination

○ CT scan

○ Carotid ultrasound

Epidemiology

The thyroid gland weighs 15–20 gm in the adult, and it is the largest endocrine gland in the body. In a 15-year Framingham, Massachusetts, study, thyroid nodules were palpable in 6.4% of women and 1.5% of men (Vander, Gaston, & Dawber, 1968). A Minnesota study reported in 1955 that thyroid nodules were noted in 57% of autopsies studied (Mortensen, Woolner, & Bennett, 1955). A prospective study to examine the prevalence of thyroid nodules showed that 67 of 100 subjects demonstrated thyroid nodules on ultrasound and palpation (Ezzat, Sarti, Cain, & Braunstein, 1994).

Common Presenting Signs and Symptoms

• Asymptomatic

• Palpable nodules

• Enlarged thyroid

• Anxiety and apprehension of cancer

• Various signs/symptoms of hypothyroidism or hyperthyroidism

• History

○ History of head and neck irradiation

○ Family history of thyroid disease

○ Presence of hyper- or hypothyroid symptoms

• Physical

○ Height and weight

○ Blood pressure

○ Thyroid exam

○ Goiter

○ Cervical adenopathy (increased risk of malignancy)

Differential Diagnoses

• Benign tumors

○ Adenomas

○ Adenomatous nodules

- Cysts
- Goitrous Hashimoto's thyroiditis
- Teratoma
- Other rare, benign tumors
- Malignant neoplasms
  - Papillary carcinoma
  - Follicular carcinoma
  - Medullary carcinoma
  - Squamous cell carcinoma
  - Lymphoma
  - Anaplastic carcinoma
  - Sarcoma
  - Metastatic neoplasms

Essential Diagnostic and Laboratory Tests

- Thyroid-stimulating hormone (TSH)
  - The single most sensitive test for hypothyroidism and hyperthyroidism
- TSH with the positive finding of thyroid nodules
  - TSH is suppressed:
    - Suspect hot nodules.
    - Obtain a thyroid scan.
  - TSH is elevated:
    - Suspect Hashimoto's thyroiditis.
    - Obtain thyroid peroxidase (TPO) antibody.
  - TSH is normal:
    - Fine-needle aspiration (FNA)
    - For all nodules over 1 cm
- Serum calcitonin level
  - Elevated
  - Suspect medullary thyroid cancer
- Fine-needle aspiration (FNA) and cytology findings
  - Benign
  - Nondiagnostic

- Suspicious
- Malignant

Management Plan

- Based on FNA cytology findings

Nonpharmacologic

- FNA cytology benign
  - Follow medically
  - Repeat FNA if nodule grows.
- Nondiagnostic: requires repeat FNA
- Suspicious
  - About a 20% risk of malignancy
  - Surgery often advised
- Malignant: surgery required

Pharmacologic

Hormone therapy is rarely recommended for benign nodules.

Patient and Family Education

- Palpable thyroid nodules should be evaluated by a physician.
- Malignant nodules are uncommon.
- References and further education
  - Health care organizations
  - Hospitals
  - Clinics

Physician Consultation

Refer all thyroid nodules or suspected nodules to an endocrinologist.

▰ RESOURCES

Web Sites

- American Diabetes Association—www.diabetes.org
- American Association of Clinical Endocrinologists—www.aace.com

- Joslin Diabetes Center—www.joslin.org
- American Association of Diabetes Educators—www.aadenet.org
- National Diabetes Education Program—www.ndep.nih.gov
- American Thyroid Association—www.thyroid.org
- Hormone Foundation—www.hormone.org
- Thyroid Foundation of America—www.tsh.org

Other Sources

Belfiore, A., Rosa, G. L., Giuffrida, D., Regalbuto, C., Lupo, L., Fiumara, A., et al. (1995). The management of thyroid nodules. *Journal of Endocrinological Investigation, 18*(2), 155.

Franklyn, J. A. (1994). Drug therapy: The management of hyperthyroidism. *New England Journal of Medicine, 330,* 1731.

Ortiz, R., Hupart, K. H., DeFesi, C. R., & Surks, M. I. (1998). Effect of early referral to an endocrinologist on efficiency and cost of evaluation and development of treatment plan in patients with thyroid nodules. *Journal of Clinical Endocrinology and Metabolism, 83,* 3803.

Torring, O., Tallstedt, L., Wallin, G., et al. (1996). Graves' hyperthyroidism: Treatment with antithyroid drugs, surgery, or radioiodine: A prospective, randomized study. *Journal of Clinical Endocrinology and Metabolism, 81,* 2986.

REFERENCES

American Diabetes Association. (2005). Retrieved February 4, 2006, from http://www.diabetes.org

Canaris, G. J., Manowitz, N. R., Mayor, G. M., & Ridgeway, E. C. (2000). The Colorado thyroid disease prevalence study. *Archives of Internal Medicine, 160,* 526–534.

Davies, T. F. (2000). Causes of thyrotoxicosis: Graves' disease. In L. E. Braverman & R. D. Utiger (Eds.), *Werner and Ingbar's the thyroid* (8th ed., pp. 518–531). Philadelphia: Lippincott Williams and Wilkins.

Davis, P. J., & Davis, F. B. (1974). Hyperthyroidism in patients over the age of 60 years. *Medicine (Baltimore), 53,* 161–181.

Ezzat, S., Sarti, D. A., Cain, D. R., & Braunstein, G. D. (1994). Thyroid incidentalomas: Prevalence by palpation and ultrasonography. *Archives of Internal Medicine, 154,* 1838–1840.

Felicetta, J. V. (2002). Thyroid disease in the elderly: When to suspect, when to treat. *Consultant,* November, 1597–1606.

Fitzgerald, P. (2005). Endocrinology. In L. Tierney, S. McPhee, S. Papadakis, & M. Lang (Eds.), *Current medical diagnosis and treatment* (44th ed., pp. 1085). New York: Medical Books/McGraw-Hill.

Harris, M. I., Flegal, K. M., Cowie, C. C., et al. (1998). Prevalence of diabetes, impaired fasting glucose, and impaired glucose tolerance in U.S. adults. The Third National Health and Nutrition Examination Survey, 1988–1994. *Diabetes Care, 21,* 518–524.

Helfand, M., & Redfern, C. C. (1998). Clinical guideline, part 2. Screening for thyroid disease: An update. *Annals of Internal Medicine, 129,* 144–158.

Hollowell, J. G., Staehling, N. W., Flanders, W. D., et al. (2002). Serum TSH, T4, and thyroid antibodies in the United States population (1988 to 1994): National Health and Nutrition Examination Survey (NHANES III). *Journal of Clinical Endocrinology and Metabolism, 87,* 489–499.

Ladenson, P. W., Singer, P. A., Ain, K. B., et al. (2000). American Thyroid Association guidelines for detection of thyroid dysfunction. *Archives of Internal Medicine, 160,* 1573–1575.

Lahey, F. A. (1931). Non-activated (apathetic) type of hyperthyroidism. *New England Journal of Medicine, 204,* 747–748.

Mortensen, J. D., Woolner, L. B., Bennett, W. A. (1955). Gross and microscopic findings in clinically normal thyroid glands. *Journal of Clinical Endocrinology and Metabolism, 15,* 1270.

National Diabetes Information Clearinghouse. (2005). Retrieved February 4, 2006, from http://diabetes.niddk.nih.gov

Resnick, B. (2005). Diabetes management: The hidden challenge of managing hyperglycemia in long-term care settings. *Annals of Long-Term Care: Clinical Care and Aging, 13*(8), 26–32.

Vander, J. B., Gaston, E. A., & Dawber, T. R. (1968). The significance of non-toxic thyroid nodules: Final report of a 15-year study of the incidence of thyroid malignancy. *Annals of Internal Medicine, 69,* 537.

White, R. D. (2004). Hyperthyroidism: Current standards of care. *Consultant, 44*(8), 1085–1090.

Wild, S., Roglie, G., Green A., et al. (2004). Global prevalence of diabetes: Estimates for the year 2000 and projections for 2030. *Diabetes Care, 27*(5), 1047–1053.

CHAPTER 9

Gastrointestinal Disorders

Eileen Simpson and Chris Butler

■ PANCREATIC CANCER

Definition

Pancreatic cancers are moderately well-differentiated mucinous adenocarcinomas originating from pancreatic duct epithelium. These cancers usually develop when malignant cells form in these tissues of the pancreas (Sial & Catalano, 2001).

Epidemiology

Pancreatic cancer is the fifth most common gastrointestinal cancer. The worldwide incidence is approximately 170,000 new cases annually with 168,000 deaths. In the United States there are 29,000 cases annually, and almost all will die within 1 year (Ahlgren, 2001). Most patients are between 65 to 80 years old at the time of diagnosis; the incidence rises sharply after age 50. There is an increased incidence in people who are diabetic or have chronic pancreatitis caused by chronic inflammation or irritation. In addition, alcohol consumption is the most common cause of chronic pancreatitis. Cigarette smoking increases the risk of developing pancreatic cancer by 30% (Sial & Catalano, 2001). There is also evidence that those who have a high intake of red meat and fat in their diet are at higher risk of developing pancreatic cancer. Seventy-five

percent of the tumors originate from the head of the pancreas, and 25% arise from the tail. In addition, most tumors arise from the exocrine duct cells. There are some patients who have a genetic predisposition to pancreatic cancer, such as those with familial breast cancer associated with the BRCA2 gene, hereditary pancreatitis, and familial atypical multiple mole-melanoma syndrome. Also, more African-Americans are afflicted with pancreatic cancer, and there is a higher incidence in men than women as well as those who are obese and lead a sedentary lifestyle (Barkin & Goldstein, 1999).

Common Presenting Signs and Symptoms

Early signs and symptoms are usually nonspecific, and when they are diagnosed it is usually too late for therapeutic intervention (Ahlgren, 2001).

- Specific signs and symptoms usually result from invasion of the tumor into structures adjacent to the pancreas.

  Those signs and symptoms are usually the following:
  - Nausea
  - Weight loss
  - Abdominal pain

○ Anorexia

○ Fatigue

○ Abdominal distention

○ Pruritis

○ Depression

○ Steatorrhea

- However, in 70% of the cases the most common presenting symptom is epigastric pain that radiates to the mid or lower back; often the pain is increased after eating (Ahlgren, 2001). This pain may be alleviated by leaning forward or sitting up straight.

- Jaundice may also be the only presenting sign.

Differential Diagnosis

- Cholelithiasis

- Acute pancreatitis

- Hepatitis

- Gastric ulcer disease

Essential Diagnostic and Laboratory Tests

- Abdominal ultrasound

- MRI/CT scan shows tumor in 80% of cases.

- Amylase and/or lipase is elevated.

- Complete blood count (CBC) shows mild anemia.

- Liver function tests

- Stool may be positive for occult blood, which indicates presence of cancer in the ampulla of Vater.

- Spiral CT scans are the most helpful in delineating the extent of the pancreatic mass.

- Endoscopic retrograde cholangiopancreatography (ERCP) involves injection of dye into the pancreatic and bile ducts.

- Endoscopic ultrasound

- Percutaneous transhepatic cholangiography (PTC)

- CA 19 = 9 used to support the diagnosis of pancreatic or hepatobiliary tumors and to monitor patient's response to treatment.

Staging of Tumors

Staging by the tumor, node, metastasis (TNM) classification:

- T1—Tumor is limited to the pancreas.

- T1a—If tumor is < 2 cm

- T1b—If tumor is > 2 cm

- T2—If tumor has extended into the duodenum, bile duct, or peripancreatic tissues

- T3—If tumor has extended into the stomach, spleen, colon, or adjacent vessels (Sial & Catalano, 2001)

Management Plan

Nonpharmacologic

For the treatment of advanced pancreatic cancer, the goal is quality of life with palliative treatment and pain control. Usually, if there is pain related to tumor invasion into the celiac plexus, the patient can be treated with ethanol ablation to relieve pain (Sial & Catalano, 2001).

- Abdominal laparotomy to attempt resection—This operation is usually attempted in 30% of patients and in those lesions strictly limited to the head of the pancreas. A radical pancreadeodectomy (Whipple procedure) may be attempted with a 1–2% efficacy of the procedure. Only 20% of patients with pancreatic cancer are surgical candidates, and less than 5% of those have a 5-year survival rate. One of the main obstacles to tumor resection is involvement of the major vessels (Sial & Catalano, 2001).

- Radiation therapy—External beam radiation therapy is helpful in achieving control of local tumor growth and pain control.

- Stents—Those patients with obstructive jaundice may get some relief with placement of a biliary stent.

- Prevention of complications—Avoid problems with glucose metabolism, jaundice, pain control, treatment of depression and metastasis.
- Consider hospice referral.

Pharmacologic

- Elderly patients may not be candidates for aggressive medical treatment or chemotherapy for pancreatic cancer because of advanced age, multiple comorbidities, and overall frail condition. An open and honest discussion with the patient and family regarding the diagnosis and prognosis of pancreatic cancer can help in avoiding the expectation of unrealistic outcomes.
- Chemotherapy—May be the only option for some patients with pancreatic cancer. Even with chemotherapy, the survival rate is one year or less. The agents most often used are fluorouracil (5-FU), mitomycin C, streptozotocin, ifosfamide, and doxorubicin. Gemcitabine has also been used in patients with advanced disease (Sial & Catalano, 2001).
- Pain control—Initially nonsteroidal anti-inflammatory drugs are used, then progressing to nonopioid pain medications. See Chapter 22, Pain Management.
- Treat for pruritis caused from excess bilirubin with Benadryl or Atarax.

Patient, Family, and Staff Education

- Discuss with patient and family treatment options and realistic treatment goals.
- Explain disease course and progression and expected symptoms with the patient and family.
- Discuss intensity-of-care issues and review advanced directive with patient and family.

Physician Consultation

- Treatment of a patient with pancreatic cancer is always done in conjunction with an oncologist and/or gastroenterologist.

- Refer to a surgeon if the patient is a surgical candidate.

◼ COLON CANCER

Definition
Colorectal cancers are almost all adenocarcinomas that tend to form bulky exophytic masses or annular constricting lesions. Approximately one half of these tumors are in the rectosigmoid area. The majority of these cancers arise from malignant transformation of adenomatous polyps (Sial & Catalano, 2001).

Epidemiology
Colorectal cancer is the most common gastrointestinal cancer in the United States. This form of cancer is the second leading cause of cancer in the country. The incidence rises sharply after the age of 50 years old. In 1999 more than 140,000 new cases of colorectal cancer were diagnosed in the United States. The average lifetime risk of developing colon cancer is 6%. Men and women are affected equally (Ahlgren, 2001).

There are high-risk groups who are more likely to develop colorectal cancer. Those individuals with a positive family history of colon cancer, adenomatous polyps, chronic ulcerative colitis, or Crohn's colitis have a higher risk for colorectal cancer. The colorectal cases are the highest in countries with a high-fat, low-fiber diet. Therefore, the United States, Canada, Argentina, Uruguay, most of Western Europe, New Zealand, and Australia have the highest incidence of colorectal cancer. Lifestyle also increases the risk of developing colorectal cancer; those who smoke, drink alcohol excessively, or are sedentary have an increased chance of developing this type of cancer (Ahlgren, 2001).

Common Presenting Signs and Symptoms

- Signs and symptoms are dependent on tumor location. Slow-growing tumors may be present several years before signs and symptoms occur.

- Iron deficiency anemia due to chronic blood loss
- Colicky abdominal pain with a change in bowel habits
- Constipation may alternate with periods of increased frequency of stools and loose stools.
- Decreased caliber of stool
- Frequent gas pain
- Bloating or fullness
- Weight loss
- Fatigue
- Vomiting
- Bright red blood in stools or maroon-colored stools
- Palpable mass in abdomen (late stages)
- Hepatomegaly (suggests metastatic spread)

Differential Diagnosis

- Irritable bowel syndrome
- Diverticulitis
- Infectious colitis
- Hemorrhoids

Essential Diagnostic and Laboratory Tests

- Complete blood count (CBC) with differential
- Liver function tests (LFTs)—If elevated may indicate metastasis
- Carcinoembryonic antigen (CEA)
- Chest X-ray to chest (to check for metastasis)
- Computerized tomography (CT) scan of the abdomen
- Colonoscopy

Staging of Tumor (After Biopsy)

Dukes Classification

- Stage 0—Carcinoma in situ
- Stage I—Tumor invades submucosa and or muscularis propria.

- Stage II—Tumor invades into subserosa or into nonperitoneal pericolic or perirectal tissues. Or tumor perforates the visceral peritoneum or directly invades other organs or structures.
- Stage III—Any degree of bowel wall perforation with lymph node metastasis, with 1–3 pericolic or perirectal lymph nodes involved. There may also be metastasis to lymph nodes along the vascular trunk.
- Stage IV—Presence of distal metastasis (Sial & Catalano, 2001)

Management Plan

Nonpharmacologic

- Surgical resection is the treatment of choice for all patients with colon cancer. However, chronically ill elderly patients residing in a long-term care facility may not be a surgical candidate or desire surgery. The clinician needs to evaluate each patient on an individual basis taking into consideration the patient's overall medical condition, comorbidities, and the patient's and the family's desire for medical or surgical treatment.
- Radiotherapy is recommended for stage II–III colorectal cancers if patient is able to tolerate and desires treatment.

Pharmacologic

Chemotherapy

- Stage I—Not warranted because of the 5-year survival rate of 80–90%.
- Stage II—Node-negative chemotherapy is usually not warranted. Five-year survival rate is between 50–75%.
- Stage III—Adjuvant chemotherapy with fluorouracil and levamisole has been shown to increase survivability. Five-year survival rate is 30–50% (Sial & Catalano, 2001).
- Stage IV—These patients have less than 5% survival rate. Systemic chemotherapy does not appear to prolong survival.

Follow-Up After Surgery

Patients are followed closely for tumor recurrence. Colonoscopy every 6 months to 1 year after surgery, then every 3 years if no tumor is found. Repeat CEA at time of surgery and then again every 3 months for the first year and then every 6 months for 3–4 years (Bond, 2000).

Patient, Family, and Staff Education

- Ensure patient and family receive detailed explanation of the risks and benefits of surgical resection of tumors, radiation therapy, and chemotherapy.
- Discuss treatment options and quality-of-life issues, especially for advanced disease.
- Advise family members of the risks they have for colon cancer. Advise screening test as necessary and recommended.

Physician Consultation

Any patient with suspected colon cancer should be referred to a gastroenterologist for further evaluation and treatment.

GASTROINTESTINAL BLEEDING

Definition

Gastrointestinal (GI) bleeding can be defined as either originating in the upper or lower GI tract. Upper GI bleeding is seen with coffee ground emesis, hematemesis, melena, or hematochezia. Lower GI bleeding is seen with hematochezia but is usually defined as bleeding arising below the ligament of Treitz, meaning the small intestine or colon, particularly in the sigmoid and anorectal region (McQuaid, 2005).

Epidemiology

There are over 350,000 hospitalizations a year in the United States due to gastrointestinal bleeding. Mortality is approximately 8–10%.

The rate can be 40% or higher in those patients with liver disease or other serious medical problems. Most deaths occur in patients who are older and have severe medical problems (Pianka & Affronti, 2001).

Upper GI Bleeding
- Posterior nasal
- Peptic ulcer disease—Accounts for half of major upper GI bleeding (McQuaid, 2005)
- Gastritis
- Duodenal ulcer
- Osler-Weber-Rendu syndrome
- Duodenitis
- Esophageal varices
- Mallory-Weiss tear
- Esophagitis
- Gastric cancer
- Gastric arteriovenous malformations
- Portal gastropathy
- Dieulafoy's lesion

Lower GI Bleeding
Small Bowel
- Angiodysplasia
- Jejunoileal diverticula
- Meckel's diverticulum
- Neoplasms or lymphomas

Large Bowel
- Diverticular disease
- Arteriovenous malformations
- Colitis
- Colonic neoplasms
- Anorectal causes
- Colonic tuberculosis

Common Presenting Signs and Symptoms

Examination should include a through cardiac, pulmonary, abdominal and rectal examination.

Upper GI Bleeding
- Hematemesis—Bright red blood or coffee ground emesis
- Melena
- Shock—Unstable vital signs (positive orthostatic vital signs indicate instability)
- Lightheadedness
- Pallor
- Bright red blood from rectum may indicate upper GI bleeding

Lower GI Bleeding
- Hematochezia
- Bright red blood from rectum
- Shock—Unstable vital signs versus orthostasis
- Lightheadedness
- Pallor

If these signs and symptoms occur, the patient should be transferred to the acute care hospital setting. However, a large bore intravenous line may be started while awaiting transport to the acute hospital.

Differential Diagnosis
Ingestion of medication or food that appear like blood in emesis or stool, such as Pepto-Bismol, iron supplements (can mimic melena), and beets can mimic bright red blood in rectum.

Essential Diagnostic and Laboratory Tests
- Complete blood count (CBC) with differential
- International normalized ratio (INR) and coagulation studies
- Chemistry 7 (sodium, potassium, glucose, blood urea nitrogen (BUN), creatinine, chloride, CO_2). BUN may be elevated due to excess protein load due to presence of blood in the intestine.
- Type and cross for potential blood transfusion
- Liver function tests—alanine aminotransferase (ALT), aspartate aminotransferase (AST), total bilirubin, alkaline phosphatase

- Amylase
- Stool for occult blood
- 12-lead EKG especially in those patients over 50 years old (loss of blood may precipitate cardiac ischemia and possible silent myocardial infarct)
- Abdominal X-rays—Acute abdominal series with a chest X-ray (to assess for free air and identify possible perforated viscus.
- Abdominal CT scan
- Nasogastric tube for upper GI bleeds
- Upper endoscopy and colonoscopy

Management Plan
Usually, the management of acute gastrointestinal bleeding is done in the acute care setting.

Nonpharmacologic—Upper GI Bleeding
- Support airway, breathing and circulation (ABCs).
- Assess volume loss; orthostatic changes and hypotension suggests a volume loss of 15–20%.
- Insert nasogastric tube.
- Serial Hgb/Hct every 2 hours during active bleeding
- Transfusion of packed RBCs to achieve a Hct of 25–30% (based on age and cardiac status; threshold to transfuse in an older patient is lower than in a younger patient).
- Transfusion of fresh frozen plasma (FFP) one unit for every 5 units of RBCs
- Consider platelet transfusion if platelet count is < 60,000/uL.
- Upper endoscopy performed after patient is hemodynamically stable.
- Surgery if bleeding is not controlled with endoscopy medications or transfusions.

Pharmacologic—Upper GI Bleeding
- IV H2 receptors antagonists—Dose sufficient to maintain intragastric pH of 4.0
  ○ Cimetidine 37.5–50 mg/hour
  ○ Ranitidine 6.25 mg/hr

○ Famotidine 1 mg/hr

○ IV proton pump inhibitors such as Prilosec, Protonix

- Octreotide IV infusion 50–100 mg/hr
- Vasopressin IV 0.2–0.6 units/min (usually reserved for patients with esophageal varices)
- Eradication of *H. pylori* infection

Nonpharmacologic—Lower GI Bleeding
- Support airway, breathing and circulation (ABCs).
- Assess volume loss as above.
- Exclude upper GI bleeding with NG tube and saline lavage.
- Anoscopy/sigmoidoscopy and possible colonoscopy (usually performed within 6–24 hours after admission)
- Possible surgical intervention—Most patients with severe lower gastrointestinal bleeding do not require surgery. Most have intermittent bleeding or can be controlled with nonsurgical techniques. Surgical intervention is required when hemodynamic instability persists.
- Transfusions and serial Hgb and Hct.

Pharmacologic—Lower GI Bleeding
- Discontinue non-steroidals (NSAIDS) and aspirin (ASA) immediately.
- Intra-arterial vasopressin or embolization angiography (the intra-arterial infusion of vasopressin may arrest bleeding in 90% of patients with active bleeding from diverticulum or vascular ectasia)

Patient, Staff, and Family Education
- Discuss the need for and the patient's/families desire for transfer back to the acute hospital.
- Discuss intensity of care issues and review advanced directive with patient and family.
- Explain that signs and symptoms of GI bleeding may include pallor, lightheadedness, dizziness, blood in stool or emesis, increased pulse, and altered mental status.
- Explain importance of holding aspirin, NSAIDS if bleeding suspected.
- Explain importance of monitoring of blood pressure and other vital signs to nursing staff.
- Explain importance of avoiding alcohol to patients and family.

Physician Consultation
- Consult physician on all cases when GI bleeding is suspected.
- Consult physician if patient requires transfer back to the acute hospital.

▰▰▰ HEPATITIS B

Definition
Hepatitis B is a viral infection of the liver caused by a virus belonging to the Hepadnaviridae family of viruses. This virus consists of double-stranded circular DNA. Acute infection is subclinical in 70% of adults and 90% of children. The incubation period after infection lasts 1–4 months. Hepatitis B can also take the form of a chronic infection. In addition, approximately 20% of those with hepatitis B go on to have chronic hepatitis B (Shapira & Yoshida, 2005).

Epidemiology
Hepatitis B causes a significant morbidity and mortality worldwide. More than 400 million persons, including 1.25 million Americans, have chronic hepatitis B (Shapira & Yoshida, 2005). Acute virus B hepatitis is a disease primarily of young people, and it is mostly seen in drug abusers, homosexuals, those with multiple sexual partners, and those who've given blood before screening of blood donors became routine. The majority of patients with hepatitis recover and clear their blood of infection. A few patients develop fulminant hepatitis, which can be fatal.

Common Presenting Signs and Symptoms

Acute Hepatitis

- Incubation period—Between 45 and 160 days, average 120 days
- Prodromal phase—General malaise, myalgia, arthralgia, easy fatigability, upper respiratory symptoms, anorexia out of proportion to degree of illness, nausea and vomiting, distaste for smoking, skin rashes, arthritis, low-grade fever, and mild abdominal pain located in the right upper quadrant. Hepatomegaly, liver tenderness, occasional splenomegaly.
- Icteric phase—Clinical jaundice may occur 5–10 days after initial signs and symptoms.
- Convalescent phase—Increased sense of well-being, return of appetite, and disappearance of jaundice; abdominal pain and fatigability also resolve.
- Course and complications: The acute illness usually subsides over 2–3 weeks.

Chronic Hepatitis

Chronic hepatitis is usually asymptomatic. (Shapira & Yoshida, 2005)

Differential Diagnosis

- Other viral illnesses
- Infectious mononucleosis
- Cytomegalovirus
- Herpes simplex
- Spirochetal diseases
- Brucellosis
- Rickettsial diseases
- Drug-induced liver disease
- Metastatic cancer

Essential Diagnostic and Laboratory Tests

- Complete blood count (CBC)
- Liver function tests—alanine aminotransferase (ALT), aspartate aminotransferase (AST), lactic dehydrogenase (LDH), total bilirubin, alkaline phosphatase
- Urinalysis
- Amylase
- Lipase
- Prothrombin Time, International Normalized Ratio (PT/PTT/INR)
- Hepatitis panel (see Table 9-1)

TABLE 9-1 Hepatitis Testing		
SEROLOGY	**APPEARANCE/DISAPPEARANCE**	**APPLICATION**
HAV-Ab/IgM	4–6 wk/3–4 mo	Acute HAV infection
HAV-Ab/IgG	8–12 wk/10 yr	Previous HAV exposure/immunity
HBeAg	1–3 wk/6–8 wk	Acute HBV infection
HBcAb	4–6 wk/4–6 yr	Acute HBV infection ended
HBsAb total	3–10 mo/6–10 yr	Previous HBV infection/ immunity indicated
HBVc-Ab/IgM	2–12 wk/3–6 mo	Acute HBV infection
HBVc-Ab total	3–12 wk/life	Previous HBV infection/ convalescent stage
HCV-Ab/IgG	3–4 mo/2 yr	Previous HCV infection
HDV Ag	1–3 days/3–5 days	Acute HDV infection
HDV-Ab/IgM	10 days/1–3 mo	Acute HDV infection
HDV-Ab total	2–3 mo/7–14 mo	Chronic HDV infection

Source: Pagana & Pagana, 1998.

- If there is a live virus and infection, either acute, chronic, or carrier, the HBsAg (hepatitis B surface antigen) test is the first to become abnormal. It rises before the onset of symptoms and returns to normal by the time jaundice resolves. If the level of this antigen persists in the blood, the patient is considered to be a carrier.

- The HBsAb (hepatitis B surface antibody) appears approximately 4 weeks after the disappearance of the surface antigen and signifies the end of the acute infection phase. The presence of this antibody also denotes immunity after the administration of hepatitis B vaccine.

- The HBcAb (hepatitis B core antibody) appears one month after infection with HBsAg. This may also be present in patients with chronic hepatitis. This level is elevated from the appearance of HBsAg and the disappearance of HBsAb.

Chronic Hepatitis B

Some patients infected with hepatitis B do not clear HBV infection; they continue to have a positive HBsAg. In most cases the chronic infection becomes nonreplicative and the patient loses HBeAg. In chronically infected individuals, the infection can switch from nonreplicative to replicative. The goal of treatment is to convert patients with chronic hepatitis B from active (replicative) (HBeAg positive) to a dormant (non-replicative) (HBeAg negative) state.

Chronic infection develops in approximately 90% of persons infected at birth and about 30% of those infected before the age of 6 years. Most persons who are infected later in life clear the infection completely; chronic HBV infection develops in only about 6% of these patients.

There are four phases of chronic HBV infection:

- Phase 1—Immune tolerant phase is secondary to perinatal transmission. Rarely occurs in patients who are infected as adolescents. This phase lasts for 10–30 years with elevated levels of HBV DNA but normal liver enzyme levels.

- Phase 2—Immune clearance phase occurs in the second to fourth decade of infections acquired at birth or early childhood. These patients have high levels of HBV DNA, fluctuating liver function tests, and presence of HBeAg. The HBV DNA levels eventually decrease, but patients are at increased risk for cirrhosis and hepatocellular carcinoma.

- Phase 3—Inactive carrier phase is characterized by low levels of HBV DNA, normal LFTs, and presence of hepatitis HBe antibody.

- Phase 4—Reactivation phase is considered reactivation of HBV replication. The patient has high levels of HBV DNA and liver function tests (LFTs) are elevated (Shapira & Yoshida, 2005).

Management Plan

Treatment goal is to achieve sustained suppression of HBV replication and remission of liver disease.

Nonpharmacologic

- Bedrest is recommended only on an as-needed basis during the acute phase of the illness.
- Gradually return to normal activity during convalescent period.
- Bland diet
- Avoid strenuous physical exertion.
- Avoid alcohol and hepatotoxic agents.
- Routine labs with serial LFTs, hepatitis panel (See Table 9-1), and coagulation tests
- Hepatitis B is a reportable disease to the local department of health.

Pharmacologic

- IV fluids as needed
- Small doses (10 mg po every 8 hours as needed) of oxazepam if needed for anxiety

- Interferon-α—5,000,000 unit SQ or IM QID for 6–12 months (monitor for signs and symptoms of depression, rashes, and abnormal blood counts)
- Ribavirin for 6–12 months used in combination with interferon. Increases the ricologic reponse.

Patient, Family, and Staff Education
- Avoid alcohol and hepatotoxic agents such as Tylenol.
- Patients with chronic HBV infection should be counseled regarding lifestyle modifications and prevention of transmission. Advise patients not share razors, toothbrushes, and other items that may transmit blood.
- Advise patient not to donate blood, plasma, organs, tissue, or sperm.

Physician Consultation
- Any patient with a diagnosis of hepatitis B should be managed along with a gastroenterologist.
- If patient shows signs of encephalopathy, severe coagulopathy, or if fulminant, then hepatic failure is suspected and hospitalization may be necessary.

▬▬ HEPATITIS C

Definition
Hepatitis C is an inflammation of the liver caused by infection with hepatitis C virus and was previously known as non-A non-B hepatitis. The hepatitis C virus (HCV) is a small enveloped virus with a single-stranded RNA genome and an associated RNA polymerase that is responsible for viral replication. It is a member of the Flavivirus family that includes West Nile virus, yellow fever virus, and Dengue virus (Butt & Jacobson, 2005a).

Epidemiology
Hepatitis C virus infection is the most common blood-borne infection. It affects approximately 1.8% of the U.S. population. Most cases of chronic HCV infection have yet to be diagnosed. Most cases are in those patients who received blood transfusions prior to 1992, injected street drugs, or shared needles with someone who was positive for hepatitis C, or who were on long-term dialysis or had multiple sex partners. 70–80% of those infected develop chronic infection, which results in cirrhosis in about 20%, typically after a 20–30-year silent period.

Common Presenting Signs and Symptoms
Patients with hepatitis C are usually asymptomatic. Incubation period is usually 6–7 weeks. Clinical illness is usually accompanied by mild signs and symptoms or none at all. Hepatitis C is usually found during routine physical exam. If signs and symptoms do occur, they usually include the following:

- Jaundice
- Right upper quadrant pain
- Fatigue
- Decreased appetite
- Pale or clay-colored stools
- Dark urine
- Pruritis
- Ascites
- Bleeding varices
- Elevated liver function tests (LFTs)

Differential Diagnosis
- Hepatitis A
- Hepatitis B, D
- Hepatitis E
- Cirrhosis

- Other viral illnesses
- Cytomegalovirus
- Metastatic cancer
- Drug-induced liver disease

Essential Diagnostic and Laboratory Tests

- Complete blood count (CBC)
- Liver function tests (LFTs), alanine amino-transferase (ALT), aspartate aminotransferase (AST), total bilirubin, alkaline phosphatase
- Hepatitis panel (see Table 9-1):
  ○ Hepatitis C RNA quantitative
  ○ Hepatitis BSAg
  ○ Hepatitis ASAb
- Alpha-feto protein
- Urinalysis
- Albumin
- BUN/creatine
- HIV
- Iron studies
- Amylase
- Prothrombin time (PT/PTT), international normalized ratio (INR)
- RUQ ultrasound to assess for liver masses or cysts
- Liver biopsy

Management Plan

The goal of treating Hepatitis C is to prevent progression of the disease.

Nonpharmacologic

- Supportive care
- Serial laboratory tests—Liver function tests, CBC, PT/PTT
- Hepatitis C is a reportable disease to the local department of health.

Pharmacologic

- Combination of treatments:
  ○ Pegylated interferon (PEG-IFN) alfa 2a or alfa 2b
  ○ Ribavirin (RBV)—This therapy is recommended for 48 weeks. If patient is still viremic. After 48 weeks prolongation of therapy for 72 weeks is recommended.
- Antidepressants for those who suffer from depression as a side effect of above treatment

Patient, Family, and Staff Education

- Instruct to avoid alcohol or liver toxic drugs such as Tylenol.
- Explain side effects of interferon therapy, which include flu-like symptoms, fatigue, arthralgia, and depression.

Physician Consultation

- Any patient with Hepatitis C should be managed along with a gastroenterologist.
- Consult with physician if patient develops side effects of treatment, such as neutropenia, thrombocytopenia, weight loss, diarrhea, thyroid dysfunction, anemia, or depression.

ACUTE PANCREATITIS

Definition

Acute pancreatitis is the onset of a sudden inflammatory process involving the pancreas and which may involve other abdominal tissues or more distant organ systems. It is usually associated with severe upper abdominal pain. However, the elderly frequently present with vague abdominal complaints, an unremarkable physical exam, and relatively normal amylase and lipase values "in spite of overt pancreatitis" (Haas & Singer, 2002). The clinician's index of suspicion should be heightened when dealing with abdominal complaints because of the high rate and early mortality associated with older age. In a Swedish study, one third of patients died in their homes from rapid, early progression of disease without being admitted to the hospital (Andersson & Andren-Sandberg, 2003). An English study came to the conclusion that patient mortality in the hospital had not improved since the 1970s, highlighting the lack of new treatments and emphasizing that pancreatitis carries a poor prognosis particularly in the acute phase (Goldacre & Roberts, 2004).

Acute pancreatitis usually leads to injury of acinar cells, fat necrosis, and or autodigestion of pancreatic cells. The interstitial form, comprising 80% of cases, is characterized by edema and inflammation within the parenchyma and microscopic necrosis. The second form, necrotizing pancreatitis, comprises 20% of cases (Haas, 2002) and can lead to macroscopic areas of necrotic damage, fat necrosis in the parenchyma, or bleeding either on the surface of the pancreas or in peripancreatic tissue (Feldman et al., 2002). It is the widespread systemic inflammatory response to acute pancreatitis that causes death in most instances (Bentrem & Joehl, 2003). Systemic complications are more likely from necrotizing pancreatitis (Feldman et al., 2002).

Epidemiology

The incidence of acute pancreatitis in England, Denmark, and the United States varies from 4.8 to 24.2 per 100,000. In women, one of the more common causes is cholecystitis; whereas, among men, alcoholic pancreatitis is a more common cause (Goldacre & Roberts, 2004). The incidence of this disease increases with age. Acute pancreatitis is three times more common among African-American males than Caucasian males. In those patients with alcoholic pancreatitis, the disease tends to manifest 5 to 10 years after commencing the heavy use of alcohol (Feldman et al., 2002).

Older patients are more likely to experience more serious forms of acute pancreatitis with a

poorer prognosis. Death may occur in 10% of all patients with acute pancreatitis experiencing severe disease even before the diagnosis is made (Feldman et al., 2002). Fifty percent of older patients who die of complications of acute pancreatitis do so within the first week of illness. The most common cause of death in that instance is adult respiratory distress syndrome (ARDS). During the second week of illness, most deaths are due to abscess, necrosis, or septicemia. Of those elders hospitalized for acute pancreatitis, 20% die as compared with 10% of hospitalized patients under the age of 50 years. This may be due in large part to the multiple medical problems usually experienced by the elderly (Hazzard et al., 2003).

Etiology

Among the elderly, gallstones are the cause of acute pancreatitis in more than 50% of cases; alcohol is the cause in 20–25%. Postoperative inflammation (postcoronary artery bypass graft [CABG] or postendoscopic retrograde cholangiopancreatography [ERCP] is another leading cause). Significantly, there are idiopathic causes reported frequently in this age group (see Table 9-2) (Hazzard et al., 2003).

Biliary sludge, common in a large segment of the elderly, is a solution of stones less than five millimeters in diameter, causing a thick solution to collect, and can be detected on sonogram. Cases like this are more likely to have a subtle presentation with fewer symptoms (Hazzard et al., 2003). Certain conditions that give rise to the potential for acute pancreatitis are shown in Table 9-2.

Pharmaceuticals may cause acute pancreatitis via toxic metabolites, which accumulate over time causing an immunologically mounted allergic reaction accompanied by rash and eosinophilia (Feldman et al., 2002).

Drugs thought to cause acute pancreatitis are considered to be causal only if other known causes of pancreatitis are not detected. If the medicine thought to be the offender is

TABLE 9-2 Conditions Predisposing to Acute Pancreatitis

- Gallstones
- Biliary sludge and microlithiasis
- Other causes of mechanical ampullary obstruction
- Alcohol
- Hypertriglyceridemia
- Hypercalcemia
- Drugs
- Infections and toxins
- Trauma
- Pancreas divisum
- Post-ERCP
- Postoperative pancreatitis
- Hereditary pancreatitis
- Structural abnormalities:
  - Duodenum/ampullary region
  - Bile duct
  - Sphincter of Oddi dysfunction
  - Main pancreatic duct

discontinued and symptoms resolve then resume again when the medicine is restarted, that implicates the drug as the offending agent. In Germany and Switzerland pancreatitis is thought to be caused by drugs in only 1.4% and 0.3% of cases, respectively. Drug-induced acute pancreatitis is more likely if the resident has additional risk factors for the disease such as hyperlipidemia, diabetes, hypothyroidism, or nephrotic syndrome. Drugs thought to cause pancreatitis include the following (Tivedi & Pitchumoni, 2005; Feldman et al., 2002):

- Thiazides
- Furosemide
- Ceftriaxone
- Nonsteroidal anti-inflammatories
- Immunosuppressive
- Sulfasalazine
- Mesalamine
- Sulfonamides
- Metronidazole
- Tetracycline
- Nitrofurantoin
- Valproic acid
- Calcium
- Estrogen
- Tamoxifen
- Beta-blockers
- ACE inhibitors
- AIDS therapy drugs

Other causes of acute pancreatitis are trauma, including iatrogenic; tumors or mechanical obstruction within the pancreas; vasculitis, which may be secondary to systemic lupus erythematosus (SLE) or polyarteritis nodosa; and emboli from cholesterol plaques after angiography, ERCP, or CABG. Metabolic causes such as hypertriglyceridemia, hypercalcemia, infection, and hereditary or structural abnormalities are additional causes of acute pancreatitis (Feldman et al., 2002).

Common Presenting Signs and Symptoms

- Presentation of acute pancreatitis in the elderly may seem vague and unimpressive to caregivers. Conversely, onset may be signaled by the sudden onset of severe pain in the upper abdomen/epigastric area and may radiate to the back or involve the whole abdomen. It may be accompanied by vomiting, epigastric tenderness, respiratory distress, or mild jaundice. It may quickly progress to a graphic picture of shock, hypothermia, multiorgan failure, and hyperglycemia (Hazzard et al., 2003).

- At autopsy, as many as 40% of older patients studied were found to have pancreatitis. These patients did not have a history of or the suspicion of pancreatitis in their medical records (Hazzard et al., 2003).

- Older people are at greater risk of developing pulmonary or renal failure and hemorrhage, rather than symptoms associated with milder and more localized presentation of acute pancreatitis (Hazzard et al., 2003).

- Systemic complications in addition to sepsis and encephalopathy include pleural effusion, myocardial depression, metabolic complications, and systemic inflammatory response syndrome (SIRS) caused by the disturbance of immune and bacteriological processes that facilitate bacterial transport via arteriovenous shunting, among other processes (Feldman et al., 2002).

- If altered, endocrine function usually returns to normal after the acute phase of pancreatitis, but exocrine function may take up to 12 months to return to normal function (Feldman et al., 2002). Other residual sequelae include scarring of the pancreas from necrosis and stricture. This can lead to malabsorption and a chronic form of pancreatitis (Feldman et al., 2002).

Essential Diagnostic and Laboratory Tests

- Abdominal flat plate may show a sentinel loop of gas filled jejunum, highlighting gallstones.

- A CT scan is the optimal choice for evaluation of the pancreas; it will likely reveal a normal gland versus the alcoholic pancreas. It may be necessary to perform a CT repeatedly before there is evidence of improvement.

- Ultrasound will assist in identifying gallstones, but is not helpful in evaluating the health of the pancreas itself (Feldman et al., 2002).

- In acute pancreatitis caused by gallstones, early ERCP and sphincterotomy have been

correlated with better outcomes among the elderly. If perforated peptic ulcer or strangulated bowel versus pancreatitis caused by gallstones are among the differential diagnoses, either requires swift surgical consultation, as might the possibilities of ischemic bowel or thrombus of the mesentery with gangrene. The latter, especially, may present clinically like an acute pancreatitis due to the pain level caused by the leakage of toxins. Perforated peptic ulcer can be excluded by means of an upper GI series using diatrizoate meglumine swallow material, not barium (Hazzard et al., 2003).

- Search for infection is a priority in the setting of pancreatic necrosis, which requires surgical intervention.

- Serum lipase should be elevated on day one of illness and stay elevated longer than amylase. Total serum amylase is a fast and inexpensive test that provides indication of acute pancreatitis about 6–12 hours after onset of symptoms. Amylase is not 100% sensitive or specific, but should remain elevated within 3–5 days of onset of symptoms (Feldman et al., 2002).

- If the workup involves ruling out perforated ulcer or hemorrhagic necrotizing pancreatitis and monitoring for infection, frequent complete blood counts will be followed closely with attention to the hematocrit and white cells/differential.

Management Plan
Surgery

If the cause of acute pancreatitis is gallstones, surgery is warranted for cholecystectomy and to clear the common bile duct of stones to prevent a recurrence (Feldman et al., 2002). Likewise, early operative debridement is required for those patients with infected necrosis, while residents with sterile necrosis or severe pancreatitis without necrosis are managed conservatively with improved outcomes (Malangoni, 2005; Hartwig et al., 2002).

Nonpharmacologic

- For nonsurgical patients the treatment is supportive: pain control, IV fluids with nothing by mouth, and close monitoring of glucose, amylase, lipase, electrolytes, and hemodynamics.

Pharmacologic

- In the past morphine sulfate and its derivatives have been avoided for treatment of pain associated with acute pancreatitis out of concern that its action increases tone in the sphincter of Oddi; however, this has come into question due to lack of clinical evidence. Meperidine, then, was the analgesia usually selected in the hospital, but this drug is usually not available in the nursing home. Furthermore, meperidine is not considered acceptable by most pain control experts, and should be avoided, particularly for the elderly.

- Proton pump inhibitors and H2 blockers and prophylactic antibiotics are not recommended in the mild form of disease. Use of nasogastric suction has not been found to impact the length of an episode of acute pancreatitis but may relieve distressing symptoms of nausea, vomiting, and abdominal distention (Friedman, 2003).

- There is a trend toward conservative management of acute pancreatitis in comparison with previous standards of care that focused on surgical intervention. The role of antibiotics is reserved primarily for those patients with infected necrosis (Feldman et al., 2002; Hartwig et al., 2002).

Patient, Family, and Staff Education

- In this setting a resident may be exposed to multiple invasive procedures and heroic measures to prolong life that may not be in line with their established goals of care. The family needs to understand the implications of the acute illness itself, and furthermore, that a hospitalization may not equal a positive outcome for the frail elderly individual.

- Educating the resident and family to the disease process, complications of disease, and the burdens and benefits of the hospital may help to minimize anxiety and alleviate concerns about the choices made regarding treatment options. Many families are anxious about the risks associated with a hospital stay. Psychological factors, such as stress, isolation, and an unfamiliar environment, may cause the resident to suffer needlessly, and the outcome of such an experience may not justify it.

- The potential to acquire a nosocomial infection could lead to dire consequences in a frail elder, so the family would be wise to give careful consideration to this and a host of other factors that should be balanced in making care decisions. The educational component that the nurse practitioner provides is critical to the quality of care that the frail elder receives and therefore has an enormous impact on the quality of life for nursing home residents during, and at the end of life.

Physician Consultation

Consult with physician on all patients suspected of having pancreatitis. In severe cases residents may be managed with the assistance of a specialist and or hospitalized. Any resident with a severe illness should be treated in accordance with goals of care previously established by the resident and family in conjunction with the primary care team. This is particularly important in the case of a resident with severe acute disease because that resident may be admitted to the ICU (Soran et al., 2000).

GASTROESOPHAGEAL REFLUX DISEASE

Definition

Gastroesophageal reflux disease (GERD) is the reverse flow of gastric material into the esophagus due to an inadequate sphincter or competent esophageal gastric junction (Langford & Thompson, 2004; Feldman et al., 2002). GERD is likely the most common condition seen in clinical practice. Because the prevalence of GERD increases with age, nurse practitioners working in long-term care must be knowledgeable in order to carefully screen and treat residents.

Patients may complain of heartburn, a substernal burning pain, acid backwash or generalized chest pain, among other complaints that might lead a clinician to consider GERD in the differential diagnosis (Hazzard et al., 2003).

Reflux esophagitis is experienced by some GERD patients, who are found to have mucosal lesions on endoscopy. Other patients with endoscopy negative GERD experience symptoms without signs of esophagitis detected on endoscopy. In some settings these patients may be diagnosed by 24-hour esophageal monitoring (Feldman et al., 2002).

Chronic GERD can cause a variety of esophageal, laryngeal, or pulmonary inflammatory injuries manifested by symptoms of pain or discomfort, cough, or wheezing (Pilotto et al., 2005). GERD can lead to pathological changes such as Barrett's esophagus (a premalignant condition), esophageal strictures, and a persistent hoarse voice, among other complications. In the western world, it is estimated that 10–20% of community dwellers report heartburn weekly (Mohammed et al., 2005).

Epidemiology

The prevalence of GERD among the elderly can be attributed to changes associated with aging, in particular, in motility and in mucosal tissue whose function is protective. Men and women experience GERD in equal numbers, but men develop esophagitis and Barrett's metaplasia in greater numbers (Feldman et al., 2002). The high incidence of esophagitis is seen on endoscopy in patients over age 50 who complain of heartburn (Hazzard et al., 2003).

An English study with a sample size of over 2000 reported that smoking, excess alcohol intake, irritable bowel syndrome, increasing body mass index (BMI), family history of gastrointestinal (GI) disease, anticholinergic and antidepressant drugs, and weight gain among other variables were associated with GERD symptoms (Mohammed et al., 2005).

A Gallup poll found that of 800 adults sampled, 20% reported over three episodes of GERD in the previous 30 days. Of those reporting symptoms, only 25% discussed the problem with a doctor (Geoff, 1999). Although the incidence of GERD is lowest in Africa and Asia, it is the number one GI complaint in the western world (Pilotto et al., 2005). Nurse practitioners in the long-term care setting must maintain a high index of suspicion in assessing nursing home residents, who may have been exposed to the irritating effects of gastric reflux for decades.

Barrett's esophagus is a consequence of untreated GERD. It is the transformation of normal esophageal mucosa to columnar epithelium or interstitial metaplasia. Barrett's esophagus is most often seen in patients between the ages of 55 to 65 years of age; 65–80% of whom are men. This disorder is rare among African-Americans. Approximately one third of Barrett's patients who present with adenocarcinoma report no history of GERD signs and symptoms (Hazzard et al., 2003).

Long-standing GERD's histopathological reactive changes to epithelium, even in the absence of endoscopic evidence of esophagitis, can lead to severe changes such as peptic strictures, pseudo diverticula, Barrett's esophagus, and inflammatory polyps. These are evidence of the body's attempt to repair injured tissue. Though rarely seen, additional complications are fistulas and perforations (Feldman et al., 2002).

Etiology

The etiology of GERD is multifactorial. Lower esophageal sphincter (LES) pressure is an important barrier to the reflux of acid into the esophagus. Its function is impaired by hiatal hernia, the irritating effects of gastric contents, decreased amplitude of esophageal peristalsis, delayed gastric emptying, certain foods, and commonly prescribed medications (Langford & Thompson, 2004).

The reflux and regurgitation of gastric contents and bile lead to irritation, corrosion, and formation of inflamed areas that form patchy surface lesions that may later extend to the whole of the esophagus. The process may advance to tissue necrosis, the transformation of normal cells to abnormal cells, scarring and narrowing of the esophageal passageway into strictures, and shortening of the esophagus (Feldman et al., 2002). Motility disorders, an ineffective acid barrier caused by a sliding hiatal hernia, and medications that increase reflux are other factors that increase the prevalence of GERD in this age group (Hazzard et al., 2003).

Nonsteroidal anti-inflammatories, thought to provoke GERD, were found to be a cause in 1 of 4 cases of reflux esophagitis in a large study of US veterans (Feldman et al., 2002). Drugs known to be contributing factors to lower esophageal sphincter (LES) incompetence are listed in Table 9-3.

Common Presenting Signs and Symptoms

- There is a lack of agreement among specialists as to what symptoms typify GERD. The nurse practitioner must be alert to an array of symptomatology that causes him or her to suspect GERD. Symptoms may range from heartburn to coughing and wheezing. Heartburn, an intermittent sign, usually presents within 60 minutes of eating (Hazzard et al., 2003). It may be the result of a meal of fatty or spicy foods, exercise, or body position.

TABLE 9-3 Factors that Contribute to LES Incompetence

DRUGS	FOODS
Alpha blockers	Chocolate
Anticholinergics	High fat content
Atropine	Mints
Calcium channel blockers	Citrus juice
Nitrites	Coffee
Theophylline	Tomato products
Valium	
Alcohol	
Nicotine	

Source: Hazzard et al., 2003.

- An atypical presentation of GERD may include hoarseness, dysphagia, nighttime cough, shortness of breath, poor dentition, jaw or ear pain, or recurrent pneumonia (Geoff, 1999). In addition to pneumonia or pneumonitis caused by aspiration, other respiratory conditions may be seen such as subglottic stenosis and laryngeal granulomas. There is also some evidence that GERD causes microaspiration leading to asthma or vagally mediated bronchospasm. Water brash, or excessive salivation, is also vagally mediated due to the presence of acid in the esophagus. It is thought to cause night cough and asthma-type symptoms (Hazzard et al., 2003).

- Based on review of the literature, there is conflicting opinion as to whether GERD is an actual cause of asthma. Experts think that GERD may be of minimal impact on pulmonary function; however, clinical data tends to support the notion that the treatment of GERD improves respiratory symptoms (Feldman et al., 2002).

- Epigastric or substernal pain are often difficult to distinguish from cardiac pain. Chest pain, dysphagia, and regurgitation are described as midcourse GERD signs. Later in the course of disease, heartburn may wane and dysphagia or bleeding may predominate (Langford & Thompson, 2004).

- In patients with such complaints, of chest pain, symptoms decreased with the use of proton pump inhibitors. This is thought to be due to lessened stimuli of afferent nerves, which are unable to distinguish between the origin of cardiac versus esophageal stimuli (Feldman et al., 2002).

- Esophagitis due to LES pressure may be caused by numerous factors including a sliding hiatal hernia or body positions that may increase intra-abdominal pressure. Residents with a history of pyloric surgery and/or a prolonged use of a nasogastric tube should be considered at risk for GERD (Langford & Thompson, 2004).

- In the older adult, the clinical picture is complicated by factors such as decreased amplitude of peristaltic action, which hampers esophageal acid clearance; the poor antireflux barrier in the setting of a hiatal hernia, and polypharmacy (Hazzard et al., 2003). Adults in a vegetative state are particularly susceptible to complications from repetitive reflux and aspiration. For example, nursing home residents who are bedridden with long-standing GERD have a greater risk of discomfort and/or complications, so are often treated with proton pump inhibitors as a precaution.

Differential Diagnosis

- Infectious esophagitis: rule out candidiasis, *H. pylori*

- Pill esophagitis

- Peptic ulcer disease

- Dyspepsia

- Biliary colic

- Coronary artery disease: rule out inferior myocardial ischemia; patients may present with what seems to be GI symptoms

- Esophageal cancer

- Esophageal motility disease

- Scleroderma, which causes impaired esophageal function (Feldman et al., 2002)

Essential Diagnostic and Laboratory Tests

- Endoscopy may be considered in the following situations, particularly as there is a lack of clarity on what constitutes "typical" GERD signs and symptoms:
  - A resident who has not responded to treatment
  - Instances where there is blood loss
  - Weight loss
  - Symptoms that are highly distressful to the resident
  - A history of Barrett's metaplasia

- Endoscopy and biopsy can detect and diagnose disease and severity. It can rule out other worrisome processes such as adenocarcinoma or Barrett's esophagus. A double-contrast barium swallow study will recognize strictures and ulcers but does not detect esophagitis or Barrett's metaplasia (Feldman et al., 2002).

- A common test for ambulatory patients, the 24-hour monitoring for pH, is impractical for long-term care residents and staff because it requires a transnasal probe and maintaining an activity journal throughout the course of the day (Feldman et al., 2002). It isn't likely that a resident will be able to tolerate a nasal tube or that a resident would be able or willing to maintain an activity journal.

Management Plan
Nonpharmacologic
Lifestyle adjustments can be helpful for those who suffer from GERD. After meals, maintaining an upright position for three hours can minimize reflux. Many find it helpful to elevate the head of the bed for sleep. Other

interventions include weight loss, wearing loose-fitting clothes, and discontinuing alcohol and cigarette smoking. These measures enhance the clearance of acid and diminish reflux (Feldman et al., 2002).

Pharmacologic

- It is reasonable to initiate a trial therapy with a proton pump inhibitor (PPI) in residents in whom you suspect have GERD. The risk is that therapy could mask peptic ulcer disease, Barrett's esophagus, or a malignancy, but if the resident and family are in agreement, a trial is appropriate. Examples of common PPIs used with usual doses are:
  - Esomeprazole (Nexium) 20–40 mg/daily
  - Lansoprazole (Prevacid) 30 mg/daily
  - Omeprazole (Prilosec) 20 mg/daily
  - Pantoprazole (Protonix) 40 mg/daily
  - Rabeprazole (AcipHex) 20 mg/daily
- The role of medications is to suppress acid. PPIs are most effective because they act on the final common pathway in acid secretion. They should be given 30 minutes before meals for optimal effect. PPIs cause rebound hypersecretion of acid when discontinued, and their effectiveness varies among individuals. Histamine (H2) blockers or receptor antagonists suppress acid production during sleep and fasting, but their disadvantage is that they cause tachyphylaxis and acid secretion stimulated by meals. Metoclopramide, an antidopaminergic agent, has a significant side effect profile, offers little benefit, and should be avoided in the elderly (Feldman et al., 2002).
- With respect to esophagitis, PPI therapy can heal approximately 80% of severe cases, but discontinuation of therapy hastens return of disease in 80% of cases, so maintenance therapy is required. For patients with nonerosive GERD, it is frequently more difficult to relieve heartburn. Studies indicate that intermittent or on-demand therapy may be

the best option. PPI therapy has been shown to decrease prevalence of peptic strictures. This therapy is not only cost effective, but enhances quality of life, given that strictures frequently require repeated dilation procedures (Feldman et al., 2002).

Patient, Family, and Staff Education

- Explain importance of eating meals in upright position.
- Explain that being overweight can increase pressure on the abdominal muscles and the stomach.
- Explain importance of discontinuing alcohol and cigarette smoking.

▒▒▒ ILEUS

Definition

Ileus is not an obstruction of the gastrointestinal (GI) tract per se but a process that causes the function of the colon to cease. There is no actual obstruction, but the clinical presentation is similar to that of an actual obstruction. Ileus then is a motility problem that is relatively common among older, inactive residents and is caused by a variety of factors. The pathophysiology of ileus is not understood; however, there seems to be agreement in the literature as to risk factors associated with it (Snape, 1999). Due to a lack of reflex nerve stimulation, probably because of a failure of electrical neurohormonal factors, peristaltic function is halted and paralysis sets in (Feldman et al., 2002).

Patients present with anorexia, cramping, nausea, and vomiting. The abdomen is distended and tympanic with varying degrees of pain. Patients often have a history of constipation and present with altered bowel habits. Fluid and gas collect above the ileus causing swelling. The resident will not be able to pass gas; with auscultation there may be high pitched or absent bowel sounds. There may be guarding or rebound tenderness, such that the patient appears to have an acute abdomen. The edematous bowel secretes fluid and electrolytes as distention builds. In a critical case pressure due to swelling can cause necrosis and lead to gangrene, compromised circulation, and hypovolemia (Langford & Thompson, 2004).

Epidemiology

The prevalence of ileus among the elderly or nursing home residents is not well documented, though intestinal obstructions account for 20% of all admission diagnoses of acute abdominal conditions in the United States (Langford & Thompson, 2004). Most of the literature deals with ileus in the postoperative setting and states that patients with other preexisting medical conditions associated with later life are predisposed to the development of ileus under the right circumstances. The nurse practitioner should maintain a high index of suspicion in residents who have a history of diabetes mellitus, cardiovascular or peripheral vascular disease, constipation, or the use of narcotics for pain control. These factors, combined with dehydration, polypharmacy, inactivity, poor bowel management, and inaccurate record-keeping on bowel movements, creates the potential for paralytic ileus among nursing home residents.

Staff may report "loose stool" or "diarrhea" that may be an indication that hard fecal material has blocked an area in the colon, allowing only liquid contents to pass through. Nurses who mistake this for diarrhea may administer antidiarrheal medication as needed and inadvertently aggravate the situation in a resident with constipation.

Etiology

The causes of acute colonic ileus may be postoperative due to inflammatory, metabolic neurogenic, or drug-related factors (see Table 9-4).

TABLE 9-4   Metabolic Causes of Ileus
• Decreased K+
• Decreased Na+
• Decreased Mg+
• Increased Mg+
• Decreased Ca+

Source: Feldman et al., 2002.

There may be intra-abdominal factors leading to the development of an ileus such as a perforated ulcer, diverticulitis, or appendicitis.

The timeframe regarding return to function in a postoperative patient is important to keep in mind, given that hospital stays are often short, and therefore nursing home residents may develop complications after transfer back to the nursing facility. Motility of the small intestine returns to baseline usually within 48 hours of surgery, or within 24 hours of a laparotomy. Large intestine motility returns in approximately 3–5 days. Signs and symptoms that warrant careful assessment of the resident are postoperative discomfort, increased metabolic demands, and prolonged immobilization (Feldman et al., 2002). After surgery the resident may complain of nausea, bloating, and show little interest in food.

Risk factors associated with abdominal surgery include incarcerated hernia, adhesions, intestinal swelling and distention, use of general anesthesia, narcotics and Lomotil, or foreign bodies (Langford & Thompson, 2004).

Inflammatory ileus may be caused by occult bleeding in the retroperitoneum, a lumbar compression fracture, trauma, pyelonephritis, acute pancreatitis, ischemia, or thrombus. Ogilvie's syndrome, a pseudo-obstructive process of the colon, is caused by inflammation and swelling from the cecum to the splenic flexure where a kink develops proximal to it (Feldman et al., 2002).

Other causes of ileus include lower rib fracture, lower lobe pneumonia, myocardial infarction and sepsis, pyelonephritis, ischemia, or mesenteric thrombus (Hazzard et al., 2003). A resident with severe constipation who develops pneumonia may present with ileus before the pneumonia is clinically apparent. Risk factors and comorbidities that increase a resident's chance of developing ileus are listed in Table 9-5.

Prescription drugs, as well as over-the-counter medicines have the potential to cause long-term complications; according to a study, 20–40% of drug-induced adverse effects are seen in the GI tract (Tolsti, 2002). Anticholinergic medications are a factor in the development of ileus. In the nursing home many medicines are ordered by providers unfamiliar with the Beers criteria, which lists medications that are dangerous for use in the elderly (see Chapter 2). Patients who are given narcotics as part of a pain regimen may have inadequate bowel regimens, increasing the likelihood that they will develop severe constipation. Examples of some of the common medications that may contribute to the development of ileus are calcium channel blockers and vitamin supplements, among others (Feldman et al., 2002).

Diabetic residents may suffer consequences of the disease such as gastroparesis or neurogenic or ischemic bowel damage to the GI tract. Nursing home residents experience constipation due to immobility, dehydration, low-fiber diet, polypharmacy, and poor toileting practices, all of which puts them at risk for ileus.

Common Presenting Signs and Symptoms

- Signs and symptoms may be subtle, such as the following:
  ○ Bloating
  ○ Nausea
  ○ Anorexia
  ○ Constipation
  ○ Diminished bowel sounds
  ○ Diffuse abdominal discomfort
  ○ Blood in the stool
- Staff may note a change in mental status or increase in confusion.
- Dramatic signs and symptoms may include the following:
  ○ Abdominal distention
  ○ Vomiting, absence of bowel sounds
  ○ Obstipation
  ○ Significant but poorly localized pain
  ○ Guarding and rebound tenderness
  ○ Residents may complain of shortness of breath, and the staff or nurse practitioner may note dyspnea or begin to suspect pneumonia or sepsis (Snape, 1999).

TABLE 9-5	Risk Factors or Comorbidities for Acute Ileus
POSTOPERATIVE	
Orthopedic procedures	Trauma
Organ transplantation	Patient > 65 years of age
Abdominal surgery	Severe heart disease
	Congestive heart failure
	Adult respiratory distress syndrome
	Pneumonia
	Mechanical ventilation
	Diabetes mellitus
	Narcotic use
	Incarcerated hernia
	Adhesions
	Renal disease
	Intestinal distention

Sources: Snape, 1999; Langford & Thompson, 2004.

Differential Diagnosis

- Diverticulitis
- Volvulus
- Intussusception

- Obstruction—The presence of severe, continuous pain that is localized suggests strangulation.
- Appendicitis
- Cholecystitis
- Pancreatitis—Sentinel loop will be seen in the epigastrium.
- Benign or malignant colonic strictures
- Adenocarcinoma
- Inflammatory bowel disease, such as Crohn's disease
- *C. difficile* infection
- Ischemic strictures
- Ulcerative colitis
- Fecal impaction (Snape, 1999; Feldman et al., 2002)

Essential Diagnostic and Laboratory Tests

- Plain abdominal radiography may reveal gas in the small intestine and colon. In a colonic ileus the bowel may be very distended with apparent gas, and the ileocecal valve prevents reflux back into the collapsed small bowel, but no obstructing lesion is detected.
- Previously, contrast barium studies were used if X-rays were unable to assist in diagnosis, but due to the tendency of barium to form a hard mass it is usually avoided.
- If the diagnosis cannot be made by radiography, computerized tomography (CT) scanning is used because it can identify other acute abdominal processes that would impact bowel function and assist in diagnosis (Feldman et al., 2002).
- Critical components of management include frequent complete blood counts (CBC) to rule out infection and electrolytes and urinalysis to rule out renal disease and to detect electrolyte abnormalities and assess hydration.

Management Plan
Nonpharmacologic
- Treatment of ileus is supportive and involves limitation of oral intake, either clear liquids or maintaining the patient with nothing by mouth (NPO). If liquids cause nausea or vomiting or bowel sounds are not evident, then NPO status is strictly maintained. Keeping residents NPO allows the bowel to rest, an important aspect of conservative treatment. Serial complete blood counts and electrolyte panels should be followed closely to rule out infection and to assist in correcting electrolytes. If residents are able to ambulate, exercise may help resolve ileus.
- Hypokalemia is most often seen, but one should continue to monitor and correct electrolytes, looking particularly for hypocalcemia, hypomagnesemia, or hypermagnesemia, among other disturbances.
- Although some nursing homes are not staffed or equipped to manage nasogastric tubes, if available, the nurse practitioner may wish to place a nasogastric tube, especially for a resident experiencing nausea and vomiting. Rectal tubes are helpful in decompression of the bowel, as an abdominal examination before and after the use of a rectal tube can illustrate. Likewise, use of a rectal tube may make the resident feel more comfortable and can be inserted on an as-needed basis two to three times a day. Frequent repositioning in bed may assist in the passage of flatus. If a patient is able, the knee to chest position may also help to expel flatus. Gentle administration of tap water enemas may help encourage bowel motility, but there is no evidence in literature to support their use.
- Medications that may contribute to causing an ileus should be stopped, and the resident's complete medication regimen should be reevaluated by the primary care team to ensure safety. A bowel regimen should be

initiated and titrated in order to promote motility and comfort.

Pharmacologic

- Administration of intravenous fluids is an important intervention in order to maintain fluid volume, hydration, and essential electrolyte balance while the resident is NPO. Electrolyte replacement may well be needed as serial labs are followed in the acute phase.

- If infection is a concern, a resident may be started on IV metronidazole. Somatostatin analogs and erythromycin have not proven to be beneficial therapies for the treatment of ileus (Feldman et al., 2002).

Patient, Family, and Staff Education

As in all changes in condition among the frail elderly who reside in the nursing home, the goals of treatment should be aligned with prior decisions made by the resident and his or her family that are documented in the plan of care. Families should be taught about the risk factors for recurrent ileus. Most cases of ileus will resolve without the need for intensive treatment in the hospital, but if invasive procedures are being considered, they should be contemplated only if they fit with the prescribed plan of care based on the resident's wishes.

Hospitalization in this group is often distressing to the patient, particularly those with dementia. It may put the resident at risk of acquiring iatrogenic infection or decubiti, so the benefits of hospitalization versus treatment in the nursing home should be thoroughly addressed.

▬ DIVERTICULAR DISEASE

Definition

Diverticulitis is the inflammation or infection of pouch-like structures, diverticula, that develop and bulge out from within the colon. Diverticula, groups of these pocket-like structures, are seen primarily in the aging colon. Their presence is described as the condition of diverticulosis, which is without symptoms (Thompson, 2005).

The individual pouches are called *diverticulum*, which refers to the structures in the singular form. They create the potential for diverticulitis if inflamed and/or infected. Given that diverticula are seen in people considered to be in good health, experts postulate that aging's effects on the colon are evidenced by changes in neuromuscular anatomy leading to the condition of diverticulosis (Hazzard et al., 2003). Both entities, diverticulosis and diverticulitis, are referred to as diverticular disease (see the NIH Web page at http://niddk.nih.gov).

The diverticula, or groups of lesions that form herniations through areas of mucosa, that project at vulnerable spots in layers of muscularis, are adjacent to blood vessels. These areas of thinned walls are susceptible to vascular damage and can give rise to micro- and macro-perforations with resulting bleeding and movement of contaminating fecal materials to other areas (Sherif & Perez, 2004).

Though diverticula can form anywhere, they are most commonly seen in the distal colon, usually in the sigmoid. The uncomplicated form, without symptoms, diverticulosis, is found in approximately 10% of the population older than age 40 (Hazzard et al., 2003). Diverticular disease is thought of principally as a disease of later life, but up to 20% of patients are younger than 50 (Sherif & Perez, 2004).

Diverticular disease is a broad category of signs and symptoms; most of the time people with diverticulosis will not have discomfort and do not seek medical attention. If symptoms are present they will range from cramps and abdominal distention to constipation. Among nursing home residents, these signs could indicate any of a variety of gastrointestinal issues; in fact, many times diverticulosis is discovered because the clinician has ordered tests to rule out another disease, like cancer (see the NIH Web page at digestive.niddk.nih.gov). Sometimes diverticulosis is described as the "innocent bystander" because the clinician discovers it by chance (Sherif & Perez, 2004).

Most diverticula are actually pseudodiverticula because not all layers of the colon's wall are involved. Changes related to the decrease in the tensile strength of the bowel due to aging, segmenting the colon into areas of high pressure, and elastin deposits are thought to lead to shortening, intraluminal narrowing, and the fibrosis that accompanies diverticular disease (Feldman et al., 2002).

Epidemiology

Diverticulitis presents equally in both sexes, and may be present in more than 50% of Americans age 60 or more. This is likewise true of other countries in the Western world, where diverticula become more common with advancing age. Diverticular disease was basically unknown prior to 1900 for the same reason that it is rarely seen in societies where the population consumes high-fiber diets. In rural Latin America, Africa, and Asia, as in early American farming and rural communities, whole grains and high-fiber fruits and vegetables were diet staples, preventing the formation of diverticula (Hazzard et al., 2003). Once refined carbohydrates became substitutes for high-fiber foods, diverticulitis became a disease entity. So, like colorectal carcinoma, diverticular disease shows an age-associated increase in the Western world. Although among Asians, diverticular disease is typically seen in the right colon (Feldman et al., 2002).

Etiology

Experts think that diverticular disease is the result of multiple factors such as intraluminal pressure, the anatomical features that charac-

terize the colon, weakness of the colonic wall due to aging, decreased fiber intake, and a diminished motor function (Feldman et al., 2002). Chronic constipation causing increased intraluminal pressure from straining to evacuate, and muscular contractions facilitate the forced penetration of areas of mucosa through the passageways where blood vessels enter the bowel wall (see the NIH Web page at http://digestive.niddk.nih.gov). Studies have implicated this relationship between hypersegmentation of the colon caused by intraluminal hypertension and the typical low-fiber diet of the Western world as the cause of diverticular disease (Feldman et al., 2002).

Common Presenting Signs and Symptoms

Symptoms of diverticulosis may be absent or minimal, such that many patients may not complain at all. However, with diverticulitis the most common sign is abdominal pain; the classic presentation being left lower quadrant pain and tenderness, fever, and leukocytosis (Friedman et al., 2003). The variety of signs and symptoms that might be expected include the following:

- Fever, chills
- Intermittent abdominal pain and tenderness
- Anorexia
- Nausea and vomiting
- Bloating, flatulence
- Local swelling and tenderness with erythema of abdomen could signal abscess
- Constipation, pellet-shaped or pencil-shaped stool
- Diarrhea, sudden or otherwise
- Irregular defecation
- Diverticula may perforate and ooze blood.
- Dysuria or urinary frequency, more likely with complicated diverticulitis in colovesicular fistula

- Purulent vaginal discharge, in colovaginal fistula (Sherif & Perez, 2004)

If a resident has a history of rectal bleeding and a barium enema has shown diverticular disease, a workup should be initiated to search for other causes, because rectal bleeding is not a common feature of uncomplicated diverticular disease. Diverticular disease and colorectal cancer may not be clinically apparent for a significant amount of time. Some clinicians think that irritable bowel syndrome, a disease of early adulthood, progresses to diverticular disease; however, there is no data to support that assumption (Feldman et al., 2002).

Diverticulitis results when there is inflammation of a diverticulum and a perforation develops. This happens in 10–25% of patients with diverticulosis. A form of uncomplicated diverticulitis is a microperforation of the colon, usually the left side, referred to as a peridiverticulitis or phlegmon (Feldman et al., 2002).

Complicated diverticulitis arises from the formation of an obstruction, abscess, fistula, or perforation resulting from inflammation due to tissue destruction and purulent drainage. The resident is likely to develop sepsis and is at risk for peritonitis if the infection spreads unchecked (Friedman et al., 2003). This is often a fatal complication requiring emergent surgery to remove the damaged colon or repair a fistula and clean out the abdomen (see the NIH Web page at http://digestive.niddk.nih.gov).

Differential Diagnosis

Diverticular Disease
- Colorectal carcinoma—Late signs of both diverticular disease and carcinoma are luminal narrowing and obstruction, fistula, and perforation.
- Conditions of altered intestinal motility, such as irritable bowel disease. To make a diagnosis of irritable bowel, there should be a long-standing history of symptoms

stemming from adulthood in an elderly individual (Feldman et al., 2002).
- Appendicitis
- Obstruction
- Sigmoid volvulus
- Ischemic colitis
- Diverticulitis in the transverse colon may mimic peptic ulcer disease (PUD), pancreatitis, or cholecystitis (Sherif & Perez, 2004).

Diverticular Bleeding
- Minor, painless diverticular bleeding can occur in 15–40% of patients with diverticulosis; major bleeding can occur in 5% of patients. Causes like colitis and carcinoma must be ruled out first before a diagnosis of bleeding due to diverticular disease is made.
- Bleeding from a right colon angiodysplasia can be a cause of large bleeds in the elderly, who may also experience bleeding diverticula in the same area (Friedman et al., 2003).

Diverticulitis
- Gastroenteritis
- Appendicitis
- Perforated colon cancer
- Inflammatory bowel disease
- Urinary tract infection, rule out fistula (Friedman et al., 2003)

Essential Diagnostic and Laboratory Tests
- Diagnosis may be primarily based on clinical skills and knowledge of resident's medical history, since laboratories may not be helpful. For example, up to 50% of patients with mild diverticulitis may not have an increase in the white cell count, also plain abdominal radiographs may appear normal with mild diverticulitis (Friedman et al., 2003).
- Barium enema is the most common test that not only makes the diagnosis of diverticulosis, but also indicates the extent and severity

of disease. Although diverticula may be seen throughout the large intestine, they are usually seen in the sigmoid in Caucasians and the right side among Asians. On radiographic studies of sacculation, retained barium within the diverticula and colonic spasms are findings indicative of diverticular disease. Barium enema is considered more accurate and reliable than colonoscopy, as it can identify areas of diverticular disease and rule out cancer. It can also identify diverticula versus polyps (Feldman et al., 2002).

- In instances in which the resident may have rectal bleeding and vomiting, serial hematocrits should be checked and electrolytes monitored to aid in diagnosis and treatment so that anemia and potassium and other electrolytes can be corrected in the plan of care.

- In severe diverticulitis, complete blood count (CBC), urinalysis (UA), computed tomography (CT) of the abdomen and pelvis with intravenous and oral contrast medium, ultrasound, and contrast enema can assist in diagnosis. CT is the clinician's test of choice and provides the most information (Friedman et al., 2003).

- For residents presenting with severe bleeding, emergent angiography is the most specific and sensitive test to determine where the bleeding originates. In a resident who is hemodynamically stable, colonoscopy will assist in finding areas of bleeding in approximately 85% of patients (Feldman et al., 2002).

Management Plan

Nonpharmacologic

High-fiber diet is the mainstay of the treatment of diverticulosis because it helps to reduce pressure in the bowel and prevents further development of diverticuli. Twenty to thirty grams of dietary fiber per day are needed to reduce colonic pressure, increase transit time of stool through the gastrointestinal tract, and increase stool weight (Feldman et al., 2002). The following are excellent sources of dietary fiber:

- Winter squash
- Apples
- Baked beans
- Bran flakes

These are examples of the highest-fiber foods among fibrous food choices and can be easily prepared and served in the long-term care facility (see the National Agriculture Web page at http://www.nal.usda.gov). In addition to helping prevent the development of diverticular disease, a high fiber diet goes a long way to preventing constipation, a common health issue among elderly in the nursing home.

Nuts, popcorn hulls, and sesame, pumpkin, and caraway seeds should be eliminated from the diet of those with known diverticulosis, but others foods, formerly thought to cause problems such as tomatoes, strawberries and raspberries, zucchini, and cucumbers are no longer considered a threat. Individuals may find certain foods cause discomfort; so maintaining a food record to help identify problematic foods may be helpful (see the NIH Web page at http://digestive.niddk.nih.gov). Because they often visit at mealtime, this would be an ideal task for a family member or friend to take on.

Most of the time diverticular hemorrhage will resolve on its own, so supportive care is given with intravenous fluids, though some patients will require treatment for coagulopathy with whole blood transfusion. For those patients who receive angiography, embolization or vasopressin may be tried, but about half those patients rebleed after vasopressin is discontinued (Feldman et al., 2002).

There is a role for surgery in a small subset of patients in general, but among the frail elderly this intervention may best be a limited one. The nurse practitioner or physician may obtain a surgeon's opinion in cases with unremitting acute disease. A resident with peritonitis may have a drain placed for an abscess via computerized tomography (CT) or ultrasound procedure, but emergent colon resection is another matter. In cases where free perforation has occurred, the general mortality rate may be as high as 30% for elective colon resection with anastomosis (Friedman et al., 2003), so the decision to proceed with surgery depends on the resident's underlying health status and his or her goals for care.

Pharmacologic
The following antibiotics are used in the treatment of diverticulitis:

- Metronidazole and ciproflaxin for 7 to 10 days along with clear liquids and bowel rest
- In severe cases, IV fluids, ampicillin sodium/sulbactam sodium, metronidazole and a cephalosporin
- If pain is an issue, morphine should be avoided because it causes an increase in intraluminal pressure.
- An important consideration to note is that experts suggest meperidine, a drug that clinicians usually avoid; it should be used in this instance for pain control (Feldman et al., 2002).

Patient, Family, and Staff Education
The health care team, family, and resident, if able, should give much thought and careful discussion to the benefits versus the burdens of surgical treatment and the hardships associated with hospitalization for a frail elderly individual. They should be made aware that diverticulitis with bleeding, if recurrent, carries a 50% increase in the risk of rebleeding after a second occurrence (Friedman et al., 2003). The resident, if unable to speak, may have already anticipated such a situation in advance directives or through verbal instructions on the limitations of

treatment. Complications of treatment should be anticipated in making a decision regarding the scope of medical care in this phase of life in the frail elderly as the individual's quality of life depends on it.

WEB SITES
- Mayo Clinic—www.Mayoclinic.com
- Hospice—www.Hospice.net
- *Merck Manual*—www.mercksource.com
- American Cancer Society—www.acs.com
- National Cancer Institute—www.nci.com
- Centers for Disease Control and Prevention—www.cdc.gov
- Liver Foundation—www.liverfoundation.org
- National Library of Medicine—www.nlm.nih.gov
- National Agriculture Library—www.nal.usda.gov
- Diverticulosis and diverticulitis—www.digestive.niddk.nih.gov

REFERENCES
Ahlgren, J. D. (2001). Gastrointestinal malignancies. *Primary Care: Clinics in Office Practice, 28*(3), 647–660.

Andersson, R., & Andren-Sandberg, A. (2003). Fatal acute pancreatitis. *Pancreatology, 3*(1), 64–66.

Barkin, J. S., & Goldstein, J. A. (1999). Diagnostic approach to pancreatic cancer. *Gastroenterology Clinics of North America, 28*(3), 709–721.

Bentrem, D., & Joehl, R. (2003). Pancreas: Healing response in critical illness. *Critical Care Medicine, 8*(Suppl.), S582–S589.

Bond, J. H. (2000). Colorectal cancer update, prevention, screening, treatment and surveillance for high-risk groups. *Medical Clinics of North America, 84*(5), 67–72.

Bounds, B. C., & Friedman, L. S. (2003). Lower gastrointestinal bleeding. *Gastroenterology Clinics of North America, 32*, 1107–1125.

Butt, A. S., & Jacobson, I. M. (2005a). Hepatitis C: Making the diagnosis. *Consultant, 45*(9), 955–959.

Butt, A. S., & Jacobson, I. M. (2005b). Hepatitis C: Latest treatment guidelines. *Consultant, 45*(9), 960–962.

Fallah, M. A., Prakash, C., & Edmunowicz, S. (2000). Acute gastrointestinal bleeding. *Medical Clinics of North America, 84*(5), 1183–1230.

Farrell, J. J., & Friedman, L. S. (2001). Gastrointestinal bleeding in the elderly. *Gastroenterology Clinics of North America, 30*(2), 377–401.

Feldman, M., Friedman, L., Sleisenger, M. (2002). *Sleisenger and Fordtran's gastrointestinal and liver disease* (7th ed.). Philadelphia: Saunders/Elsevier Science.

Friedman, S., McQuaid, K., & Grendell, J. (2003). *Current diagnosis and treatment in gastroenterology* (2nd ed.). New York: Lange Medical/McGraw-Hill.

Gladwin, M., & Trattler, B. (1997). *Clinical microbiology made ridiculously simple* (2nd ed.). Miami, FL: Med Master Inc.

Geoff, H. (1999). GERD pharmacotherapeutic management in the senior patient. *American Society of Consultant Pharmacists Annual Meeting*. Retrieved November 7, 2005, from http://www.medscape.com/viewarticle/425044

Goldacre, M., & Roberts, S. (2004). Hospital admission for acute pancreatitis in an English population. 1963–98. *British Medical Journal, 328*(7454), 1466–1469.

Haas, S., & Singer, M. (2002). Differential diagnosis of acute pancreatitis. *Schweizerische Rundschau fur Medizin Praxis, 91*(39), 1595–1602.

Hartwig, W., Maksan, S., Foitzik, T., Schmidt, J., Herfath, C., & Klar, E. (2002). Reduction in mortality with delayed surgical therapy of severe pancreatitis. *Journal of Gastroenterointestinal Surgery, 6*(3), 481–487.

Hazzard, W., Blass, J., Halter, J., Ouslander, J., & Tinetti, M. (2003). *Principles of geriatric medicine and gerontology* (5th ed.). New York: McGraw-Hill.

Howden, C. (2005). *Practical solutions for challenging GERD cases*. Retrieved November 7, 2005, from http://www.medscape.com/viewarticle/481811_23

Langford, R., & Thompson, R. M. (2004). *Mosby's handbook of diseases* (3rd ed.). St. Louis, MO: Elsevier Mosby.

Lin, K. W., & Kirchner, J. T. (2004). Hepatitis B. *American Family Physician, 69*(1), 75–82.

Manning-Dimmitt, L. L., Dimmitt, S. G., & Wilson, G. R. (2005). Diagnosis of gastrointestinal bleeding in adults. *American Family Physician, 71*(7), 1339–1345.

McQuaid, K. (2005). Alimentary tract. In L. M. Tierney, S. J. McPhee, & M. A. Papadakis (Eds.), *Current medical diagnosis and treatment*. Stamford, CT: Appleton & Lange.

Mitchell, S. H., Schaffer, D. C., & Dubagutta, S. (2004). A new view of occult and obscure gastrointestinal bleeding. *American Family Physician, 69*(4), 875–881.

Mohammed, I., Nightengale, P., & Trudgill, N. J. (2005). Risk factors for gastroesophageal reflux disease symptoms: A community study. *Alimentary Pharmacology and Therapeutics, 21*(7), 821–827.

Pagana, K. D., & Pagana, T. J. (1998). *Manual of diagnostic & laboratory tests*. St. Louis, MO: Mosby Inc.

Pianka, J. D., & Affronti, J. (2001). Management principles of gastrointestinal bleeding. *Primary Care: Clinics in Office Practice, 28*(3), 557–571.

Pilotto, A., Franscheschi, M., & Paris, F. (2005). Recent advances in treatment of GERD in the elderly: Focus on proton pump inhibitors. *Internal Journal of Clinical Practice, 59*(10), 1204–1209.

Shapira, S. C., & Yoshida, E. M. (2005). Hepatitis B: Latest treatment guidelines. *Consultant, 45*(6), 605–610.

Sherif, A., & Perez, N. (2004). Diverticulitis. Retrieved January 11, 2006, from http://www.emedicine.com/med/topic578.htm

Sial, S. H., & Catalano, M. F. (2001). Gastrointestinal tract cancer in the elderly. *Gastroenterology Clinics of North America, 30*(2), 565–589.

Snape, W. J. (1999). Pathogenesis, diagnosis and treatment of acute colonic ileus. Retrieved November 26, 2005, from http://www.medscape.com/viewarticle/407936

Soran, A., Chelluri, L., Lee, K., & Tisherman, S. (2000). Outcome and quality of life of patients with acute pancreatitis requiring intensive care. *Journal of Surgical Research, 91*(1), 89–94.

Thompson, G. (2005). *Diverticula, diverticulosis, diverticular disease: What's the difference?* Retrieved December 6, 2005, from http://www.iffgd.org

Tilman, K., & Counselman, F. (2005). Interpreting abnormal liver function tests. *Emergency Medicine, 37*(5), 31–38.

Tivedi, C., & Pitchumoni, C. (2005). Drug-induced pancreatitis: An update. *Journal of Clinical Gastroenterology, 39*(8), 709–716.

Tolstoi, L. G. (2002). Drug-induced gastrointestinal disorder. *Medscape Pharmacotherapy, 4*(1).

Ward, R. P., Kugelmas, M. & Libsch, K. D. (2004). Management of hepatitis C: Evaluating suitability for drug therapy. *American Family Physician, 69*(6), 1429–1436.

CHAPTER 10

Genitourinary and Renal Disorders

BENIGN PROSTATIC HYPERTROPHY

Definition

Benign prostatic hyperplasia (BPH) is the benign enlargement of the prostate gland. There is an increased growth of epithelial and stromal cells in the periurethral area of the prostate that tends to cause lower urinary tract symptoms. The prostate gland is the only organ that has new growth as it ages.

Epidemiology

BPH is the most common benign tumor in men. The incidence of BPH rises with age. By age 60, prevalence is greater than 50%, and by age 80 approximately 90% of men have microscopic evidence of BPH. About half of these men have noticeable enlargement, and half of that group will progress to clinical symptoms needing treatment (Agency for Health Care Policy and Research, 1994).

Common Presenting Signs and Symptoms

- An enlarged prostate gland is determined by digital rectal exam (DRE). The normal size of a prostate is that of a walnut with the consistency of a pencil eraser. It is important to note that the size of the prostate does not necessarily relate to the severity of symptoms or the degree of obstruction.

- Patient initially presents with lower urinary tract symptoms. These symptoms include the following:
  ○ Hesitancy to initiate voiding
  ○ Weak urinary stream
  ○ Sensation of incomplete bladder emptying
  ○ Pushing or straining to urinate
  ○ Up two or more times at night
  ○ Urgency and frequency

- More severe symptoms of BPH include the following:
  ○ Chronic urinary retention with a post-void residual of > 150 cc
  ○ Frequent UTI including difficult resolution with antibiotics due to retention
  ○ Bladder stones
  ○ Hematuria
  ○ Hydronephrosis
  ○ Chronic kidney disease

Differential Diagnosis

- Impaired detrusor contractility related to neurogenic, myogenic, or psychogenic bladder problems
- Detrusor instability/hyperreflexia from inflammatory or infectious conditions such as prostatitis or UTI
- Other causes of bladder outlet obstruction including prostate cancer, urethral obstruction, or vesical neck obstruction

Essential Diagnostic and Laboratory Tests

- Digital rectal exam (DRE)
- Uroflowmetry used to measure urinary flow rate. Can help rule out BPH in patients with prostatism.
- Postvoid residual per bladder scan. Avoid catheterization if possible
- CBC, serum electrolytes, BUN, creatinine
- PSA; do before DRE more specific for cancer
- Urinalysis
- Transrectal ultrasound of prostate along with biopsy if cancer suspected
- Ultrasound of abdomen or intravenous pyelogram used only to confirm upper tract pathology such as hydronephrosis, stones, or renal mass.

Management Plan

The goal in treating patients with BPH is to alleviate symptoms that interfere with quality of life or cause significant complications of the urinary tract.

Nonpharmacologic

Watchful waiting is a strategy where no medical or surgical intervention is chosen for treatment of the disease. This approach is appropriate for men with minimal to mild symptoms including minimal or no interference with quality of life, no recurrent UTI, no recurrent gross hematuria, no urinary retention, no bladder stones, no renal insufficiency related to BPH, peak flow rates greater than 15 cc/second and relatively low postvoid residual urine (Issa & Marshall, 2004).

Pharmacologic

- Alpha-1 adrenergic receptor blockers relax the smooth muscle of the bladder neck and prostate. The purpose in prescribing these drugs is to increase urine flow and decrease lower urinary tract symptoms.
  - Flomax (tamsulosin) 0.4, 0.8 mg (0.4 mg is usual dose)
  - Uroxatral (alfuzosin) 10 mg
  - Hytrin (terazosin) 1, 2, 5, 10 mg (titrated)
  - Cardura (doxazosin) 2, 4, 8 mg (titrated)

  Side effects include postural hypotension, dizziness, syncope, fatigue, upper respiratory symptoms, and insomnia.

- 5-alpha reductase inhibitors block conversion of testosterone to dihydrotestosterone. These drugs affect the epithelial component of the prostate resulting in reduction in the size of the gland and subsequent improvement in symptoms. These drugs are used as combination therapy with alpha blockers.
  - Proscar (finasteride) 5 mg every day
  - Avodart (tutasteride) 0.5 mg every day

  Side effects include sexual related events (impotence, loss of libido, and ejaculatory disorders) and gynecomastia. Effectiveness of this drug class begins around 6 months after start of therapy. Improvement of symptoms, including increased flow rate, irritative bladder symptoms, and further reduction in prostate size continue for 48 months (Debruyne et al., 2004).

- Phytotherapy are herbal preparations used as far back as 1899 by Native Americans to relieve genitourinary symptoms, specifically lower urinary tract symptoms. They are known to reduce swelling and inflammation of the prostate and in turn improve flow rates and decrease lower urinary tract symptoms, including nocturia. Some short-term studies indicate similar efficacy for Flomax (Wilt et al., 1998)

- ○ Saw palmetto berry (*Serenoa repens*)
- ○ Red stinkwood or African plum (*Pygeum africanum*)
- In patients with symptoms of both bladder outlet obstruction and concomitant detrusor instability, the use of Flomax (tamsulosin) 0.4 mg and Detrol LA 4 mg (tolterodine) has been shown to be effective in resolving both problems (Athanasopoulos et al., 2003)

Surgical Therapy—Minimally Invasive
- Transurethral needle ablation
- Laser therapy
- Transurethral electrovaporization of the prostate
- Hyperthermia
- High-intensity focused ultrasound
- Intraurethral stents
- Transurethral balloon dilation of the prostate

Conventional Surgical Therapy
- Transurethral resection of the prostate
- Transurethral incision of the prostate
- Open simple prostatectomy, suprapubic or retropubic approach

Patient, Family, and Staff Education
- Observe urine output.
- Teach patient to use crede catheter after voiding to prevent retention.
- Avoid sudden diuresis with diuretics and/or large ingestion of caffeine.
- Inform patient to report any difficulty with voiding.

- Avoid all drugs causing urinary retention.

Physician Consultation
Refer to urology if any of the following occur:
- Watchful waiting is no longer acceptable.
- Medication is not controlling symptoms.
- Patient is incurring more serious side effects from enlarged prostate.
- Patient desires invasive treatment.
- Impending renal failure

CHRONIC RENAL FAILURE

Definition
Chronic renal failure (CRF) and the signs and symptoms of such are a direct result of a decrease in the glomerular filtration rate resulting in a reduced clearance of certain solutes. The net result is irreversible damage to the renal parenchymal mass. The progression of the disease can be over months or years. Secondary problems such as infection, dehydration, or hypertension tend to result in end-stage renal failure (ESRF) if not assessed, evaluated, and treated in a timely manner.

Epidemiology
The incidence of CRF is on the rise. The number of patients treated with dialysis or transplantation is projected to increase from 340,000 in 1999 to 651,000 in 2010 (Johnson et al., 2004). CRF affects people of all ages. Treatment, including dialysis, is on the rise for older adults. With so many advances in medical treatment, the severity and rapidity of the development of uremia is unpredictable. Unfortunately, patients with declining renal function are initially asymptomatic. Progression of CRF is most often discovered in the evaluation of another subset of contributing problems or by accident with routine laboratory testing.

Common Presenting Signs and Symptoms

- Initially, asymptomatic
- Slow, with the progression of the disease:
  - Generalized malaise, lassitude, easy fatigability
  - Nausea
  - Pruritis
  - Forgetfulness, shortened attention span
- Blood pressure (BP) fluctuates depending on concomitant conditions, such as volume overload; renal salt losing tendencies: normal or low.
- High pulse and respiratory rates due to anemia and metabolic acidosis
- Profound anemia (normochromic, normocytic)
- Symptoms of multisystem disorders may be present coincidentally, e.g., lupus erythematous.
- Later stages:
  - Subtle myoclonus, restlessness, hiccough, flapping tremors, muscle jerks, cramps, and tics
  - Coma, convulsions, and death

Differential Diagnosis

- Be aware of the presentation of acute renal failure (ARF). Treat conditions that are treatable.
- Know patients' history:
  - Do they have hypertension, diabetes mellitus, polycystic kidney disease, chronic glomerulitis, or history of acute kidney injury?
  - How long?
  - These patients may experience symptoms over a long period of time until renal function finally fails them. They no longer can adapt to biochemical changes that have been ongoing for quite some time.

- Rapid progression of CRF may occur after removal of cancerous kidneys or acute obstructive disease.

Essential Diagnostic and Laboratory Tests

- Urinalysis
  - Volume—Normal in polycystic and interstitial forms of failure. Low when GFR falls below 5% of normal; then look for sodium retention.
  - Protein—Can be variable, however 1+ consistently noted on dipstick should prompt a 24-hour urine specimen to quantify proteinuria. Normal adult excretion is < 160 g/day, and creatinine clearance normally is 120 mL/minute.
  - Mononuclear white cells (leukocytes) may be present.
  - Occasional casts—Type of cast can give a clue as to where in the kidney it was formed.
- Blood studies
  - CBC—Anemia
  - Chemistry—Multiple factors contribute to the variation in electrolytes and other metabolites based on the origin and current state of the disease.
- Diagnostic imaging—Renal sonogram
  - Measures size of kidney and cortical thickness
  - A good guide for localizing tissue for biopsy
  - Shows cystic disease
  - Detects hydronephrosis
- Kidney, ureter, bladder (KUB)
  - Helps detect presence of kidney stones
  - Indicates size of kidney
  - May discover any masses
  - Downside—Presence of free air in the bowel may obstruct views.

- Avoid *all* contrast studies in patients with reduced renal function. Consult nephrologist.
- Kidney biopsy
  - Advantage is in detecting specific type of renal disease, such as interstitial fibrosis versus glomerulosclerosis
  - Biopsies in end-stage shrunken kidneys are associated with a high incidence of hemorrhage and patient morbidity.

Management Plan

The treatment goal for patients with CRF is to attempt to meet quality-of-life issues and effectively recognize ongoing resultant complications and treat accordingly to prevent disease progression.

- Attempt conservative measures first.
- Consult with a dietician to accomplish the following:
  - Restrict dietary protein (0.5 g/kg/day), potassium, and phosphorus.
  - Maintain sodium balance in the diet to prevent sodium depletion or expansion.
  - Ensure adequate caloric intake
- Review medications with pharmacist that could potentiate kidney failure. Reduce and eliminate as able.
- Monitor patient's weight—A good indicator of sodium retention.
- Monitor blood pressure—Hypertension aggravates all forms of CRF.
- Monitor acid base balance—Moderate acidemia can be treated with bicarbonate (sodium bicarbonate tablets or Shohl's solution).
- Anemia can be treated with recombinant erythropoietin. Iron is also critical to the successful treatment of anemia. Iron availability will make erythropoietin stimulate proteins more efficiently and therefore is less costly to use (Tangalos, 2004). Both ferrous gluconate and iron sucrose are very safe intravenous drugs for the timely correction of iron deficiency. Watch for hypertension as a potential side effect of this combination therapy.
- Chronic peritoneal dialysis can be used when vascular access is limited. Nursing support and knowledge is essential in long-term care to support this therapy. Nephrology will determine dosage of fluid instilled and number of treatments.
- Chronic hemodialysis—Used more frequently in long-term care. Need vascular access. Advances in medical treatment provide more accurate exchange. Treatment is intermittent, generally 3–5 hours, 3 times per week. Place of treatment options include a kidney center, satellite unit, or in the home depending on needed resources. Infection, wasting syndrome, cardiomyopathies, polyneuropathies, and renal osteodystrophy (defective bone development) are common complications. After discontinuation of dialysis, death usually occurs within 7–10 days because of increased potassium and resultant cardiac arrest.
- Renal transplantation—Dependent on availability of organs, patient age, and state of morbidity.

Patient, Staff, and Family Education

- Knowledge of the disease progression and possible complications as well as family roles
- Financial considerations need to be recognized if dialysis is started.
- Psychological support for the patient and family should be provided for the following reasons:
  - Dealing with death and dying is a daily reality.
  - Determining when to stop dialysis weighs heavily on the minds of patient and family.

- Consult with the social worker to ensure advanced directives have been completed according to the patient's wishes.
- Patience and understanding is needed for the family and patient as they work through very difficult decisions.
- The time will come when patient and family will need to weigh the benefits versus the burden of hemodialysis.

- Provide physical and emotional comfort for the dying patient.

Physician Consultation

Due to multiple system failures and complicated management, a nephrologist should be consulted regarding the original management plan and regularly thereafter as changes in condition occur.

The patient's primary care physician can be a helpful source with ongoing management of day-to-day progression of the disease.

ACUTE RENAL FAILURE

Definition

Acute renal failure (ARF) is a condition in which there is a rapid decrease in the glomerular filtration rate causing an abrupt rise in BUN and creatinine. ARF may or may not be accompanied by oliguria. Rarely there is no output at all (anuria) in ARF. Acute renal failure can occur over a period of hours to days. Causes are many and dependent on the location of failure, either prerenal, intrinsic renal, or postrenal. Knowledge of baseline renal function is paramount in making a timely diagnosis.

Epidemiology

The elderly population is especially prone to ARF because of the number of medications they take and comorbidities coupled with normal aging changes in the kidney and reduced renal function.

ARF is fairly common among hospitalized patients. Prospective studies have demonstrated that 2–5% of all patients admitted to a general medical-surgical hospital unit will develop ARF (Nolan & Anderson, 1998).

Acute tubular necrosis (ATN) marks the highest cause of ARF (45%), followed by prerenal (21%), acute-on-chronic renal failure (13%), urinary tract obstruction (10%), glomerulitis-vasculitis (4%), acute interstitial nephritis (2%), and atheroembolic renal disease (1%) (Liann & Pascual, 1996). Identifying the type of ARF is critical as it directs timely treatment.

Common Presenting Signs and Symptoms

Dependent upon cause, but generally can include those of dehydration:

- Thirst
- Poor skin turgor
- Collapsed neck veins
- Dry mucous membranes
- Dizziness
- Orthostatic hypotension
- Overt fluid loss and subsequent weight loss
- Patient may or may not be oliguric.

Differential Diagnosis

Prerenal Failure

- Volume depletion due to vomiting, diarrhea, nasogastric suction, osmotic diuresis as with hyperglycemia and congestive heart failure, surgical hemorrhage
- Drug induced—Angiotensin-converting enzyme inhibitors (ACE), nonsteroidal anti-inflammatories, cyclosporine, and tacrolimus
- Vascular collapse due to third spacing or sepsis, frequently after surgery or trauma
- Compromised vascular situation due to atheroembolism, dissecting arterial aneurysm, malignant hypertension, or renal artery stenosis

Intrinsic Renal Disease

- Acute tubular necrosis—Decrease in glomerular filtration rates and renal ischemia
- Acute interstitial nephritis, most often induced by drug therapy
- Toxic nephropathies—Radiocontrast agents especially in patients with diabetes or myeloma
- Infectious process

Postrenal Failure

- Generally caused by an obstruction in the lower urinary tract manifested by pain and possibly a large postvoid residual per catheterization
- Urethral or bladder neck obstruction can cause renal failure especially in elderly men (BPH).

Essential Diagnostic and Laboratory Tests

See Table 10-1 for tests useful in evaluating acute renal failure.

Management Plan

The treatment goal for ARF is finding the cause and preventing fluid and metabolic complications.

- Obtain important lab values: serum electrolytes, BUN, creatinine, CBC.
- If the patient is dehydrated, start a fluid challenge to increase central venous pressure. Inadequate fluid management can cause further insult to the kidneys. Rapid intravenous administration of 300–500 mL of physiologic saline is the usual initial treatment (Amend & Vincenti, 2004). Watch for fluid overload and hyperkalemia.

TABLE 10-1   Tests Useful in Evaluating Acute Renal Failure

TEST	PRERENAL	INTRARENAL	POSTRENAL
Urinalysis (UA) 24 hour urine	• Volume usually decreased. • Increased specific gravity > 1.025 • Urine osmolality > 600 Osm/kg. • Nothing abnormal on routine UA	• UA shows active sediment, many white cells, plus multiple types of granula and cellular casts • Eosinophiluria is present in 75% of patients with the exception of AIN secondary to NSAID therapy • Specific gravity usually low or fixed 1.005–1.015 range. • Urine osmolality low • Urine may be muddy brown	• Not usually helpful • May have occult blood or hematuria with obstructive stone
Lab findings	• Elevated BUN with dehydration • Elevated creatinine • Hyperkalemia • Hyperphosphatemia • Metabolic acidosis	• Serum creatinine initially rises then gradually falls with recovery • Hyperkalemia • Hyperphosphatemia • Metabolic acidosis	• Elevated BUN and creatinine gradual or acute with total obstruction • Hyperkalemia • Hyperphosphatemia • Metabolic acidosis
Other		Avoid dye studies.	• Renal scans used to avoid radiocontrast-induced ARF and provides information on kidney size, thickness of the cortex, and presence of obstruction • Cystoscopy • Catheterization

- Send urine for analysis and 24-hour creatinine clearance.
- Review medications for nephrotoxicity. Discontinue diuretics, antihypertensives, especially angiotensin-converting enzyme inhibitor drugs and nonsteroidal anti-inflammatories. These measures in themselves may correct prerenal failure.
- Identify presence of infection and treat accordingly. Infectious complications, due to altered immune response and use of invasive treatment procedures, are the most common cause of death in patients with ARF.
- Check postvoid residual (PVR) per catheterization for possible postrenal causes.
- Order appropriate diagnostic testing to rule out renal obstruction. Dye studies should be avoided; therefore, renal sonography is the best option.
- Watch for signs of uremia including anorexia, nausea, and vomiting, pruritis, and changes in cognition.
- Consider plasmapheresis to eliminate toxic materials and drugs.
- Initiation of supportive dialysis may be necessary.

Patient, Staff, and Family Education

- Explain the acute and chronic course of renal failure in understandable terms.
- Discuss need for physician specialists.
- Review treatment options including hospitalization and dialysis.
- Provide emotional support to family.

Physician Consultation

- Danger levels of lab reports
- Prioritization of appropriate diagnostic testing
- Rapid decline
- Acute hospitalization

- Referral to a nephrologist or urologist
- Need for cystoscopy
- Initiation of plasmapheresis
- Use of dialysis

▓▓▓   PROSTATE CANCER

Definition

Prostate cancer (CaP) is an abnormal growth of cells in the prostate gland. They can be benign or malignant. Over 95% of the cancers of the prostate are adenocarcinomas (Presti, 2004). Most CaP cells grow very slowly and never cause a problem. The vast majority of men, 3 out of 100 Americans die *with* CaP versus *from* it (Michigan Cancer Consortium Prostate Cancer Action Committee, 2003).

Epidemiology

In American men, CaP is the most common cancer (other than skin cancer), and it is the second leading cause of cancer deaths in men, following lung cancer (Jemal et al., 2004). However, if the cancer is found early enough, survival rate is very high. The incidence of CaP increases with age. Prostate cancer has a wide range of virulence and growth activity. "This broad spectrum of biological activity can make decision making for individual patients difficult" (Presti, 2004).

Screening for CaP generally begins at age 50 unless there is a family history. This continues to be a controversial topic generating much discussion, especially regarding when to stop the screening. There is some consensus that screening should stop when a person has a life expectancy of 10 years or less. However, this should be a resident and family decision (Gerared, 1998). This decision should be based on a thorough knowledge of the progression of CaP, existing comorbidities, and the recognition that CaP with or without treatment has almost identical outcomes in men more than 70 years old (Lu-Yao et al., 2003). It should also be noted that patients aged 80 years and older are less likely to respond to aggressive therapy and generally die of comorbid or unrelated causes (Sung et al., 2000).

Common Presenting Signs and Symptoms

- Most men with early CaP experience no bladder or prostate symptoms.
- Abnormal prostate digital rectal exam (DRE)
  - Presence of nodules
  - Enlarged prostate
  - Lack of symmetry of right and left prostate lobes
  - Firmness or rocklike feeling with palpation
- Voiding dysfunction occurs as the prostate becomes abnormal and causes irritative bladder symptoms.
  - Hesitancy
  - Urgency
  - Slow, sometimes interruptive urinary stream
  - Frequency
  - Nocturia
- With advanced or metastatic disease the resident may experience bone pain, lower extremity weakness, and lymphedema, as well as spinal cord compression, which can in turn also cause problems of fecal and urinary incontinence.

Differential Diagnosis

An elevated prostate specific antigen (PSA) can be due to the following:

- Prostatitis
- Instrumentation of the urethra
- BPH
- Infection
- Prostatic massage

Staging Prostate Cancer

Determination of the extent of CaP is called *staging*. A chest X-ray, bone scan, CT scan, MRI, and/or other lab tests can help determine the stage. There are two systems used for staging. The TNM stage uses these letters that stand for tumor, node, and metastases. The other system used is the A, B, C, D or Whitmore-Jewett system. If the cancer is stage A or B, or if it is a T1 or T2, then it has not spread beyond the prostate. If a cancer is a stage C or D, or if it is a T3 or T4 (or N+ and/or M+), then the cancer has spread beyond the prostate (Oesterling & Moyad, 1998).

The grade of the cancer gives a good idea how fast the cancer is growing. This is determined by examining the prostate cells under the microscope. The higher the grade, the more aggressive the cancer. This grading is called the Gleason score and ranges from 2–10. The lower the score, the more responsive the cancer will be to treatment.

Essential Diagnostic and Laboratory Tests

- Digital rectal exam (DRE)
- Prostate specific antigen (PSA)—As men age "normal" values for the PSA rise due to a natural progression of enlargement of the prostate. Screening for CaP in the oldest males is controversial. According to the American Urologic Association, the normal PSA values for men ages 70–79 are 0–5.5 ng/mL for African-Americans, 0–5.0 ng/mL for Asians, and 0–6.5 ng/mL for Caucasians (American Urologic Association, 2000). The PSA is an important marker when it comes to diagnosing CaP. As the level increases to 2.6–10 ng/mL, the likelihood of CaP increases to moderate. Greater than 10 ng/mL generally indicates a higher level of suspicion for CaP (Gretzer & Partin, 2003). In the absence of prostate cancer it should be emphasized that PSA screening is not recommended in men over the age of 75 (Lu-Yao

et al., 2003). Men being treated for prostate cancer will have different interval PSA testing periods depending on the type of treatment they are undergoing. This should be at the discretion of his urologist. For those treated with radical prostatectomy, the PSA should continue to be undetectable. If not, cancer may still be present and additional studies and/or therapy may be necessary, if the patient wishes. After radiation therapy, there is some level of PSA that is still slightly detectable (below 1 ng/mL) many years after therapy. Treatment with hormonal therapy generally drops the PSA level below 5 to 10 ng/mL within 3 months. Those patients choosing watchful waiting will generally see their PSA rise over time. Work closely with the urologist to maintain both the requests of the patient and the plan of care from the urologist.

- Prostate biopsy is done after DRE and PSA indicate suspicion for CaP. It is an office procedure that is quick with minimal discomfort. This is the only way to diagnose CaP. There may be some blood in the bowels, semen, or urine that should resolve after a few weeks.

- Transrectal ultra sonography (TRUS) is used in conjunction with biopsy to view and guide the needle into the prostate to take tissue from several positions, on average 6–8 different areas.

- Other lab work includes the following:

  ○ Creatinine will increase if kidney function has been compromised from an enlarged prostate causing obstructive problems.

  ○ Hemoglobin/hematocrit—Anemia if below normal range

  ○ Alkaline phosphatase—Increased in the presence of bone metastasis

  ○ Serum acid phosphates—Indicates disease outside the prostate when elevated

Management Plan

To determine proper treatment, comprehensive assessment and relevant disease staging information must be available. This helps determine the best approach emphasizing quality of life. Curative strategies must be compatible with theoretical, curative treatment indications (Terret et al., 2004).

Pharmacologic

- Hormone therapy is used in conjunction with microscopic lymph node involvement, radiation therapy, or with recurrence of metastatic disease to induce androgen deprivation. Hormone therapy works best with prostate cancer cells that are "hormone sensitive" (Oesterling & Moyad, 1998). The goal is to decrease a patient's testosterone level to zero. This is palliative treatment and not intended as a cure.

  LHRH agonists (luteinizing hormone-releasing hormone)—Most common are Lupron (1-, 3-, or 4-month IM injection), Eligard (1-, 3-, or 4-month subcutaneous injection (planning to come out with 1-year injection), Zoladex (every 28 days, subcutaneous injection) and Viadur (one 65 mg subcutaneous implant annually)

- Estrogen therapy

  ○ DES (diethylstilbestrol) 3 mg daily

  ○ As effective as LHRH therapy

  ○ Decreases testosterone levels as effectively as LHRH agonists, but takes two weeks before levels begin to drop.

  ○ Side effects are similar to LHRH agonists except for hot flashes, and the additional risk of heart disease

- Combination therapy is used in conjunction with LHRH or orchiectomy for complete ablation of testosterone. This combination therapy helps shut down the extra 10% of testosterone that is believed to be excreted from the adrenal glands as well as the production of other types of male hormones that activate CaP. It is used in locally advanced CaP or that which has spread to other parts of the body. Most common antiandrogen drugs are Eulexin (flutamide) or Casodex (bicalutamide). Multiple side effects have been reported in > 5% of patients (see package insert). They also interfere with long-term anticoagulant therapy. Prothrombin times should be closely monitored in patients already receiving coumarin anticoagulants who are started on antiandrogen drugs. Adjustment of the anticoagulant dose may be necessary (PDR, 2005). It should be noted that eventually hormone insensitive cells take over, and hormonal therapy is no longer effective. Chemotherapy may help for a short while. Combination therapy is known to increase life expectancy for only a short time.

- Palliative treatment of bone metastasis from prostate cancer can be accomplished with Zometa, an intravenous bisphosphonate used to treat patients with bone metastasis in conjunction with advancing CaP after treatment with at least one hormonal therapy. Zometa increases bone density and therefore helps prevent fractures and controls bone pain.

- Pain management—It is important for patients to receive adequate pain control.

Surgical

- Radical prostatectomy—Choosing this treatment option is less clear for older men who are likely to have more postoperative side effects (incontinence and impotence) and who may exhibit more underlying medical problems that can cause potential surgical complications such as infection, pneumonia, and blood clots (Calabrese, 2004).

- Brachytherapy is done through implantation of radioactive seeds into the prostate gland. Like any radioactive procedure to the prostate, postoperative side effects can include irritative voiding symptoms of frequency, urgency, and dysuria. These symptoms can be treated with alpha-blockers (see BPH) and/or anticholinergics (see urinary incontinence). Urinary retention is an infrequent problem that is generally temporary and can be treated with intermittent catheterization.

- Cryotherapy is the freezing of the prostate. The morbidity of cryosurgery is significant, and the long-term results are unknown (Presti, 2004).

- Bilateral orchiectomy (surgical castration) is best used in men who are symptomatic or asymptomatic with local advancing CaP or cancer that has spread to other parts of the body. The procedure is not reversible. Same side effects as the LHRH agonists.

Patient, Family, and Staff Education

- Resident and family should be involved with all discussions regarding initial and ongoing treatment for CaP.

- Be aware of educating residents and family members regarding comorbidities that influence treatment choices and why.

- Maintain a keen awareness that hearing and seeing deficits exist in the older man and that information may not always be heard or seen the way it was intended.

- Support residents and families with their decisions regarding treatment.

- Explain the side effects and possible outcomes of each treatment choice and what treatment is available to combat them.

- Involve a social worker in helping care for the spouse or family member who may need help coping with the diagnosis.

- If the resident has memory problems, repeat the information as needed.

- Offer educational materials to supplement one-on-one teaching.
- If the CaP results in a terminal diagnosis, help the family and resident search end-of-life options (Forest, 2004).

Physician Consultation

The physician must be involved in all discussions related to initial and ongoing treatment, especially the urologist, as necessary. Side effects from treatment should be relayed to the MD to decide on next steps.

■■■ URINARY INCONTINENCE

Definition

The International Continence Society (ICS) defines urinary incontinence (UI) as "the complaint of any involuntary leakage of urine" (Abrams et al., 2002). There should be an awareness that UI is not uniformly defined in studies, which makes the studies difficult to compare because most studies define UI by frequency of urine loss.

Epidemiology

Urinary incontinence is a major reason why people are admitted to a nursing home. It is associated with substantial morbidity and cost. Approximately 55% of all long-term care residents are incontinent. In facilities where there is a higher case mix of more complicated residents, incontinence can be as high as 70% (Watson et al., 2003). Staffing considerations can determine outcomes of treatment. Generally, residents with urinary incontinence have several issues that need resolving, including observation and tenacious care levels with dedicated staff in order to succeed in accomplishing resident goals toward continence.

Morbidity and mortality are associated with greater levels of incontinence although concomitant frailty, functional impairment, and higher illness severity among these residents

may be the reason (Holroyd-Ledue, 2004). Urinary incontinence has also been shown to be associated with increased depression, skin breakdown, and the number of falls and fall risks (Ouslander, 1995b).

Centers for Medicare and Medicaid Services (CMS) require nursing homes to provide an assessment of the incontinent problem as well as an interdisciplinary approach to treatment and management. The Minimum Data Set (MDS) documents the amount and severity of the incontinence, and the Resident Assessment Profile (RAP) for urinary incontinence guides the provider in the assessment and care of the resident with incontinence.

Common Presenting Signs and Symptoms

- Stress incontinence is the involuntary loss of urine during coughing, sneezing, laughing, or other physical activities that increase intra-abdominal pressure, in the absence of a detrusor contraction or an overdistended bladder.
- Overactive bladder (OAB)
  - ○ Urgency—The complaint of a sudden compelling desire to pass urine, which is difficult to defer.
  - ○ Frequency > 8 micturitions per day plus > 2 at night
  - ○ Urge incontinence is the complaint of involuntary leakage accompanied by or immediately preceded by urgency
- Mixed incontinence is a combination of stress and urge incontinence.
- Overflow incontinence is involuntary loss of urine associated with overdistension of the bladder. May present as frequent or constant dribbling or as urge or stress incontinence symptoms. Postvoid residual is abnormally high, generally > 150 cc.
- Functional incontinence is urine loss that may be caused by factors outside the lower

urinary tract such as chronic impairment of physical or cognitive function, or both. Diagnosis must be made by that of exclusion. Common causes are environmental, inaccessible toilet, lack of help, depression, hostility, anger, dementia, pain, or limited mobility.

Differential Diagnosis

- Identify any problems that may be causing only transient incontinence:

  ○ Delirium—Resident may be temporarily confused due to medication, infection, or environment.

  ○ Infection—Urinary tract infection, prostatitis, or BPH can cause frequency, urgency, and urge incontinence.

  ○ Atrophic vaginitis or urethritis

  ○ Medications—Some medications can cause urinary retention that in turn causes overflow incontinence. Diuretics can cause frequency and urge incontinence.

  ○ Excessive flow—Metabolic problems and congestive heart failure can cause increased urine flow that is unable to be controlled by the resident. Uncontrolled diabetes can cause bladder irritability as the resident spills sugar through his or her urine.

  ○ Restricted mobility—Residents using walkers, canes, or wheelchairs may not be able to get to the bathroom in time or their strength to transfer may be impaired.

  ○ Pain—Residents do not want to move when they are in pain and would rather wet in their peri-pad.

  ○ Constipation or stool impaction—Due to the close proximity of the rectum and bladder, stool in the rectum and colon can cause pressure on the bladder that might in turn cause bladder irritability or OAB as well as stress incontinence

due to sphincter instability or pelvic floor dysfunction.

  ○ Abnormal lab values—Elevated blood glucose or blood calcium can cause bladder irritability and in turn incontinence.

- Other causes of incontinence include the following:

  ○ Neurologic conditions, such as stroke or Parkinson's disease

  ○ Disorders of the brain and spinal cord

  ○ Urethral obstruction, such as stones or cancer of the bladder or prostate

  ○ Other chronic diseases—Cardiac, pulmonary, or dementia

Common Presenting Signs and Symptoms

- Focused history based on the frequency of urination, amount of leakage, nocturia, and ability to control urge. It is also important to determine when leakage occurs, such as with cough, sneeze, laugh, change in position, or if it is a constant leak and if resident is unaware of the leakage. How long has resident had UI, and did anything in particular cause it, such as surgery, trauma, childbirth, and so on? Was there prior treatment? Other questions can be asked based on the initial findings, especially determining the importance of the problems of UI to the resident.

- Targeted physical exam. Include at minimum the following:

  ○ Assess strength in upper and lower extremities to determine ability to toilet self.

  ○ Check sensation in lower extremities to determine ability to know when bladder is full.

  ○ Check edema in lower extremities, This fluid needs to be redistributed prior to bedtime by elevating legs in the late afternoon to promote fluid elimination and thereby decreasing nocturia.

○ Listen for bowel sounds for hypoactivity that may signal constipation.

○ Palpate abdomen for suprapubic fullness, urinary retention, tenderness, or presence of mass.

○ Perform perineal examination to include vaginal inspection for prolapse, atrophic vaginitis and skin condition in females,

stress test (urinary leakage with Valsalva or cough), and rectal exam (presence of impaction can cause pressure on the bladder).

Essential Diagnostic and Laboratory Tests

• Urinalysis—Rule out any abnormalities. See Table 10-2.

DETERMINATION	NORMAL VALUE	CLINICAL SIGNIFICANCE
	Macroscopic Analysis	
Color	Pale yellow to dark amber	Very pale: diabetes insipidus, excess fluid intake, chronic renal disease, nervousness. Very amber: dehydration. Note: medications may alter color.
Appearance	Clear to slightly hazy	Cloudy, turbid: presence of bacteria; WBCs or RBCs
Odor	Faintly aromatic	Fetid odor: bacterial infection Ammonia: urea breakdown by bacteria
Specific gravity	1.017–1.028	Decreased: overhydration: diabetes insipidus; diet (NA, protein restriction) Elevated: decreased fluid intake; fever; diabetes mellitus Note: lower maximum value in the elderly
pH	4.5–8.0	> 8.0: bacterial infection due to *Pseudomonas* or *Proteus*, chronic renal failure; < 4.5: metabolic/respiratory acidosis, starvation
Protein	Negative	Increased: renal disease, cardiac failure, febrile states, hematuria, amyloidosis
Glucose	Negative	Positive: uncontrolled diabetes mellitus, pituitary disorders, increased intracranial pressure. Renal threshold for glucose rises after age 50 in the female > in the male.
Ketones	Negative	Positive: uncontrolled diabetes mellitus, prolonged vomiting, fasting
Blood	Negative	Positive: infection, renal calculus
Bilirubin	Negative	Positive: liver dysfunction
Nitrite	Negative	Positive: bacterial infection
Leukocyte esterase	Negative	Positive: pyuria
	Microscopic Analysis	
RBCs	Rare per high-power field	Increased: renal genitourinary disorders
WBCs	0–4 per high-power field	Increased: bacterial infection—not always a reliable indicator of infection in the elderly; if clinically asymptomatic, is not significant
Epithelial cells	0–3	Increased: probable perineal contamination
Casts	Rare per high-power field	Increased: renal disease
Bacteria	< 105 colonies/mL	Increased: bacterial infection—significance is dependent upon specimen collection technique and specific gravity of sample

Source: Brazier & Palmer, 1995.

- Postvoid residual
  - Bladder scan all residents (if scanner available).
  - 20% +/- accuracy, meaning the result of the scan can indicate 20% more or less of actual residual that has been determined by Diagnostic Ultrasound (the manufacturer) validation testing. Scanning can also be skewed by obese abdomens, scars, or ostomies.
  - Rescan residents who:
    - Experience a change in condition
    - Begin to dribble
    - Start a new medication and new incontinence
    - Are unable to void
    - Output is noted to be abnormally low in relationship to intake
    - Complain of frequent urination or urge to void
  - If a scanner is not available, obtain a postvoid residual (PVR) by in-and-out catheterization to determine proper treatment for the type of incontinence (ICI, 2001)
  - No consensus on abnormal PVR. However, > 200 cc needs attention and treatment.
- Bladder records (see Table 10-3)
  - Purpose is to identify patterns of incontinence that can help determine appropriate interventions for the incontinent resident.
  - Comparison of three full days of documentation is important to determine patterns or lack thereof.
- Interdisciplinary involvement includes the following:
  - Social worker: Mini Mental State Exam to determine level of cognition and Geriatric Depression Scale to rule out depression as a transient cause

  - Dietician—Determine fluid balance and dietary fiber needs to prevent constipation and avoid unnecessary laxatives.
  - Pharmacist—Review medications that may contribute to incontinence.
  - PT/OT—Assess mobility/dexterity for toileting and feeding.

Management Plan

The treatment goals for residents with urinary incontinence must be individualized and developed with the resident's wishes in mind. They may range from being completely continent during the day, continent at night, decreased incontinent episodes, incontinence containment with incontinent products, incontinent when going out, to being completely dry. For some residents, continence is not possible. Their goals should be that they are odor free and that their skin remains intact.

Nonpharmacologic
- Begin with behavioral management. Minor changes can make a world of difference when treating incontinence.
  - Avoid bladder irritants including caffeine, artificial sweeteners, grapefruit/grapefruit juice, tomatoes and tomato products, spicy foods, citrus drinks, excessive milk, and alcohol.
  - Fluid management—6–8 cups per day in a balanced distribution with and between meals is all that is necessary. Avoid fluids after supper except when necessary. Minimal fluid intake not only increases bladder irritability but also puts the resident at risk for dehydration (Simmon, 2001).
  - Weight loss—Excessive abdominal pressure causes increased stress and urge incontinence.
  - Stop smoking if your facility still allows smoking.
- Pelvic muscle rehabilitation
  - Kegel exercises have been shown to be quite effective in both stress and urge in-

TABLE 10-3   Bladder Record

Instructions: Collect data for a minimum of 3 days. Compare the days and develop a plan for prompt voiding, habit training or bladder retraining. Also determine fluid modifications as well as other interventions that would be helpful in maintaining continence. Utilize all recorded information for an individualized approach to continence care. This form should be completed by all staff toileting residents.

TIME	DID RESIDENT URINATE IN TOILET? Y = YES N = NO	WAS THE URGE TO URINATE PRESENT? Y = YES N = NO	WAS THERE A LEAKING EPISODE? Y = YES N = NO	ACTIVITY AT THE TIME OF LEAKING	AMOUNT AND TYPE OF FLUID INTAKE	DIURETIC ADMINISTERED. NOTE TIME AND NAME WITH DOSAGE
6–7 am						
7–8 am						
8–9 am						
9–10 am						
11–12 am						
12–1 pm						
1–2 pm						
2–3 pm						
3–4 pm						
4–5 pm						
5–6 pm						
6–7 pm						
7–8 pm						
8–9 pm						
9–10 pm						
10–11 pm						
11 pm to 6 am						

Number of pads used today: _____
(please make slash mark every time a new pad is put on)
Number of times resident changed clothes/underwear today: _____
(please make a slash mark whenever clothes or underwear were changed due to wetness)

NOTES/COMMENTS: _____

_____

continence (Burgio et al., 2002). Residents can be taught proper technique with a simple vaginal exam with one finger. Have resident squeeze that finger without moving her abdomen or rest of the body. Isolation of the muscle as well as proper technique is important when it comes to success. This should be taught to cognitively intact residents.

○ Kegel exercises with the ball can be performed in a group or in private. Place a 4-inch ball or large roll of toilet paper between the knees. With toes pointed inward, have resident squeeze the ball. This technique contracts the pelvic floor muscles (Hulme, 1997).

○ Kegel exercises with biofeedback can be done by an advanced practice nurse or therapist in the community or in the facility if the equipment is available. This technique is also very effective (Burgio et al., 2002). Resident must be cognitively intact.

○ Kegel exercises with pelvic floor stimulation is generally done by an advanced practice nurse or therapist. If available, pelvic floor stimulation is an excellent technique for the cognitively intact resident who cannot identify his or her pelvic floor muscle.

• Toileting techniques

○ Urge reduction techniques for residents with urgency and urge incontinence. When the resident feels the urge to urinate, have him or her stop what they are doing, take a deep breath and do 2–3 quick Kegel exercises. Relax and try distraction until someone can come to help. Going to the bathroom while having an urge will result in leakage every time.

○ Bladder emptying techniques are for residents with higher postvoid residuals and for those who dribble after they urinate. When the resident is finished voiding,

have them move side to side or partially stand, sit back on the toilet, press over the bladder, lean forward, and relax. Excessive urine should evacuate. Men should do the same except add a Kegel exercise to empty the urethra.

• Bladder training

○ Retraining the bladder gradually increases voiding time intervals. It is used for frequency and urgency. The resident is encouraged to delay or postpone voiding, practice urge reduction inhibition, and urinate according to a timetable.

○ Prompt voiding, especially in long-term care is very effective in maintaining dryness (Ouslander, 1995a). A specific behavioral protocol is developed, such as contact resident every 2 hours. Toileting assistance at this time is offered. Positive feedback for dryness is given as well as for successful toileting. This technique provides social interaction and verbal feedback.

○ Habit training is voiding according to one's schedule. Use the bladder diaries as a guideline (Pfister, 1999).

• Miscellaneous interventions include the following:

○ Environment—Cold increases urge. Make sure there is bathroom access.

○ Toileting substitutes—Condom catheters at night or when going out. Bedside commode.

○ Garments—Adaptive clothing

○ Use proper incontinent products. Avoid larger products for small leaks.

○ Skin care for prevention of excoriated areas and skin ulcers

• Treating contributory problems:

○ Constipation—Consult with dietician for increases in dietary fiber.

○ UTI—Treat symptomatic residents. Refer to UTI section.

○ Vaginal prolapse—Fit for pessary or refer to gynecologist or other provider who fits pessaries.

• Nocturia—This is very difficult to treat in a long-term care facility because of the limited numbers of staff in attendance on the night shift. Other shifts can help by avoiding all fluid overload to be processed and excreted at night. The general consensus is to not wake the resident at night to toilet. It is normal for an elderly person to void 1–2 times at night. Kidneys generally manufacture more urine at night. Dependent fluid circulates when supine. It would be helpful for the afternoon staff to lay the resident to rest for 45–60 minutes prior to dinner to help elevate edematous extremities to improve circulation and help eliminate excess fluid at that time. Bedpans generally do not help in the elimination process unless the resident is sitting upright. Encourage use of bedside commode or get resident up to the bathroom when he or she awakens. Giving diuretics at noon will sometimes help "dry out" the bladder prior to bedtime if the resident is not going to bed too early. Staff should not have any greater expectations than five uninterrupted hours of sleep for each resident. Tranquilizers and sedatives contribute to UI by relaxing the bladder at night. Waking residents at night should be reserved for those who request it. There is no evidence that proves prompted voiding at night improves continence (Ouslande et al., 2001). Provide proper protection and skin care.

• Cognitively impaired residents can be dry. All medical and transient possibilities for UI must be treated. Residents can easily be toileted on a prompt voiding schedule and will do well if treated according to dementia guidelines.

• Catheters:

○ Intermittent catheterization should be used for residents with abnormally high postvoid residuals, such as > 200 cc (ICI, 2002) or neurogenic bladders. Proper cleansing, skin care, and lubrication are important to prevent trauma and infection. If the retention and/or incontinence is not able to be managed with intermittent catheterization, a Foley catheter may be appropriate (Centers for Medicare and Medicaid Services [CMS], 2005).

○ Condom catheters can be used on men at night or when going out. Apply and change according to manufacturers' recommendations. Proper skin care is critical to prevent skin breakdown and UTI (Lekan-Rutledge et al., 2003)

○ Foley catheter should be used when the positives outweigh the negatives. When there is a concomitant stage III or IV pressure ulcer that needs healing in an area where voiding would prevent that, a Foley is a good temporary choice. Foley catheters can also be used to rest a bladder in cases where overdistention has caused decreased elasticity of the bladder walls causing inability of the detrusor muscle to contract. Terminal illness or severe impairment that makes movement extremely painful can also warrant a Foley catheter. In instances where there are symptomatic UTIs causing renal function impairment characterized by an inability of the bladder to empty properly, a Foley catheter would be a proper choice (CMS, 2005).

■ Irrigation of Foley catheters is not recommended except for removal of clots or mucus due to obstruction. Disrupting the closed system causes the highest concern for infection. Long-term catheter use is not recommended because of the multiple complications it can cause. Reassess resident periodically to determine the potential for catheter removal

○ Suprapubic catheters are used for residents who need long-term catheterization when intermittent catheterization is not an option. They are contraindicated for residents with intrinsic sphincter deficiency or chronic unstable bladders. This is a surgical procedure. Periodic changing of the catheter can be done in the skilled facility by a nurse as ordered by the provider.

Pharmacologic

- There are currently no FDA-approved medications for stress urinary incontinence. Some medications have been used off label, but none of them have proven effectiveness nor are they free from side effects, especially in the elderly (Gray, 2004).

- Urgency and urge incontinence are treated with anticholinergic and antimuscarinic medications. These medications carry with them side effects of dry mouth, constipation, dry eyes, and some central nervous system (CNS) effects of confusion and dizziness that can be exacerbated by coexisting diseases, especially dementia. They are contraindicated in residents with narrow-angle glaucoma and GERD (gastroesophageal reflux disease). Alzheimer patients who are taking cholinergic agents are not good candidates for these drugs (Roe et al., 2002). Furthermore, if a resident has detrusor hyperactivity with impaired contractility, urinary retention can become a problem. The antimuscarinic agents are better tolerated and generally have no CNS side effects (see Table 10-4).

- For men with lower urinary tract symptoms caused by BPH, alpha blockade is the first line of therapy. It has recently been shown that residents with BPH and lower urinary tract symptoms can increase their quality of life by adding an anticholinergic agent, preferably Detrol LA. This combination has

been shown to be safe and effective. Together they have not affected the quality of urine flow nor caused any urinary retention (Athanasopoulos et al., 2003).

- Vaginal estrogens have had mixed reviews in the research literature, but have been notably effective in case reports. It is a known fact that estrogen receptors reside in the urethra as well as vaginal tissues. Its role is unclear in stress and urge incontinence but is known to improve it. (Robinson & Cardozo, 2003). Vaginal estrogens come in three different preparations: cream, Vagifem suppositories, or Estring. Creams (Estrace and Premarin) are dosed at 2 gm nightly for 2–3 weeks, then twice weekly. The Vagifem suppositories are dosed similarly. An Estring is placed in the vagina for 3 months and then changed. No other care is needed. Even though there is minimal systemic absorption of topical estrogens, for women on long-term therapy, breast cancer is still a remote possibility. Vaginal estrogen therapy also reduces vaginal burning and itching thereby increasing comfort and decreasing agitation.

Surgical

- Urethral bulking agents are indicated for patients with stress urinary incontinence with intrinsic sphincter insufficiency. It is a simple, office-based procedure. Only local anesthesia is necessary. Symptomatic improvement is generally seen. However, the procedure must be repeated anywhere from every 6 months to 2 years, and it should be noted that some women with repeat injections (40%) continued to have unresolved incontinence (Winters et al., 2000).

- The tension-free vaginal tape (TVT) procedure is a simple, outpatient procedure that is relatively painless but does require general, but minimal, anesthesia and recovery time. It offers about an 85–90% cure rate for residents with stress incontinence (Haab et al., 2001), but that decreases to 74% in residents

TABLE 10-4   Medications for Incontinence

MEDICATION	DOSAGES	ADVERSE EVENTS (> 5%) *DOSE	DRUG-DRUG INTERACTIONS	HALF-LIFE	COMMENTS
Detrol LA (Tolterodine)	2 mg or 4 mg* QD Immediate release Also available, given BID	Dry mouth 23% Headache 6% Constipation 6%	None	8 hours	No dosage adjustments needed for elderly residents unless renal, hepatic impairment Research available on elderly (Zinner, 2002) for safety, efficacy, and adverse events
Ditropan XL (Oxybutynin)	5 mg, 10 mg* or 15 mg, QD Available in tablet or syrup 5 mg/5 mL Available generic, immediate release	Dry mouth 29% Diarrhea 7% Constipation 7% Headache 6%	Studies not conducted	12 hours	Likely to cross blood-brain barrier (Kay, 2005) May have significant cognitive effects
Enablex (Darifenacin)	7.5 mg* or 15 mg QD	Constipation 20.9% Dry mouth 18.7% Headache 6.7%	Digoxin, ketoconazole, itraconazole, ritonavir, nelfinavir, clarithromycin and nefazodone (see package insert for details)	13–19 hours	Highest percentage of constipation of all drugs in the class
Oxytrol (Oxybutynin)	3.9 mg* patch Change twice weekly (every 3-4 days)	Site pruritis 14% Site erythema 8.3%	Studies not conducted	7–8 hours	Geriatric effectiveness no different than younger people. 49% of patients in original study were >65 years old Likely to cross blood-brain barrier More convenient mode of delivery. Much fewer GI side effects
Sanctura (Trospium chloride)	20 mg* BID	Dry mouth 20.1% Constipation 9.6%	None	20 hours	Needs to be taken on an empty stomach or 1 hour before meals In residents > 75 years, dosage may be decreased to 20 mg. QD based on tolerability
VESIcare (Solifenacin)	5 mg* or 10 mg QD	Dry mouth 10.9% Constipation 5.4%	None	45–68 hours	No CNS side effects Favorable tolerability profile

• Do not administer these drugs to residents with controlled narrow-angle glaucoma, significant bladder outflow obstruction, GI obstructive disorders, or renal or hepatic dysfunction.
•• All information provided is from package inserts or advertised company literature.
••• Effectiveness similar in all drugs.

with incontinence secondary to intrinsic sphincter deficiency (Rezapour et al., 2001). It is important to perform preoperative urodynamics and urologic examination to determine proper diagnosis.

- In-office microwave procedures may be appropriate for men with BPH and lower urinary tract symptoms. Several types are available (see the section titled "Surgical Therapy—Minimally Invasive" in this chapter). Qualification includes size of prostate, no cancer, and ability of patient to tolerate the procedure.

- Other surgical procedures are available, but not likely appropriate for residents in long-term care. They are artificial sphincters, sling procedures, reconstructive vaginal procedures, and prostate resection and/or removal.

Patient, Family, and Staff Education

- Demystify all myths regarding urinary incontinence:
  - *It is a normal part of aging:* it is not a normal part of aging. Normal aging processes may contribute to incontinence, but they do not inevitably cause it.
  - *There are no effective treatments for nursing home residents:* explain that many different interventions have improved outcomes for long-term residents as proven through research.
  - *Incontinence is not manageable in residents with dementia:* bladder training programs have been shown to be effective in both cognitively intact as well as impaired residents (Palmer et al., 1997)
  - *Total dryness is the only successful outcome:* many residents are happy to sleep through the night, have dry days, fewer episodes of incontinence resulting in the use of fewer products, ability to go out with family without wetting, toilet less frequently, and have a greater percentage of dry time in a 24-hour period.

  - Foley catheters are the only way to control intractable incontinence: a critical review of both negative and positive reasons why someone may need a Foley catheter should be done if one is being considered. Foley catheters should be used only under extreme circumstances and must be closely monitored and cared for to prevent infection.
- Reinforce preventive and behavioral interventions.
- Encourage participation in bladder training programs.

Physician Consultation

To ensure proper care and treatment of residents with complex urological problems, it is prudent to refer to an urologist in the following situations (Kane et al., 1994):

- History of recent lower urinary tract or pelvic surgery or irradiation
- Relapse or rapid recurrence of a symptomatic UTI
- Marked pelvic prolapse
- Severe stress incontinence not treatable by behavioral treatments
- Marked prostatic enlargement and/or suspicion of cancer causing severe hesitancy, straining, and/or interrupted urinary stream
- Postvoid residual volumes > 200 mL
- Difficulty passing a #14 French catheter
- Hematuria—Greater than five red blood cells per high-power field on microscopic exam in the absence of infection
- Uncertain diagnosis after complete history and physical exam

■ URINARY TRACT INFECTIONS

Definition

The term *urinary tract infection* (UTI) refers to an inflammation in the urinary tract. Such infections can range from an asymptomatic presence of bacteria in the urine to severe infection in the kidney. In any event, a microbial pathogen is present in the urinary tract associated with bacteriuria and pyuria. Symptomatic urinary tract infections can be complicated or uncomplicated (Blais, 2004). Complicated symptomatic UTI can involve the upper urinary tract, be catheter related, pertain to frequent UTIs, or just be the presence of bacteremia. Generally they are caused by a wider spectrum of organisms showing resistant pathogens or multiple pathogens. UTIs also occur in people with bladder prolapse, neurogenic bladder, or underlying structural and functional genitourinary abnormalities. Uncomplicated UTI is a lower tract infection occurring most frequently in women. Localized symptoms versus systemic symptoms are present. Organisms are usually *E. coli*, *Staphylococcus*, *Klebsiella*, and *Proteus* (Shua-Haim & Ross, 2000).

Epidemiology

Urinary tract infection is the most common infection in elderly residents of long-term care facilities. The identification, monitoring, and treatment of UTI, especially with asymptomatic bacteriuria, becomes challenging due to the atypical presentations of symptoms in the elderly. Left untreated, UTI can contribute to grave complications including sepsis and renal and perirenal disease such as pyelonephritis and subsequent increased morbidity.

Incidence varies among the institutionalized elderly. Urinary tract infections are usually asymptomatic, with a high prevalence of asymptomatic bacteriuria ranging between 15–30% in men and 25–50% in women. Men with external collection devices have twice the evidence. The incidence of symptomatic infection varies from 0.1–2.4 episodes per 1000 resident days (Nicolle, 2002a).

Risk factors for UTI in the elderly in long-term care include the following:

- Urinary retention
  - Men—Prostatic hypertrophy
  - Women—Anterior vaginal prolapse

- Any form of instrumentation, especially catheterization
- Recent surgery and/or hospitalization
- Cognitive impairment
- Incontinence
- Immunosuppression
- Noncircumcised male

Common Presenting Signs and Symptoms

- In the young adult, UTIs generally present with dysuria, urgency, and frequency.
- The elderly patient presents with atypical symptoms. Generally there is an increase in incontinence, a new incontinence, urinary frequency, nocturia, loss of appetite, a decline in cognition or functional status, or fever. Less than 10% of episodes of fever are attributable to invasive UTI (Orr et al., 1996).
- Upper tract infection presents with flank pain, chills, fever and costovertebral angle (CVA) tenderness, headache, and malaise.
- Change in the character of urine is common: cloudy, bloody, or malodorous.

Differential Diagnosis

- Determine:
  - Asymptomatic versus symptomatic
  - Lower urinary tract versus upper tract
- Prostatitis—Urinary frequency, dysuria
- Atrophic vaginitis—Pain with urination, itching, vaginal bleeding
- Urinary calculi—Pain and hematuria
- Bladder cancer—Frequency, urgency, hematuria (gross or microscopic)

Essential Diagnostic and Laboratory Tests

Urinalysis
Urine dipstick is a screening tool. Procedure must be followed exactly to achieve reliable

test results. See package insert for specific sensitivity issues. Leukocyte esterase (indicative of pyuria or presence of WBCs) and nitrite can be easily detected by urine dipstick and are more reliable when the bacterial count is greater than 100,000 colony-forming units (CFU) per milliliter (Smith, 2004). They are not recommended for general screening due to the high incidence of bacteriuria already present in this patient population. All skilled nursing residents should have a baseline urine profile to compare in determining presence or absence of UTI.

Voided specimens have a high probability of contamination especially in the elderly woman.

For patients with chronic UTIs, or those unable to give a clean catch, midstream urine specimen (obese, demented, or incontinent patients), a catheterized specimen is the most accurate testing tool. Clear patient and staff instruction is critical for collection of a good specimen.

Urine Culture and Sensitivity

The gold standard for identification of UTI is the quantitative culture of urine for specific bacteria (Smith, 2004) and sensitivity testing to determine proper treatment. Sources of bacterial infection include *Escherichia coli*, *Proteus, Mirabilis, Klebsiella pneumoniae*, and the *Pseudomonas, Enterococcus*, and *Staphylococcus* species, both gram-positive and gram-negative cocci (McCue, 2000).

Consensus on criteria for presence of infection is mixed. Generally, 10^5 colony-forming units (CFU) of a uropathogen per mL of urine is the standard for determination of the presence of infection.

Other Tests

- CBC if systemic symptoms are present
- Blood cultures with severely ill elderly presenting with elevated WBCs and fever
- Consider other diagnostic studies after consultation with physician.
- Centers for Medicare and Medicaid Services (CMS) requires the following criteria

for treatment of symptomatic UTIs (Centers for Medicare and Medicaid, 2005):

○ Residents without a catheter should have at least three of the following signs and symptoms:

- Fever—Increase in temperature of > 2°F (1.1°C) or rectal temperature > 99.5°F (37.5°C) or single measurement of temperature > 100°F (37.8°C)

- New or increased burning pain on urination, frequency, or urgency

- New flank or suprapubic pain or tenderness

- Change in character of urine (e.g., new bloody urine, foul smell, or amount of sediment) or as reported by the laboratory (new pyuria or microscopic hematuria)

- Worsening of mental or functional status (e.g., confusion, decreased appetite, unexplained falls, incontinence of recent onset, lethargy, decreased activity)

○ Residents with catheter should have at least two of the following signs and symptoms:

- Fever or chills

- New flank pain or suprapubic pain or tenderness

- Change in character of urine (e.g., new bloody urine, foul smell, or amount of sediment) or as reported by the laboratory (new pyuria or microscopic hematuria)

- Worsening of mental or functional status. Local findings such as obstruction, leakage, or mucosal trauma (hematuria) may also be present.

Management Plan

The treatment goals for patients with UTIs are to alleviate symptoms, identify causative organism(s) and treat accordingly, and prevent further urinary tract problems.

Nonpharmacologic

- Identify causative pathogens. After obtaining a urine culture and sensitivity, the report will guide treatment. See Table 10-5 for treatment guidelines for common genitourinary pathogens.

- Scan bladder or quick cath to determine postvoid residual (PVR) to rule out chronic retention. If abnormal PVR, refer to urologist. Stagnant urine in the bladder harboring pathogens must be removed either by indwelling catheter, use of bladder-emptying techniques, or correction of outlet obstruction. This is especially problematic in the elderly male patient and the female patient with large anterior bladder prolapse.

- Assess for adequate fluid intake. Baseline of 1200–1500 cc would ensure the bladder is adequately flushed (Blais, 2004). Increase water intake to 8–10 cups per day at first sign of infection.

- Review personal hygiene techniques, women wiping front to back and men pulling foreskin back for cleansing.

- Implementation of bowel program if fecal incontinence present.

Pharmacologic

- Medical treatment is indicated only if patient is symptomatic or at risk for developing further complications (Melillo, 1995). Unless there is an actual urinary tract obstruction there is no convincing evidence that asymptomatic bacteriuria causes renal insufficiency or can lead to premature death (Gleckman, 1994). Still, some researchers favor drug therapy for long-term care residents who may be immunosuppressed by diabetes, leukopenia, and steroid therapy.

- According to a consensus panel (Loeb et al., 2001), the following minimum criteria must be present prior to treatment for UTI:
  - Without indwelling catheter:

    - Acute dysuria by itself, *or*
    - Fever > 37.9°C with at least one of the following: new or worsening urgency, frequency, suprapubic pain, gross hematuria, costovertebral angle tenderness, or new or worsening urinary incontinence
  - With indwelling catheter:
    - Presence of any one of the following: fever, new costovertebral angle tenderness, rigors with or without identified cause, or new onset delirium

- Medication type, duration, and strength will depend on simple versus complex UTI, source/type of infection, and prophylactic usage.

- Intravaginal estrogen—Use as directed to initially estrogenize vagina. Types may include Estrace cream, Vagifem suppositories, or an Estring.

- Cranberry pills, 1–2 up to BID, are used as a preventative measure. It prevents bacteria from adhering to the bladder walls. Cranberry pills *do not* cure bacterial bladder infections.

Patient, Family, and Staff Education

- Discuss treatment plan and rationale.
- Monitor vital signs, especially temperature and pulse, during the initial stages of treatment.
- Assist in encouraging resident to increase fluid intake.
- Good perineal hygiene including timely changing of incontinent products

Physician Consultation

- Report any patients with complicated UTIs (i.e., more than one organism or systemic manifestations).
- Infections with unusual organisms
- Upper tract involvement (pyelonephritis)

TABLE 10-5   Treatment Guidelines for Common Genitourinary Pathogens

UTI TYPE	PATHOGEN	CHOICE OF ANTIBIOTIC	DOSE	DURATION OF TX	COMMENTS
Asymptomatic bacteremia	Escherichia coli Staphylococcus saprophyticus Proteus mirabilis Klebsiella pneumoniae				Treatment not recommended (McCue, 2000; Nicolle, 2002) May give prophylactic, one dose of fluoroquinolone with genitourinary invasive procedures.
Simple, symptomatic UTI	Escherichia coli Proteus mirabilis Klebsiella pneumoniae Staphylococcus Saprophyticus	Trimethoprim-sulfamethoxazole (TMP-SMX) double strength (DS) Nitrofurantoin (Macrobid) Fluoroquinolone Amoxicillin	160/800 mg BID 100 mg BID Depends on drug 250 mg every 8 hours	3–7 days 7–10 days 1–3 days 7 days	Follow sensitivity chart for all bacteria for proper treatment. If gram-negative organism, oral fluoroquinolone If gram-positive, amoxicillin or amoxicillin/clavulanate
Complicated UTI	Escherichia coli Proteus mirabilis Klebsiella pneumoniae Serratia Providencia Enterobacter Pseudomonas Candida	Trimethoprim-sulfamethoxazole (TMP-SMX) double strength (DS) Nitrofurantoin (Macrobid) Fluoroquinolone Amoxicillin 3rd-generation cephalosporin	160/800 mg BID 100 mg BID Depends on drug 250 mg every 8 hours 7–10 days Depends on drug	7–10 days 10 days 3–10 days 7 days	Follow sensitivity chart for all bacteria for proper treatment. If gram-negative organism, oral fluoroquinolone If gram-positive, amoxicillin or amoxicillin/clavulanate
Catheter-associated UTI	Escherichia coli Proteus mirabilis Klebsiella pneumoniae Serratia Providencia Enterobacter Pseudomonas Candida Multiple organisms	Fluoroquinolone	Depends on drug	10–14 days	Replace catheter prior to treatment. Follow sensitivity chart for all bacteria for proper treatment. If gram-negative organism, oral fluoroquinolone If gram-positive, amoxicillin or amoxicillin/clavulanate

continued

TABLE 10-5 (*continued*)

UTI TYPE	PATHOGEN	CHOICE OF ANTIBIOTIC	DOSE	DURATION OF TX	COMMENTS
Acute pyelonephritis	Escherichia coli Proteus Klebsiella Enterobacteria	Fluoroquinolone, 3rd-generation cephalosporin Beta-lactamase inhibitor Ampicillin, aminoglycosides	Depends on drug	10–14 days Oral therapy 7–10 days, IV therapy	IV drugs if febrile. Maintain IV while fever persists Continue 7–10 days after fever gone with bacteremia
Prophylactic treatments	Escherichia coli Staphylococcus saprophyticus Proteus mirabilis Klebsiella pneumoniae	TMP-SMX* Nitrofurantoin* Cephalexin*	160/800 mg, ½ tablet at bedtime 50–100 mg at bedtime 250 mg at bedtime	Minimum of 3–6 months	Use prophylaxis if more than three documented UTIs in one year. Drugs can also be used postcoital.* Can also consider every other day dosing.* If breakthrough UTIs occur, can alternate TMP-SMX and nitrofurantoin every other month.

Note: Drugs do not necessarily correspond to specific pathogen on chart. Always utilize culture and sensitivity as a guide in treating urinary tract infections. Also note that there is only general consensus on length of treatment, but that too depends on circumstances.

- Recurrent, symptomatic UTIs—3–4 in the past year
- Men with elevated PVR and/or outlet obstruction
- Women with grade III–IV cystocele
- Patients who are refractory to treatment

▄▄ WEB SITES

- National Kidney and Urologic Diseases Information Clearinghouse—www.kidney.niddk.nih.gov/about/index.htm
- National Institute on Aging—www.nia.nih.gov
- The National Kidney Foundation—www.kidney.org
- Prostate Cancer—www.PROSTATEinfo.com
- Us Too! International, Inc.—www.ustoo.org
- Prostate Cancer Resource Network—www.pcrn.org
- Prostate Cancer Research and Education Foundation—www.prostatecancer.com
- American Foundation for Urologic Disease—www.incontinence.org
- Simon Foundation for Continence—www.simonfoundation.org.html
- National Association for Continence (NAFC)—www.nafc.org
- National Institute of Diabetes and Digestive and Kidney Diseases—www.niddk.nih.gov
- National Institute on Aging—www.nia.nih.gov
- National Kidney and Urologic Diseases Information Clearinghouse—www.kidney.niddk.nih.gov/about/index.htm
- Centers for Medicare and Medicaid—www.cms.hhs.gov/providers/snfpps

▄▄ REFERENCES

Abrams, P., Cardozo, L., Fall, M., Griffiths, D., Rosier, P., Ulmsten, U., et al. (2002). The standardisation of terminology of lower urinary tract function: Report from the standardisation sub-committee of the International Continence Society. *Neurology and Urodynamics, 21*, 167–178.

Agency for Health Care Policy and Research. (1994). Benign prostatic hyperplasia: Diagnosis and treatment. Clinical practice guideline No. 8 (DHHS Publication No. 94–0582). Rockville, MD: U.S. Department of Health and Human Services.

Amend, W., & Vincenti, F. (2004). Oliguria: Acute renal failure. In E. A. Tanagho & J. W. McAninch (Eds.), *Smith's general urology* (16th ed., pp. 538–542). New York: Lange Medical Books/McGraw-Hill.

American Urologic Association. (2000). *AUA prostate specific antigen (PSA) best practice policy*. Linthicum, MD: Author.

Athanasopoulos, A., Gyftopoulos, K., Giannitsas, J., Fisfis, P., Perimenis, P., & Barbalias, G. (2003). Combination treatment with an a-blocker plus an anticholinergic for bladder outlet obstruction: A prospective, randomized, controlled study. *Journal of Urology, 169*(6), 2253–2256.

Blais, D. (2004). Urinary tract infections among the institutionalized older adult. *Perspectives, 28*(2), 23–34.

Bostwick, D., Crawford, E. D., Higano, C., & Roach, M. (2005). *Complete guide to prostate cancer*. Atlanta, GA: American Cancer Society.

Brazier, A., & Palmer, M. (1995). Collecting clean catch urine in the nursing home: Obtaining the uncontaminated specimen. *Geriatric Nursing, 16*(2), 219.

Burgio, K. L., Goode, P. S., Locher, J. L., et al. (2002). Behavioral training with and without biofeedback in the treatment of urge incontinence in older women: A randomized controlled trial. *Journal of the American Medical Association, 288*, 2293–2299.

Burgio, K. L., Locher, J. L., Goode, P. S., et al. (1998). Behavioral versus drug treatment for urge urinary incontinence in older women: A randomized controlled trial. *Journal of the American Medical Association, **280***: 1995–2000.

Calabrese, D. (2004). Prostate cancer in older men. *Urologic Nursing, 24*(4), 258–269.

Centers for Medicare and Medicaid, U.S. Department of Health and Human Services. (2005). *CMS manual system: Pub. 100-7 state operations: Provider certification*. Retrieved September 25,

2006, from http://www.cms.hhs.gov/transmittals/downloads/R8SOM.pdf

Centers for Medicare and Medicaid Services, U.S. Department of Health and Human Services. (2005). *CMS online manual system.* Retrieved September 25, 2006, from http://www.cms.hhs. gov/ Manuals

Chow, D. (2001). Benign prostatic hyperplasia: Patient evaluation and relief of obstructive symptoms. *Geriatrics, 56*(3), 33–38.

Debruyne, F., Barkin, J., vanErps, P., Reis, M., Tammela, T. L. J., & Roehrborn, C. (2004). Efficacy and safety of long-term treatment with the dual 5a-reductase inhibitor dutasteride in men with symptomatic benign prostatic hyperplasia. *European Urology, 46,* 488–495.

Duffield, P. (1997). Urinary tract infections in the elderly a common complication. *ADVANCE for Nurse Practitioners,* April, 30–32.

Eriksen, P. S., & Rasmussen, H. (1992). Low-dose 17 beta-estradiol vaginal tablets in the treatment of atrophic vaginitis: A double-blind placebo controlled study. *European Journal of Obstetric, Gynecologic, and Reproductive Biology, 44,* 137–144.

Fanti, J. A., Newman, D. K., Colling, J., et al. (1996). Clinical practice guidelines, No. 2, Update: Urinary incontinence in adults. Acute and chronic management (AHCPR Publication No. 96–0682). Rockville, MD: U.S. Department of Health and Human Services, Public Services Agency for Health Care Policy and Research.

Fleischmann, N. B. (2004). The diagnosis, management, and treatment of geriatric urinary incontinence. *Issues in Incontinence,* Spring/Summer, 1–7.

Forest, P. (2004). Being there: The essence of end-of-life nursing care. *Urologic Nursing,* Aug. 24, 270–280.

Gerared, M., & Frank-Stromborg, M. (1998). Screening for prostate cancer in asymptomatic men: Clinical, legal, and ethical implications. *Oncology Nursing Forum, 25*(9), 1561–1569.

Gleckman, R. (1994). Urinary tract infections in nursing home residents. *Long-term Care Forum, 4*(3), 10–14.

Gray, M. (2004). Myth, misconceptions, and other impediments to the diagnosis and treatment of stress urinary incontinence. *American Journal for Nurse Practitioners,* May (Suppl.), 15–22.

Gretzer, M., & Partin, A. (2003). PSA and PSA molecular derivatives. *Campbell's Updates, 1*(1), 1–12.

Haab, F., Ciofu, C., & Traxer, O. (2001). The tension-free vaginal tape technique: Why an unusual concept is so successful. *Current Opinion in Urology, 11,* 293–297.

Hazard, W. R., & Bierman, E. L. (1994). *Principles of geriatric medicine and gerontology* (3rd ed.). New York: McGraw-Hill.

Holcomb, S. (2005). Evaluating chronic kidney disease risk. *The Nurse Practitioner, 30*(4), 12–27.

Holroyd-Leduc, J. M., Mehta, K., & Covinsky, K. (2004). Urinary incontinence and its association with death, nursing home admission, and functional decline. *Journal of the American Geriatrics Society, 52,* 712–718.

Hulme, J. (1997). *Beyond Kegels.* Missoula, MT: Phoenix Publishing.

Issa, M., & Marshall, F. (2004). *Contemporary diagnosis and management of diseases of the prostate* (2nd ed.). Newtown, PA: Handbooks in Health Care Co.

Johnson, C. A. J., Levey, A. S., Coreshl, J., et al. (2004). Clinical practice guidelines for chronic kidney disease in adults: Part 1. Definition, disease stages, evaluation, treatment, and risk factors. *American Family Physician, 70*(5), 869–876.

Kane, R., Ouslander, J., & Abrass, I. (1994). *Essentials of clinical geriatrics* (3rd ed., pp. 145–196). New York: McGraw-Hill.

Kay, G., & Granville, L. (2005). Antimuscarinic agents: Implications and concerns in the management of overactive bladder in the elderly. *Clinical Therapeutics, 27*(1), 127–138.

Lekan-Rutledge, D., Doughty, D., Moore, K., & Saltzstein-Wooldridge, L. (2003). Promoting social continence: Products and devices in the management of urinary incontinence. *Urologic Nursing, 23*(6), 416–428.

Liann, E., & Pascual, J. (1996). Epidemiology of acute renal failure: A prospective, multi-center, community based study. Madrid Acute Renal Failure Study Group. *Kidney International, 50,* 811–818.

Loeb, M., Bentley, D. W., Bradley, S., et al. (2001). Development of minimum criteria for the initiation of antibiotics in residents of long-term care facilities: Results of a consensus conference. *Infection Control and Hospital Epidemiology, 22,* 120–124.

Lowance, D. (2002). Withholding and withdrawal of dialysis in the elderly. *Seminars In Dialysis, 15*(2), 88–90.

Lu-Yao, G., Stukel, T., & Yao, S. L. (2003). Prostate-specific antigen screening in elderly men. *Journal of the National Cancer Institute, 95*(23), 1792–1797.

McCue, J. (2000). Complicated UTI: Effective treatment in the long-term care setting. *Geriatrics, 55*(9), 48–61.

Melillo, K. (1995). Asymptomatic bacteriuria in older adults: When is it necessary to screen and treat? *Nurse Practitioner, 20*(8), 50–66.

Michigan Cancer Consortium Prostate Cancer Action Committee. (2003). Making the choice: Deciding what to do about early stage prostate cancer. A guide for patients. Michigan Cancer Consortium (MCC). Ann Arbor, MI: University of Michigan, Comprehensive Cancer Center, Health Media Research Laboratory.

Midthun, S. (2004). Criteria for urinary tract infection in the elderly: Variables that challenge nursing assessment. *Urologic Nursing 24*(3), 157–170.

Nicolle, L. (2002a). Resistant pathogens in urinary tract infections. *Journal of the American Geriatrics Society, 50,* S230–S235.

Nicolle, L. (2002b). Urinary tract infection in geriatric and institutionalized patients. *Current Opinion in Urology, 12,* 51–55.

Oesterling, J., & Moyad, M. (1998). *The ABC's of prostate cancer. The book that could save your life.* Lanham, MD: Madison Books.

Orr, P., Nicolle, L. E., Duckworth, H., Brunka, J., Kennedy, J., Murray, D., et al. (1996). Febrile urinary infection in the institutionalized elderly. *American Journal of Medicine, 100,* 71–77.

Ouslander, J., Al-Samarrai, N., & Schnelle, J. (2001). Prompted voiding for nighttime incontinence in nursing homes: Is it effective? *Journal of the American Geriatrics Society, 49,* 706–709.

Ouslander, J., & Schnelle, J. (1995). Incontinence in the nursing home. *Annals of Internal Medicine, 122*(6), 438–449.

Ouslander, J., Schnelle, J., Uman, G., Fingold, S., Nigam, J., Tuico, E., et al. (1995). Predictors of successful prompted voiding among incontinent nursing home residents. *Journal of the*

American Medical Association, 273(17), 1366–1370.

Palmer, M. H., Czarapata, B. J., Wells, T. J., & Newman, D. K. (1997). Urinary outcomes in older adults: Research and clinical perspectives. *Urologic Nursing, 17*(1), 2–9.

Pfister, S. M. (1999). Bladder diaries and voiding patterns in older adults. *Journal of Gerontological Nursing,* March, 36–41.

Presti, J. (2004). Neoplasms of the prostate gland. In E. A. Tanagho, & J. W. McAninch (Eds.), *Smith's general urology* (16th ed., pp. 367–385). New York: Lange Medical Books/McGraw-Hill.

Retik, A., Vaughan, E., & Wein, A. (Eds.). (2002). *Campbell's urology* (8th ed.). Philadelphia: Saunders.

Rezapour, M., Falconer, C., & Ulmsten, U. (2001). Tension-free vaginal tape (TVT) in stress incontinent women with intrinsic sphincter deficiency (ISD)—a long term follow up. *International Urogynecology Journal and Pelvic Floor Dysfunction, 12,* S12–S14.

Robinson, D., & Cardozo, L. D. (2003). The role of estrogens in female lower urinary tract dysfunction. *Urology, 62,* 45–51.

Roe, C. M., Anerson, M. J., & Spivack, B. (2002). Use of anticholinergic medications by older adults with dementia. *Journal of the American Geriatrics Society, 50,* 836–842.

Schnelle, J., Cadogan, M., Grbic, D., Bates-Jensen, B. M., Osterweil, D., Yoshii, J., et al. (2003). A standardized quality assessment system to evaluate incontinence care in the nursing home. *Journal of the American Geriatrics Society, 51,* 1754–1761.

Shua-Haim, J., & Ross, J. (2000). Urinary tract infections in the elderly: A practical approach. *Clinical Geriatrics, 22,* 1–15.

Smith, J. M. (2004). Indwelling catheter management: From habit-based to evidence-based practice. *Ostomy Wound Management, 49*(12), 34–45.

Specht, J. K. P. (2005). 9 Myths of incontinence in older adults. *American Journal of Nursing, 105*(6), 58–69.

Speight, J., & Roach, M. (2004). Radiotherapy of urologic tumors. In E. A. Tanagho, & J. W. McAninch (Eds.). *Smith's general urology* (16th ed., pp. 416–434). New York: Lange Medical Books/McGraw-Hill.

Sung, J., Kabalin, J.W., & Terris, M. (2000). Prostate cancer detection, characterization, and clinical outcome in men aged 70 years and older referred for transrectal ultrasound and prostate biopsies. *Urology, 56*(2), 295–301.

Tanagho, E.A., & McAninch, J. W. (2004). *Smith's general urology* (16th ed.). New York: Lange Medical Books/McGraw-Hill.

Tangalos, E. (2004). Treatment of kidney disease and anemia in elderly, long-term care residents. *Journal of the American Medical Directors Association, 5*(4 Suppl.), H1–H6.

Tannenbaum, C., & Lepage, C. (2002). Practical management of urinary incontinence in the long-term care setting. *Annals of Long-Term Care, 10,* 26–34.

Terret, C., Albrand, G., & Droz, J. P. (2004). Geriatric assessment in elderly patients with prostate cancer. *Clinical Prostate Cancer*, March, 236–240.

Vaughn, K. (1998). The prostate cancer screening in perspective. *Cleveland Clinic Journal of Medicine, 65*(9), 459–462.

Walmsley, K., Gjertsen, C., & Kaplan, S. (2004). Medical management of BPH—an update. *Campbell's Urology Updates, 2*(2), 1–12.

Watson, N., Brink, C., Zimmer, J., & Mayer, R. (2003). Use of the agency for health care policy and research urinary incontinence guideline in nursing homes. *Journal of the American Geriatrics Society, 51,* 1779–1786.

Wilt, T. J., Ishani, A., Stark, G., MacDonald, R., Lau, J., & Mulrow, C. (1998). Saw palmetto extracts for treatment of benign prostate hyperplasia: A systematic review. *Journal of the American Medical Association, 280,* 1604–1609.

Winters, J. C., Chiverton, A., Scarpero, H. M., & Prats, L. J., Jr. (2000). Collagen injection therapy in elderly women: Long-term results and patient satisfaction. *Urology, 55,* 856–861.

Zinner, N., Mattiasson, A., & Stanton, S. (2002). Efficacy, safety, and tolerability of extended-release once-daily tolterodine treatment for overactive bladder in older versus younger patients. *Journal of the American Geriatrics Society, 50,* 799–807.

CHAPTER 11

Hematology/Oncology

Julie Eggert

ACUTE LEUKEMIA

Definition

Acute leukemia is a rapidly growing malignant proliferative disease with blast cells from the myeloid or lymphoid cell lines. These nonfunctional cells accumulate in the bone morrow and peripheral blood.

Epidemiology

Acute Lymphocytic Leukemia (ALL)

Though very small, since 1998 the incidence of acute lymphocytic leukemia (ALL) has increased in male Caucasians over the age of 65. There are no known risk factors for this acute leukemia. Higher rates of ALL are found in more developed countries and in higher socioeconomic groups.

Acute Myelogenous Leukemia (Monocytic [AMoL] and Myelocytic [AMyL])

Acute myelogenous leukemia (AML) is the most common type of acute leukemia in older adults. The most recent Surveillance Epidemiology and End Results (SEER) data (1975–2003) indicates a median age at diagnosis of 67 years of age with 55.4% diagnosed after the age of 65 (National Cancer Institute [NCI], 2005). There is an overall decrease in incidence of 6.7% in all races of males and 9.6% in all races of females. However, the mortality has increased for all races of males and females.

Risk factors include exposure to high doses of radiation or radiation therapy, exposure to benzene, and previous treatment for cancer with an alkylating agent. The greatest risk factor is increasing age. Some types of myelodysplastic syndromes convert to AML.

Common Presenting Signs and Symptoms

- Insidious with progressive weakness, pallor, altered sense of well-being, and delirium
- Acute onset of malaise and high fever
- Enlarged liver, spleen, and lymph nodes
- Bleeding or easy bruising, if associated with thrombocytopenia

Acute Lymphocytic Leukemia (ALL)

- Mediastinal mass

Acute Myelocytic Leukemia (AML)

- Symptoms due to decreased levels of normal blood cells
- New cardiac symptoms or exacerbation of known cardiac disease

- Fever that may or may not be associated with infection
- Shortness of breath due to pulmonary infiltration of blast cells

Differential Diagnosis

- Leukocytosis
  - Eosinophilic (see also Hodgkin's lymphoma)
    - Asthma
    - Allergic skin diseases
    - Drug reaction
  - Monocytosis (see chronic leukemia)
- Lymphocytosis (see chronic leukemia)
  - Chronic immune stimulation
  - Epstein-Barr virus
  - Cytomegalovirus
  - Thyrotoxicosis
  - Tertiary syphilis
- Acute or chronic infection
- Endotoxemia
- Hypoxemia
- Glucocorticoid use

Essential Diagnostic and Laboratory Tests

Acute Lymphocytic Leukemia

- Peripheral white blood cell count > 20,000/mL
- Bone marrow aspiration shows evidence of leukemic cells.
- Histochemical stains, immunophenotypic and cytogenetic examination

Acute Myelocytic Leukemia

- Peripheral white blood cell counts can be high, low, or normal.
- CBC reveals anemia and low platelet count.
- Bone marrow aspiration shows evidence of leukemic cells.

- Histochemical stains, immunophenotypic and cytogenetic examination

Management Plan

Refer to a hematology oncologist or hematology specialist.

Nonpharmacologic

- Collaborate with the oncology specialists to provide a continuum of care.
- Monitor for signs and symptoms of bone marrow depression. This includes bleeding, anemia, and infection.
- Prevent trauma in order to limit bleeding and bruising.
- Promote careful hand washing and other interventions to prevent infection.

Pharmacologic

Acute Lymphocytic Leukemia

- Combination chemotherapy with vincristine, prednisone, anthracycline, and asparaginase. Typically this is poorly tolerated by older adults who usually have a relapse within one year. There is no salvage therapy for older adults, and bone marrow transplant is usually not an option for patients older than 65 years.
- Survival rate is 59% at 5 years for adults. Complete remission rates after induction are 60–90%. Maintenance therapy may be offered for up to 2 years (Magrath et al., 2005).

Acute Myelogenous Leukemia

- Several induction regimens are available to push the patient's bone marrow into remission. The use of blood products, antibiotics, and colony-stimulating factors yields a 30–50% rate of remission in persons over 60 years of age with a median relapse free survival of 9–12 months. The use of consolidation and maintenance therapy for the elderly is being studied. Like ALL, bone marrow transplant is usually not an option for patients older than 65 years (Seiter, 2002).

- Unfavorable cytogenetic profiles in the elderly reveal an increased prevalence of the multidrug resistance gene (MDR1) causing a decreased sensitivity to chemotherapy.
- For promyelocytic leukemia the patient may receive all-*trans*-retinoic acid as an oral agent to induce differentiation and put the patient in remission. The outcome is questionable, and chemotherapy may still be used.

Patient, Family, and Staff Education

- After referral and consultation with the specialist, support the patient and family in their decision for treatment.
  - Monitor for the side effects of chemotherapy.
  - Discuss interventions for anemia, neutropenia, and thrombocytopenia.
- After referral and consultation with the specialist, support the patient and family in their decision for no treatment and the goal of patient comfort using hospice and palliative care.
- Support the patient and family in the knowledge that the life span after a diagnosis of acute leukemia in elderly patients is usually 1–2 years. There is very little addition to the life expectancy even with aggressive chemotherapy.

Physician Consultation

If the peripheral blood smear has blast cells the patient should be referred to a hematology oncologist or hematology specialist for bone marrow aspiration to confirm the diagnosis.

CHRONIC LEUKEMIAS

Definition

Chronic leukemia is a slow growing malignant proliferative disease with mature cells from the myeloid or lymphoid cell lines. The cellular defect causing chronic leukemia is characterized by a failure of malignant cells to stop dividing at maturity causing a larger pool of abnormal dividing cells. Because this collective change found with chronic leukemias develops over a lifetime, the symptoms are manifested slowly.

Epidemiology

The chronic leukemias account for almost 40% of the leukemias diagnosed in adulthood (Huether & McCance, 2004). Both chronic myelogenous leukemia (CML) and chronic lymphocytic leukemia (CLL) occur more frequently after the age of 67. CLL involves the B-cell more than 95% of the time (Leukemia & Lymphoma Society, 2004). Neither leukemia has causative risk factors; however, CML does have a translocation between chromosomes 9 (ABL) and 22 (BCR). This has been identified as the "Philadelphia chromosome."

Chronic Lymphocytic Leukemia (CLL)

Men develop this proliferative disorder twice as frequently as women. There is a slight increased incidence of CLL, < 2.5%, for Caucasians of both sexes and African-American females (NCI, 2003). Because CLL tends to be diagnosed in multiple generations of a family, it is believed this leukemia has a genetic link. Families with this disease also tend to have other immunosuppressive disorders. Viruses may have a role as a risk factor, but research indicates no link between ionizing radiation and CLL (Beers, 2005).

Chronic Myelogenous Leukemia (CML)

CML is a rare disorder with only African-American women showing an increase (> 7.5%) in diagnosis between the years 1998 and 2002 (NCI, 2003). CML has a chronic phase, an accelerated phase, and blast crisis. During the chronic phase it is slow growing. When the cells begin to transform and become more blast (immature) they can transform into either a lymphoid or a myeloid leukemia.

Common Presenting Signs and Symptoms

CLL

- Often asymptomatic
- Fatigue
- Malaise
- Exercise intolerance
- Anemia and thrombocytopenia due to marrow replacement
- Night sweats

CML

- In chronic phase, symptoms similar to CLL
- Accelerated phase
  - Anemia
  - Thrombocytopenia
  - Basophilia in peripheral blood
- Later stages include the following:
  - Dragging sensation in abdomen due to splenomegaly
  - Nonspecific bone pain
  - Bleeding problems
  - Mucus membrane irritation
  - Frequent infections
  - Pallor and anemia
  - Lymphadenopathy
  - Fever
  - Night sweats

Differential Diagnosis

- Leukocytosis
  - Eosinophilic (see also Hodgkin's lymphoma)
  - Basophilic
    - Myeloproliferative disease (e.g., CML)
- Monocytosis
  - Chronic infections
  - Collagen vascular diseases
  - Inflammatory bowel diseases
- Lymphocytosis

Essential Diagnostic and Laboratory Tests

Because these are leukemias with mature cells, there is no screening test. Patients are typically diagnosed during a routine physical examination and a CBC with differential.

CLL

- CBC with differential
  - Absolute lymphocyte count > 4800 per µL
  - Cells appear mature and tend to smudge.
  - Normocytic normochromic anemia
- Coombs' test
- Bone marrow aspiration shows evidence of leukemic cells.
- Histochemical stains, immunophenotypic and cytogenetic examination

CML

- CBC with differential
  - Small proportion of very immature cells (leukemic blast cells and promyelocytes)
  - Larger proportion of maturing and fully matured white cells (myelocytes and neutrophils)
- Bone marrow aspiration shows evidence of leukemic cells.
- Histochemical stains, immunophenotypic and cytogenetic examination
  - Philadelphia chromosome

Patients with CML may relapse quickly and convert to acute leukemia. These persons may require the following:

- Cardiac scan to determine function
- Lumbar puncture if neurologic symptoms are present

Management Plan

Refer to a hematology oncologist or hematology specialist.

Nonpharmacologic
- Collaborate with the oncology specialists to provide a continuum of care.
- Protect against infection, anemia, and easy bruising or bleeding.

Pharmacologic
Treatment with chemotherapy depends on the stage of the disease. Because the malignant clones in chronic leukemias do not multiply significantly faster than normal cells, they are resistant and difficult to treat.

CLL
Gamma globulin may be administered for hypo- or agammaglobulinemia with CLL.

CML
- Gleevec (imatinib mesylate) is used during the chronic phase. It inhibits the tyrosine kinase receptors for *bcr-abl*, platelet-derived growth factor, and stem cell factor.
- Bone marrow transplant is not typically used for the elderly.

Patient, Family, and Staff Education
- Reinforce to the patient and family that the patient may live for years or decades with a chronic leukemia but it can still cause death.
- Support the patient and family in the treatment decision, and be knowledgeable about the rationale for the different management approaches.
- Educate patient, family, and staff about how to prevent infection.
- As the disease progresses, support the patient and family and reinforce the goal of patient comfort using hospice and palliative care. Help patients verbalize their desires, and assist families in preparing for the death.

Physician Consultation
Refer to a hematology oncologist or hematology specialist.

▆▆ MULTIPLE MYELOMA

Definition
Multiple myeloma is an overproduction of abnormal plasma cells. This results in excessive production of an atypical monoclonal immunoglobulin (M-protein) and the Bence-Jones protein. As the disease progresses the characteristic "punched-out lesions" in bone matrix begin to form and can be found on X-rays.

Epidemiology
There are no known risk factors for multiple myeloma. However, the research suggests a correlation with radiation exposure, cholecystitis, osteomyelitis, allergies requiring injections, rheumatoid arthritis, hereditary spherocytosis, and Gaucher's disease. Some occupations such as farming; the petroleum industry; persons who work with leather, wood, or paint; and cosmetologists all seem to have an above average chance of developing multiple myeloma. History of exposure to herbicides, insecticides, petroleum products, heavy metals, plastics, and various dusts including asbestos may also be risk factors for the disease. As individuals age there is an increase in incidence after the age of 50, with a peak between the ages of 50 and 60. African-Americans are at highest risk, especially males. There are reports in the literature of familial clusters of multiple myeloma, so genetic factors may play a role in this hematological malignancy. Genetic profiling is available as prognostic and therapeutic markers. Multiple myeloma accounts for approximately 10% of all hematological malignancies.

Common Presenting Signs and Symptoms
- Bone pain, especially low back and ribs
- Signs of thrombocytopenia
- Repeated infections
- Cold sensitivity and urticaria
- Chronic kidney disease or pyelonephritis

- Hypercalcemia
- Neurologic symptoms with compression of the spinal cord and peripheral neuropathy
- Hyperviscosity of blood
- Bleeding problems due to coagulopathy

Differential Diagnosis
- Normocytic normochromic anemias
- Osteoporosis, involutional

Other Problems to Be Considered
- Hyperparathyroidism
- Toxicity, thyroid hormone
- Toxicity, vitamin
- Metastases
- Acute lymphatic leukemia
- Nodular histiocytic lymphoma
- Chronic lymphatic leukemia
- Waldenström macroglobulinemia

Essential Diagnostic and Laboratory Tests
- CBC with differential
- Chemistry metabolic panel
- Urinalysis
- X-ray of bone at area of focused pain
- Serum protein electrophoresis with immuno-fixation
- Urine immunoelectrophoresis with immuno-fixation (24-hour urine for M-protein looking for Bence-Jones protein)
- Bone marrow aspiration with biopsy
- Beta-2 microglobulin
- Serum immunoglobulins
- Skeletal survey looking for bone disease
- Albumin (new prognostic scoring looks at albumin and beta-2 microglobulin)

Management Plan
Refer to a hematology oncologist or hematology specialist.

Nonpharmacologic
- Collaborate with the oncology specialists to provide a continuum of care.
- Encourage activity to prevent demineralization of the bone and resulting hypercalcemia.
- Encourage fluids up to 2–3 L/day.
- Monitor for hyperviscosity syndrome, hyperuricemia, and hypercalcemia.

Pharmacologic
- The most common treatments for elders are intermittent melphalan with prednisone or low-dose continuous melphalan. If the patient is eligible for transplant, this chemotherapy would not be used because it damages the bone marrow.
- Radiation therapy may be used for the osteolytic lesions in the bone.
- Autologous bone marrow transplant for persons up to age 78
- Discontinue calcium supplements and multiple vitamin supplements containing Vitamin D
- Stool softeners should be added to relieve constipation.
- Signs of hypercalcemia should be treated aggressively with etidronate disodium (Didronel), pamidronate (Aredia), or gallium nitrate (Ganite).
- Analgesics as appropriate for control of neuropathic bone pain
- Aredia, Zometa for bone strengthening
- There are many more options available for stable older patients with multiple myeloma. These can include thalidomide, Vincristine, Adriamycin, and dexamethasone. Bone marrow transplant can be an option for older patients into their 70s.

Patient, Family, and Staff Education
- Drink fluids (as much as 3 L per day) until the urine is a light yellow.
- Small, frequent feedings to help with nausea.

- Provide assistive devices to prevent falls and injury.
- Discuss the importance of activity to prevent calcium loss from bone. However, activity needs to be carefully monitored depending on where the lytic lesions are in the bone. These could place the patient at risk for pathologic fractures.
- Notify provider for increased signs and symptoms of disease, increasing bone pain, signs of infection, new or worsening confusion, fatigue, and failure to eat or drink.

Physician Consultation

Refer to a hematology oncologist or hematology specialist.

MYELODYSPLASTIC SYNDROMES

Definition

Myelodysplastic syndromes (MDS) are a group of diseases in which the clonal stem cells in the bone marrow are immature, causing clonal hematopoiesis of one or more cell lines. The abnormalities arise from the myeloid cell line as a result of excessive proliferation of cells and decreased apoptosis. There is an increased risk of transformation to acute myelogenous leukemia in certain types of MDS. It is also known as "smoldering leukemia" or preleukemia.

Epidemiology

MDS has two causes. The first is idiopathic and develops insidiously in persons over age 50. The second is a complication of previous treatment (t-MDS) with genotoxic drugs (e.g., alkylating agents) or radiation. Benzene is also considered a risk factor. Like the leukemias, this disease occurs primarily in men.

Common Presenting Signs and Symptoms

- Asymptomatic
- Insidious cytopenia
- Pallor with anemia contributed to aging
- Fatigue
- Decreased exercise tolerance

Differential Diagnosis

- Agranulocytosis
- Anemia
- Aplastic anemia
- Bone marrow failure
- Chronic myelogenous leukemia
- Hairy cell leukemia
- Megaloblastic anemia
- Myelophthisic anemia
- Myeloproliferative disease

Essential Diagnostic and Laboratory Tests

- CBC with differential
- Bone marrow aspiration with cytogenic studies
- Kidney panel to rule out anemia due to kidney disorders and lack of erythropoietin
- Splenic ultrasound, as 10% of the patients present with splenomegaly

Management Plan

Refer to a hematology oncologist or hematology specialist.

Nonpharmacologic

- Collaborate with the oncology specialists to provide a continuum of care.
- Monitor for low blood counts.
- Supportive therapy with the following:
  - Transfusions of cells that are depleted (e.g., platelets or RBCs).
  - Antibiotics—More patients die of bleeding and infection than conversion to AML.
- Monitor renal function and other side effects if prescribing Vidaza.
- Monitor for hematopoietic response.

Pharmacologic

- Persons with chronic or stable disease may not be treated.
- Growth factors
  - Procrit, Aranesp
  - Neupogen, Leukine
- Azacitidine (Vidaza) is approved for MDS.
  - The recommended starting dose is 75 mg/m², daily for 7 days, every 4 weeks. Dose should be adjusted for elders with impaired renal function. Premedicate for nausea and vomiting.
  - Repeat the cycle every 4 weeks. Increase the dose to 100 mg/m² if there are no results after two treatments. Treat for a minimum of four cycles and continue as long as the patient has some benefit.
- Revlimid for low-risk MDS in patients with 5q- abnormalities

Patient, Family, and Staff Education

- Discuss implications of MDS and the disease process. Reinforce the likelihood of AML transformation.
- Prepare the patient and family for potential signs and symptoms and for what to monitor (e.g., due to thrombocytopenia or anemia).

Physician Consultation

Refer to a hematology oncologist or hematology specialist.

▰▰▰ HODGKIN'S LYMPHOMA

Definition

Hodgkin's lymphoma (HL) is a localized or disseminated lymphoproliferative disorder with a characteristic sign of painless lymphadenopathy, most commonly in the supraclavicular, cervical, or mediastinal sites.

Epidemiology

HL accounts for less than 1% of all new cancer cases (Jemal et al., 2005). It has a bimodal peak of incidence, with the second occurring between ages 50 and 80. Men have a slightly higher incidence than women. The etiology is unknown, but there is a questionable association with the Epstein-Barr virus. Persons with immunodeficiencies or autoimmune disease are at higher risk. Other correlations include taking hydantoin drugs (such as phenytoin), woodworking as an occupation, or persons having a higher socioeconomic status. The presence of the Reed-Steinberg cell distinguishes HL from the other types of lymphoma.

Common Presenting Signs and Symptoms

The elderly tend to present with stage IV disease, atypical signs and symptoms, and the following unfavorable prognostic indicators (Beers, 2005):

- Painless swelling of supraclavicular, cervical, axillary, or groin lymph nodes. Spreading occurs to adjacent lymph nodes. Drinking alcohol makes the lymph nodes painful.
- Fever
- Night sweats
- Weight loss >10% of body weight
- Diffuse adenopathy with spleen, liver, bone marrow, or lung involvement

Differential Diagnosis

- Non-Hodgkin's lymphoma
- Benign lymphoproliferative diseases (e.g., infectious mononucleosis)
- Cytomegalovirus
- Lung cancer, oat cell (small cell)
- Rheumatoid arthritis
- Serum sickness

- Syphilis
- Systemic lupus erythematosus
- Toxoplasmosis
- Tuberculosis

Essential Diagnostic and Laboratory Tests

- CBC
- Erythrocyte sedimentation rate
- Liver function tests
- Chemistry profile for uric acid, serum calcium, serum protein, and LDH
- Chest X-ray
- Computerized tomography (CT) of the chest, abdomen, and pelvis
- Liver and spleen scan
- Intravenous pyelogram (IVP)
- Biopsy of an enlarged lymph node
- Positron emission tomography (PET) scan
- Bone marrow, to rule out involvement

Management Plan

Refer to medical oncologist.

Nonpharmacologic

- Collaborate with the oncology specialists to provide a continuum of care.
- Gastrointestinal side effects of chemotherapy seem to be worse in the elderly, so these should be monitored carefully.
- Screen for breast cancer as this is a high-risk group.
- Monitor thyroid function annually.

Pharmacologic

Treatment depends on the stage of the disease. Chemotherapy and radiation therapy are used in combination for the early stages (I and II) and intermediate (IIIA) HL. For the later stages, chemotherapy is the primary modality. Regimens for the elderly include Mustargen, Oncovin, procarbazine, and prednisone (MOPP), British MOPP, or adriamycin, bleomycin, Velban and dacarbazine (ABVD) for 6–8 months.

Patient, Family, and Staff Education

- Depending on the lymphoma grade and treatment, discuss the disease progression and treatment. Focus on the importance of controlling the side effects caused by treatment.
- Discuss the long-term effects of treatment.
- Encourage small, frequent meals of favorite foods.
- Encourage fluid intake.

Physician Consultation

Refer to medical oncologist.

▬▬ NON-HODGKIN'S LYMPHOMA

Definition

Non-Hodgkin's lymphomas (NHL) are a group of cancers originating in cells of the lymphatic system. There are multiple types that are classified based on their aggressive nature, development, and how they respond to treatment.

Epidemiology

NHLs are the sixth most commonly diagnosed cancer excluding the basal and squamous cell skin cancers. Although the risk factors are unknown, there is an increased incidence in persons who are immunosuppressed or have an abnormally high immune function, such as collagen-vascular disease; have a history of viral infections (e.g., Epstein-Barr or HTLV-1); taking hydantoin drugs; have occupation exposures (e.g., benzene, pesticides, or herbicides) or more than 20-years exposure to dark hair dyes;

or a history of *Helicobacter pylori* infection (Beers, 2005, Itano & Taoka, 2005). NHL frequently develops in persons with HIV.

Common Presenting Signs and Symptoms

- Painless swelling of lymph nodes in neck, underarm, or groin
- Fever
- Night sweats
- Fatigue
- Itching
- Recurring infections
- Symptoms caused by mediastinal tumor infringement (e.g., periorbital edema, dyspnea, and chest pain)

Differential Diagnosis

- Hodgkin's lymphoma
- Benign lymphoproliferative disorders, such as mononucleosis
- Metastatic cancer, unknown primary site
- Sarcoidosis
- Mycobacterial infections
- Fungal infections (histoplasmosis in the acute phase)

Essential Diagnostic and Laboratory Tests

- CBC
- Erythrocyte sedimentation rate
- Liver function tests
- Chemistry profile for uric acid, serum calcium, serum protein, and LDH
- Chest X-ray
- CT of the chest, abdomen and pelvis
- Liver and spleen scan
- IVP
- Biopsy of an enlarged lymph node

- PET scan
- Bone marrow, to rule out involvement

Management Plan

Refer to medical oncologist.

Nonpharmacologic

Collaborate with the oncology specialists to provide a continuum of care.

Pharmacologic

- Treatment depends on the grade of the NHL. Low grade will receive minimal or no treatment, and intermediate and high-grade lymphomas will most likely receive chemotherapy. Elderly patients with these higher-grade lymphomas may receive aggressive treatment if their functional status is good. The most likely regimen includes cyclophosphamide, doxorubicin, procarbazine, bleomycin, vincristine, and prednisone (CAP/BOP).
- B-cell lymphomas are treated with Rituxan alone or in combination with chemotherapy

Patient, Family, and Staff Education

- Discuss the disease progression and treatment. Focus on the importance of controlling the side effects caused by treatment.
- Encourage small, frequent meals of favorite foods.
- Encourage fluid intake.

Physician Consultation

Refer to medical oncologist.

▉ WEB SITES

- American Cancer Society—www.cancer.org
- The Leukemia and Lymphoma Society—www.leukemia.org/hm_lls
- National Cancer Institute—www.nci.nih.gov

- National Comprehensive Cancer Network, Clinical Practice Guidelines in Oncology: Senior Adult Oncology—www.nccn.org/professionals/physician_gls/PDF/senior.pdf
- CML links—cml.tlls.org
- International Myeloma Society—www.myeloma.org
- Multiple Myeloma Association—www.webspawner.com/users/myelomaexchange
- Multiple Myeloma Research Foundation—www.multiplemyeloma.org

REFERENCES

Argiris, A., & Kaklamani, V. (2004). *Hodgkin's lymphoma*. Retrieved July 28, 2005, from http://www.emedicine.com/med/topic1022.htm

Beers, M. H. (Ed.). (2005). Hematologic malignancies. In *Merck manual of geriatrics* (3rd ed.). Retrieved July 26, 2005, from http://www.merck.com/mrkshared/mmg/sec9/ch73/ch73f.jsp#ind09–073–4878

Berenson, J. R., & Miguel, J. (n.d.). *Introduction to multiple myeloma*. Retrieved July 28, 2005, from http://www.multiplemyeloma.org/about_myeloma

Breccia, M., Gentile, G., Martino, P., Petti, M. C., Russo, E., Mancini, M., et al. (2004). Acute myeloid leukemia secondary to a myelodysplastic syndrome with t (3; 3) (q21; q26) in an HIV patient treated with chemotherapy and highly active antiretroviral therapy. *Acta Haematology, 111*(3), 160–162.

Gajra, A., & Vajpayee, N. (2005). *Lymphoma B-cell*. Retrieved July 28, 2005, http://www.emedicine.com/med/topic1358.htm

Greipp, P. R., San Miguel, J., Durie, B. G., Crowley, J. J., Barlogie, B., Blade, J., et al. (2005). International staging system for multiple myeloma. *Journal of Clinical Oncology, 23*(15), 3412–3420.

Grund, S. (2004). *Acute myelogenous leukemia*. Retrieved July 26, 2005, from http://www.nlm.nih.gov/medlineplus/ency/article/000542.htm

Huether, S., & McCance, K. (2004). *Understanding pathophysiology* (3rd ed.). St. Louis, MO: Mosby.

Itano, J., & Taoka, K. (2005). *Core curriculum for oncology nursing* (4th ed.). Philadelphia: W. B. Saunders.

Jemal, A., Murray, T., Ward, E., Samuels, A., Tiwari, R. C., Ghafoor, A., et al. (2005). Cancer statistics, 2005. *CA: A Cancer Journal for Clinicians, 55*, 10–30.

Khan, A. N., & Rajiah, P. R. (2005). *Non-Hodgkin's lymphoma, thoracic*. Retrieved July 28, 2005, http://www.emedicine.com/radio/topic477.htm

Kumar, V., Abbas, A. K., & Austo, N. (2005). *Robbins & Cotarn pathologic basis of disease* (7th ed.). Philadelphia: Elsevier Saunders.

Landgren, O., Linet, M. S., McMaster, M. L., Gridley, G., Hemminki, K., & Goldin, L. R. (2006). Familial characteristics of autoimmune and hematologic disorders in 8,406 multiple myeloma patients: A population-based case-control study. *International Journal of Cancer, 118*, 3095–3098.

Leigh, C., Kopecky, K., Godwin, J., McConnell, T., Slovak, M., Chen, I., et al. (1997). Acute myeloid leukemia in the elderly: Assessment of multidrug resistance (MDR1) and cytogenetics distinguishes biologic subgroups with remarkably distinct responses to standard chemotherapy. *Blood, 89*(9), 3323–3329.

Leukemia and Lymphoma Society. (n.d.). *Leukemia facts and statistics: Leukemia, lymphoma, myeloma*. Retrieved July 28, 2005, from http://www.leukemia-lymphoma.org/all_page?item_id=9346#_incidencebyage

Lynch, H., Sanger, W., Pirruccell, S., Quinn-Laquer, B., & Weisenburger, D. (2001). Familial multiple myeloma: A family study and review of the literature. *Journal of the National Cancer Institute, 93*(19), 1479–1483.

Magrath, I., Shanta, V., Advani, S., Adde, M., Anya, L. S., Banavali, S., et al. (2005). Treatment of acute lymphoblastic leukemia in countries with limited resources: Lessons from use of a single protocol in India over a twenty year period. *European Journal of Cancer, 41*(11), 1570–1583.

McFadden, M. E., Guicio, T., & Boyle, D. (2004). Treating the older patient with leukemia, lymphoma, and myeloma. *ONS News, 19*(9 Supplement), 77–78.

Meredith, P. V., & Horan, N. M. (2000). *Adult primary care*. Philadelphia: W. B. Saunders.

National Cancer Institute. (2003). *Surveillance, epidemiology, and end results (SEER): Fast facts.* Retrieved August 28, 2006, from http://seer.cancer.gov/faststats/sites

National Comprehensive Cancer Network. (2005). *Clinical practice guidelines in oncology: Senior adult oncology.* Retrieved January 29, 2006, from http://www.nccn.org/professionals/physician_gls/PDF/senior.pdf

National Comprehensive Cancer Network. (2006). *Clinical practice guidelines in oncology: Acute myeloid leukemia.* Retrieved January 29, 2006, from http://www.nccn.org/professionals/physician_gls/PDF/aml.pdf

National Comprehensive Cancer Network. (2006). *Clinical practice guidelines in oncology: Multiple Myeloma.* Retrieved August 28, 2006, from http://www.nccn.org/professionals/physician_gls/PDF/myeloma.pdf

Novartis Pharmaceuticals Company. (2005). *Gleevec.* Retrieved November 25, 2005, from http://www.gleevec.com/hcp/page/consider

Rosenbloom, B. E., Weinreb, N. J., Zimran, A., Kacena, K. A., Charrow, J., & Ward, E. (2005). Gaucher disease and cancer incidence: A study from the Gaucher Registry. *Blood, 105*(12), 4569–4572.

Seiter, K. (2002). Treatment of acute myelogenous leukemia in the elderly patient. *Clinical Geriatrics, 10,* 1070–1389.

Shaughnessy, J., Jr., Zhan, F., Barlogie, B., & Stewart, A. K. (2005). Gene expression profiling and multiple myeloma. *Best Practice and Research Clinical Haematology, 18*(4), 537–552.

CHAPTER 12

Infectious Diseases

Bethsheba Johnson

DIARRHEA

Definition

Diarrhea is a symptom defined by the patient that may include changes in bowel movement frequency, consistency, urgency, and continence. Each of these definitions of diarrhea is based on the patient's prior experience. Diarrhea is a change in bowel habits that is distressing in terms of the physiologic consequences. It can involve the following:

- The number of bowel movements per day
- Increased volume of stool with a single bowel movement
- Increased fluid content of the stool
- The onset of urgency

It is important to characterize the patient's symptoms in each of these categories to help establish a differential diagnosis. For example, fecal incontinence is often perceived as diarrhea, even when the stool volume and the consistency of the stool would be considered normal. In this instance, the patient is describing the inability to maintain continence from the time of sensing an impending bowel movement to the actual passage of stool. Therefore, allowing the patient to define diarrhea is a useful tool.

For the clinician a more objective criterion is used to define diarrhea. Diarrhea is defined as more than 200 g or 200 mL of stool per 24 hours while consuming a typical Western diet (Park & Giannella, 1993; Donowitz, Kokke, & Saidi, 1995). Recently, as many individuals have increased their dietary fiber, 250 g or 250 mL has become the normal value.

Epidemiology

There are five classifications for the etiology or pathophysiology of diarrhea: (1) osmotic diarrhea, (2) secretory diarrhea, (3) motility dysfunction, (4) mucosal inflammation, and (5) absorption defect.

Osmotic diarrhea occurs in response to the change in the osmotic gradient from the vascular space to the intestinal lumen. It prevents the absorption of tissue water or draws tissue water out of the bloodstream into the colonic lumen. There are three main causes of osmotic diarrhea: (1) ingestion of solutes that are difficult to absorb (e.g., saline purgatives), (2) maldigestion of nutrients (e.g., disaccharidase deficiency), and (3) failure of mucosal transport mechanisms (e.g., glucose–galactose malabsorption). The characteristic clinical feature of osmotic diarrhea is cessation when the patient fasts or stops ingesting the offending substance.

Secretory diarrhea occurs when normal absorptive mechanisms are stopped or when there is net luminal secretion of water and electrolytes. In most patients with secretory diarrhea both mechanisms of action are active. Patients with secretory diarrhea, in contrast to those with osmotic diarrhea, may have an increase in stool volume when fasting, because severe secretory diarrhea often has an osmotic component that further worsens the condition. Causes of secretory diarrhea include enterotoxin-induced secretions (*Escherichia coli*, *Vibrio cholerae*), pancreatic cholera syndrome (vasoactive intestinal polypeptide syndrome), carcinoid syndrome, medullary carcinoma of the thyroid, Zollinger-Ellison syndrome, and bile acid-induced secretion.

Motility dysfunction is the accelerated gastric emptying or small bowel transit that may decrease the time for absorption of nutrients and fluid that can occur at any level of the gastrointestinal tract. Additionally, disturbed colonic motility may accelerate the transit from the cecum to the rectum. Abnormal motility of the sigmoid colon, rectosigmoid junction, or rectum may result in a feeling of urgency and/or fecal incontinence. Although altered motility can be a cause of rapid intestinal transit leading to diarrhea, poor motility or intestinal stasis can also lead to diarrhea due to bacterial overgrowth. Examples of diseases with motility dysfunction include irritable bowel syndrome (IBS), carcinoid syndrome, medullary carcinoma of the thyroid, VIPoma (tumor secreting vasoactive intestinal peptide), Zollinger-Ellison syndrome (dumping syndrome), and giardiasis. The most common disorder in this classification that clinicians encounter seems to be IBS.

Absorption defect can be caused by pancreatic insufficiency, which may lead to diarrhea related to maldigestion of fat and other nutrients. Thus, food passes undigested through the gastrointestinal tract to the colon. Voluminous nutrient loss may predispose to the production of toxic bacterial products from degradation of the nutrient-rich colon contents, resulting in osmotic diarrhea. If the small bowel surface area is reduced, malabsorption may also occur. The best example of an absorption defect is gluten-sensitive enteropathy (celiac disease). Gluten sensitivity induces an inflammatory reaction, with subsequent loss of mucosal surface area that results in steatorrhea and malnutrition.

Mucosal inflammation is most commonly associated with infection including *Clostridium difficile*, although it can occur with autoimmune diseases such as Behçet's syndrome or idiopathic inflammatory bowel disease such as ulcerative colitis or Crohn's disease. Mucosal inflammation may induce dysmotility of the circular and longitudinal muscle, resulting in excessive contractility in response to luminal distention. Distal colonic inflammation can cause both diarrhea and constipation. Diarrhea is related to spasm of inflamed distal colon segments associated with decreased compliance. Constipation occurs due to inhibition of motility in the colon proximal to active inflammation. The diarrhea is often characterized as relatively scant fluid and inflammatory exudates. When stool passes into the inflamed colonic segment, poor compliance activates motility and may provoke fecal incontinence. Inflammatory changes in the small bowel or colon may also lead to malabsorption of fluid and nutrients, resulting in loose stools.

Clostridium difficile

Clostridium difficile (*C. difficile*) is the prominent mucosal inflammatory, nosocomial cause of diarrheal disease in hospitals and long-term care facilities, with increasing numbers now being reported in the community (Dial, Delaney, Barkun, & Suissa, 2005). Although the incidence of *C. difficile*-associated disease (CDAD) in the community is much lower than in the hospital setting, the absolute number of cases in the community could be significant as *C. difficile*-colonized persons move through the community to hospitals and long-term care facilities.

In the United States, the reported rate of infection is 3.4 to 8.4 cases per 1000 hospital admissions. In intensive care units and long-term care facilities approximately 30% of the patients who receive antibiotics are colonized but never develop CDAD (Kyne, Warny, Qamar, & Kelly, 2000).

C. difficile is a spore-forming, gram-positive, anaerobic bacteria. Spores are shed in feces and can survive outside the body on environmental surfaces such as hands, furniture, stethoscopes, toilets, and other equipment found in healthcare settings. When spores are ingested and colonize the gastrointestinal tract, active infection may occur resulting in diarrhea and possibly pseudomembranous colitis with toxic megacolon and death. Colonization alone does not produce infection.

Risk factors for CDAD development include advanced age, immunocompromise, comorbid conditions, gastrointestinal surgery or manipulation, prolonged stay in any closed healthcare environment such as a hospital or nursing home, and recent antimicrobial therapy. Antibiotic therapy that alters the balance of flora in the gastrointestinal tract allows the overgrowth of *C. difficile* in susceptible individuals and is the major cause of CDAD. Studies have indicated that there is a high degree of *C. difficile* resistance to broad-spectrum antibiotics such as ampicillin and amoxicillin; clindamycin, cephalosporins, erythromycin, trimethoprims; and fluoroquinolones (Moyenuddin, Williamson, & Ohl, 2002). The organism, at this time, has demonstrated no or little resistance to metronidazole, or vancomycin.

Gastric acidity is a major defense mechanism against ingested pathogens, and loss of the normal stomach pH has been associated with colonization of the normally sterile upper gastrointestinal tract. Proton pump inhibitors and H2-receptor antagonists raise the gastric Ph. Proton pump inhibitors have also been shown to affect leukocyte function.

Nonsusceptible hosts likely develop antibodies to the *C. difficile* toxins or may become asymptomatic carriers of the bacteria. In a susceptible host *C. difficile*-associated diarrhea is mediated by exotoxins A and B of pathogenic *C. difficile* strains (Moyenuddin, Williamson, & Ohl, 2002; Oldfield, 2004). Toxins A (enterotoxin) and B (cytotoxin) cause the release of cytokines in the colonic mucosa that produce an inflammatory response and if not treated effectively eventually cause pseudomembranes to form in the intestinal tract from purulent and necrotic debris. Pseudomembranous colitis (PMC) produces severe diarrhea and abdominal pain, tenderness and peritoneal signs, usually without the bloody stools of inflammatory bowel disease, ischemic bowel, or infection with other bacteria such as *Salmonella, Shigella,* or *C. jejuni*. Complications of PMC include severe dehydration, electrolyte imbalances, hypotension, hypoalbuminemia, and toxic megacolon.

Recent reports suggest that the rate and severity of *C. difficile*-associated disease in the United States are increasing and that the increase may be associated with the emergence of a new strain of *C. difficile* with increased virulence, resistance, or both (McDonald et al., 2005; Oldfield, 2004). It can produce larger quantities of toxins A and B and is more resistant to fluoroquinolones (CDC, 2005a). The new strain cannot currently be selectively identified with stool testing. Healthcare providers are urged to be judicious in following existing treatment guidelines in order to treat it.

Common Presenting Signs and Symptoms

- Increase in stool frequency, urgency, volume
  - Watery diarrhea is common in *C. difficile* infection
  - History of other abdominal pain, ileus, and minimal diarrhea may make a diagnosis of *C. difficile* more difficult.
  - *C. difficile* diarrhea should be suspected in any nursing home patient with a history of recent antibiotic therapy.

○ In the elderly, symptoms of *C. difficile* may not occur until several weeks after antibiotic therapy (Simor et al., 2002).

- Abdominal cramps and pain (right lower quadrant)
- Fever
- Cramping abdominal pain and tenderness
- Peritoneal signs (pseudomembranous colitis)
- Loss of appetite and weight loss
- Dehydration
- Blood in stool
- Leukocytosis

Differential Diagnosis

Base the approach to the differential diagnosis and management of a patient with diarrhea on the duration (acute or chronic), severity, and public health implications of the illness. Evaluation of diarrhea can be complex. The most important tool is obtaining a history of the current illness and review of systems at the time of the initial evaluation. History and systems review can generally divide the disease into acute or chronic. The acute illnesses are most always infectious in origin.

- Acute diarrhea (bacterial, viral, or protozoal)
  ○ *Salmonella*
  ○ *Shigella* species
  ○ *Campylobacter jejuni*
  ○ *Escherichia coli* 0157:H7 (enterohemorrhagic *E. coli*)
- Acute diarrhea (spore-forming protozoa)—Usually found in contaminated public drinking water, beef, fruits, and vegetables
  ○ *Cryptosporidium*—Most common cause of diarrhea; often not diagnosed because it is typically serious only in immunocompromised patients.
  ○ *Giardia*
  ○ *Microsporida*

○ *Isospora*
○ *Cyclospora*
- Diarrhea associated with hyperthyroidism, diabetic neuropathy
- IBS (diagnosis by exclusion)
- Dietary causes of diarrhea
  ○ Nonabsorbable carbohydrates (sorbitol- or mannitol-containing products)
  ○ High methylxanthine and caffeine
- Lactose intolerance
- Gluten-sensitive enteropathy
- Microscopic and collagenous colitis
- Pancreatic insufficiency
- Antibiotic-induced (especially fluoroquinolones) diarrhea—This is a very complex differential diagnosis that many believe is attributed to *C. difficile*. Although *C. difficile* is an important part of the differential diagnosis, there are other necessary considerations. Antibiotic-induced diarrhea may occur through the following three mechanisms (Collings & Miner, 2002):
  ○ Chemical effects—Mucosal injury, impaired absorption, stimulation of secretion, or a change in motility. Erythromycin, for example, enhances gastrointestinal motility and may change gastrointestinal transit.
  ○ Known antibiotic effects—Suppression (bacteriostasis) or eradication (bactericide) of bacteria. The most common cause of antibiotic-associated diarrhea is impaired carbohydrate salvage. Decreased intestinal bacteria also reduces metabolism of colonic carbohydrate. The resulting osmolarity of the carbohydrates draws fluid into the colon. This mechanism explains more than 50% of the cases of antibiotic-induced diarrhea.
  ○ Changed colonic flora with opportunistic overgrowth of other bacteria or fungi—

C. difficile proliferates in the altered environment provided by antibiotic therapy. The toxins activate mucosal injury leading to diarrhea, colitis, and pseudomembrane formation. This can also lead to the proliferation of other opportunistic bacteria or fungi that may cause diarrhea.

Essential Diagnostic and Laboratory Tests

- With a recent history of antibiotic therapy or other risk factors, assess stool for toxin A and toxin B produced by *C. difficile*. Enzyme-linked immunosorbent assays (ELISA) for toxins A, B, or both are the most cost effective and rapid of the available tests but have less sensitivity than some other tests (CDC, 2005a). Clinical judgment should override negative results.

- Complete blood count with differential and erythrocyte sedimentation rate to confirm inflammation and/or infection. Low lymphocyte counts may indicate HIV/AIDS-associated diarrhea.

- Blood tests to identify fluid and electrolyte abnormalities and to assess nutritional consequences of diarrhea (electrolytes, serum albumin, blood urea nitrogen, serum creatinine). Additional blood tests may be indicated to rule out other causes of diarrhea, including (Collings & Miner, 2002):
  - Thyroid panel to assess for hyperthyroidism
  - Fasting blood glucose to assess for diabetes mellitus and diabetic diarrhea
  - Cholesterol: low in significant malabsorption syndromes
  - Vitamin B_{12}: low in severe ileal disease, bacterial overgrowth, pancreatic insufficiency, pernicious anemia
  - Blood cultures to assess for sepsis

- In patients with acute bloody diarrhea obtain a stool culture for enteric pathogens and check samples for fecal leukocytes. Also culture stool if acute diarrhea does not resolve in 3 to 5 days. Testing for ova and parasites may not be necessary in nursing home settings. Additional stool tests may be performed if other differential diagnoses need to be ruled out, such as (Collings & Miner, 2002):
  - Occult blood to assess for gastric or duodenal mucosal inflammation or ulceration, carcinoma, Zollinger-Ellison syndrome
  - Fecal alpha-1 antitrypsin: elevated in protein-losing enteropathy
  - Qualitative and quantitative fat to assess for fat malabsorption or maldigestion
  - Bacterial culture for enteric pathogens
  - 24-hour stool volume/weight: increases with diarrheal disorders due to increased stool frequency and liquidity
  - Osmotic gap: differentiates between osmotic and secretory diarrhea. Normally serum and stool osmolality are similar (290 mOsm/kg) due mostly to sodium and potassium concentrations. Unabsorbable solute in osmotic diarrhea decreases electrolyte concentrations. The gap in osmotic diarrhea is greater than 50 mOsm/kg.

- Radiographic testing
  - Plain films of the abdomen may indicate colonic distention and distorted haustral markings.
  - CT scan—Can show thickening of the colon, segmental Vs pancolitis, ascites, or colonic dilation. Findings will depend on timing in the disease process, and may be within normal limits in early *C. difficile* disease.
  - Colonoscopy may indicate pseudomembranous plaque, which is often in the right colon.
  - Other tests that may be considered in ruling out differential diagnoses include

barium enema, enteroclysis, transit studies, scintigraphy, arteriography, esophagogastroduodenoscopy, and endoscopic retrograde cholangiopancreatography.

Management Plan

The goals for treating diarrhea are to prevent the spread of infectious diseases, correct fluid and electrolyte imbalances, and reduce morbidity and mortality.

Nonpharmacologic

- Initiate a minimum of enteric isolation precautions during acute disease. Single room isolation or cohort isolation may also be used.

- Most patients with acute diarrhea do not benefit from antimicrobial therapy because the conditions are self-limiting. Decreasing unnecessary antibiotic use may decrease the carrier rate in some cases of antibiotic-resistant strains of bacteria.

- Treatment for diarrhea should include oral replacement therapy (ORT) for fluid and electrolyte losses, if the patient can drink an electrolyte replacement without nausea and vomiting, and has only moderate signs of dehydration (mild orthostasis, tachycardia, pliable skin, dry mouth, urinary specific gravity < 1.025, and blood urea nitrogen < 20). In many patients with diarrhea, electrolyte imbalance results because of the severity of the diarrhea. This occurs frequently with secretory diarrhea, during which there is a profound loss of electrolytes.

- Administer intravenous fluids to patients with signs of severe dehydration (three liter fluid loss). Severe dehydration is defined as orthostatic hypotension, tenting of abdominal skin, dry mucous membranes, dry tongue with longitudinal furrowing, BUN > 20, and urinary specific gravity ≥ 1.025.

- Consult with the registered dietician to manage diet and fluids during and after a diarrheal episode.

- Consider hospitalizing a patient with diarrhea and dehydration, blood loss, temperature > 103°F (39.4°C), or electrolyte imbalance.

Pharmacologic

- Studies indicate the need for judicious use of antibiotics in long-term care facilities, hospitals, and the community in order to prevent infection and the development of further virulent strains of *C. difficile*.

- Since *C. difficile* is associated with the use of broad-spectrum antibiotics the first step is to remove the offending antibiotic, if possible (Fekety, 1997). Except for Clindamycin, there are limited reports of success with this strategy (Sunenshine & McDonald, 2006).

- Use antidiarrheals such as loperamide (Imodium) or diphenoxylate HCL/atropine sulfate (Lomotil) cautiously in infectious diarrhea. Antiperistaltics can decrease the duration of diarrhea but do not affect the amount of fluid loss. They can also have adverse effects because they allow the pooling of infectious material within the intestine delaying its expulsion from the body. These antidiarrheals have been shown to increase the severity and duration of invasive diarrheal diseases and have led to pseudomembranous colitis and toxic megacolon in patients with *C. difficile* (Sunenshine & McDonald, 2006).

- Narcotic analgesics may also slow colonic transport and contribute to complications in CDAD and should be avoided, if possible.

- Treat *C. difficile* diarrhea with the following:
  - Metronidazole—This is considered first-line therapy. For mild diarrhea treat with 250 mg four times daily or 500 mg three times daily, by mouth, for 10–14 days.
  - Vancomycin—For moderate disease associated with systemic symptoms (fever, abdominal pain, leukocytosis) treat with vancomycin 125–500 mg four times daily, by mouth, for 10–14 days. If patients are unable to take oral drugs, IV formulation

is recommended in an acute care setting. Vancomycin has also been delivered via the intracolonic route

○ Some authorities recommend following antibiotic therapy with 7 days of a bile acid-binding agent such as colestipol or cholestyramine (Moyenuddin, Williamson, & Ohl, 2002). The bile acid-binding agents block the toxin and allow reequilibrium with nonpathogenic, normal colonic flora.

○ Prophylactic administration of probiotics for patients receiving antibiotics has not proved effective in preventing CDAD, to date, in the nursing home setting (Simor et al., 2002). Probiotics such as *Saccharomyces boulardii* (nonpathogenic yeast) and lactobacilli have been used with some success in conjunction with standard treatment in an attempt to reestablish normal intestinal flora. *S. boulardii* should not be used in immunosuppressed patients.

○ Follow-up with the patient is made by assessing the resolution of diarrhea. A stool culture is not recommended for *C. difficile* as patients may remain colonized with toxin-producing strains (Sunenshine & McDonald, 2006).

○ Relapse rates are approximately 20% to 25% after successful treatment (Moyenuddin, Williamson, & Ohl, 2002; Oldfield, 2004). This phenomenon cannot be solely explained by antibiotic resistance but may involve sporulation, which leads to relapse within 4 weeks after therapy. If relapses occur first-line therapy is to repeat the course of metronidazole for another 10 days. Vancomycin is usually reserved for metronidazole therapy failure. Further relapses may be treated with a variety of drug regimens (see Table 12-1). There is limited research on the effectiveness of these combinations in long-term care settings.

TABLE 12-1	Therapeutic Options for Recurring *Clostridium difficile* Infection
Initial therapy:	Repeat: Metronidazole 250–500 mg 3–4 times daily, by mouth, for 10–14 days *or*
Alternate therapies:	Vancomycin 125 mg 4 times daily, by mouth, for 10–14 days Tapering regimen Week 1: Vancomycin 125 mg 4 times daily, by mouth, for 7 days Week 2: Vancomycin 125 mg 2 times daily, by mouth, for 7 days Week 3: Vancomycin 125 mg daily, by mouth, for 7 days Week 4: Vancomycin 125 mg every other day, by mouth, for 7 days Week 5/6: Vancomysin every 3rd day, by mouth, for 14 days
Bile sequestrants:	Cholestyramine 4 grams 3–4 times daily for 14 days *plus* Vancomycin 125–250 mg 4 times daily, by mouth, for 14 days
Antibiotic combination:	Vancomycin 125–250 mg 4 times daily, by mouth, for 14 days *plus* Rifampin 150–300 mg 2 times daily, by mouth, for 14 days *or* Bacitracin 25,000 U 4 times daily, by mouth, for 14 days
Alternate probiotics:	Vancomycin 125 mg 4 times daily, by mouth, for 10–14 days *plus* *Saccharomyces boulardii* 500 mg 2 times daily, by mouth, for 28 days *or* *Lactobacillus* GG (Lactinex) 1 gram packet, 4 times daily, by mouth after vancomycin regimen

Source: Joyce & Burns, 2002.

Patient, Family, and Staff Education

Infection Control

Prevention of the transmission of organisms to patients is essential. Patients, family caregivers, and staff should understand the principles of disease prevention including the following:

- Hand washing is essential for patients, families and staff before and after every patient contact to prevent transmission of organisms. Alcohol-based gels are not recommended with *C. difficile* because alcohol does not effectively kill the spores.

- Staff should wear disposable gloves when in contact with stool, and change gloves before leaving the room or caring for another person in the same room.

- Use isolation gowns if soiling of clothes is likely. Remove gown upon leaving the room.

- All surfaces should be carefully disinfected where spores may be present (Loo et al., 2005). Hypochlorite (bleach) solutions appear to be effective.

- Patients with enteric infections should be placed in private rooms, if possible. Alternately, infected patients can be grouped in a designated area (cohorted).

- Dedicated or single-use equipment should be used for infected patients.

- Reinforce to staff the need for prompt reporting of persistant diarrhea.

Health Promotion

- Explain to the patient that it will be necessary to avoid dietary factors that induce or worsen diarrhea such as caffeine, alcohol, dairy products, sorbitol (sugar-free candies or drinks), gluten, or products such as magnesium-containing antacids.

- Drink prescribed electrolyte solutions or commercial sports drinks to help the body retain fluid. These drinks contain sugars and salts that pull water out of the intestines and reduce diarrhea.

- Advise families and/or staff traveling to developing areas, to seek information about risks, prevention, and treatment of travelers' diarrhea from the Centers for Disease Control and Prevention (CDC).

- Avoid using antidiarrheal agents such as Imodium when diarrhea is accompanied by blood or high fever.

- Clean and avoid injuring the perineum (the skin between the genitals and the anus) during acute diarrhea. The perineum can be damaged by digestive products and bacterial by-products in the feces. Frequent wiping can remove the skin's natural oils. Avoid physical damage to the perineum by "patting dry" rather than wiping.

Physician Consultation

- Consult or refer when a properly diagnosed disease fails to respond to conventional therapy (e.g., recurrent *C. difficile* infection).

- Consult with the medical director and infection control nurse for persistent diarrheal outbreaks.

- Consult or refer for unexplained diarrhea lasting longer than 2 weeks that requires specific evaluation, specific testing, or an expanded differential diagnosis.

- Consult or refer to a gastroenterologist for management of bloody diarrhea, secretory diarrhea with dehydration, fecal incontinence, or IBD.

- Consult the health department in the city or state in which you practice when an epidemic is present in the community or when an infectious diarrhea needs to be reported.

▰▰▰ HERPES ZOSTER VIRUS (HZV; SHINGLES)

Definition

Herpes zoster is defined as an acute infection caused by the reactivation of the latent varicella zoster virus (VZV or human herpes virus 3) (Anderson, Anderson, & Glanze, 1998).

Epidemiology

The transmission of the varicella virus can occur through the following methods of contact: (1) direct contact with respiratory secretions and/or fluids from the vesicles of the patient (primary zoster), and (2) airborne contact through inhalation of small particle aerosols from nasopharyngeal secretions from an infected patient followed by localized replication at an undefined site. This leads to the seeding of the reticuloendothelial system and viremia. After this, localization and replication of the viral particulate in the skin produces the onset of the classic zoster rash.

The incubation period for the zoster is 10 to 21 days, and if the varicella-zoster immune globulin was administered the incubation period is 28 days. Twenty-four to 48 hours before the onset of lesions until they crust completely is called the infectious period.

During the primary infection of varicella zoster (chicken pox) the virus spreads from the lesions to the skin and mucous membranes into the sensory nerve endings (Wallace & Oxman, 1997). The virus travels towards the brain to the dorsal ganglion cells where it enters a latent state. At this stage it is no longer infectious, but it retains the ability to reactivate fully and cause secondary viremia (McCary, Severson, & Tyring, 1999). The mechanism(s) underlying VZV reactivation are not fully understood. It has been postulated that VZV is reactivated as a result of a decline in T lymphocyte proliferation in response to the VZV antigen. When reactivated, VZV replicates and spreads within the ganglion, where it causes neuronal necrosis and inflammation that is characterized by severe prodromal neuralgic pain (Wallace & Oxman, 1997). The virus then travels down the sensory nerve and is released at the nerve endings in the skin where it causes lesions (Wallace & Oxman).

Herpes zoster (HZ) is becoming more frequent. It is currently estimated in the United States that 600,000 to one million cases of HZ occur annually. These numbers indicate that approximately 10% to 20% of the population will experience herpes zoster in their lifetimes (CDC, 1999). Although HZ can affect people of all ages, the risk increases with advancing age. Two thirds of cases are reported in individuals older than 50. HZ is rare in children. The incidence of HZ per 1000 persons per year rises from 0.74 among children under 9 years of age, to 5.09 among people aged 51 to 79, and 10.1 among those over age 80. Persons who are immunosuppressed are at the greatest risk for HZ. Nursing home patients are especially susceptible to HZ because of an age-related decrease in cell-mediated immunity associated with conditions such as HIV, malignancy, chemotherapy, radiation therapy, and chronic corticosteroid use. Caregivers of patients should also be indirectly assessed for stress that may increase the risk of HZ.

Common Presenting Signs and Symptoms

- *Acute neuralgia* coupled with *paresthesia* in the involved dermatome
- Rash—One to three days after the neuralgia and paresthesia a rash develops that appears as a grouping of vesicles that vary in size. Look for a rash that is unilateral and dermatomal in distribution and does not cross the midline of the body. The rash of herpes zoster begins as closely grouped, erythematous maculopapules of various sizes that form vesicles within 12 to 24 hours and spread to involve all or part of a single dermatome. HZ usually appears in the dermatome where the varicella lesions were more abundant in the primary infection. HZ usually affects the spinal sensory ganglia from T1 to L2 but it may also involve the ophthalmic division of the trigeminal nerve (Wallace & Oxman, 1997). Approximately

50% of patients present with lesions outside of the affected dermatome (Ferri, 1999). Within three to four days the various-sized vesicles turn into pustules, which will umbilicate or rupture before forming a crust over the next 7 to 10 days. Within the next four weeks, and once the underlying skin has reepithelialized, the crusts fall off. Resolution is usually complete, although scarring may result (either hyperpigmentation or hypopigmentation, particularly in people with darker skin hues) (Whitley, 2000). Clinical involvement is more extensive and inflammatory in older adults and immunocompromised patients (e.g., HIV) (Habif, 1996).

- Patients usually have hyperesthesia (increased sensitivity to stimuli) and hyperpathia (increased subjective response to painful stimuli) in the affected dermatome. Pain will accompany the rash in approximately 60% to 90% of immunocompetent patients (Wallace & Oxman, 1997). Pain can be described as mild itching, tingling and burning, to deep boring, sharp, stabbing and lancinating. It can be constant or intermittent. Commonly in older adults transient motor neuropathies affect about 5% of persons whose HZ involves an extremity. Approximately 75% of those affected will make a complete recovery (Habif, 1996).

- Lesions on the side or tip of the nose (Hutchinson's sign) and ipsilateral eyelid edema can indicate *ophthalmic zoster*. Ophthalmic zoster is associated with a high rate of complications such as blindness and can be fatal. Ophthalmic HZ is characterized by a vesicular rash that is distributed over the skin served by cranial nerve V, the ophthalmic division of the trigeminal nerve. The ophthalmic division has three branches, the frontal, lacrimal, and nasociliary nerves (Habif, 1996). The distribution of the rash can cover the eye level to the vertex of the skull. Common signs include contralateral eyelid edema and follicular conjunctivitis (Miedziak & O'Brien, 1999). Approximately half of pa-

tients with ophthalmic HZ develop ocular complications and postherpetic neuralgia (PHN) (Habif, 1996; Miedziak & O'Brien, 1999). Ninety-three percent of patients with ophthalmic HZ develop acute neuritis localized to the affected dermatome and proportional to the severity of the rash. It remains in at least 31% of patients 6 months after the rash first appears (Habif, 1996).

- Complications of HZ can be peripheral *facial palsy* in combination with a *painful ear*. The presence of vesicles on the pinna and external auditory canal is indicative of Ramsay Hunt syndrome. Other signs of this condition include a unilateral loss of taste on the anterior two thirds of the tongue due to facial nerve VII involvement, tinnitus, deafness, and vertigo due to involvement of auditory nerve VIII (Habif, 1996). Sometimes the characteristic vesicles of HZ can be absent which is a condition called "zoster sine herpete" or can appear after the onset of facial palsy (Murakami et al., 1998). Delayed diagnosis, misdiagnosis (Bell's palsy), and consequent treatment without antiviral medications until the vesicles appear can increase the likelihood of hearing loss (Whitley, 2000).

- *Constitutional symptoms* such as fever, headache, and malaise, as well as regional lymphadenopathy, may be present.

Differential Diagnosis

- Herpes simplex virus, which differs from herpes zoster due to its manifestation of uniform vesicles

- Other acute eczematous eruptions including erythema multiforme, and cellulitis (with its characteristic edematous or urticarial-like inflamed plagues)

- Bell's palsy

- Trigeminal neuralgia

- Other acute pain syndromes when prodromal herpes zoster virus is suspected such as acute myocardial infarction, pulmonary embolism, pleuritis, pericarditis, and renal colic

Essential Diagnostic and Laboratory Tests

- Diagnosis of herpes zoster is generally by history and physical examination

  ○ Characteristic dermatomally distributed rash, usually accompanied by pain especially in older adults, with unexplained severe pain and tenderness that is localized to a dermatome and is not usually accompanied by systemic manifestations.

  ○ Prodromal herpes zoster can be diagnosed retrospectively based on certain clinical features. Herpes zoster should be suspected in an older adult who presents with recent acute onset of unexplained severe pain (stabbing, burning, itching) or localized skin tenderness (hyperalgesia). Prodromal herpes zoster should also be suspected when a patients who presents with unexplained extreme ear pain (especially if associated with unilateral facial paralysis, deafness, vertigo, or tinnitus) or unexplained acute eye pain.

- Viral culture and a Tzanck smear can reveal multinucleated giant cells and epithelial cells in atypical presentations of HZ. The Tzanck smear is only 55% sensitive and not specific enough to be definitive (McCary et al., 1999).

- If the disease is recurrent or clinically indeterminate a more invasive procedure is indicated. Consider obtaining a tissue culture or a direct immunofluorescence (DIF) or polymerase chain reaction (PCR) test to confirm a clinical diagnosis. A tissue culture is more specific than the Tzanck smear, but it is not always positive because varicella is a labile, highly cell-associated virus (McCary et al., 1999; Zirn, Tompkins, Huie, & Shea, 1995).

Management Plan

The goals for treatment are to relieve pain, estimate the risk of postherpetic neuralgia (Table 12-2) that is thought to result from damage to the neural tissues of the affected dermatome during the prodromal and acute phases of herpes zoster (Wallace & Oxman, 1997), and prevent transmission of the virus to

TABLE 12-2 Determining Risk for Postherpetic Neuralgia	
FACTORS	**RISK CATEGORY**
Age less than 50 years with any number of lesions	Risk category 1: Very low risk
Age 50 or greater with no or mild pain, < 47 lesions	Risk category 2: Small risk, great likelihood of fast resolution of pain (~ 15 days)
Age 50 or greater with: No or mild pain, > 47 lesions Moderate pain, 21 to 46 lesions Severe or incapacitating pain, < 47 lesions	Risk category 3: Moderate to high risk, time to resolution of pain ~ 73 days; likely to return to usual activities[a]
Age 50 or greater with: Severe or incapacitating pain, > 47 lesions Compromised immunity due to HIV infection, connective tissue disorder, or organ transplant Herpes rash located on face	Risk category 4: High risk, time to resolution of pain ~ 180 days or longer; unlikely to return fully to usual activities[a]

[a] Includes quality-of-life factors such as ability to sleep uninterrupted and cessation of analgesic use.

Source: Choo et al., 1997; Whitley & Gnann, 1999.

susceptible individuals who are at high risk from exposure (Whitley, 2000).

Nonpharmacologic

- Cool tap water compresses for 20 minutes several times a day to macerate the herpes zoster vesicles, remove serum and crusts, and help suppress secondary bacterial infections such as *Streptococcus pyogenes* or *Staphylococcus aureus.*

- Tepid showers or baths twice daily with the use of a soap-free cleansing bar or dermatologic cleansing fluid (except antiseptics) may also prevent superinfections (Peyramond et al., 1998).

- Wear loose clothing to avoid irritating the affected skin.

Pharmacologic

Initiate therapy within 72 hours of rash eruptions to reduce the frequency or shorten the duration of postherpetic neuralgia (see Table 12-3) (Whitley, 2000).

Pharmacologic Prevention

According to Oxman et al. (2005), the zoster vaccine decreased the burden of illness due to herpes zoster by 61.1% and reduced the incidence of herpes zoster and PHN by 51.3% and 66.5% respectively. A Food and Drug Administration advisory panel in January 2006 recommended approval of a herpes zoster vaccine, Zostavax, for adults 60 years of age and older for the prevention of outbreaks and for the prevention or lessening of the severity of postherpetic neuralgia. At time of publication, the interim vaccine information statement (VIS) (CDC, 2006) recommended administration of a single dose of the vaccine for adults 60 years of age and older, *except* those with a history of:

- Life-threatening allergic reaction to gelatin, neomycin, or other vaccine components

- Moderate or severe illness

- Active, untreated tuberculosis
- Weakened immune system due to:
  - ○ HIV/AIDS
  - ○ Treatment with drugs that affect the immune system, including steroids
  - ○ Cancer treatment including radiation or chemotherapy
  - ○ Cancer affecting bone marrow or the lymphatic system

Pharmacologic Treatment

- Acyclovir 800 mg five times per day for 7 days for acute herpes zoster, or

- Famciclovir 500 mg three times per day for 7 days, or

- Valacyclovir 1000 mg three times a day for 7 days

- Concomitant administration of Prednisone 60 mg daily for 7 days; 30 mg daily for 7 days; and 15 mg daily for 7 days, in divided doses, for severe pain in patients over the age of 50 years who have no contraindications.

- IV acyclovir 10 mg/kg every 8 hours for 7 days for immunocompromised patients

- Burow's solution wet compresses for 20 minutes several times a day to macerate the vesicles, remove serum and crusts, and help suppress secondary bacterial infections such as *Streptococcus pyogenes* or *Staphylococcus aureus.*

- Treat with oral analgesics (aspirin, acetaminophen) and/or narcotics (oxycodone, acetaminophen with codeine) as needed. Prescribe analgesics on a regular schedule rather than "as needed" to assure better pain control

Postherpetic Neuralgia

Treatment options may include the following:

- Capsaicin (Zostrix) to affected areas 3–5 times daily. Initial burning should subside in several days.

TABLE 12-3 Pharmacologic Approaches to Managing Herpes Zoster

PATIENT CHARACTERISTICS	MEDICATIONS/DOSE	COMMENTS
No modifying factors, up to 50 years of age	ASA Acetaminophen Oxycodone hydrochloride Acetaminophen/codeine	Pain usually resolves spontaneously; only symptomatic treatment is required. Titrate dose as needed.
No modifying factors, over 50 years of age	Oral acyclovir (Zovirax), 800 mg 5 times a day for 7 days Oral famciclovir (Famvir), 500 mg 3 times a day for 7 days Oral valacyclovir (Valtrex), 1000 mg 3 times a day for 7 days In individuals who present with severe pain, consider a 3-week course of prednisone (if not contraindicated by hypertension; diabetes; or osteoporosis): 60 mg daily for 7 days; 30 mg daily for 7 days; 15 mg daily for 7 days.	Greater bioavailability and more convenient dosing favor newer agents over acyclovir to reduce duration, and possibly prevalence, of PHN. Begin treatment within 72 hours of rash onset. Recent data show that concomitant antiviral-corticosteroid therapy may favorably affect quality-of-life factors[a] in older patients without contraindications
Postherpetic neuralgia (PHN)	Topical lidocaine, 5%; Capsaicin cream Oral amitriptyline, 50 mg to 75 mg daily for 2–3 weeks. Nortriptyline 10–25 mg at bedtime, increase gradually to a maximum of 125 mg day Gabapentin 900 mg to 3600 mg (maximum) daily	Anticholinergic effects of tricyclic antidepressants may deter use in the elderly. Gabapentin and other anticonvulsants (e.g., carbamazepine) reduce neuropathic pain, but can cause significant morbidity.
Ophthalmic zoster, all ages	Oral acyclovir (Zovirax), 800 mg 5 times a day for 7 days Oral famciclovir (Famvir), 500 mg 3 times a day for 7 days	Increased risk for PHN may favor use of famciclovir over acyclovir for ophthalmic zoster. Begin treatment within 72 hours of rash onset.
Immunocompromised, all ages	IV acyclovir, 10 mg/kg every 8 hours for 7 days	No conclusive data exists on newer agents. Thrombotic, thrombocytopenic purpura, hemolytic anemia syndrome, and mortality have been reported in patients with advanced HIV disease taking valacyclovir for HSV.
HIV+ with acyclovir resistance, all ages	Foscarnet, 40 mg/kg IV every 8 hours for 10 days or until lesions are healed	Acyclovir resistance is common among severely immunocompromised patients receiving prolonged (e.g., prophylactic) oral acyclovir therapy; look for dermatomal or disseminated hyperkeratotic verrucous papules and plaques. Cross-resistance among acyclovir, famciclovir, and valacyclovir is likely.

[a] Quality-of-life factors include return to usual activities, ability to sleep uninterrupted, and total cessation of analgesic use.

Source: Miedziak & O'Brien, 1999; Rico et al., 1997; Wallace, 1997; Whitley & Gnann, 1999.

- Lidocaine patch to affected area every 4–12 hours

- Tricyclic antidepressants—Use cautiously due to anticholinergic side effects. Nortriptyline (Pamelor) may be an appropriate choice for older adults. Order 10–25 mg at bedtime with increases of 25 mg every 2–4 weeks to a maximum dose of 125 mg daily. Tricyclic antidepressants also require several weeks to

reach therapeutic effects, which may make them a second-line drug.

- Anticonvulsants such as gabapentin 100–300 mg at bedtime with gradual increase to a maximum dose of 300–900 mg three times daily

- Complementary therapies such as transcutaneous electrical nerve stimulation (TENS)

Patient, Family, and Staff Education

- Explain to patient and/or family that uncomplicated herpes zoster usually resolves within 10 days, although it can take up to 4 weeks for the skin to return to normal.

- Herpes zoster may recur, because the virus stays in the nerve cells of the dorsal root ganglia for decades.

- Explain to the patient, family, and staff the need to avoid direct contact with susceptible individuals until all lesions have crusted over.

- Use prescribed analgesics, as needed, for pain.

- Notify healthcare provider if pain persists more than 30 days, or if new pain arises 30 or more days after the initial diagnosis of herpes zoster.

- Watch for adverse effects from antiviral medications including gastrointestinal upset, headache, dizziness, fatigue, rash, itching, and renal failure.

- For long-term facility staff:

  ○ Patients infected with HZ should be placed on contact isolation until the lesions crust over. Roommates, healthcare workers, and visitors with a history of chickenpox do not need to take further precautions. Healthcare workers and visitors without previous history of varicella should not enter the room until lesions have crusted over, or observe both airborne and contact isolation procedures.

  ○ Roommates without previous history of varicella should be moved to another room and placed on airborne and contact precautions for 10–21 days postexposure or 28 days if given VZIG.

  ○ Patients with varicella should be placed in strict or airborne isolation, depending on the classification nomenclature of the institution, and in negative pressure rooms, if available. If the resident is given VZIG, extend precautions to 28 days.

  ○ Immunocompromised hosts with disseminated zoster should also be placed in strict isolation (Campos, 1994).

  ○ Restrict nonimmune healthcare workers and/or visitors from contact with the patient until lesions have crusted unless wearing gown, gloves, and mask.

  ○ After exposure to varicella or shingles, nonimmune staff should be placed on leave for 10–21 days or until the 28th day if VZIG is given. If varicella develops, the worker cannot return until lesions have crusted over. Varicella vaccine is also a choice if given within 3–5 days postexposure.

  ○ All healthcare workers should have established immunity to varicella zoster by history or vaccination.

  ○ New employees should be screened for varicella antibodies and immunized if seronegative.

Physician Consultation

- Refer patients with ophthalmic zoster to an ophthalmologist because it can cause acute and serious complications. Preferably the patient should be referred within *3 days* of rash eruption.

- Refer or consult with primary physician for patients with HZ who are severely immunocompromised.

- Refer patients with persistent severe pain that is unresponsive to conventional treatment for sympathetic nerve blocks.

- Consider a neurosurgical consult for patients with severe pain that does not respond to conventional pharmacologic therapy for possible rhizotomy (surgical section of the nerve root).

WEB SITES

- Centers for Disease Control and Prevention (CDC), *Clostridium difficile* infections—www.cdc.gov/ncidod/dhqp/id_Cdiff.html
- CDC, Advisory Committee on Immunization Practices—www.cdc.gov/nip/ACIP
- CDC, Vaccines and Immunizations—www.cdc.gov/node.do/id/0900f3ec8000e2f3
- Immunization Action Coalition: Vaccine Information for Healthcare Professionals—www.immunize.org

REFERENCES

Anderson, K. N., Anderson, L. E., & Glanze, W. D. (Eds.). (1998). *Mosby's medical, nursing, & allied health dictionary* (5th ed.). St. Louis, MO: Mosby-Yearbook, Inc.

Campos, A. J. C. (1994). Varicella zoster infections. In American Academy of Pediatrics, *Red book: Report of the committee on infectious diseases* (23rd ed., pp. 511–517). Elk Grove Village, IL: Author.

Centers for Disease Control and Prevention (CDC). (1999). Prevention of varicella. Updated recommendations of the Advisory Committee on Immunization Practices (ACIP). *Morbidity and Mortality Weekly Report, 48*(RR-6), 1–5.

Centers for Disease Control and Prevention (CDC). (2005a). *Information about a new strain of* Clostridium difficile. Retrieved December 28, 2005, from http://www.cdc.gov/ncidod/dhqp/id_CdiffFAQ_newstrain.html

Centers for Disease Control and Prevention (CDC). (2006). *Shingles vaccine.* Retrieved October 1, 2006, from http://www.cdc.gov/nip/publications/VIS/default.htm#shingles

Choo, P. W., Galil, K., Donahue, G. K., Walker, A. M., Spiegelman, D., & Platt, R. (1997). Risk factors for postherpetic neuralgia. *Archives of Internal Medicine, 157*, 1217–1224.

Collings, K. L., & Miner, P. B. (2002). Diarrhea. *Best practices in medicine.* Retrieved December 28, 2005, from http://www.merckmedicus.com/pp/us/hcp/frame_micromedex.jsp?pg=http://merck.micromedex.com/index.asp?page=bpm

Dial, S., Delaney, J. A. C., Barkun, A. N., & Suissa, S. (2005). Use of gastric acid-suppressive agents and the risk of community-acquired *Clostridium difficile*-associated disease. *Journal of the American Medical Association, 294*, 2989–2995.

Donowitz, M., Kokke, F. T., & Saidi, R. (1995). Evaluation of patients with chronic diarrhea. *New England Journal of Medicine, 332*, 725–729.

Fekety, R. (1997). Guidelines for the diagnosis and management of *Clostridium difficile*—associated diarrhea and colitis. American College of Gastroenterology Practice Parameters Committee. *American Journal of Gastroenterology, 92*, 739–750.

Ferri, F. F. (1999). Herpes zoster. In: F. F. Ferri (Ed.), *Clinical Advisor* (p. 228). St. Louis, MO: Mosby-Yearbook, Inc.

Guerrant, R. L., Van Gilder, T., Steiner, T. S., Thielman, N. M., Slutsker, L., Tauxe, R.V., et al. (2002). Practice guidelines for the management of infectious diarrhea. *Clinical Infectious Diseases, 32*, 331–351.

Habif, T. P. (1996). Herpes zoster. In T. P. Habif (Ed.), *Clinical dermatology: A color guide to diagnosis and therapy.* (3rd ed. pp. 351–360). St. Louis, MO: Mosby-Yearbook, Inc.

Joyce, A. M., & Burns, D. L. (2002). Recurrent *Clostridium difficile* colitis. *Postgraduate Medicine Online, 112.* Retrieved March 3, 2006, from http://www.postgradmed.com/issues/2002/11_02/joyce3.htm

Kyne, L., Warny, M., Qamar, A., & Kelly, C. P. (2000). Asymptomatic carriage of *Clostridium difficile* and serum levels of IgG antibody against toxin A. *New England Journal of Medicine, 342*, 390–397.

Loo, V. G., Poirier, L., Miller, M. A., Oughton, M., Libman, M. D., Michaud, S., et al. (2005). A predominantly clonal multi-institutional outbreak of *Clostridium difficile*–associated diarrhea with high morbidity and mortality. *New England Journal of Medicine, 353*(23), 2442–2449.

McCary, M. L., Severson, J., & Tyring, S. K. (1999). Varicella zoster virus. *Journal of the American Academy of Dermatology, 41*(1), 1–14.

McDonald, L. C., Killgore, G. E., Thompson, A., Owens, R. C., Kazakova, S. V., Sambol, S. P., et al. (2005). An epidemic, toxin gene-variant strain of *Clostridium difficile. New England Journal of Medicine, 353*(23), 2433–2341.

Miedziak, A. I., & O'Brien, T. P. (1999). Ocular infections: Update on therapy. Therapy of varicella-zoster ocular infections. *Ophthalmologic Clinics of North America, 12*(1), 51–62.

Moyenuddin, M., Williamson, J. C., & Ohl, C. A. (2002). *Clostridium difficile*-associated diarrhea: Current strategies for diagnosis and therapy. *Current Gastroenterology Reports, 4*(4), 279–286.

Murakami, S., Honda, N., Mizobuchi, M., Nakashiro, Y., Hato, N., & Gyo, K. (1998). Rapid diagnosis of varicella zoster virus infection in acute facial palsy. *Neuropathy, 51*, 172–180.

Oldfield, E. C. (2004). *Clostridium difficile*-associated diarrhea: Risk factors, diagnostic methods and treatment. *Review of Gastroenterology Disorders, 4*(4), 186–195.

Oxman, M. N., Levin, M. J., Johnson, G. R., Schmader, K. E., Strauss, S. E., Gelb, L. D., et al. (2005). A vaccine to prevent herpes zoster and postherpetic neuralgia in older adults. *New England Journal of Medicine, 352*, 2271–2284.

Park, S. I., & Giannella, R. A. (1993). Approach to the adult patient with acute diarrhea. *Gastroenterology Clinics of North America, 22*(3), 483–497.

Peyramond, D., Chidiac, D., Lucht, F., Perronne, C., Saimot, A. G., Soussy, J. C., et al. (1998). Management of infections due to the varicella-zoster virus. 11th concensus conference on anti-infectious therapy of the French-speaking Society of Infectious Diseases (SPILF). *European Journal of Dermatology, 8*, 397–402.

Rico, M. J., Myers, S. A., Sanchez, M. R., and the Guidelines/Outcomes Committee, American Academy of Dermatology. (1997). Guidelines of care for dermatologic conditions in patients infected with HIV. Guidelines/Outcomes Committee. American Academy of Dermatology. *Journal of the American Academy of Dermatology, 37*(Pt 1.1), 450–472.

Simor, A. E., Bradley, S. F., Strausbaugh, L. J., Crossley, K., Nicolle, L. E., The SHEA Long-Term-Care Committee. (2002). *Clostridium difficile* in long-term care facilities for the elderly. *Infection Control and Hospital Epidemiology, 23*, 696–703.

Sunenshine, R. H., & McDonald, L. C. (2006). *Clostidium difficile*-associated disease: New challenges from an established pathogen. *Cleveland Clinic Journal of Medicine, 73*(2), 189–197.

Wallace, M. S., & Oxman, M. N. (1997). Pain: Nociceptive and neuropathic mechanisms. Acute herpes zoster and postherpetic neuralgia. *Anesthesiology Clinics of North America, 15*, 371–405.

Whitley, R. (2000). Herpes zoster. *Best practice of medicine.* Retrieved December 28, 2005, from http://merck.micromedex.com/index.asp?page=bpm_brief&article_id=BPM01IDM10

Whitley, R. J., & Gnann, J. W., Jr. (1999). Therapeutic approaches to the management of herpes zoster. *Advanced Experiments in Medical Biology, 458*, 159–165.

Zirn, J. R., Tompkins, S. D., Huie, C., & Shea, C. R. (1995). Rapid detection and distinction of cutaneous herpesvirus infections by direct immunofluorescence. *Journal of the American Academy of Dermatology, 33*(Pt. 1), 724–728.

▆ BIBLIOGRAPHY

Bartlett, J. G., & Perl, T. M. (2005). The new *Clostridium difficile*—what does it mean? *New England Journal of Medicine, 353*(23), 2433–2441.

Centers for Disease Control and Prevention (CDC). (2005b). Severe *Clostridium difficile*-associated disease in populations previously at low risk in four states, 2005. *Morbidity and Mortality Weekly Report, 54*, 1201–1205.

Cunningham, R., Dale, B., Undy, B., & Gaunt, N. (2003). Proton pump inhibitors as a risk factor for *Clostridium difficile* diarrhea. *Journal of Hospital Infection, 54*, 243–245.

Gold, R. (1988). Overview of the worldwide problem of diarrhea. *Drugs, 36*(S4), 1–5.

Kapikian, A. Z. (1996). Viral gastroenteritis. In *Cecil textbook in medicine* (20th ed., pp. 1793–1797). Philadelphia: W. B. Saunders.

Joyce, A. M., & Burns, D. L. (2002). Recurrent *Clostridium difficile* colitis. *Postgraduate Medicine, 112*(5). Retrieved December 28, 2005, from http://www.postgradmed.com/issues/2002/11_02/joyce3.htm

Kowlessar, O. D. (1995). Antibiotic-associated diarrhea and colitis. In W. B. Abrams, M. H. Beers, & R. Berkow (Eds.), *The Merck manual of geriatrics* (2nd ed., pp. 669–671). Whitehouse Station, NJ: Merck Research Laboratories.

Muñoz, P., Bouza, E., Cuenca-Estrella, M., Eiro, J. M., Perez, M. J., Sanchez-Somolinos, M., et al. (2005). *Saccharomyces cervisiae* fungemia: An emerging infectious disease. *Clinical Infectious Diseases*, 40(11), 1625–1634.

Powell, D. W. (1999). Approach to the patient with diarrhea. In T. Yamaya, D. H. Alpers, C. Owyang, and D. W. Powell, *Textbook of Gastroenterology* (3rd ed., pp. 858–909). Philadelphia: Lippincott, Williams & Wilkins.

Stankus, S. J., Dlugopolski, M., & Packer, D. (2000). Management of herpes zoster (shingles) and postherpetic neuralgia. *American Family Physician, 61*, 2437–2444, 2447–2448.

CHAPTER 13

Musculoskeletal Disorders

David Casey and Deborah Truax

GOUT AND PSEUDOGOUT

Definition

Gout and pseudogout are illnesses characterized by an inflammatory response to deposits of crystalline material in joints. In gout there is a precipitation of monosodium urate crystals, in pseudogout there are findings of calcium pyrophosphate dihydrate (CPPD) crystals in the joints and surrounding tissues.

Epidemiology

The prevalence of gout has approximately doubled over the past 2 decades in the United States, associated with marked increases in people older than age 65. Those older than the age of 75 have undergone the most dramatic increases in prevalence of gout. Gouty arthritis in many of these patients is difficult to manage because of comorbid conditions, including advanced chronic kidney disease, diabetes mellitus, and renal intolerance to nonsteroidal anti-inflammatory drugs (NSAIDs) (Terkeltaub, 2006).

An elevated uric acid (hyperuricemia) is frequently noted in gout, but normal uric acid levels have been found in up to 2% of cases of proven gout. Urate is the end product of purine metabolism. Purines are eliminated via the kidneys and the gastrointestinal tract. When purines are either overproduced or underexcreted, the stage is set for hyperuricemia and gout (McTigue, 2005). Urate deposits are common in distal and proximal interphalanges (DIPs and PIPs) in the hand.

There is usually no sequela from an initial acute gout attack. The attack resolves, and the patient is without symptoms in approximately 90–95% of cases. The remaining 5–10% are subject to a pattern of recurrent acute episodes. Although the disease is quiescent in this phase, hyperuricemia is still present, and the disease continues to advance unless the disease is diagnosed and treated. If the underlying hyperuricemia is poorly controlled, chronic arthritis is the major manifestation often associated with tissue deposition of urate crystals (tophi) (McTigue, 2005).

Pseudogout is found primarily in elderly women and frequently seen in conjunction with calcification of cartilage (chondrocalcinosis) on X-ray. It can be associated with trauma to affected joint, hyperparathyroidism, and hemachromatosis.

Common Presenting Signs and Symptoms

- In both gout and pseudogout there is usually a sudden onset of pain, swelling, heat, and redness of the affected joint. The most common joint involved in gout is the first metatarsal phalangeal joint (MTP).

- Tophi may be seen in the external ears, hands, feet, olecranon, and prepatellar bursas.

- Pseudogout most frequently affects the knee and occasionally the wrist joints.

- Long-term diuretic use in patients with hypertension or congestive heart failure, chronic kidney disease, prophylactic low dose aspirin, and alcohol abuse are factors associated with the development of hyperuricemia and gout in the elderly (Fam, 1998). Gout can also follow minor trauma and medical illness (Campbell, 1988). An acute attack of gout can also be induced by general anesthesia for a major surgery.

- Pseudogout is often associated with trauma and occasionally with hyperparathyroidism or hemachromatosis.

Differential Diagnosis

- The most important consideration in a patient who presents with acute arthritis is to consider and evaluate for septic arthritis. The most common joint involved in septic arthritis is the knee.

- Rheumatoid arthritis may be difficult to distinguish from chronic gout or pseudogout arthropathy, particularly in women.

- Osteoarthritis

- Psoriatic arthritis

- Reactive arthritis—A clinical tetrad of arthritis, urethritis, conjunctivitis, and mucocutaneous lesions

- Cellulitis

Essential Diagnostic and Laboratory Tests

- Examination of synovial fluid for crystalline structures is the only specific test for these diseases. Hyperuricemia is usually present in gout, but an elevated uric acid level may be present for other reasons, including use of diuretics. See Table 13-1 for evaluation of crystal arthropathies.

- Pseudogout is often seen in the presence of chondrocalcinosis, but may occur without the X-ray finding. Cystic changes and well-defined erosions with overhanging bony edges (Martel's sign) associated with soft tissue calcified masses are characteristic radiographic features of chronic tophaceous gout. However, similar signs can be observed in erosive osteoarthritis and rheumatoid arthritis.

Management Plan

Nonpharmacologic

- For acute attacks, bed rest is indicated and should be continued until 24 hours following an attack.

- Immobilization of affected joint using splints

- Local application of cold pack to affected joint has been shown to reduce pain during bouts of an acute episode of gout (Schlesinger et al., 2002).

- Dietary consultation for low-purine diet. Avoid high-purine foods such as organ meats, yeast products, beans, peas, oatmeal, and spinach.

Pharmacologic

- Drugs to lower the level of uric acid should be started only after subsidence of the acute attack. Prophylactic doses of colchicine should also be provided at the same time to prevent flare up of the disease; these should be continued for at least a year after normalization of serum uric acid. Unfortunately, there is no proven therapy to prevent attacks

TABLE 13-1   Crystal Arthropathies

CHARACTERISTICS	GOUT	PSEUDOGOUT
Sex ratio: male to female	2–3:1	1:2
Peak age	40–50	> 60
Most common joint	1st MTP	Knee
Serum urate	High	Normal
Radiology		
Calcification	Absent	Chondrocalcinosis
Erosions	Often characteristic	Often degenerative change
Crystals	Needle-shaped	Rod-shaped
	Negative birefringent	Positive birefringent
Initiating factor	Obesity, alcohol abuse, trauma, stress	Trauma, stress, infection
Treatment		
Acute	NSAIDs, colchicine, corticosteroids	NSAIDs, corticosteroids
Chronic	Normalize serum uric acid with allopurinol or probenecid	Look for complication conditions (e.g., hyperparathyroid or hemochromatosis)

Note: MTP, metatarsophalangeal.

of pseudogout, but a search for secondary causes and prompt initiation of NSAIDs are important. Joint aspiration with or without intra-articular corticosteroids can reduce the severity of the attack.

- In both acute gout and pseudogout, non-steroidal anti-inflammatory drugs (NSAIDs) may be helpful for symptom relief of pain. See osteoarthritis section for NSAIDs.

- Colchicine has been used for more than three centuries and is effective in gout though it has significant side effects when used in large doses. It is currently used in acute gout only when NSAIDs are contraindicated. The usual dose is 0.6 mg twice a day. Reduce dose in patients with chronic kidney disease or heart failure. Common side effect is diarrhea. Prophylactic doses of colchicine 0.6 mg twice daily should be provided to prevent flare of the disease and be continued for at least a year after normalization of serum uric acid.

- Rapid reduction of pain and swelling may be accomplished in both diseases by intra-articular corticosteroid injection and oral corticosteroids. Triamcinolone 10–40 mg depending on the size of the joint may be injected or corticosteroids may be given IV or methylprednisolone 40 mg/day tapered or oral prednisone 40–60 mg tapered.

- For recurrent attacks of gout it is necessary to use drugs to reduce hyperuricemia to < 300 μmol/liter (6.0 mg/dL). This may be accomplished by either promoting renal excretion of uric acid with uricosuric drugs such as probenecid 200 mg twice daily, increasing gradually to 2 grams to maintain serum uric acid < 6.0 mg/dL. Use probenecid only in patients with normal renal function. Allopurinol is most commonly used to reduce uric acid starting with 100 mg initially then increasing to 300 mg daily as required. If there is chronic kidney disease present, reduce dose; e.g., 50 mg/daily for creatinine clearance < 10 mL. Allopurinol interrupts the metabolic pathway of uric acid production. The most serious side effect is skin rash progressing to epidermal necrolysis especially in patients with chronic kidney disease.

- Asymptomatic hyperuricemia is not treated; however, an attempt to identify and treat the cause should be made (check for chronic kidney disease or alcohol abuse).

Patient, Family, and Staff Education

- Explain importance of compliance with prophylactic treatment with colchicine and hypouremic therapy for control of symptoms of gout. Explain that gout can be effectively treated and in most cases prevented if the patient complies with the drug regime.
- Explain triggering factors such as obesity, excess alcohol use, systemic infections, and trauma.

Physician Consultation

- Consult physician on any patient with suspected new diagnosis of gout.
- Refer to rheumatologist for evaluation of synovial fluid to search for crystals and to evaluate for any suspected infection.
- Consult rheumatologist on those patients who do not improve or respond to initial treatment.

▒ LOW BACK PAIN

Definition

Low back pain (LBP) is classified by the anatomic structures affected along with the clinical symptomatology. The most common origin of LBP is from the musculoligamentous structures. Pain is usually localized to the low back and buttock areas but occasionally radiates to the lower leg with nerve root irritation or with lumbar canal stenosis. Serious underlying disorders such as infection, cancer, and fractures are uncommon causes of LBP (Vogt et al., 2005). Low back pain can be defined as either acute or chronic. Acute low back pain typically lasts less than one month, and chronic or persistent low back pain lasts longer than 3 months. Back pain

is a frequent complex symptom for a myriad of processes afflicting the lumbar spine and paraspinal tissues, and for this reason the nurse practitioner must carefully consider and exclude a large number of potential spinal disorders in the workup of the patient with LBP. Patients experiencing LBP who can benefit from short-term rehabilitation and pain management may be admitted to a skilled nursing facility (SNF).

Epidemiology

Low back pain is experienced at some time by up to 80% of the population (Hellmann, Stone, & Tierney, 2005). In most cases of low back pain, patients recover within a few weeks of the onset of symptoms, although recurrences are common and low-grade symptoms are often present years after an initial episode. Acute low back pain is the fifth most common reason for all physician visits. It is responsible for direct health care expenditures of more than $20 billion annually and as much as $50 billion per year when indirect costs are included (Patel & Ogle, 2000).

Among patients over 65 years of age, the diagnosis probability of cancer, compression fractures, spinal stenosis, and aortic aneurysms become more common (Deyo & Weinstein, 2001).

Risk factors for the development of disabling chronic or persistent low back pain (usually defined as lasting > 3 months) include preexisting psychological distress, disputed compensation issues, other types of chronic pain, and job dissatisfaction (Carragee, 2005).

Common Presenting Signs and Symptoms

- For the patient presenting with LBP a focused medical history and physical exam are critical. The primary purpose is to seek medical history responses or physical exam findings suggesting a serious underlying condition such as fracture, tumor, infection, or cauda equina syndrome (red flags). In the absence of red flags, special tests are not usually required within one month of low back symptoms because most patients recover from their activity limitations.

○ Red flags for spinal fracture
  ▪ History of trauma/fall
  ▪ Prolonged use of steroids
  ▪ Age > 70 years
○ Red flags for cancer or infection
  ▪ History of cancer
  ▪ Unexplained weight loss
  ▪ Immunosuppression
  ▪ Urinary infection
  ▪ Intravenous drug use
○ Red flags for cauda equina syndrome and severe spinal compromise
  ▪ Acute onset of urinary retention or incontinence
  ▪ Loss of anal sphincter tone or fecal incontinence
  ▪ Saddle anesthesia
  ▪ Global or progressive motor weakness in lower limbs

• Other key questions on the medical history should include the following:
○ Constitutional symptoms and the presence of night pain or morning stiffness
○ Any neurological symptoms such as numbness, weakness, radiating pain, bowel and bladder dysfunction
○ Duration of symptoms
○ Rating of pain; 0–10 scale, face scale
○ Onset, location, description of pain
○ Aggravating factors
○ Alleviating factors
○ Patient's work and activities of daily living
○ Previous and present treatments

• *Radiating back pain* down the buttock and below the knee suggests a nerve root impingement as source of pain. Other conditions occur such as sacroiliitis, facet joint degenerative arthritis, spinal stenosis, myofascial trigger points in lumbar and gluteal areas with referred pain to the lower extremities.

• *Nocturnal low back pain* unrelieved or increased by bed rest or the supine position suggests the possibility of a malignancy or a cauda equina tumor. Similar pain can be caused by compression fractures.

• Low back pain that worsens with rest and improves with activity is characteristic of rheumatoid arthritis or inflammatory spondyloarthropathy.

• Most degenerative back disease produces pain with activity; rest alleviates the pain.

• Spinal range of motion may be limited in spinal infections; otherwise, it has been found to be of limited diagnostic value (Frymoyer et al., 1988).

• Fever suggests the possibility of spinal infection. Vertebral tenderness has sensitivity for infection but not specificity.

Physical Examination

• The basic elements of a physical examination should include inspection, palpation, range of motion testing, strength testing, and reflexes.

• Have the patient point to the area of maximal pain.

• Inspection should include posture, body habitus, skin discoloration, masses, and asymmetry. Ask the patient to bend forward as though to touch the toes. Observe flexibility versus rigidity in the lumbar spine. Observe the patient's gait, sitting, and standing. Does the patient limp or guard when walking? Does the patient sit and stand gingerly?

• Perform range of motion (ROM) of the hips, especially internal rotation to rule out hip disease as a cause of back pain.

• Palpate the cervical spine, neck and upper back, elbow/forearms, wrists, thumbs for tenderness, spasm, and myofascial trigger points.

- Straight leg raising with the patient sitting as well as supine helps reveal irritability of the nerve roots. Pain on active and passive dorsiflexion of the foot may provide further evidence of radiculopathy. Hold the patient's leg straight and cup the heel with the other hand. An elevation of less than 60 degrees is abnormal. A positive test reproduces the symptoms of sciatica, with the pain that radiates below the knee, not merely back or hamstring pain.

- Neurological examination should include ankle and great toe dorsiflexion strength (S1), ankle and knee reflexes (S1 and L4), and dermatomal sensory loss. The L5 and S1 nerve roots are involved in approximately 95% of lumbar disc herniations (Deyo & Weinstein, 2001). Biceps, triceps, and brachioradialis reflexes should also be checked.

- Rectal examination to assess sensation and tone if cauda equina syndrome suspected and to rule out rectal mass or enlarged prostate.

- Palpate abdomen for aortic aneurysm and listen for bruits. Aortic aneurysm should be suspected among older adults with coronary artery disease or multiple risk factors. Some aneurysms are detected by physical examination although ultrasonography, CT, or MRI is often necessary.

Differential Diagnosis

Causes of low back pain can be divided into *extraspinal* and *spinal*.

Extraspinal causes of low back pain include the following:

- Aortic aneurysm
- Pancreatitis
- Ruptured viscus
- Retroperitoneal tumor
- Hip disease

Spinal causes of back pain include the following:

- Tumor
- Infection
- Fractures
- Inflammation
- Degenerative disc disease
- Spondylolisthesis
- Spinal stenosis
- Herniated nucleus pulposus
- Cauda equina syndrome

Psychosocial Risk Factors for Delayed Recovery

Many studies have found an association between depression and other types of psychological distress (Hurwitz, Morgenstern, & Yu, 2003). Attention to psychological and socioeconomic problems in the patient's life is important since nonphysical factors can complicate the treatment plan. Factors include the following:

- Previous history of disability
- Inconsistent findings and abnormal pain behavior
- Inconsolable
- "Secondary gain" (litigation, work unhappiness, excessive attention from family member)
- Preference for bed rest
- Depression
- Chemical dependency
- History of patient being abused

Essential Diagnostic and Laboratory Tests

- Low back pain lasting less than one month generally does not require any imaging studies.

- Regular radiographs of the spine give limited information. Plain films can be useful in evaluating spinal infection, spondylolysis, metastatic disease, and fractures. Obtain anterior posterior (AP), lateral, and oblique views. Plain radiographs have a very low sensitivity and specificity for disc disease.

- Computed tomography (CT) and magnetic resonance imaging (MRI) should be reserved for patients for whom there is a strong clinical suggestion of underlying infection, cancer, or persistent neurological deficit. Disc and other abnormalities are common among asymptomatic adults. Degenerated, bulging, and herniated discs are frequently incidental findings. The strengths and weaknesses of CT are the following:

  - Produces detailed pictures of the bony architecture of the vertebral, facet, and sacroiliac joints

  - Fewer problems with claustrophobia

  - CT myelogram involves injection of a contrast medium into the spinal canal. May be performed for the planning of surgery.

  - Provides less information than MRI because it does not visualize soft tissue and nerve roots well.

- The strengths and weaknesses of MRI include the following:

  - Useful to clarify the diagnosis in patients with chronic pain that has not responded to physical therapy and other conservative measures

  - Used to plan intervention such as injections or surgery

  - Used to monitor the regression of disc herniations treated without surgery

  - Ability to scan the entire lumbar spine and vertebral canal and to visualize malignant tumors, rare abnormalities within the vertebral canal, impingement of nerve roots, bulging or herniated discs, enlargement of the ligamentum flavum, and degenerative changes in the facet joints.

  - Essential for diagnosing inflammatory conditions, including metabolic arthropathies and infections

  - More expensive than CT

- For patients who have a history of cancer, imaging is recommended.

- Bone scanning can be useful when radiographs of the spine are normal but the clinical findings are suspicious for osteomyelitis, bony neoplasm, or occult fracture. Early diagnosis and treatment of spinal metastasis are needed to prevent complications such as pain, pathological fracture, weakness, sensory loss, paralysis, and bowel and bladder dysfunction.

- Radionuclide bone scanning has limited utility. It is most useful for early detection of vertebral body osteomyelitis or osteoblastic metastases.

- Simple laboratory tests, including complete blood count (CBC) and erythrocyte sedimentation rate (ESR), alkaline phosphate, and calcium can be done as initial tests when there is a suspicion of back-related tumor or infection. Leukocyte count may be increased with infection. ESR may be increased in malignancy, infections, and connective tissue disorders. It is also useful to assess the response to therapy.

- Electrodiagnostic assessments such as needle electromyography and nerve conduction studies are useful in differentiating peripheral neuropathy, radiculopathy, or myopathy.

Management Plan

Nonpharmacologic

- Bed rest is generally not recommended for the treatment of low back pain or sciatica for more than 1–2 days, and a rapid return to normal activities is usually the best course.

- PT for modalities and exercises. See Rehabilitation chapter.

- Use of lumbar supports such as a corset for a short period (a few weeks) may be indicated in patients with osteoporotic compression fractures.

- Referral to "back school" on an outpatient basis when patient discharged.

- Consider adjunct therapies such as therapeutic massage or acupuncture.

Pharmacologic
- Guidelines for the treatment of LBP developed by the Agency for Health Care Policy and Research (AHCPR, 1994) with other groups recommend that nonopioid analgesics including acetaminophen and NSAIDs be used first in treatment of mild or moderate LBP. See Osteoarthritis section for NSAIDs.

- Opioid drugs may be required for short duration; 1–2 weeks. See Osteoarthritis section for opioid medication.

- Skeletal muscle relaxants such as methocarbamol (Robaxin) 500 mg two to three times daily or cyclobenzaprine hydrochloride (Flexeril) 10 mg twice daily can be used as adjunct therapy for spasms.

- Epidural corticosteroid injections can provide short-term relief of sciatica.

Patient, Family, and Staff Education

Successful treatment depends on the patient's understanding of the disorder and his or her role in avoiding reinjury. Referral to outpatient classes on weight loss and healthy lifestyle choices can be helpful.

Physician Consultation
- Any patient with LBP that does not respond to initial treatment or who has symptoms that worsen despite treatment.

- Any patient with suspected cauda equina lesions requires immediate surgical evaluation.

- Surgical evaluation is also indicated in patients with worsening neurological deficits such as bowel or bladder incontinence or intractable pain.

- Consider physical medicine consultation in cases where pain is severe and unresponsive to the standard PT measures.

- Referral to pain clinic in acute cases for possible epidural injection.

- Referral to pain clinic for chronic pain management program.

▆▆▆ OSTEOARTHRITIS

Definition

Osteoarthritis is the most common disease of the joints. It is a degenerative disorder affecting many joints, especially the hands and large weight-bearing joints. It is characterized by pain, deformity and enlargement of the joints, limitation of movement, and frequently new bone growth in the joint margins (osteophytes).

Epidemiology

Osteoarthritis affects more than 20 million Americans and accounts for 60–70% of joint diseases in older persons. Almost all persons aged 65 to 74 years have radiographic osteoarthritis of the hands; one third of those aged 63 to 93 years have findings indicative of osteoarthritis on knee radiographs. Most osteoarthritis is idiopathic and can be linked to advancing age, obesity, occupational overloading of joints, and familial type II collagen gene polymorphisms. In some patients osteoarthritis is secondary and may develop at varying intervals after trauma, infection, osteonecrosis, or congenital malalignment, or in the setting of metabolic disease. These changes result in fibrillation and denudation of articular cartilage, variable degrees of secondary inflammation, decreased synovial fluid viscosity, and altered joint biomechanics. These pathologic processes culminate in impaired joint function, pain, and reduced quality of life (Grober & Thethi, 2003).

This can be particularly significant for the elderly person residing in a skilled nursing facility who may already be experiencing a loss of independence and require assistance with activities of daily living (ADLs).

Risk Factors

- Age
- Female sex
- Race
- Genetic factors
- Major joint trauma
- Repetitive stress
- Obesity
- Congenital and developmental defects
- Prior inflammatory joint disease
- Metabolic or endocrine disorders

Common Presenting Signs and Symptoms

- Joint pain that slowly progresses, worsens with use, and improves with rest.
- In advanced disease, pain may be constant. Many patients with moderate to severe osteoarthritis (OA) complain of nocturnal pain.
- Many patients experience morning stiffness that lasts usually less than 30 minutes.
- Joints commonly involved are the hips, knees, cervical spine, lumbar spine, first carpometacarpal (CMC) or basilar thumb joints, proximal and distal interphalangeal joints (PIPs and DIPs) of the hands, and midfoot joints. DIP and PIP joint involvement resulting in Heberden's and Bouchard nodes is more common in women.
- Consider one of the secondary causes of OA if a patient has pain and or swelling in the wrist, shoulder, elbow, or metacarpophalangeal (MCP) joints.
- Joint affected by OA may be minimally or not swollen at all. Tenderness on palpation is characteristic. In most cases, erythema or warmth over the joint does not occur; however, an effusion may be present. Crepitus is common as well as reduced passive and active ranges of motion. Angular deformity may be present in advanced disease.
- Limited joint motion or muscle atrophy around a more severely affected joint may occur.

Differential Diagnoses

- Rheumatoid arthritis
- Gout
- Tendonitis
- Bursitis

Essential Diagnostic and Laboratory Tests

- The diagnosis of OA is made based on a thorough history, physical examination, and radiographs. See Table 13-2 for diagnostic criteria for OA (American College of Rheumatology, 2000).
- Radiographic hallmarks of OA are asymmetric narrowing of joint spaces, osteophyte formation, and subchondral sclerosis.
- There are no practical specific laboratory markers for OA.
- Arthrocentesis of the affected joint can help exclude inflammatory arthritis infection or crystal arthropathy.

TABLE 13-2   Diagnostic Criteria for Osteoarthritis
Joint pain
Osteophytes or bone spurs on X-ray and *one of the following*:
Age older than 50 years
Stiffness usually less than 30 minutes
Crepitus on physical examination

Source: American College of Rheumatology, 2000.

Management Plan

There is no cure for OA, but treatment tailored to the individual patient can reduce its impact. *The treatment goals of OA management include pain relief, optimal joint function, and maximal overall quality of life.*

Nonpharmacologic

- In 1995, the American College of Rheumatology (ACR) published guidelines for the nonpharmacologic management of OA of the hip and knee; these were most recently updated in 2000. The guidelines focus on a combination of patient education, follow-up, and support to ensure patient compliance. They include the following:
  - ○ Weight loss
  - ○ Physical and occupational therapies
  - ○ Judicious use of exercise
  - ○ Use of adaptive equipment and bracing

- Rest when pain is severe. Increase activity gradually as soon as patient can tolerate.

- Avoid repetitive movements that aggravate symptoms.

- Weight loss if overweight to reduce stress on the affected joints such as the knees and hips

- Physical therapy for range of motion exercises, strengthening exercises, and assistive devices for ambulation. Joint unloading in certain joints such as the knee or hip. Occupational therapy for joint protection and energy conservation techniques, assistive devices for activities of daily living. Splints can rest and protect affected small joints in the hands. It is important to prevent contractures from occurring.

- Thermal modalities such as heat or cold applied for 10–15 minutes.

- Therapeutic ultrasound can be helpful when there are adhesions or contractures present.

- Consider acupuncture for pain control as an adjunct therapy (Lie, 2004).

Pharmacologic

Categories of drugs used to treat OA include nonsteroidal anti-inflammatory drugs (NSAIDs), COX-2 selective drugs, acetaminophen, and opiates.

- Start with acetaminophen up to 1 gm three times daily (3,000 mg/day). This is the first choice for pain relief because it is safer than NSAIDs and often effective. May put patients at risk for liver disease, especially if alcohol is consumed (Hochberg et al., 1995). Avoid in those patients with known liver disease and alcohol abuse.

- If response is inadequate, use NSAIDs and selective COX-2 inhibitors. See Table 13-3 for commonly used medications to treat pain in OA. Individuals response to these drugs varies greatly, and several may be tried before relief is obtained. The lowest possible dose should be used. The most common side effect is GI upset which often occurs without evidence of ulceration or bleeding and may require discontinuance of the drug. Unfortunately, ulceration and bleeding do not correlate with subjective symptoms; thus bleeding can occur without warning. Taking these medications with food may help minimize GI symptoms. In addition, NSAIDs can cause acute renal failure and should be used with caution in the elderly particularly in those who have renal disease, heart failure, volume depletion or liver disease. See Table 13-4 for risk factors for NSAID-induced complications.

- If patient is at risk for upper GI tract bleeding or peptic ulcer disease, add a proton pump inhibitor (PPI) or misoprostol.

- Tramadol 50–100 mg every 4–6 hours not to exceed 400 mg/day can be used in patients whose symptoms are not controlled with NSAIDs. Tramadol is a nonnarcotic analgesic.

- Use of opiate analgesics may be effective in certain individuals and for those with severe pain that have not responded well to

TABLE 13-3   Commonly Used Medications Used to Treat Pain in Osteoarthritis

Nonacetylated salicylates

Choline magnesium trisalicylate (Trilisate)	500–1000 mg twice daily
Diflunisal (Dolobid)	250–500 mg every 8–12 hr
Sodium salicylate (Disalcid)	500–1000 mg twice daily after meals

NSAIDs

Diclofenac (Voltarin)	50–75 mg twice daily
Etodolac (Lodine)	200–400 mg 2–3 times daily ER 400–1200 daily
Fenoprofen (Nalfon)	300–600 mg every 6 hrs
Flurbiprofen (Ansaid, Ocufen)	50–100 mg 3–4 times daily
Ibuprofen (Motrin)	200–800 mg 3 times daily
Indomethacin (Indocin)	25–50 mg three times daily SR 75 mg 1–2 daily
Ketoprofen (Orudis)	25–75 mg 2–3 times a day ER 100–200 mg daily
Meloxicam (Mobic)	7.5 mg daily
Nabumetone (Relafen)	500 mg by mouth daily to start; maximum dose 2000 mg daily
Naproxen (Naprosyn)	250–500 mg every 6–8 hrs
Oxaprozin (Daypro)	1200 mg daily
Piroxicam (Feldene)	20 mg daily
Sulindac (Clinoril)	150–200 mg twice a day
Tolmetin (Tolectin)	200–600 mg three times a day

Nonselective COX inhibitor/misoprostol

Diclofenac/ misoprostol	50–200 mg daily

Selective COX-2 inhibitors

Celecoxib	100 mg daily

Notes: COX, cyclooxygenase; ER, extended release; OA, osteoarthritis; SR, sustained release.

TABLE 13-4   Risk Factors for NSAID-Induced Complications

History of gastroduodenal ulceration or gastrointestinal bleeding
Age older than 60 years
Concomitant anticoagulant or corticosteroid use
Multiple or high-dose NSAIDs
Major organ impairment
Arthritis-related disability
Possible risks may include *Helicobacter pylori*, alcohol consumption, cigarette use

NSAIDs or COX-2 selective agents. Tolerance, dependency, and adverse reactions may occur. See Table 13-5 for opiate medications. Stool softeners should be added to avoid constipation from opiates.

- Local injections of glucocorticoids, methylprednisolone acetate, and triamcinolone acetonide have been used with success in relieving pain.

- Intra-articular hyaluronan injections have been shown to be effective for pain relief. Consider in patients who have not responded to a nonpharmaceutical program or in those patients for whom NSAIDs and COX-2 inhibitors are contraindicated (Kotz & Kolarz, 1999).

- Capsaicin cream applied directly to affected area can provide temporary relief. Start with lower concentration 0.025% or 0.075%. Avoid contact with any open skin or mucous membranes.

- Glucosamine and chondroitin 500 mg twice daily with food. Benefit should be noted

TABLE 13-5   Opiate Analgesics Used to Treat Osteoarthritis

DRUG	DOSE
Oxycodone (OxyContin)	10 mg every 12 hrs, maximum. dose 40 mg every 12 hrs
Morphine sulfate (Oramorph, MS Contin)	15 mg by mouth every 12 hrs to start; titrate as needed. Oral solution 10 mg/5 mL
Oxycodone/aspirin (Percodan)	5/325 mg, 1–2 tabs every 4–6 hrs as needed
Oxycodone/ acetaminophen (Percocet)	5/325 mg, 1–2 tabs by mouth every 4–6 hrs as needed
Hydrocodone/ acetaminophen (Vicodin)	5/500 mg, 1–2 tabs by mouth every 4–6 hrs as needed
Acetaminophen/ codeine	(#3) 300/30 mg, 1–2 tabs every 4–6 hrs; maximum 12 tabs/24 hrs (#4) 300/60 mg, 1–2 tabs every 4-6 hrs
Fentanyl (Duragesic)	25 μg/hr patch, topical every 72 hrs; maximum 100 μg/hr

within 3 months. Glucosamine stimulates production of glycosaminoglycans, leading to increased synthesis of cartilage. Chondroitin may help maintain articular fluid viscosity and stimulate cartilage repair (Bulletin on the Rheumatic Diseases, 2001).

Patient, Family, and Staff Education

- Explain natural history and management options for OA.
- Explain benefit of exercise and activity programs.
- Educate on importance of weight reduction, if indicated.
- Explain risks and benefits associated with medications used to treat OA.

Physician Consultation

- If effusion is significant and results in pain and/or affects activities of daily living, refer to physician for further evaluation to rule out infection or for possible aspiration and injection of intra-articular corticosteroid.
- If patient is a candidate for surgery, refer to orthopedic surgeon for joint surgery (arthrodesis, osteotomy, arthroplasty, or arthroscopy).
- Consider referral to rheumatologist if joint pain persists or response to treatment inadequate.

▰▰ OSTEOPOROSIS

Definition

The World Health Organization (WHO) consensus conference defines *osteoporosis* as "a disease characterized by low bone mass and microarchitectural deterioration of bone tissue leading to bone fragility and a consequent increase in fracture risk" (Consensus Development Conference, 1993). *Osteopenia* is a less advanced state of low bone mineral density (Nguyen et al., 1993). By the time the diagnosis

of osteopenia is made radiographically, significant and irreversible bone loss has already occurred (Masud, 2000).

Epidemiology

Osteoporosis is a major public health problem; 44 million Americans have or are at risk for osteoporosis; 10 million people have osteoporosis, and another 34 million more are at risk of developing osteoporosis and consequent fractures. Approximately 40–50% of women ages 50 or older will have an osteoporosis-related fracture in their lifetime. The prevalence of osteoporosis is expected to increase with the aging of our population (U.S. Department of Health and Human Services, 2004). By the year 2040, the incidence of hip fractures may double or triple (Cummings, Black, & Thompson, 1998).

Osteoporosis is a particular health concern for women in long-term care facilities, who face a 3–8% annual risk of hip fracture; 5–10 times greater than that of their community-dwelling counterparts. Osteoporosis is responsible for more than 1.5 million fractures annually, among them more than half a million vertebral fractures, 300,000 hip fractures, 200,000 wrist fractures, and 300,000 other sites. Approximately 37,000 people die each year from complications related to osteoporotic fractures. Osteoporosis combined with dependency, impaired mobility, delay or loss of usual protective action, and a high fall rate render the long-term care population particularly vulnerable to fractures. Expenditures for care of patients with these fractures for 2001 were estimated at $17 billion, a figure that is expected to rise as the population continues to age (AMDA, 2003).

The overall prevalence of osteoporotic fractures rises dramatically in menopausal women. Bone loss is more abrupt for the first decade after the onset of menopause, followed by more gradual loss thereafter. The frequency of hip fractures increases exponentially with age, particularly after age 70, and is more commonly seen in Asian and Caucasian women. Osteoporosis is less common in men for several reasons including men have larger skeletons, their bone loss starts later in life and progresses more slowly, and they do not experience the rapid bone loss that affects women when their estrogen production drops as a result of menopause. Despite this men can experience a marked loss of bone as they age. It is estimated that one-fifth to one-third of all hip fractures occur in men. Seventeen percent of men who reach age 90 have had a hip fracture in their lifetime. Men are also much more likely than women to die or experience chronic disability after a hip fracture. It is estimated the number of men older than 70 will double between 1993–2050 according to the U.S. National Osteoporosis Foundation (Masud, 2000).

Classification of Osteoporosis

Osteoporosis may be categorized as either a primary or secondary form. *Primary* osteoporosis is the more common form and is due to the typical age-related loss of bone from the skeleton. It is classified as type 1 and type 2. *Secondary* osteoporosis results from the presence of other diseases or conditions that predispose to bone loss and is classified as type 3 (Masud, 2000).

- *Primary type 1*—Occurs in 5–20% of postmenopausal women, with a peak incidence in the 60s and early 70s. Estrogen deficiency is thought to be the cause of this form of osteoporosis, rendering the skeleton more sensitive to parathyroid hormone (PTH), resulting in increased calcium resorption from bone.
- *Primary type 2*—Occurs in women or men greater than 70 years of age and usually is associated with decreased bone formation along with decreased ability of the kidney to produce 1,25(OH)2D3. The vitamin D deficiency results in decreased calcium

absorption which increases PTH level and therefore bone resorption. Both cortical and trabecular bone is lost, primarily leading to increased risk of hip, long bone, and vertebral fractures.

- *Secondary*—Occurs more commonly in men than women. The most commonly reported secondary causes of osteoporosis in men include hypogonadism and malabsorption syndromes, including gastrectomy. Medications that have been shown to adversely affect bone mineral density (BMD) include glucocorticoids, excess thyroid supplement, anticonvulsants, methotrexate, cyclosporine, and heparin (Prestwood & Kenny, 1998). See Table 13-6 for secondary causes of osteoporosis.

Common Presenting Signs and Symptoms

- Usually asymptomatic
- Bone pain, especially the spine
- Postural changes (kyphosis), and loss of height (> 1.5 inches) may indicate vertebral fractures.
- Minimally traumatic fractures may suggest a low bone density. Vertebral fractures suggest

TABLE 13-6 Causes of Secondary Osteoporosis

Hormonal: Cushing's syndrome, diabetes
Cancer: Multiple myeloma, leukemia, lymphoma
Gastrointestinal disorders: Inflammatory bowel disease, chronic liver failure
Drug use: Corticosteroids, cancer chemotherapy drugs, anticonvulsants, heparin, excessive aluminum-containing antacids
Chronic kidney disease
Hyperthyroidism or excessive thyroid replacement
Hypogonadism
Inflammatory arthritis: Rheumatoid arthritis
Poor nutrition: Eating disorders, vitamin D deficiency
Immobilization, paralysis
Osteogenesis imperfecta

the diagnosis of osteoporosis as well as rib, pelvic, and wrist fractures. Vertebral fractures are underdiagnosed (not being identified on X-rays), underreported, and undertreated (Gehlback, 2000) (see Table 13-7).

Differential Diagnoses

- Osteomalacia
- Myeloma
- Metastatic bone disease

Essential Diagnostic and Laboratory Tests

- By the time the diagnosis osteopenia is made radiographically, significant and irreversible bone loss has occurred.
- World Health Organization (WHO) defines osteoporosis in terms of bone mineral density (BMD) that is > 2.5 standard deviations (T-score) below a young adult. BMD is measured by dual energy X-ray absorptiometry (DEXA), which is the gold standard. (Femoral neck is the best predictor of hip fracture.) See Table 13-8 for DEXA scores to measure BMD. One major obstacle in diagnosing osteoporosis is that DEXA is not readily

available in the LTC setting. In addition, patients may have difficulties with the positioning and motion control necessary for central DEXA testing. Newer, portable technologies such as ultrasonography and peripheral DEXA are simpler alternatives for BMD testing in this population. However nonavailability of DEXA should not be a deterrent to treat. The postacute patient who is at the SNF for short-term rehabilitation who has not had a prior BMD assessment, and performance of the test is not feasible during his or her stay at the facility, can be referred to their primary care provider at the time of discharge.

- A workup may not be indicated if the patient has a terminal disease or end-stage condition, if the information obtained is unlikely to change management, or if the patient does not wish to consider treatment. The burden of the workup must always be weighed against the benefit to be obtained from treatment (AMDA, 2003).

- Disagreement exists about which women should be screened and when they should be screened. Both the United States Preventive Services Task Force (USPSTF) and the National Osteoporosis Foundation's recommendations to measure BMD agree on screening women age 65 and older and those at high risk starting at age 60. Risk factors include low body weight < 70 kg or body mass index

TABLE 13-7 Risk Factors for Osteoporosis and Related Fractures

Advanced age	Female
Low body weight (< 70 kg)	Tobacco use
Family history in first-degree relative	Previous fracture history
Low physical activity	Low conitive function/ dementia
Caucasian/Asian	Estrogen deficiency
Use of oral corticosteroid therapy for > 3 months	Low calcium intake
Alcohol excess (> 2 drinks/day)	Poor health status/frailty/ low physical activity
Impaired vision	Recent falls

Source: National Osteoporosis Foundation, 2003.

TABLE 13-8 DEXA/T-Scores to Measure BMD

T-SCORE	DIAGNOSIS
Equal to or above –1	Normal range
Between –1 and –2.5	Osteopenia
Equal to or below –2.5	Osteoporosis
Equal to or below –2.5 + fracture	Severe osteoporosis

Source: World Health Organization, 1994.

(BMI) and no current use of estrogen. No studies have evaluated the optimal intervals for repeated screening. A minimum of 2 years may be needed to reliably measure a change in bone mineral density; however, longer intervals may be adequate for repeated screening to identify new cases of osteoporosis. There are no data to determine the appropriate age to stop screening and few data on osteoporosis treatment in women older than 85 years.

- Currently, there are no recommendations when to measure BMD in men. However, screening men 65 and older or those men who have conditions associated with bone loss such as heavy alcohol or tobacco use, hyperparathyroidism, hypogonadism, glucocorticoid therapy, kidney stones with hypercalciuria, fracture with low trauma, osteopenia on radiographs, and presence of vertebral deformities should be considered.

- Routine laboratory evaluation should include the following:
  - Complete blood count
  - Renal/liver function
  - Serum chemistries
  - Thyroid-stimulating hormone (TSH)
  - 25 hydroxyvitamin D
  - 24-hour urine for calcium and creatinine
  - Parathyroid hormone

- Specialized laboratory testing for secondary osteoporosis should include the following:
  - Urine-free cortisol or overnight dexamethasone suppression test if considering Cushing's syndrome
  - Serum calcium phosphorus, alkaline phosphatase, albumin, and creatinine
  - Serum protein electrophoresis (SPEP), Urine protein electrophoresis (UPEP), and IEP if anemia, high ESR, protein or calcium

  - Tissue transglutaminase AB IgA and small bowel biopsy if malabsorption, low iron, or vitamin D
  - Serum iron and ferritin if malabsorption or hemachromatosis
  - Serum testosterone level in males

Management Plan

Because osteoporosis is usually asymptomatic, education of patients about the disease and its long term consequences is critical. *Goals include the following*:

- *Prevention of fractures/reduction in falls*
- *Optimization of skeletal development and maximization of peak bone mass*
- *Prevention of age-related and secondary causes of bone loss, preservation of the structural integrity of the skeleton*
- *Improvement in quality of life*
- *Decreases in morbidity and mortality*
- *Optimize diet*

Nonpharmacologic

- Hip protectors in patients at high risk for falling. Low use of hip protectors may include cost, patient noncompliance, discomfort and/or self-image and lack of support among clinicians and facility administrators. Studies have shown effectiveness in preventing hip fractures when used (Lauritzen, Petersen, & Lund, 1993; Kannus, Parkkari, & Niemi, 2000; Meyer, Warnke, & Bender, 2003).

- Regular physical exercise reduces risk of osteoporosis. Exercise improves overall physical fitness, muscle strength, coordination and balance, and reduces depression. The goal of increasing activity may be facilitated through the use of restorative programs. Regular weight-bearing and muscle-strengthening exercises are recommended (National Osteoporosis Foundation, 2003).

- Smoking cessation

- Limit alcohol intake to two or less drinks daily.

- Provide safe environment and reduce risk of falls. Remove clutter, proper shoes, adequate lighting, use of walker or cane for ambulation if indicated. If balance is poor, determine etiology.

- Evaluate patient for polypharmacy and use of medications such as psychotropics and sedatives that could lead to falls.

- Address patient's concerns about side effects of medication used to treat osteoporosis.

Pharmacologic

- National Osteoporosis Foundation (NOF) guidelines (2003) for treatment of postmenopausal women are the following:

  ○ Treat if T-score less or equal –1.5 SD and risk factors present.

  ○ Treat if T-score less or equal –2.0 SD if risk factors not present.

  ○ Treat in the presence of a fragility fracture.

- Adequate dietary intake of vitamin D and calcium are required throughout life to maintain peak bone mass and reduce the risk of subsequent osteoporosis. Vitamin D deficiency is common and can occur secondary to aging or inadequate exposure to sunlight. Vitamin D may preserve muscle strength and reduce the risk of falls (Montero-Odasso & Duque, 2005). Many elderly persons have a vitamin D deficiency due to age-related decreases in synthesis of vitamin D and a decreased intestinal absorption of calcium. A recent study showed that 400 IU/daily of vitamin D is not sufficient for fracture prevention. Vitamin D 700–800 IU/daily was found to reduce risk (Holick, 2002). Calcium plays a role in muscular, neural, and most metabolic processes as well as bone strength. Most postmenopausal women lack sufficient dietary calcium intake. Serum determination of

25-hydroxyvitamin D should be obtained on any patient with an abnormally low bone density.

- Bisphosphonates are agents that reduce bone resorption and increase BMD (antiresorptive agents). This includes alendronate (Fosamax), risedronate (Actonel), and ibandronate (Boniva). Several well-designed trials have confirmed the potent antifracture efficacy of bisphosphonates. Patients must be able to stand or sit upright for 30 minutes after ingestion of these medications. The most common complaint is gastrointestinal upset (Follin & Hansen, 2003). Pamidronate (Aredia) is a parenteral bisphosphonate that can be given every 3 months to patients who cannot tolerate the oral bisphosphonate preparations. Bisphosphonates are indicated for prevention and treatment of osteoporosis. They are contraindicated in patients with achalasia or esophageal stricture and in patients with hypocalcemia or who cannot remain upright for dosing purposes. Bisphosphonates should not be taken at the same time as other medications including calcium. Bisphosphonates can cause muscle and joint pain, and a rare but serious adverse reaction is osteonecrosis of the jaw.

- Calcitonin nasal spray (Miacalcin) has been shown to decrease bone pain in the setting of an acute fracture and reduce vertebral fractures. Studies in postmenopausal women with low BMD have demonstrated increases in spine BMD of 1–3% after therapy with 200 IU of calcitonin nasal spray. Significant changes in hip BMD have not been seen (Follin & Hansen, 2003).

- Raloxifene (Evista), a selective estrogen receptor modulator (SERM), can be used by postmenopausal women in place of estrogen for prevention of osteoporosis and has been shown to increase bone density and reduce risk of spine fracture by 55% in women without a prior history of fracture and a 30% reduction of new fractures in women with a previous history of vertebral fracture (Ettinger et al., 1999). Raloxifene is indicated for prevention and treatment of osteoporosis. Raloxifene increases hot flashes and may cause leg cramps, and there is an increased risk of thromboembolic events. There is no increase in the incidence of endometrial or breast cancer with its use.

- While hormone therapy (HT) has a positive effect on bone mineral density, it is no longer considered first line therapy for postmenopausal osteoporosis. Its primary indication is for improvement of menopausal symptoms such as vaginal atrophy, hot flashes, and mood changes. For maximum prevention of postmenopausal osteoporosis, HT should begin at the time of menopause or oophorectomy. Start at the lowest dose and use for the shortest duration. Women with intact uteruses should be prescribed both estrogen and progestrone, and women without uteruses should be prescribed estrogen alone. The use of HT should be determined on an individual basis. Risk of breast cancer, uterine cancer, and venous thromboembolic events need to be considered when choosing this option for treatment.

- Prescription drugs approved for osteoporosis treatment in men include alendronate (Fosamax), risedronate (Actonel), and teriparatide (Forteo).

- Teriparatide (Forteo), a form of parathyroid hormone, is FDA-approved for the treatment of men with primary or hypogonadal osteoporosis who are at high risk for fracture, and for the treatment of osteoporosis in women who are at high risk for fracture. Teriparatide decreases bone resorption, improves bone density, and decreases risk of spine fractures. Studies have shown that after 9 months of therapy, teriparatide increases lumbar spine BMD by 9.7 percent in women and 5.8 percent in men. In women, it was shown to reduce the risk of new vertebral fractures by 65 percent and reduce non-vertebral fractures by 53 percent (Orwoll et al., 2003).

Teriparatide should not be prescribed for patients who are at increased baseline risk for osteosarcoma including those with Paget's disease, or unexplained elevations of alkaline phosphatase, open epiphyses, or prior external beam or implant radiation therapy involving the skeleton, multiple kidney stones, or patients with primary or secondary hyperparathyroidism. See Table 13-9 for FDA-approved medications used for the prevention and treatment of osteoporosis.

- Glucocorticoid-induced osteoporosis is the most common cause of secondary osteoporosis. More than one half of all patients treated chronically with glucocorticoids will develop osteoporosis. Rapid bone loss occurs in the first six months of treatment. Currently FDA-approved therapies for glucocorticoid-induced osteoporosis are alendronate and risedronate.

- Persistence with long-term osteoporosis therapy can be poor due to the following:
  - Multiple concomitant diseases and other treatments
  - Cost and availability of medications
  - Advanced age of patient
  - Denial, lack of understanding
  - Fear of real or perceived adverse effects

- Adjust potentially hazardous medications such as psychoactives, antihypertensive medications, and polypharmacy that can contribute to falls.

Patient, Family, and Staff Education

- Educate on the importance of lifestyle changes: discontinuing smoking, limiting alcohol consumption, and exercising to improve gait, balance, and strength to help reduce fall risk.

- Educate on importance of proper diet and calcium and vitamin D supplements.

- Explain risks and benefits, side effects, and costs of medications.

TABLE 13-9   FDA-Approved Medication Used to Treat Osteoporosis

DRUG	P/T	USUAL DOSE	SIDE EFFECTS/CONCERNS
Calcium carbonate or citrate with vitamin D	P/T	1000–1200 mg with 700–800 IU vitamin D/orally, daily	Constipation
Hormone therapy (HT)	P	1. Oral conjugated estrogen, 0.625–1.25 mg daily without uterus 2. Oral estrogen plus progestin-estrogen plus medroxyprogesterone, 5–10 mg daily by mouth 10–14 days/month or estrogen plus medroxy-progesterone 2.5 mg daily with uterus 3. Transdermal estradiol patch, 0.05 mg patch/24 hours	Endometrial hyperplasia, uterine bleeding, breast tenderness Increased risk of breast cancer and venous thrombus
Bisphosphonates • Alendronate (Fosamax)	P/T	35–70 mg orally weekly	Precautions: Active gastritis, duodenitis, or ulcer Esophageal stricture, hypocalcemia, poor pill swallowing ability
• Risedronate (Actonel)	P/T	35 mg orally weekly	Do not use if the following present: CrCl < 30 mL/min, hypocalcemia
• Pamidronate (Aredia)	P/T	60–90 mg slow IV infusion every 2–3 months	Nausea, vomiting, generalized pain, fever
• Ibandronate (Boniva)	P/T	2.5 mg orally daily OR 150 mg orally monthly	GI upset, diarrhea
SERMs • Raloxifen (Evista)	P	60 mg orally daily	Hot flashes and leg cramps Increased risk of thromboembolic event (rare but serious)
• Calcitonin (Miacalcin)	T	One puff nasally daily, alternate nares, 0.09% mL, 200 IU	Runny nose, nasal dryness, irritation, sinusitis, and headache
• Teriparatide (Forteo)	T	20 mg subcutaneous daily for no more than 2 years per lifetime	Contraindicated in Paget's disease, unexplained elevations of alkaline phosphatase, open epiphyses, or prior external beam or implant radiation therapy involving the skeleton.

Notes: P, prevention of osteoporosis; SERMS, selective estrogen receptor modulators; T, treatment of osteoporosis.

Physician Consultation

Patients with conditions associated with secondary osteoporosis should be referred to a specialist for evaluation and treatment.

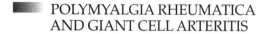

POLYMYALGIA RHEUMATICA AND GIANT CELL ARTERITIS

Definition

Polymyalgia rheumatica (PMR) and giant cell arteritis (GCA) are closely related inflammatory conditions that affect persons of middle age and older and frequently occur together (Cornelia & Goronsy, 2003). PMR is a clinical diagnosis based on pain and stiffness of the shoulder and pelvic girdle areas. It can occur in the absence of GCA (Hellmann et al., 2005). In giant cell arteritis (GCA) there is demonstrable vasculitis of large and medium-sized vessels, particularly the cranial arterial vessels including the temporal arteries (Cornelia & Goronsy, 2003).

Epidemiology

The annual incidence rate of PMR in individuals 50 years of age and older is 52 per 100,000; it increases with age. The pathophysiology is unclear, but PMR is thought to be a synovitis characterized by T-cell and macrophage infiltration (Murphy et al., 2005). It occurs almost exclusively in individuals older than 55 years. It is far more common in women than in men and is rare in African-Americans. Features of GCA are found in 15–20% of cases of biopsy-proven PMR (Swannell, 1997).

GCA rarely presents below the age of 50. The incidence is 15–25 per 100,000 in at-risk populations. The disease is most common in Caucasians, particularly those of Scandinavian descent and is rare in Hispanic persons. Women are more susceptible than men. The single most important risk factor is age (Cornelia & Goronsy, 2003). About 50% of patients with GCA also have PMR (Hellmann et al., 2005).

Common Presenting Signs and Symptoms

- Pain often arises abruptly and persists for at least 2 months. It is associated with generalized malaise and morning stiffness. There may also be associated fever malaise, fatigue, anorexia, and weight loss (Salvarani et al., 2002).

- In PMR there is diffuse myalgias and joint stiffness that predominately affects the pelvic and shoulder girdles in patients over 50 years of age. Limitation of activity from the myalgias and joint stiffness also leads to disuse and atrophy. See Table 13-10 for diagnostic criteria for PMR (Salvarani et al., 2002).

- On examination, limitation of active and often passive movements of the shoulders due to pain.

- As with most geriatric syndromes, assessing impact on function is crucial. Functional impairments are among the most convincing evidence for a diagnosis of PMR. Patients

TABLE 13-10 Diagnostic Criteria for Polymylagia Rheumatica
Age 50 years of age or older
At least one month of pain and morning stiffness in two of the following areas:
• Shoulders and upper arms • Hips and thighs • Neck and torso
Erythrocyte sedimentation rate (ESR) > 40 mm/hrs (typically elevated greater than age of patient)

Source: Salvarani et al., 2002.

may report that they are having difficulty getting out of bed because of morning stiffness.

- GCA frequently has all of the previous symptoms, but in addition fever tends to be more common and headache occurs in the majority of patients and tends to be located over the temporal and occipital areas. There is frequently tenderness, thickening, and nodularity of the superficial temporal arteries. Pain on chewing (jaw claudication) occurs in almost half of the patients. The most feared complication is permanent or partial loss of vision that can progress to total blindness. Once blindness develops, it is usually permanent (Hellmann et al., 2005).

- Screen for depression, which can accompany PMR. See the chapter on psychological disorders for treatment of depression.

Differential Diagnoses

- Rheumatoid arthritis (RA) can be difficult to distinguish from PMR and GCA, especially in RA patients who are seronegative for rheumatoid factor.

- Systemic lupus erythematous (SLE) in the elderly may sometimes present as PMR.

- Bacterial endocarditis and cancers may also present with a constellation of symptoms that can mimic PMR.

- Fibromyalgia can be confused with PMR though it typically affects a younger population and is not associated with elevated ESR.
- Polymyositis and dermatomyositis. Muscle weakness is more prominent in these two diseases, and creatine kinase (CK) is elevated strongly suggesting the diagnosis. A classic rash on the forehead, neck, shoulders, and trunk in dermatomyositis rules out PMR.

Essential Diagnostic and Laboratory Tests

- An elevated erythrocyte sedimentation rate (ESR) usually about 40 mm/hr is almost always found in both conditions but may be normal in a small percentage of cases.
- Complete blood count (CBC)—A normochromic, normocytic anemia is commonly seen.
- In patients who present with signs and symptoms most consistent with GCA, a temporal artery biopsy is necessary and is diagnostic in 60–80% of patients with arteritis (Swannell, 1997).
- C-reactive protein, a marker of inflammation is generally elevated.
- EMG, serum creatine kinase (CK) levels, and muscle biopsy are normal in patients with PMR.

Management Plan

Nonpharmacologic

Regular exercise particularly emphasizing range of motion (ROM) and stretching are important to maintain mobility and strength and to prevent muscle atrophy. Consider referral to physical therapy.

Pharmacologic

- Prednisone in doses of 10–20 mg/day usually provides rapid relief of symptoms within a few days in PMR. If GCA is suspected, then the initial dose of prednisone should be 40–60 mg/day for 1 month followed by a gradual tapering to a maintenance dose of 7.5–10 mg daily. Therapy should be continued for 1 to 2 years. The ESR can be a useful indication of inflammatory disease and in monitoring and tapering therapy. It is vital to start corticosteroids quickly especially to prevent catastrophic complications such as blindness. It has been shown that such early use of corticosteroids will not significantly alter biopsy results if the biopsy is performed expeditiously. In patients with clear evidence of PMR and no signs of GCA, temporal artery biopsy is not usually indicated.
- If a flare occurs shortly after the corticosteroids are tapered, a slower rate of tapering is recommended.
- Start osteoporosis prevention for patients on chronic steroid therapy. See osteoporosis section.
- Add aspirin 81 mg/daily to steroid to reduce risk for CVA and visual loss.

Patient, Family, and Staff Education

- It is very important to give patients and families information regarding the similarities between PMR and GCA and to be vigilant regarding reporting any visual changes, headaches, or jaw claudication.
- Explain importance of continuing medications as prescribed.
- Explain need for osteoporosis treatment when corticosteroids are prescribed.

Physician Consultation

- Physician consultation should be obtained on any patient suspected of having PMR or GCA. GCA is considered to be a medical emergency and prompt referral is necessary.
- Refer to rheumatologist if there is pain, stiffness, or swelling of a joint that is unresponsive to initial treatment.

- Referral to rheumatologist should be made if GCA is suspected and temporal artery biopsy is needed.

▬ RHEUMATOID ARTHRITIS

Definition

Rheumatoid arthritis (RA) is an autoimmune inflammatory disease of unknown etiology. It is characterized by symmetric polyarthritis and often associated with extra-articular features including anemia, skin ulcers, pulmonary, cardiac and ophthalmologic problems. RA has a chronic fluctuating disease course, and if left untreated, results in progressive joint destruction, deformity, disability, and premature death.

Epidemiology

About 1.2 million people, or 1% of the US adult population have rheumatoid arthritis. RA occurs in all races and ethnic groups. The disease often begins in middle age and occurs with increased frequency in older people; however, young adults and children may also develop it. RA occurs much more frequently in women than in men; about two to three times as many women as men have the disease. Susceptibility to RA is genetically determined. Most patients have a class 2 human leukocyte antigen (HLA) with an identical five-amino acid sequence. Although RA was once considered to be a relatively benign disorder, it is now known to be a disease with a strong tendency to shorten life and cause severe disability (Hellmann et al., 2005).

Functional disability often occurs early in RA and usually increases if disease control is inadequate. RA is responsible for more than 250,000 hospitalizations per year. The most common reason for hospitalization is total joint arthroplasty (Savage et al., 2005). Early and aggressive treatment, often with drugs used in combination, is preferred when treating RA.

Common Presenting Signs and Symptoms

- The clinical manifestations of RA are highly variable. The onset of articular signs of inflammation is usually insidious, with prodromal symptoms of malaise, weight loss, and vague periarticular pain or morning stiffness.

- There is characteristically symmetric joint swelling with associated stiffness, warmth, tenderness, and pain. Stiffness persisting for over 30 minutes is prominent in the morning and subsides during the day. Stiffness may reoccur after daytime inactivity and may be more severe after strenuous activity.

- RA may also arise explosively with severe pain, swelling of joints, and marked fatigue and weakness. An acute onset may be triggered by infection, surgery, trauma, or emotional strain.

- Although any joint may be affected in RA, the proximal interphalangeal (PIPs) and metacarpophalangeal joints (MCPs) of the fingers as well as the wrists, knees, ankles, and toes are most often involved. Grip strength is decreased because of pain and mechanical derangement.

- After months or years deformities may occur; the most common are ulnar deviation of the fingers, boutonniere deformity, "swan-neck" deformity and valgus deformity of the knee.

- Knee arthritis is common and is occasionally a primary manifestation in early RA. Swelling and thickening of the synovium and effusions may be present. There can also be atrophy of the muscles around the knee, especially the quadriceps, with resultant weakness.

- Extra-articular manifestations are common and include the following:
  - Rheumatoid nodules are the most common extra-articular manifestation and are present in about 15% of patients.

There is no specific therapy (ACP Medicine, 2004).

○ Eye—The sicca syndrome, which is part of Sjogren syndrome, is the most frequent ocular manifestation of RA. Symptoms include sensations of grittiness, accumulation of dried mucoid material, and decreased tear production.

○ Lungs—The most common form of lung involvement in RA is pleurisy with effusions. Clinical features include gradual onset and variable degrees of pain and dyspnea. Progressive, symptomatic interstitial pulmonary fibrosis that produces coughing and dyspnea in conjunction with radiographic changes of a diffuse reticular pattern is usually associated with high titers of rheumatoid factor.

○ Heart—Cardiac involvement in RA is common but rarely symptomatic. Pericardial effusion or thickening has been found in about one third of patients studied. Other findings include rheumatoid nodules, healed or active pericarditis, myocarditis, endocarditis, and valvular fibrosis.

○ Blood—Mild anemia of chronic disease is characteristic of active RA. Although iron levels are not reduced in RA, administration of erythropoietin alleviates anemia (ACP Medicine, 2004).

○ The constellation of RA with splenomegaly and leukopenia is known as Felty syndrome. The mean serum leukocyte count in patients is usually 1500 to 2000/mm, and the mean granulocyte count is 500 to 1000/mm. Other findings in Felty syndrome include hepatomegaly, lymphadenopathy, and chronic cutaneous infections (Rashba, Rowe, & Packman, 1996).

○ Vasculitis in small synovial vessels is a hallmark of early RA, but more widespread vascular inflammation of medium-sized muscular arteries also occurs in older men with advanced disease, rheumatoid nodules, and high titers of rheumatoid factor. Treatment usually requires high-dose corticosteroids or cyclophosphamides, which still may not be effective (ACP Medicine, 2004)

• The American Rheumatism Association has developed criteria for the classification of rheumatoid arthritis (Arnett et al., 1988). See Table 13-11.

TABLE 13-11   The American Rheumatism Association Revised Criteria for the Classification of Rheumatoid Arthritis

Morning stiffness—Morning stiffness in and around the joints lasting at least 1 hour before maximal improvement
Arthritis of three or more joint areas—Joint areas with simultaneously soft tissue swelling or fluid. The joint areas include proximal interphalangeal (PIP), metacarpophalangeal (MCP), wrist, elbow, knee, ankle, and metatarsophalangeal (MTP) joints.
Arthritis of hand joint—At least one joint area swollen as above in wrist, MCP, or PIP
Symmetrical arthritis—Simultaneous involvement of the same joint areas on both sides of the body
Rheumatoid nodules—Subcutaneous nodules over bony prominences or extensor surfaces or in juxta-articular regions that are observed
Serum rheumatoid factor—Demonstration of abnormal amounts of serum rheumatoid factor by any method that has been positive in fewer than 5% of normal control subjects
Radiographic changes—Radiographic changes typical of rheumatoid arthritis on posteroanterior hand and wrist X-rays, which must include erosions or unequivocal bony decalcification localized to or most marked adjacent to the involved joints (osteoarthritis changes alone do not qualify)

Source: Arnett et al., 1994.

Differential Diagnoses

- In its classic presentation, RA is easily diagnosed, but it may be confused with a host of other illnesses in its atypical form. RA must be differentiated from a number of common subacute or chronic polyarthritic diseases and painful syndromes that may mimic chronic polyarthritides. Conditions to be considered are the following:
  - Polyarticular gout
  - Degenerative joint disease
  - Osteoarthritis
  - Polymyalgia rheumatica
  - Systemic lupus erythematosus
  - Bacterial arthritis—Can be distinguished by chills and fever as well as localized painful joint or joints. Consider bacterial arthritis whenever a patient with RA has one joint inflamed out of proportion to the rest.
  - Ankylosing spondylitis
  - Psoriatic arthritis
- In its earliest manifestations before the onset of actual joint swelling, RA may be confused with fibromyalgia.

Essential Diagnostic and Laboratory Tests

There are several tests that are helpful in diagnosing RA, but no one test is diagnostic:

- Rheumatoid factor (RF) is common and may eventually be found in about 80% of patients with RA. Anticyclic citrullinated peptide (anti-CCP) is proving to be a test that is more specific than RF and may be detectable in RA patients who do not demonstrate RF.
- Measurement of systemic inflammation such as erythrocyte sedimentation rate (ESR) and C-reactive protein (CRP) are helpful in measuring disease activity. A highly elevated value indicates a likelihood of inflammation, infection, or malignancy; however, up to 40% of patients have normal ESR or CRP. Therefore, a normal ESR or CRP does not exclude RA.
- CBC to evaluate for anemia. Anemia of chronic disease with normocytic, normochromic RBC, and a low reticulocyte count is frequently seen in RA.
- Radiographs may be very helpful in distinguishing RA from other forms of arthritis. The earliest changes occur in the wrists or feet and consist of soft tissue swelling and juxta-articular demineralization. Later, changes of uniform joint space narrowing and erosions develop. Diagnostic changes also occur in the cervical spine with C1-2 subluxation but take years to develop. The value of MRI in early diagnosis is not established.

Management Plan

The primary goals in treating RA are reduction of inflammation and pain, preservation of function, and prevention of deformity. Often drugs used in combination are necessary (Hellmann et al., 2005).

Nonpharmacologic

- It is essential that patients with RA be counseled regarding appropriate exercises including range of motion exercises. Both physical and occupational therapy can be very helpful in directing the treatment. At the same time it is important for appropriate rest to be included in the therapeutic prescription.
- Occupational therapy can be helpful in setting appropriate goals, in testing patients in their activities of daily living, and for joint protection.
- Locally applied heat and cold can be used to help relieve pain.
- Splints can be applied for a short period if needed and should be removed several times a day for range of motion exercises.

- Assistive devices such as a raised toilet seat, grab bar, cane, or walker may be helpful for patients with arthritis in the knees or hips.

- Indications for surgical intervention include intractable pain and impaired function. Total joint replacement has allowed patients to gain or maintain independence. RA is a chronic condition that has a global effect on daily life. It is important to screen patients for depression and refer to mental health professional to help deal with these emotional concerns.

Pharmacologic
- For initial therapy patients are usually treated with NSAIDs, and their course is carefully monitored over the next several weeks to few months. In certain patients, moderate to severe joint pain and swelling may prompt the addition of low-dose corticosteroids (prednisone 5 to 10 mg day orally). Systemic corticosteroids given even in small doses are associated with accelerated bone loss. All patients receiving chronic corticosteroid therapy should be on medication for osteoporosis prevention. See osteoporosis section.

- There is now clear recognition that early and aggressive treatment with disease-modifying antirheumatic drugs (DMARDs) is necessary to inhibit the progression in RA. Most rheumatologists initiate DMARD therapy within 3–6 months or as soon as possible after the diagnosis has been established to prevent the development of joint damage. Rheumatologists are increasingly using 2 or 3 DMARD drug combinations to obtain superior clinical responses. See Table 13-12 for drugs used to treat RA.

- Methotrexate has been used successfully for many years to induce and sustain remission in RA and is the most common disease-modifying anti-inflammatory drug (DMARD) in use today. At least 80% of patients show improvement with methotrexate. All patients treated with methotrexate should also take folic acid 1 mg which has been shown to reduce the likelihood of toxicity (Morgan, Baggott, & Vaughn, 1994). Other DMARDs that have been used in combination with methotrexate include hydroxychloroquine (Plaquenil), sulfasalazine (Azulfidine), and leflunomide (Arava).

- Periodic laboratory monitoring is important for early detection of toxicity caused by certain DMARDs. Liver function tests (LFT) and a complete blood count (CBC) are recommended every 4 to 8 weeks in patients taking methotrexate and leflunomide (Arava). In general, DMARDs should be continued indefinitely to control inflammation.

- A major recent advance in rheumatology has been the development of biological agents that are directed against tumor necrosis factor (TNF). These drugs have been shown to slow the progression of RA. Three examples of this class of drugs are infliximab (Remicade), etanercept (Enbrel), and adalimumab (Humira). All must be given parenterally. The main toxicity in this class of drugs is lowered resistance to infection. Therefore, before starting a patient on these drugs, a search should be made for active or latent infection, particularly tuberculosis or other granulomatous diseases. Chest X-ray or skin test should be done. The use of biological agents is limited in part by substantial costs of these medications.

- Abatacept (Orencia) is first in a new class of agents called selective costimulation blockers. It is used to treat RA patients with moderate to severe disease who have failed therapy with one or more DMARDs. It should not be used with TNF alpha antagonists. It is administered by intravenous infusion.

- Rituximab (Rituxan) is a monoclonal antibody that was developed for the treatment of B Cell Lymphoma and found to be efficacious in treating RA. It is indicated in patients who have failed one or more DMARDs but should

TABLE 13-12   Drugs Used for Rheumatoid Arthritis

DRUG	DOSE	MOST COMMON SIDE EFFECTS
NSAIDs (see osteoarthritis section)	Varies	Gastrointestinal Fluid retention Renal impairment
DMARDs Hydroxychloroquine (Plaquenil)	200 mg daily twice daily	Gastrointestinal Blood dyscrasia Ocular damage
Sulfasalazine (Azulfidine)	500–1000 mg twice daily	Gastrointestinal Hematologic Cutaneous
Leflunomide (Arava) Cyclosporine Minocycline	10–20 mg daily	Diarrhea Hepatic Nausea Fetal damage
Methotrexate	7.5–20 mg weekly	Hepatic Mucocutaneous Pneumonitis (rare)
Corticosteroids Prednisone	5–20 mg daily to control acute inflammation. Taper as soon as possible.	Weight gain Osteoporosis Easy bruising Decreased resistance to infection
Anti-tumor necrosis factor/TNF agents Etanecept (Embrel)	25 mg 2 times a week or 50 mg weekly	Reduced resistance to infection Hematologic changes are rare but may include anemia and leukopenia.
Adalimumab (Humira)	40 mg every other week	Same
Infliximab (Remicade)	3–10 mg/kg every 4–8 weeks IV. Should be given with methrotrexate	Same plus acute infusion reaction

Notes: DMARDs, disease-modifying anti-rheumatic drugs; NSAIDs, non-steroidal anti-inflammatory drugs.

not be used with TNF alpha antagonists. It is administered by intravenous infusion.

- Intra-articular corticosteroid injections may help control isolated joint inflammation.
- Alternative and complementary therapies including special diets, vitamin supplements, and other alternative approaches have been suggested for the treatment of RA. Although many of these approaches may not be harmful, controlled scientific studies either have not been conducted or have found no definite benefit to these therapies. Some alternative or complementary approaches

may help the patient cope or reduce some of the stress associated with living with a chronic illness. The Arthritis Foundation publishes material on alternative therapies at www.arthritisfoundation.com.

Patient, Family, and Staff Education

- Provide explanation of the disease process of RA, emphasizing the chronicity of this illness and the need for frequent monitoring, especially for drug toxicity.
- Explain importance of balancing rest and exercise. Counsel family members about

the importance of providing emotional support to the patient.

- Discuss benefits, risks, and costs of medications.

Physician Consultation

- All patients with RA should be managed in conjunction with a rheumatologist for optimal treatment results.

- Consult physician for any abrupt change in the patient's condition as it could relate to a flare of the disease, extra-articular complications, and may require a search for underlying infectious diseases of the joints.

- Refer to physician if intra-articular corticosteroid is being considered.

████ WEB SITES

- The Arthritis Foundation—www.arthritis foundation.com

- Primer on the rheumatic diseases—www. primerontherheumaticdisease.com

- American Back Society—www.american backsoc.org

- National Institute of Neurological Disorders and Stroke—www.ninds.nih.gov/ disorders/backpain

- American Academy of Physical Medicine and Rehabilitation—www.aapmr.org

- Spinehealth.com, Wholistic Health Center— www.spinehealth.com

- American College of Rheumatology—www. rheumatology.org

- National Institute of Arthritis and Musculoskeletal and Skin Diseases—www.niams. nih.gov

- The Arthritis Society (Canada)—www. arthritis.ca

- National Osteoporosis Foundation—www. nof.org

- International Osteoporosis Foundation— www.osteofound.org

- The Osteoporosis Center—www.endocrine web.com/osteoporosis

- U.S. Preventive Services Task Force—www. USPSTF.com

- National Institutes of Health, Osteoporosis and Related Bone Diseases, National Resource Center—http://www.niams.nih.gov/ bone

████ REFERENCES

ACP Medicine. (2004). *Rheumatoid arthritis.* Retrieved September 26, 2005, from http://www. webmd.com

Agency for Health Care Policy and Research. (AHCPR). (1994). *Quick reference guide for clinicians. Acute low back pain problems in adults: Assessment and treatment* (Publication No. 95–0643). Washington, DC: Department of Health and Human Services.

Agency for Healthcare Research and Quality. (2002). *Recommendations and rationale: Screening for osteoporosis in postmenopausal women. U.S. Preventive Task Force. Guide to clinical preventive services.* Retrieved September 26, 2006, from http:// www.ahrq.gov/clinic/uspstf/uspsoste.htm

American College of Rheumatology Subcommittee on Osteoarthritis. (2000). Recommendations for the medical management of osteoarthritis of the hip and knee: 2000 update. *Arthritis and Rheumatism, 43,* 1905–1915.

American Medical Directors Association (AMDA). (n.d.). *Osteoporosis, clinical practice guideline.* Retrieved September 26, 2006, from http://www. amda.com/tools/cpg/osteoporosis.cfm

Arnett, F. C., Edworthy, S. M., Block, D. A., et al. (1988). The American Rheumatism Association 1987 revised criteria for the classification of rheumatoid arthritis. *Arthritis and Rheumatism, 31,* 315.

Arthritis Foundation. (2001). Glucosamine and condroitin for osteoarthritis? *Bulletin of the Rheumatic Diseases, 50*(7), 1–4.

Campbell, S. M. (1988). Gout: How presentation, diagnosis, and treatment differ in the elderly. *Geriatrics, 43*(11), 71–77.

Cassessa, M., & Gorevic, P. D. (2004). Crystal arthritis. Gout and pseudogout in the geriatric patient. *Geriatrics, 59*(9), 25–30.

Consensus Development Conference. (1993). Diagnosis, prophylaxis, and treatment of osteoporosis. *American Journal of Medicine, 94*(6), 646–650.

Cornelia, W., & Goronsy, J. (2003). Giant-cell arteritis and polymyalgia rheumatica. *Annals of Internal Medicine, 139*(6), 505–515.

Cummings, S. R., Black, D. M., & Thompson, D. E. (1998). Effect of alendronate on risk of fracture in women with low bone density but without vertebral fractures: Results from the Fracture Interventions Trial. *Journal of the American Medical Association, 280*, 2077–2082.

Deyo, R., & Weinstein, J. (2001). Primary care: Low back pain. *New England Journal of Medicine, 344*(5).

Ettinger, B., Black, D., & Mitlak, B. (1999). Reduction of vertebral fracture risk in post-menopausal women with osteoporosis treated with raloxifene: Results from a 3-year randomized clinical trial. Multiple outcomes of raloxifene evaluation (MORE) investigators. *Journal of the American Medical Association, 282*, 637–345.

Fam, A. G. (1998). Gout in the elderly. Clinical presentation and treatment. *Drugs and Aging, 13*(3), 229–243.

Follin, S., & Hansen, L. (2003). Current approaches to the prevention and treatment of post-menopausal osteoporosis. *American Journal of Health-System Pharmacy, 60*(9).

Frymoyer, J. W. (1988). Back pain and sciatica. *New England Journal of Medicine, 318*, 291–300.

Gehlback, S. H. (2000). Recognition of vertebral fracture in a clinical setting. *Osteoporosis International, 11*, 577–582.

Grober, J., & Thethi, A. (2003). Osteoarthritis: Practical nondrug steps to successful therapy. *Consultant, 43*(1), 53–60.

Hellmann, D., Stone, J., & Tierney, L. (2005). Low back pain. In L. Tierney, S. McPhee, & M. Papadakis (Eds.), *Current medical diagnosis and treatment* (44th ed., pp. 791–793, 801–803, 818–821). New York: Lang Medical Books/McGraw-Hill.

Hochberg, M., Altman, R., Brandt, K., Clark, B., Dieppe, P., & Griffin, M. (1995). Guidelines for the medical management of osteoarthritis, Part 1. *Arthritis Rheumatology, 38*, 1535–1540.

Holick, M. F. (2002). Recommendations for treatment of vitamin D deficiency. *Current Opinions in Endocrinology and Diabetes, 9*, 87–98.

Hurwitz, E., Morgenstern, H., & Yu, F. (2003). Cross-sectional and longitudinal associations of low back pain and related disability with psychological distress among patients enrolled in the UCLA low back pain study. *Journal of Clinical Epidemiology, 56*, 663–471.

Kannus, P., Parkkari, J., & Niemi, S. (2000). Prevention of hip fracture in elderly people with use of a hip protector. *New England Journal of Medicine, 343*, 1506–1513.

Kotz, R., & Kolarz, G. (1999). Intra-articular therapy in osteoarthritis. *American Journal of Orthopedics, 83*(29, Suppl. 1), 5–7.

Lauritzen, J. B., Petersen, M. M., & Lund, B. (1993). Effect of external hip protectors on hip fractures. *Lancet, 341*, 11–13.

Lie, D. (2004). Acupuncture may improve symptoms of knee osteoarthritis. *Annals of Internal Medicine, 141*, 901–910.

Masud, M. (2000). Osteoporosis: Epidemiology, diagnosis and treatment. *Southern Medical Journal, 93*(1).

McTigue, J. (2005). Current concepts in managing gout. *Arthritis Practitioner, Sept/Oct*, 22–27.

Meyer, G., Warnke, A., & Bender, R. (2003). Effect on hip fractures of increased use of hip protectors in nursing home: Cluster randomized controlled trial. *British Medical Journal, 326*, 76.

Montero-Odasso, M., & Duque, G. (2005). Vitamin D in the aging musculoskeletal system: An authentic strength preserving hormone. *Molecular Aspects of Medicine, 26*(3), 203–219.

Morgan, S. L., Baggott, J. E., Vaughn, W. H., et al. (1994). Supplementation with folic acid during methotrexate therapy for rheumatoid arthritis: A double blind, placebo-controlled trial. *Annals of Internal Medicine, 12*, 833.

National Osteoporosis Foundation. (2003). *Fast facts on osteoporosis*. Retrieved September 26, 2006, from http://www.nof.org/osteoporosis/diseasefacts.htm

Nguyen, T., Sambrook, P., Kelly, P., Jones, G., Lord, S., & Freund, J. (1993). Prediction of osteoporotic fractures by postural instability and bone density. *British Medical Journal, 307*, 1111–1115.

Orwoll, E., & Scheel, W. (2003). The effect of teriparatide therapy on bone mineral density in men with osteoporosis. *Journal of Bone and Mineral Research, 18*, 9–16.

Patel, A., & Ogle, A. (2000). Diagnosis and management of acute low back pain. *American Family Physician, 61*(6).

Prestwood, K., & Kenny, A. (1998). Osteoporosis: Pathogenesis, diagnosis, and treatment in older adults. *Clinics in Geriatric Medicine, 14*(3).

Rashba, E. J., Rowe, J. M., & Packman, C. H. (1996). Treatment of neutropenia of Felty syndrome. *Blood Review, 10*, 177.

Salvarani, C., Cantini, F., Boiardi, L., & Hunder, G. (2002). Polymyalgia rheumatica and giant-cell arteritis. *New England Journal of Medicine, 347*(4), 261–217.

Schlesinger, N., Detry, M. A., Holland, B. K., Baker, D. G., Beutler, A. M., et al. (2002). Local ice therapy during bouts of acute gouty arthritis. *Journal of Rheumatology, 29*(2), 331–334.

Stitik, T., Yonclas, P., Foye, P., & Schoenherr, L. (2006). Osteoarthritis: Practical nondrug steps to successful therapy. *Consultant, 45*(12), 1248–1258.

Swannell, A. J. (1997). Fortnightly review: Polymyalgia rheumatica and temporal arteritis: Diagnosis and management. Clinical review. *British Medical Journal, 314*(7090), 1329–1332.

Terkeltaub, R. (2006). Rheumatology. *Medscape Rheumatology, 8*(1).

U.S. Department of Health and Human Services. (2004). *Bone health and osteoporosis: A report of the Surgeon General.* Retrieved September 26, 2006, from http://www.surgeongeneral.gov/library/bonehealth

Vogt, M., Kwoh, K., Cope, D., Osial, T., Culyba, M., & Starz, T. (2005). Analgesic usage for low back pain: Impact on health care costs and service use. *Spine, 29*(9), 1075–1081.

World Health Organization. (1994). *Assessment of fracture risk and its application to screening for postmenopausal osteoporosis: Report of a WHO study group.* Retrieved September 29, 2006, from http://whqlibdoc.who.int/trs/WHO_TRS_843.pdf

CHAPTER 14

Neurological Disorders

Marianne McCarthy

PARKINSON'S DISEASE

Definition

In 1817, a British physician, James Parkinson, reported his observations about a neurological illness consisting of resting tremor and an unusual form of progressive motor disability (Samii, Nutt, & Ransom, 2004). The illness, now known as Parkinson's disease (PD), is a common neurological disorder caused primarily by the degeneration of dopaminergic cells in the substantia nigra. It is a persistently progressive, degenerative central nervous system (CNS) disease characterized by slow and decreased movement, muscular rigidity, resting tremor, and postural instability. The cause of PD is enigmatic in most individuals. In the past 10 years, great strides have been made in the understanding and treatment of PD, which is now recognized to involve cognition, behavior, and mood as well as the nigrostriatal dopamine system.

Epidemiology

The crude prevalence of PD among all age groups in the United States is about 100 cases per 100,000. The prevalence of PD is about 50% lower among African Americans and Asians than among Caucasians. The incidence among all age groups is 10 to 20 per 100,000. The incidence of PD increases dramatically with age. Among persons in their 70s and 80s, the incidence is about 200 cases per 100,000 in the United States. Interestingly, it is about 2000 per 100,000 in other countries such as Iceland, India, Scotland, and Australia (Beers & Berkow, 2000).

Idiopathic PD, the most common type, begins most often in people between the ages of 45 to 65 years. The average age at onset had been thought to be 55 years, but it is now believed to begin in the early to middle part of the sixth decade. Eighty-five percent of patients with PD are more than 65 years old (Mayeux et al., 1995; Samii & Ransom, 2004). PD tends to be progressive over one to two decades, leading to ultimate incapacity and death.

People of all ethnic origins and all socioeconomic classes can be affected. Men are slightly more prone to PD than women, with a 3:2 ratio of men to women (Rajput, 1992). In people with young-onset PD, the initial symptoms can arise between age 20 and 40 years. Young-onset PD affects 5–10% of patients (Golbe, 1991). The first symptoms in juvenile-onset disease occur before the age of 20 years (Samii & Ransom, 2004).

PD progression is heterogeneous, but mean life expectancy is 14.6 years. In general, prognosis seems better in patients whose primary manifestation is tremor. Risk factors for rapid disease progression include older age at onset (> 50), concomitant major depression, dementia, and presentation with akinetic rigid symptoms. Patients with PD have a two-fold to five-fold increased mortality risk as compared to nondemented, healthy older adults (Rajput, 1992).

Parkinsonism is any disorder that manifests the symptoms of PD. Parkinsonism is divided into four categories: idiopathic, symptomatic, Parkinson-plus syndromes, and other heredodegenerative diseases in which parkinsonism is a manifestation. People with idiopathic Parkinson's disease (IP) make up the largest subgroup, representing 78% of the affected population (Rhoades, 2001).

Pathologically, the disorder is characterized by the presence of cytoplasmic inclusions (Lewy bodies) and selective degeneration of the nigrostriatal dopaminergic pathway. As a consequence, dopamine is depleted in the neostriatum, leading to the symptoms that are observed in people with Parkinson's disease. Despite decades of intense research, the etiology of sporadic PD and the mechanism underlying the selective neuronal loss remains unknown (Beers & Berkow, 2000). The pathogenesis is thought to be multifactorial, resulting from a combination of genetic predisposition and exogenous and endogenous toxins. The evidence regarding the role of heredity is conflicting. A positive family history is reported in approximately 15% of cases (Rhoades, 2001).

There are many theories regarding the role of environmental factors in the development of PD. One theory has suggested increased vulnerability of "old" neurons to environmental toxins. The late onset and slow-progressing nature of the disease has prompted the consideration of environmental exposure to agrochemicals, including pesticides, as a risk factor. Moreover, increasing evidence suggests that early life occurrence of brain inflammation, as a consequence of either brain injury or exposure to infectious agents, may play a role in the pathogenesis of PD. Most important, there may be a self-propelling cycle of an inflammatory process involving brain immune cells that drives the slow yet progressive neurodegenerative process. A summary of suspected risk factors are listed in Table 14-1.

Common Presenting Signs and Symptoms

The features of PD become apparent after a 70–80% loss of nigral neurons (Wiederholt, 1995). The three cardinal features include tremors, rigidity, and bradykinesia. They generally present asymmetrically and then gradually involve both sides of the body. Postural instability, sometimes judged a cardinal symptom, is nonspecific and usually absent in early disease, especially in the younger patient. Although motor features define the disorder, various nonmotor symptoms are typically seen. These include autonomic dysfunction, cognitive and psychiatric changes, sensory symptoms, and sleep disturbances. Because of the importance of the three cardinal features, it is imperative to be familiar with their presentation.

TABLE 14-1   Suspected Risk Factors for Parkinson's Disease

- Advanced age
- Positive family history
- Early head trauma
- Industrial exposure to heavy metals
- Drinking well water
- Exposure to pesticides
- Drug-induced parkinsonism
- Rural living
- Infections
- Free radical-oxidative stress

Resting Tremor

- First sign in 75% of patients and the most visible manifestation (Minteer, 2006)

- Occurs at a rate of 4 to 6 Hz and is described as a pill-rolling tremor with characteristic motion of the thumb and forefinger

- Maximum at rest, diminishes during voluntary movement but reemerges as the limb resumes position

- Stress and fatigue worsen tremors.

- Absent during sleep

- Usually begins in one finger or hand (pill rolling), and then spreads up the arm

- Resting tremor of the hands increases when the person is walking and may be an early sign of PD before other signs are visible

- Typically, the tremor then spreads ipsilaterally before bilateral involvement occurs

- Usually, the hands, arms, and legs are most affected in that order.

- Jaw, tongue, and eyelids may also be affected, but the voice escapes the tremor

- Tremor often becomes less prominent as the disease progresses

- In the clinical setting, tremor can be elicited by assigning the patient a task that requires concentration, or a motor task using the contralateral extremity, such as fisting and unfisting of the hand.

- In rare cases, the tremor occurs as the only manifestation of PD, particularly in early stages.

- Postural tremor may be a manifestation of PD or of essential tremor; thus, it is important to inquire about family history of tremor without PD.

Rigidity

- Rigidity is described as uniform resistance to passive flexion and extension throughout the range of motion.

- Rigidity can have a cogwheel quality, be ratchet-like, or be a rhythmic contraction upon passive stretching even without tremor.

- Rigidity is equal in all directions.

- It is usually more pronounced in the tremulous hand.

- In some patients only rigidity occurs and tremor is absent.

- Rigidity is enhanced by contralateral motor activity or mental task performance.

Bradykinesia

- Described as slowness of movement and is the most disabling symptom of PD

- Initially manifests by difficulties with fine motor movements

- Blinking slows and patient may seem to stare

- The ability to change facial expression diminishes and the person assumes a mask-like facies (hypomimia)

- Speech becomes softer (hypophonia) and slurred (dysarthria) or stuttered; characteristically monotonous with stuttering dysarthria

- Reduced swallowing allows saliva to pool in the mouth and increases the risk of aspiration

- Fine motor impairment may hinder dressing or buttoning of clothes, cutting food, brushing teeth, or handling coins

- Handwriting becomes small (micrographia) and eventually not legible

- As rigidity progresses and movement becomes decreased (hypokinesia), patient finds it difficult to initiate (akinesia) movement

- Rigidity and hypokinesia may contribute to muscular aches and sensations of fatigue

- Patients may complain of feeling weak, tired, or unable to get out of a chair, initiate walking, or turning in bed.

- Can be tested by finger tapping, alternating forearm pronation and suppination, foot tapping, and fist clenching and unclenching

Secondary manifestations are common in PD and include the following:

Gait Disturbances
- Postural instability is usually a later sign of PD.
- Postural instability refers to the gradual development of poor balance, leading to increased risk of falls.
- Posture becomes stooped as rigidity progresses and the center of gravity changes, causing forward flexion of the neck and trunk and flexion of the arms—pushing the patient forward and downward
- Arms flex to the waist and do not swing with the stride.
- Patient finds it difficult to initiate walking and gait becomes shuffling with short steps
- Steps may inadvertently quicken, and the patient may break into a run to keep from falling (festinating).
- Freezing phenomenon, also called motor block, is the transient inability to perform active movements.
  - Legs are most often affected, but it may also involve eyelid opening, speaking, and writing
  - Freezing is transient and occurs suddenly; typically occurs when a person begins to walk (start-hesitation), attempts to turn while walking, or approaches a destination (target-hesitation).
  - The person may be fearful about the ability to handle perceived barriers such as elevator doors and heavily trafficked streets.
- Turning requires multiple steps with a characteristic *en bloc* appearance, where the person turns without twisting the torso.

- The tendency to fall forward (propulsion) or backward (retropulsion) when the center of gravity is displaced results from loss of postural reflexes.
- Postural instability refers to the gradual development of poor balance, leading to increased risk of falls.
- Postural instability can be evaluated by the "pull test"—having the patient stand with arms hanging loose. Explain that the patient should try to remain still, as you pull from behind. With your hands on the patient's upper arms, gently pull backward—ready to catch him/her, if necessary. Patients with mild instability will need to step back to regain balance; those with severe instability will fall into your arms.

Autonomic Sensory Disturbances
- Excessive perspiration as a result of a disorder of the hypothalamic heat-regulating mechanism and impairment of perspirational controls
- Constipation secondary to hypomotility of the gastrointestinal tract
- Orthostatic dizziness and hypotension as a result of deterioration of the peripheral autonomic system
- Seborrhea is common, for example at the hairline and nasolabial folds
- Erectile dysfunction frequently occurs.
- Urinary dysfunction may affect up to 70% of patients (Samii, Nutt, & Ransom, 2004).
  - Urinary hesitation and retention secondary to autonomic dysfunction
  - Nocturia, the earliest and most common symptom, may be followed by incomplete bladder emptying and daytime frequency and urgency.
- Persons may also complain of sensory dysfunctions such as pain, burning, and tingling. Sensory symptoms may decrease when the patient moves.

Neuropsychological Symptoms

- More than half of patients with PD meet the criteria for major depression; depression may precede motor symptoms.

- Patients with anxiety frequently report a sensation of internal tremor or generalized restlessness.

- Sleep disturbance is common in PD and has many different causes including nocturnal stiffness, nocturia, depression, restless leg syndrome, and REM sleep behavior disorder (Stacy, 2002).

- Behavioral changes are commonly seen.

- Personality changes reflect increased fearfulness, dependency, and anxiety.

- Passivity, lack of motivation, and decreased attention span are common.

- Psychosis, agitation, and mania related to activation of the dopamine receptors in the nonstriatal regions is common in patients who take dopaminergic drugs.

- Dementia is a late manifestation and occurs in about 20% of patients (Ben-Shlomo, 1997). If it occurs early, providers should consider alternative diagnoses.

- Cognitive dysfunction includes slow information processing, altered personality with apathy or depression, forgetfulness, impaired facial recognition, and poor visuospatial memory.

Differential Diagnoses

The differential diagnosis is not always clear and as many as 15% of patients seen for presumed PD in specialty clinics have some other disorder (Paulson, 1993). Patients may manifest extrapyramidal features as part of a totally different process, such as late-stage Alzheimer's disease. Conversely, PD remains undiagnosed for years in cases that present without tremor. Idiopathic PD must be differentiated from other types of parkinsonism (symptomatic, Parkinson-plus syndromes, and other heredodegenerative

diseases). Additional disorders that may be considered when persons exhibit parkinsonian-like symptoms include the following:

- Essential tremors
- Progressive supranuclear palsy
- Normal pressure hydrocephalus
- Frontal lobe tumors
- Lewy body dementia
- Alzheimer's disease with parkinsonism
- Drug-induced (reversible) parkinsonism, especially with phenothiazine, metoclopramide, reserpine, carbon monoxide, and manganese poisoning
- Hypothyroidism
- Wilson's disease
- Multiple system atrophy (Shy-Drager syndrome)
- Depression
- Huntington's disease
- Cerebrovascular accident
- Toxin-induced parkinsonism

Essential Diagnostic and Laboratory Tests

The diagnosis of PD is purely clinical, based upon signs and symptoms that can be obtained from a detailed history focusing on clinical symptoms, a limited physical examination, and in some cases, the patient's response to medication. PD is usually asymmetric and responsive to dopaminergic treatment, with no historical or examination clues to suggest an alternate cause for symptoms. Pathological findings show that nigral dopamine neurons are greatly diminished, and Lewy bodies are present in the remaining neurons. Thus, to obtain a definite diagnosis of idiopathic Parkinson's disease, autopsy is needed.

Fortunately, a patient's history and examination conducted by skilled clinicians can predict the pathological findings with fairly high assurance. Primary care providers should be able to make an accurate diagnosis in about 85% of cases (Beers & Berkow, 2000).

- Collection of historical and physical information is focused on teasing out the presence of cardinal signs and symptoms and other features associated with PD.
- Baseline information regarding a person's functional and cognitive abilities is crucial for establishing a parameter from which subsequent data can be prepared to both evaluate the person's response to treatment as well as to track progression of the disease itself.
- Imaging or laboratory techniques are useful to rule out other disorders but are not required to make a diagnosis of PD. There are many clinical and laboratory clues that suggest that a person with parkinsonism may have some form of the syndrome other than PD itself.
  - CT scan and MRI of the brain may be performed to exclude structural brain lesions but not to demonstrate pathologic changes indicative of PD.
  - A serum calcium level may be drawn to exclude hypoparathyroidism.
  - A positron emission tomography (PET) scan with 18F-6 fluorodopa can be used to assess changes in striatal dopamine and to detect subclinical nigral pathology (Rhoades, 2001).

Management Plan

Treatment is life-long and the goal is to keep the patients with PD functioning independently as long as possible.

Treatment of PD may require an interdisciplinary team approach and both pharmacologic and nonpharmacologic modalities should be implemented. Nothing has yet been proven to be neuroprotective for PD. There is no drug or surgical approach currently available that prevents the progression of the disease. Once patients develop functionally disabling symptoms, they need to start symptomatic therapy. Because

there is no single right choice for treatment for patients with PD and because each patient has a unique set of signs, symptoms, and responses to medications, treatment must be individualized according to the following criteria:

- Type and severity of symptoms
- Degree of functional impairment
- Degree of cognitive impairment
- Associated disease processes
- Risk-benefit ratio

General therapeutic considerations are outlined in Table 14-2.

TABLE 14-2   General Therapeutic Considerations for the Management of Parkinson's Disease

- Treatment decisions are based upon the degree of disability caused by symptoms.
- The proper combination of exercise and medication is essential.
- Discontinue all drugs that cause/aggravate symptoms such as neuroleptics, sedatives, and metoclopramide.
- No single drug is ideal for initial therapy.
- Treat symptomatically with lowest effective doses.
- Keep therapeutic drug regimen simple.
- In general, the risk of adverse effects is lower when one or two drugs are given at higher doses than when multiple drugs are given at lower doses.
- Try one drug at a time in modest doses then consider adding drugs from different classes to control symptoms.
- Abrupt withdrawal of any medication may worsen symptoms (abnormal involuntary movements [AIMS], on-off phenomenon)
- Monitor progression of disease and effectiveness of treatment by clinical and functional assessments (consider videotaping).

Nonpharmacologic

- The importance of exercise cannot be over-stressed. Patients should be encouraged to engage in a regular exercise program.

- Therapeutic massage may be a useful strategy to promote relaxation and pain relief (Paterson, Allen, Browning, Barlow, & Ewings, 2005).

- Acupuncture can provide temporary relief from stiffness.

- Dietary carbohydrate-protein balancing as well as meal timing and frequency has been shown to influence L-dopa's effect. Patients with advanced disease are advised to take L-dopa with a high carbohydrate meal and delay protein intake until the final meal of the day in order to maximize the drug's therapeutic efficacy (Caspi & Thomson, 1999; Parkinson's Disease Study Group, 1995).

- The following rehabilitation services may provide additional approaches to help patients maintain as much independence as they can for as long as possible.

  - Physical therapy may assist in restoring confidence in walking and maintaining balance; may help patients develop simple means of managing unpredictable and disabling freezing episodes; and can provide additional training as mobility problems progress.

  - Occupational therapy may be indicated to train patients in strategies for carrying out daily activities and in the use of adaptive equipment to simplify tasks.

- Institution of bowel and bladder programs is essential to address problems inherent in the disease as well as the treatment.

- Fall assessments and strategies to prevent falls should be instituted.

- Guidance for immunizations must be provided to decrease risk of mortality from influenza and pneumonia.

- Clinicians must remember that patients with PD also have social and emotional needs to be considered:

  - Provide anticipatory guidance and counseling for patients and families.

  - Patients should be routinely assessed for physical, functional, cognitive, and emotional health.

  - Refer patients and families to support groups as deemed appropriate.

- Patients with severe symptoms such as tremors that are refractory to medications may require referral to a movement disorder neurologist or neurosurgeon for evaluation. Options include ablative therapies (pallidotomy and thalamotomy) and augmentive therapies (deep brain stimulation). Restorative therapies are also being investigated (tissue transplantation and gene therapy). Candidates for ablative and augmentive therapies must be responsive to L-dopa because surgery tends to benefit only those patients.

Pharmacologic

Treatment decisions are challenging in patients with PD because, in addition to managing symptoms and complications, the clinician is often faced with the occurrence of side effects associated with an expanding arsenal of pharmacologic and surgical options. Drug therapy for PD is challenging whether the disease is newly diagnosed or advanced and requires careful timing and selection of agents. Drug efficacy declines over the course of the disease, and the therapeutic response can be blunted by improper timing or by medication choice.

The major goal of pharmacologic intervention is to maximize function and quality of life with as few adverse effects as possible. Treatment must be individualized, beginning as soon as symptoms interfere with function or well-being.

The *major principles* for medication management are the following:

- Treat the chief complaint first.
- Start low and go slow.
- Add one new agent at a time, and adjust one medication at a time.
- Focus on the dosing interval, not just the dose.
- Stay alert for red flags such as confusion and psychosis, particularly when treating older patients.

There are several classes of drugs that are commonly prescribed for the management of PD, including the following:

- Anticholinergic drugs
  - Antihistamines
  - Antidepressant agents
- Antiviral agents
- Dopaminergic agents
  - Dopamine precursors
  - Dopamine agonists
- Monoamine oxidase type B inhibitors
- Catechol-*o*-methyltransferase (COMT) inhibitors

Anticholinergic Agents
These are centrally acting drugs that have been used to treat symptoms of PD for many years. They specifically act against cholinergic excitation. Many anticholinergic agents are available, and all are similar in effects and side effects. In general, anticholinergics are used less often now than in the past because of potential side effects including constipation, urinary retention, memory impairment, hallucinations, and confusion, which are especially problematic in older adults. Anticholinergics are more typically used in younger patients, age 60 years or less, in whom tremor is the predominant feature but in whom cognitive function is preserved.

Although there is no proof that initial therapy with anticholinergics is better than levodopa for amelioration of tremor, the addition of an anticholinergic does often dampen the tremor of a patient who is already receiving a dopamine precursor. In addition to decreasing tremor, anticholinergics usually provide some reduction in rigidity and can be used to manage significant drooling. Examples of medications that are prescribed in the treatment of PD for their anticholinergic properties and usual daily doses include the following (Selma, Beizer, & Higbee, 2005):

- Centrally acting anticholinergics
  - Benztropine (Cogentin) 2 mg to 6 mg by mouth two times daily
  - Trihexyphenidyl (Artane, Trihexy), 2 mg by mouth three times daily
  - Procyclidine (Kemadrin), 5 mg by mouth twice daily
  - Biperiden (Akineton), 2 mg by mouth twice daily
- Antihistamines (with anticholinergic action; useful for treating tremors)
  - Diphenhydramine (Benadryl), 25 mg by mouth three times daily
  - Orphenadrine (Norflex), 100 mg by mouth once daily
- Antidepressant/anticholinergic tricyclic agents are useful adjuvants to levodopa:
  - Amitriptyline (Elavil, Endep), 25 mg by mouth at bedtime
  - Doxepin (Adapin, Sinequan), 50 mg by mouth at bedtime

Dopaminergic Agents
Although dopamine is deficient in PD, the dopaminergic receptors may still respond to dopamine that is supplied by several mechanisms. Agents that probably act through their effect on these preceptors include amantadine HCL, the dopamine receptor agonists, and dopamine precursors. Unfortunately, the dop-

aminergic receptors deteriorate with the progression of PD, and all of these medications become less effective with time.

The antiviral agent, amantadine HCl (Symmetrel), is thought to release dopamine from intact dopaminergic terminals that remain in the substantia nigra and perhaps from other sites. It is recommended as first-line monotherapy in patients younger than 60 years and in older patients with milder symptoms. The effect of amantadine as initial therapy is measured in days or months. The benefit may be modest, and side effects are occasionally noted. In higher doses, amantadine may cause some of the same problems seen with other antiparkinson drugs, including hallucinations or confusion. Amantadine is generally innocuous. Skin rash, ankle edema, exacerbation of heart failure, and livedo reticularis have been noted with amantadine in rare cases. *The usual dose of amantadine is 100 mg to 200 mg twice daily* (Selma, Beizer, & Higbee, 2005). Amantadine is also recommended to augment the effects of levodopa later in the disease. Its mechanism of action is uncertain. It often loses its effect in a period of months when used alone.

Dopamine Receptor Agonists

These are ergot alkaloids that directly activate dopamine receptors in the basal ganglia. Presumably, these agents do not require metabolic conversion to an active product in order to exert effects. They have been suggested as initial therapy by some, particularly by those who feel that the initial use of an agonist tend to delay the development of dyskinesia and other fluctuations characteristically seen after prolonged use of levodopa. Dopamine agonists are usually not as beneficial as levodopa (L-dopa), but their action is longer, and they cause less dyskinesia.

For most "parkinsonologists," however, agonists are not used alone in the early stages of PD but as an additional medication with levodopa/carbidopa, often in low dosages. Dopamine agonists may offer an L-dopa sparing effect, allowing lower dosages of L-dopa

to be used. There is little data suggesting that a trial shift from one agonist to another is desirable, particularly if the patient tolerates the first one well. Adverse reactions associated with these agents include nausea, somnolence, dizziness, dyskinesia, dystonia, fluctuation of symptoms, and the potentiation of alcohol and other CNS depressants. Examples of dopamine receptor agonists commonly used and their usual recommended dose include the following (Selma, Beizer, & Higbee, 2005):

- Bromocriptine (Parlodel), 30 mg to 90 mg by mouth three times a day

- Pergolide (Permax), 2 mg to 5 mg by mouth three times a day

- Praxipexole (Mirapex), 1.5 mg to 4.5 mg by mouth three times a day

- Ropinirole (Requip), 0.75 mg to 24 mg by mouth three times a day

Levodopa

L-dopa provides the most benefit in terms of improving the motor manifestations of PD relative to its central nervous system effects. L-dopa, first introduced in the 1960s, yields an 80% improvement of symptoms in most patients. L-dopa is the metabolic precursor of dopamine. It crosses the blood-brain barrier into the basal ganglia where it is decarboxilated to form dopamine, replacing the missing neurotransmitter.

In the United States, levodopa is used almost exclusively with carbidopa. It is usually given in combination to reduce gastrointestinal symptoms and to permit lower L-dopa dosing. Coadministration of the peripheral decarboxalase inhibitor, carbidopa lowers dosage requirements by preventing levodopa catabolism, thus decreasing side effects and allowing more efficient delivery of levodopa to the brain.

Use of L-dopa as initial therapy is not unreasonable, particularly if the therapy goal is to treat bradykinesia and rigidity. As initial therapy, the effect may be smooth improvement, and patient acceptance is excellent. The correct dose of L-dopa is the lowest dose that provides satisfactory response. Carbidopa/levodopa (Sinemet, Sinemet CR, Atamet) is available in fixed-ratio preparations of 10/100, 25/100, 25/250, and in a controlled released tablet 50/200. Most patients require 400 mg to 1000 mg/day of levodopa in divided doses every 2 to 5 hours with at least 100 mg/day of carbidopa to minimize peripheral side effects. Some may require up to 2000 mg/day of levodopa with 200 mg of carbidopa. The usual daily dose is 50/200 mg to 200/2000 mg by mouth two or three times a day for controlled release (Selma, Beizer, & Higbee, 2005).

Bradykinesia and rigidity are the symptoms helped the most with L-dopa, although tremor is often substantially reduced as well. Levodopa is clearly the most effective treatment, on the average, for managing the symptoms of PD. Withholding levodopa to try to achieve better effects later or to assure a longer period during which therapy works well is understandable, but this strategy is not based on firm clinical data. Long-acting levodopa compounds have been found to be particularly useful both initially and in patients who develop fluctuations. These sustained-release formulations seem to be more physiologic and more protective than pulsatile therapy with regular L-dopa, and provide patients with a smoother control of symptoms.

Monoamine Oxidase Type B Inhibitors
Selegiline (Eldepryl) is the most popular type B monoamine oxidase (MAO-B) inhibitor. MAO-B inhibits one of the two major enzymes that break down dopamine in the brain. It also works to reduce oxidative metabolism of dopamine in the brain, slowing the neurodegenerative process. In this regard, Selegiline may be considered neuroprotective. At doses of 5 mg to 10 mg/day it does not cause hypertensive crisis, common with nonselective MAO-A inhibitors that block the A and B isoenzymes.

Used as an initial treatment, selegiline may delay the initiation of levodopa for about nine months. It also may potentiate residual dopamine in the brain of patients in later stages of the disease thereby prolonging the action of individual doses of L-dopa. After several days on selegiline, L-dopa dosage may be reduced by 10% to 30%. Adverse effects of selegiline include nausea, dizziness, confusion, hallucinations, and dry mouth. Care must be taken when combining selegiline with L-dopa because in combination, selegiline can increase dopaminergic effects and contribute to dopamine toxicity and worsening of dyskinesia in some patients. The usual daily dose of selegiline is 5 mg by mouth twice daily with breakfast and lunch or 10 mg by mouth in the evening (Selma, Beizer, & Higbee, 2005).

Catechol-O-Methyltransferase (COMT) Inhibitors
COMT inhibitors, such as tolcapone (Tasmar) and entacapone (Comtan), inhibit the breakdown of dopamine and ensure the duration of action of both levodopa and dopamine. They are useful adjuncts to L-dopa therapy in patients who experience "wearing-off" symptoms at the end of a dosing interval. Most common side effects associated with entacapone include orthostatic hypotension, dyskinesias, hallucinations, and diarrhea. Tolcapone has proven beneficial in both early and late PD. Its most common side effects are diarrhea, nausea, vomiting, orthostasis, dyskinesias, hallucinations, and fatigue. A rare complication is fulminate hepatic necrosis. Liver function tests are required every 2 weeks during the first year of therapy and then monthly thereafter. Patients should give written consent before initiating therapy with tolcapone (Selma, Beizer, & Higbee, 2005). Usual dosages for the COMT inhibitors are as follows:

• Tolcapone (Tasmar), 300 mg to 600 mg by mouth three times daily
• Entacapone (Comtan), 200 mg by mouth with each dose of levodopa/carbidopa (maximum daily dose is 1600 mg/day)

Patient, Family, and Staff Education

In the later stages of PD, all aspects of care may have to be assumed by someone other than the patient. Teaching needs include the following:

- Education about the disease, what can exacerbate symptoms and how to manage them
- Use of medications, including side effects, dosage, timing, and desired effects
- Importance of recognizing and reporting medication side effects to the provider
- Maintaining adequate fluid intake
- Importance of balancing activities to include relaxation and fun activities
- Need for balanced diet
- Range of motion (ROM) exercises
- Safety factors to prevent falls and injuries
- Positioning to prevent contractions and pressure ulcers
- Importance of skin inspection and procedures
- Importance of avoiding temperature extremes
- Awareness of mood changes and importance of reporting them to provider

Physician Consultation

- Referral to a specialist should be made based upon the practitioner's knowledge level and comfort treating PD and on the severity of symptoms
- As the disease progresses, especially in the area of tremor, it may become necessary to refer the patient to a movement disorder neurologist for evaluation.
- Refer patients approaching the end of life to hospice.

▐▬▬ MULTIPLE SCLEROSIS

Definition

Multiple sclerosis (MS) is the most common cause of disability among young adults. It is a recurrent, occasionally progressive, inflammatory demyelination of the white matter of the brain and spinal cord resulting in multiple and varied neurological signs and symptoms. The disease results from an autoimmune attack on the myelin that envelops the axons in the brain and spinal cord. Typical symptoms include unilateral visual loss, diplopia that lasts for days or weeks, and hemiparesis that has an insidious or slow onset.

Multiple sclerosis has a significant impact on patients, potentially leading to considerable disability in terms of fatigue, mobility, cognitive function, bowel and bladder function, and depression and other mood problems. Because symptoms of MS wax and wane over time, unless they affect function, such as gait, patients may not initially seek medical evaluation. Because most of the initial presenting symptoms resolve over brief periods (days to weeks), the diagnosis may be delayed for years (Hess & Hughes, 2005a).

Epidemiology

The prevalence of MS is approximately 2.5 million worldwide and 400,000 in the United States where the cost of the disease is estimated to be $41,000 per patient per year (Pryse-Phillips & Costello, 2001; Whetten-Goldstein, Sloan, Goldstein, & Kulas, 1998). It is about two to three times as common among women as among men and usually begins in the second or third decades of life. The predominant age of onset is between 16 to 40 years. Onset before age 10 and after age 60 is rare. MS is more common in Caucasians than in African-Americans or Asians (Rollins & Corboy, 2005).

Multiple sclerosis is almost unknown in parts of Africa and is extremely rare in Japan. The disease is more common in higher latitudes in both the northern and the southern hemispheres. In general, MS is most common among persons of Scandinavian or Northern European descent. There are also geographic pockets of MS, the most notable being the Orkney Islands off the coast of Scotland (Hess & Hughes, 2005a).

The National Multiple Sclerosis Society's Long-Term Care Committee (2003) estimates that about 5–10% of persons with multiple sclerosis require nursing home care. These individuals present unique characteristics that set them apart from most residents including the following:

- Younger age
- More mentally alert
- More physically dependent
- More symptoms of depression
- Longer length of stay

The cause of MS is unknown. Nevertheless, several popular theories of causation have been proposed. Based on twin studies, familial cases, and an association with specific HLA antigens, a likely one theorizes that there is a genetic susceptibility to the disease. There is also a viral theory that is supported by increasing incidence of disease at higher altitudes, clusters of cases within families, geographical clusters, and animal studies of infectious diseases of the myelin. Many viruses have been implicated; the most recent is the human herpes virus 6 (HHV-6). This virus can cause a latent infection in the central nervous system. However, there is still no convincing evidence that a specific virus causes MS (Soldan et al., 1997). A combined theory has also been posited and is the most widely accepted hypothesis explaining the disease as a genetic predisposition for an autoimmune disorder, triggered by environmental exposure to a toxin or virus early in life (Smith, 2006). Several risk factors have been identified. They include living in the temperate zone, being of Northern European descent, and having a family history of the disease.

Common Presenting Signs and Symptoms

There are four clinical subtypes of MS: (1) relapsing-remitting (RR), (2) secondary progressive (SP), (3) progressive relapsing (PR), and (4) primary progressive (PP). The RR and SP subtypes account for about 85% of cases (Lublin & Reingold, 1996). Patients with RRMS initially experience a relapsing and remitting disease course, meaning that they have attacks followed by a partial or complete recovery. The average attack rate for untreated patients is approximately 1 to 2 per year. The RR course is the most common and carries the best prognosis. However, although symptoms remit, there is usually a mild residual deficit. Over time, these deficits produce disability.

Following an RR phase that lasts about 6 to 10 years, a significant number (30–40%) of patients transition into an SP phase. This phase is characterized by a slow progression of the disease, with a clear period of remission. Relapses may be superimposed on a background of functional decline (Rollins & Corboy, 2005).

The transition from the RR to the SP phase is generally retrospectively noted when a patient's neurologic status has begun to worsen between attacks. Spastic paraparesis generally develops in patients with SPMS, eventually requiring the use of a wheelchair. Significant bowel and bladder dysfunction may develop during the SP phase. Historically, many authors have thought that this change in clinical phase may signify a transition between the earlier, inflammatory phase of the disease and a later, degenerative phase (Rollins & Corboy, 2005). However, recent data suggest that this distinction is not necessarily correct (Fillippi et al., 2003).

About 5% to 10% of patients present with PPMS, a disease type characterized by the absence of relapses, with a steady decline in multiple aspects of neurologic function. A rare, acute form of MS often called Marburg syndrome, has an explosive course from the beginning and causes the rapid onset of disability and often death (Hess & Hughes, 2005a).

A variety of symptoms are associated with MS including ataxia, cognitive dysfunction, diplopia, fatigue, gait disorders, optic neuritis, numbness or paresthesias, poor bladder or bowel control, slowed or slurred speech, spasticity, tremor, and weakness (Hess & Hughes,

2005a). Some symptoms are commonly observed during the initial presentation of the disease. Others are demonstrated by persons experiencing RR disease, SP disease, and PP disease. Examples of these symptoms are detailed in Table 14-3.

Differential Diagnoses

A long list of disorders can account for the signs and symptoms observed in MS. A list of these are detailed in Table 14-4.

Essential Diagnostic and Laboratory Tests

MS is a clinical diagnosis of inclusion, characterized by a typical clinical history of neurologic symptoms separated in time, supported by laboratory tests. MRI and inspection of cerebrospinal fluid for oligoclonal banding are most commonly used to aid in diagnosing MS. Taken together these data must satisfy requirements for dissemination of CNS inflammation given that other possible causes must be appropriately ruled out. When patients present with clinical symptoms typical of demyelination but have a clinical history of only one neurologic attack, they are said to have a clinically isolated syndrome (CIS).

MRI studies are only supportive of a diagnosis of MS, and no MRI finding is pathognomonic for it. However, normal imaging results are unusual in patients with MS. MRI studies have consistently shown that 50% to 75% of

TABLE 14-3 Symptoms and Signs of MS Featured Throughout the Disease	
Common initial presentation	• Symptoms may disappear after a few days or weeks, although examination often reveals a residual deficit. • Weakness, numbness, tingling or unsteadiness in a limb • Spastic paraparesis • Retrobulbar neuritis • Diplopia • Dysequilibrium • Sphincter disturbance, such as urinary urgency or hesitancy
Relapsing-remitting (RR) disease	• Symptoms occur months or years after initial presentation. • Eventually relapse and usually incomplete remissions lead to increasing disability, with weakness, spasticity and ataxia of the limbs, impaired vision, and urinary incontinence • The findings on examination commonly include optic atrophy, nystagmus, dysarthria, and pyramidal, sensory, or cerebellar deficits in some or all of the limbs.
Secondary progressive (SP) disease	• The clinical course changes to steady deterioration, unrelated to acute relapses in some of the relapsing-remitting patients.
Primary progressive (PP) disease	• Less common • Symptoms steadily progress from their onset. • Disability develops at a relatively early stage. • Diagnosis cannot be made unless the total clinical picture indicates involvement of different parts of the CNS at different times. • A number of factors (infection, trauma) may precipitate or trigger exacerbations. • Relapses are also more likely during 2 to 3 months following pregnancy.

Source: Adapted from Aminoff, 2006c; Hess & Hughes, 2005a; O'Riordan et al., 1998; Smith, 2006.

TABLE 14-4 Differential Diagnosis for Multiple Sclerosis

- Acute disseminated encephalomyelitis
- Foramen magnum lesion
- Progressive multifocal leukoencephalopathy
- Pernicious anemia
- Spinal cord tumor
- Vasculitis
- Neurosyphilis
- Lyme disease
- Syringomyelopathy
- HIV-associated myelopathy
- Amyotrophic lateral sclerosis
- Bechet's disease
- Brain stem tumors
- CNS infections
- Cerebellar tumors
- Hereditary ataxias

patients who present with a CIS during an initial neurologic attack have brain abnormalities on MRI scan consistent with MS, suggesting that these lesions are either concurrent or have preceded the clinical attack. In long-term follow-up studies, 88% of these patients ultimately experience second clinical attacks consistent with MS. Of the patients with a CIS and an otherwise normal MRI scan, MS developed in only 19% (Brex et al., 2002). Therefore, the clinical diagnosis of MS relies on the following:

- At least two attacks in which two areas of the CNS were involved

- Neurological signs that reflect at least two separate areas of CNS involvement

- No disease that can better explain the signs and symptoms

Other important points that should be considered when diagnosing MS include the following:

- Bilateral internuclear ophthalmoplegia (INO) in a young person is virtually diagnostic of MS.

- Be alert to depression in patients with MS. Several studies have found that more than one third of MS patients experience a major depressive episode (Hess & Hughes, 2005a).

- If you first diagnose MS in a patient over 50 years of age, diagnose something else (Tierney, Saint, & Whooley, 2005)

- If you are fairly certain of the diagnosis of MS by the clinical picture, and if the MRI scan confirms the clinical impression, a lumbar puncture is unnecessary.

Management Plan

Treatment of MS falls into three broad categories. Goals of treatment are related to the category of treatment (Hess & Hughes, 2005b):

- Disabling symptoms are treated with a variety of symptomatic therapies, with the goal of improving quality of life.

- Acute attacks are treated with therapies designed to reduce inflammation and shorten the duration of the disabling attack.

- For the long-term treatment of MS, there are now five FDA-approved therapies, the goals of which are to reduce attacks and to prevent the accumulation of new brain lesions, as well as to slow progression of disability.

Nonpharmacologic

The role of rehabilitation in MS has been increasingly defined in the past few years. Although MS is a chronic, progressive disorder, functional gains can be made through aggressive rehabilitation after acute events. Rehabilitation should also be considered for those patients who are experiencing an insidiously progressive decline in functioning. Aggressive symptom management combined with rehabilitation can improve quality of life and help patients regain their independence.

Surveys have revealed that up to 80% of patients with MS use complementary and alternative medicine, such as high-dose vitamins, bee sting therapy, and marijuana. It is vital to open the lines of communication with patients so they feel comfortable with disclosing their entire treatment regimen (Bowling, 2001).

Pharmacologic
Symptom Relief
There are many available therapies that offer patients at least partial relief from symptoms of MS such as fatigue, bladder problems, spasticity, and depression. Table 14-5 shows a range of approaches that can help patients who have MS.

TABLE 14-5 Management Strategies for Treatment of Symptoms in MS

SYMPTOM	MANAGEMENT
Spasticity, painful spasms	• Muscle relaxants such as baclofen (Lioresal) start at 5 mg 2 to 3 times/day and titrate up to 80 mg; withdraw by titration if no benefit is reported • Consider intrathecal baclofen for select patients • Tizanidine (Zanaflex) start at 4 mg and titrate to a maximum daily dose of 24 mg in three divided doses; be alert to sedation • Botulism toxin for focal spasticity
Urinary incontinence, detrusor hyperreflexia, urinary retention	• Anticholinergics such as oxybutynin XL (Ditropan XL), 5 mg to 20 mg or tolterodine (Detrol) 2 mg twice daily for small bladder capacities and detrusor hyperreflexia • Tamsulosin (Flomax) 0.4 mg daily 30 minutes after meals; may increase to 0.8 mg to relax the sphincter • Large-capacity bladders: frequent catheterization; watch for urinary tract infections
Fatigue	• Lifestyle adjustments, education of patient and family, heat avoidance, regular exercise balanced with rest periods • Amantadine (Symmetrel), 100 mg two to three times daily, can be tried • Modafinil, 100 mg in the morning and midday • Stimulants, such as methylphenidate 10 mg 2–3 times daily up to 60 mg/day
Depression	• Counseling, including marriage and vocational issues • SSRI antidepressants
Tic douloureux	• Carbamazepine 100 mg twice daily to 200 mg four times daily • Gabapentin 900–3600 mg in 2–3 divided doses • If poorly tolerated or ineffective, phenytoin, valproic acid, or baclofen can be tried • Surgical exploration of posterior fossa in refractory cases • Radiofrequency ablation useful in some cases
Cognitive dysfunction	• Strategic use of memory aids • Aggressive management of contributing factors, such as fatigue • Identification and treatment of contributing medical disorders, such as hypothyroidism • Avoidance, as much as possible, of medications that have cognitive side effects, such as antispasmodics • Administration of interferon-beta-1a (Avonex) 30 µg intramuscular once weekly • Trials of cholinesterase inhibitors, such as donepezil
Fever	• Use antipyretic agents liberally in febrile patients because fever may worsen preexisting signs and symptoms of MS

- Significant *fatigue* occurs in about 67% of MS patients (Krupp et al., 1988). Several studies have shown a modest benefit from symptomatic treatment with amantidine and modafinil (Zifko et al., 2002).

- Fifty percent to 90% of patients with MS report *urinary symptoms*, which commonly include urinary frequency, urgency, and urge-related incontinence. Incomplete bladder emptying, hesitancy, and recurrent urinary tract infections (UTIs) are also common complaints, the last of which is a common cause of worsening MS symptoms. Symptoms of urinary urgency, frequency, and urge incontinence are suggestive of detrusor hyperreflexia and can be at least partly alleviated by anticholinergic medications such as oxybutynin. Urinary frequency, UTI, straining, and hesitancy are often symptoms of urinary retention and can be treated with agents such as tamsulosin (Flomax) to relax the sphincter. Patients who do not respond to these treatments or whose symptoms have an unclear cause should be referred for urodynamic studies. In addition, patients with urinary retention may need to perform intermittent self-catheterization to empty the bladder.

- *Muscle spasticity* can produce a variety of symptoms, including pain or a "tight" feeling in the affected muscles, decreased dexterity of fine motor movements, spasms, and contractures. Patients should be encouraged to exercise and participate in physical therapy to maintain flexibility, strength, and coordination. In addition, these symptoms are often treated with muscle relaxants and with certain benzodiazepines.

- *Major depression* has a lifetime frequency of 50% among patients with MS (Sadovnick et al., 1996). This is probably a result of both direct CNS damage and the psychological toll of the diagnosis and symptoms of MS. Depression also can arise as a side effect of some of the medication used to treat MS. Generally, selective serotonin reuptake inhibitors (SSRIs) are the first-line treatment for depression in any setting, unless a patient has a contraindication to these medications. The SSRIs tend to be effective in MS-related depression. As in any clinical setting, if a patient has mood symptoms that are severe or refractory to standard treatment, he or she should be referred to a mental health provider who has experience treating patients with neurological disorders.

Acute Relapses

Not all relapses need to be treated. Clinicians should target those that affect function, such as vision or gait. Moreover, when considering whether or not to treat a patient for an acute relapse, it is important to distinguish between a true *new* attack (exacerbation) and a "pseudoattack." It is common for patients with MS to transiently reexperience symptoms from an older attack when they become fatigued or overheated or develop an infection. A true *new* attack consists of novel symptoms or a significant worsening of older ones.

Recovery from acute relapses may be hastened by corticosteroids, but the extent of recovery is unaffected. Therefore, the goal of treatment during acute relapses is to shorten the duration and severity of the attack. A high dose (prednisone, 60 to 80 mg by mouth) is given daily for 1 week. Medication is then tapered over the following 2 to 3 weeks (Aminoff, 2006c). The gold standard for treating acute disabling relapses in MS is to precede treatment with oral corticosteroids with methylprednisolone, 1 gram daily, intravenously for 3 to 5 consecutive days (Beck et al., 1992; Rollins & Corboy, 2005). Although several studies support this treatment recommendation, the best data are from the Optic Neuritis Treatment Trial (Beck et al., 1992) that found that intravenous methylprednisolone with an oral taper was significantly better than oral prednisone or placebo for patients with optic neuritis in terms of time to recovery, symptom recurrence, and the experience of further neurologic events leading to the diagnosis of MS. Table 14-6 provides several corticosteroid regimens recommended for the

TABLE 14-6 Corticosteroid Regimens for the Treatment of Acute Relapse in MS

- Methylprednisolone sodium succinate, 1 g IV per day for 3 days; then prednisone, 1 mg/kg/day for 11 days, then 20 mg for 1 day, then 10 mg/day for 2 days, then discontinue (Beck et al., 1992)

- Methylprednisolone, 500 mg by mouth per day for 5 days; then a dose tapered over 10 days—400 mg, 300 mg, 200 mg, 100 mg, 64 mg, 48 mg, 32 mg, 16 mg, 8 mg, 8 mg, on successive days (Sellebjerg et al., 1998)

- Dexamethasone, 96 mg by mouth per day for 5 days; then a dose tapered over 10 days—72 mg, 64 mg, 48 mg, 24 mg, 12 mg, 6 mg, 4 mg, 2 mg, 1 mg, 1 mg, on successive days (Hess & Hughes, 2005b)

treatment of acute relapse in MS. It is also important to note that long-term treatment with corticosteroids provides no benefit and does not prevent further relapses. Similarly, there is little evidence that plasmapheresis, another commonly used strategy, enhances any beneficial effects of immunosuppression in MS (Aminoff, 2006c).

Long Term Therapies

Unfortunately, there are currently no approved therapies for PPMS. However, three classes of drugs have been found to be of benefit in modifying the course of MS. Two forms of recombinant interferon beta are FDA approved for use in MS. IFN-beta-1a (Avonex) is approved for use in RRMS, and IFN-beta-1b (Betaseron) is approved for use in both SPMS and RRMS. Glatiramer acetate (Copaxone), a myelin-like polypeptide, has been approved for treatment of RRMS. Lastly, mitoxantrone (Novantrone), an anthracenedione with both anti-inflammatory and immunomodulating properties, has most recently been approved for the treatment of worsening RRMS, SPMS, and PRMS. In addition, the FDA approved natalizumab (Tysabri), an antiadhesion molecule drug, for RRMS in November 2004. However, as of February 28, 2005, natalizumab has been voluntarily suspended from use by the manufacturer after reports of two cases of progressive multifocal leukoencephalopathy in patients treated for more than 2 years with a combination of IFN-beta-1a and natalizumab (Jacobs et al., 2000; PRISMS, 1998; Rollins & Corboy, 2005).

A summary of drugs approved by the FDA for long-term treatment of MS is available in Table 14-7. Other considerations to facilitate

TABLE 14-7 Summary of Drugs Approved by the FDA for Long-Term Treatment of MS

	INTERFERON BETA-1A (AVONEX, REBIF)	INTERFERON BETA-1B (BETASERON, BERLEX)	GLATIRAMER ACETATE (COPAXONE)	MITOXANTRONE (NOVANTRONE)
Dose and frequency	30 µg intramuscular once weekly (Avonex) 44 µg subcutaneous three times weekly	250 µg every other day 3 times a week (high dose)	20 mg daily	12 mg/m² every three months
Route	Intramuscular	Subcutaneous	Subcutaneous	Intravenous
Efficacy	Reduces relapse frequency and severity, slows disability progression in RRMS, slows brain atrophy and cognitive dysfunction (Avonex)	Reduces relapse frequency and severity, slows disability progression in both SPMS and RRMS	Reduces relapse rate	Reduces relapse rates and severity and slows disability progression for SPMS and RRMS
Adverse effects	Flulike symptoms, injection site reactions, fever, muscle spasms	Flulike symptoms, redness at injection site, fever, muscle spasms; depression and suicidal ideation	Postinjection reaction with flushing, palpitations for < 20 minutes; injection site reactions	Nausea, vomiting, fatigue, hair thinning, menstrual abnormalities; leukemia and cardiotoxicity
Effect on MRI lesions	Reduces	Reduces	Reduces	Reduces

patient adherence when prescribing these agents include the following:

- Premedication and dose titration enhance the tolerability of the interferons.
- Acetaminophen or an NSAID, combined with diphenhydramine (Benadryl), taken 30 minutes before the injection attenuates flu-like symptoms that frequently accompany therapy.
- Interferon beta is titrated by starting the drug at one quarter of the full dose for 1 to 2 weeks, then half the dose for 1 to 2 weeks, then three quarters of the dose for another 1 to 2 weeks, then finally the full dose.
- Although glatiramer is generally well tolerated, about 5% of injections are associated with a benign systemic reaction that consists of tachycardia and dyspnea. Failure to warn patients about the reaction may lead to unnecessary emergency department visits (Hess & Hughes, 2005b).

Patient, Family, and Staff Education

Teaching is important for both patients, significant others, and staff. In the later stages of MS, all aspects of care may have to be assumed by someone other than the patient. Teaching needs include the following:

- Education about the disease, what can exacerbate symptoms and how to manage them
- Use of medications, including side effects, dosage, timing, and desired effects
- Importance of recognizing and promptly reporting medication side effects to provider
- Importance of maintaining adequate fluid intake
- Importance of balancing activities to include relaxation and recreational activities
- Need for a balanced diet
- Range of motion (ROM) exercises
- Safety factors to prevent falls and injuries

- Positioning to prevent contractions and pressure ulcers
- Importance of skin inspection and procedures
- Importance of avoiding temperature extremes
- Awareness of mood changes and importance of reporting them to provider

Physician Consultation

- If confirmation of diagnosis is needed
- If disease is progressive despite standard therapy
- For expertise in the use of immunotherapy

■ SPINAL STENOSIS

Definition

Spinal stenosis is a common spine pathology that is described as a narrowing of the spinal canal or neuronal foramen to such an extent that pressure is exerted on nerve roots and occasionally, the cord itself. This narrowing is due to structural bone changes that result in bulging and herniation of the vertebral body and ultimately, a narrowing of the spinal canal. The resulting compression of neural structures limits vascular supply to nerve roots so that symptoms associated with spinal stenosis are predominately those of neural ischemia.

Stenosis can occur anywhere along the spine. The most serious form of spinal stenosis is cervical spondylotic myelopathy (CSM), which occurs as a consequence of cervical cord compression by osteophytes, ligamentum flavum, or intervertebral discs. With disc degeneration, osteophytes develop posteriorly and project into the spinal canal, compressing the cord and its vascular supply.

Fortunately, a less serious form of spinal stenosis is also the most frequently occurring. The lumbar spine is the site of involvement in most cases of stenosis. Lumbar spinal stenosis (LSS) can involve either central or lateral spinal recesses. With lateral recess stenosis, the patient experiences compression of the nerve roots and may experience radicular symptoms of varying severity, including numbness in the toes with exercise. With central stenosis, compression of the spinal cord occurs and the patient will be more likely to fall, complaining of a sensation that his or her "legs go out" with physical activity or exercise. LSS is dynamic and is affected by movement. Both the neural canal and the neural foramen are narrowed when the spine is extended, and they are opened when the spine is in flexion. Therefore, the pain associated with the compression is most often temporary. Fortunately, in cases of LSS, the pain associated with the nerve compression induces patients to change positions and relieve nerve pressure generally before permanent neurologic damage can be done (Lieberman, 2004).

Epidemiology

Low back pain resulting from degenerative disease of the spine is a major cause of morbidity, disability, and lost productivity. Up to 90% of the US population may have significant low back pain at some point during their lifetime and approximately 5 million people are incapacitated as a result of lower back pain on a daily basis. According to Borenstein (2001), mechanical disorders of the spine cause more than 90% of all episodes of back and neck pain. The financial impact in terms of health care dollars and lost work hours reaches billions of dollars each year in this country. Moreover, with the aging of our population and a continually expanding number of people entering middle and later lives, the problem of back pain is reaching ever-increasing proportions.

In general, spinal stenosis is typically a disorder of older persons. Spinal stenosis affects men with slightly higher frequency than women. Although CSM is the most common form of spinal cord dysfunction in individuals older than 55 years of age, it is not the most common form of stenosis. Instead, about 75%

of cases of spinal stenosis occur in the lumbar area. Although symptomatic spinal stenosis is usually a disease of the middle-aged and the elderly, younger persons may also be affected.

Causes and Risk Factors

Narrowing of the spinal canal has many potential causes. A classification scheme proposed by Verbiest (1990), categorizes the multiple causes of lumbar stenosis into two major types: (a) conditions that lead to progressive bony encroachment of the lumbar canal, including developmental, congenital, acquired, and idiopathic, or (b) stenosis produced by nonosseous structures such as ligaments, intervertebral discs, and other soft tissue masses. For practical purposes, however, the etiologies of lumbar stenosis generally are divided into congenital or acquired forms.

Younger persons who develop spinal stenosis are usually those with congenitally narrow spinal canals. Narrowed or "shallow" spinal canals may be a result of congenitally short pedicles, thickened lamina and facets, or excessive scoliotic or lordotic curves. These anatomic changes often lead to clinically significant stenosis if additional elements such as herniated intervertebral discs or other space-occupying lesions further narrow the canal and contribute to the compression. However, few forms of spinal stenosis are truly congenital.

Although there are other potential causes for spinal stenosis, the most common is associated with age-related changes that affect the spine itself. With aging, the spinal ligaments and facet joints thicken, spurs may develop on the bones and protrude into the spinal canal, and vertebral disks may begin to deteriorate. Other causes include the following:

- Tumors of the spine
- Trauma
- Paget's disease of bone
- Osteoarthritis
- Rheumatoid arthritis
- Fluorosis

Common Presenting Signs and Symptoms

Spinal stenosis has an insidious onset. Symptoms may appear slowly and get worse over time and vary depending on the site of narrowing of the spinal canal. Spinal stenosis can occur at single or multiple levels, causing radiating lower extremity pain when walking or standing. Neurologic examination may reveal motor, sensory, or reflex abnormalities when the person is exercised to the point of developing neurogenic claudication.

Lumbar spinal stenosis is generally asymptomatic and not associated with neurologic abnormalities. However, LSS can also cause chronic low back pain, frequently lasting more than 12 weeks. Progression of the disorder causes increased narrowing of the spinal canal, resulting in stenosis and compression of neural elements. The clinical manifestation of spinal stenosis is neurogenic claudication, sometimes referred to as "pseudoclaudication." Symptoms of pseudoclaudication include leg and buttock pain brought on with activity that is alleviated by rest or maneuvers that increase spinal canal dimension, such as stooping forward to walk or resting a foot on a raised platform. The common denominator is changing the position of the spine from extension to flexion. Additional symptoms may include the following:

- Foot-slapping gait
- Frequent falling, clumsiness
- Lower extremity numbness, tingling, hot or cold feelings in the legs
- Weakness or a heavy and tired feeling in the legs
- Reflexes may be decreased, absent or normal, depending on the chronicity of the caudal root compression
- Hyperreflexia, clonus, and positive Babinski's sign in the lower extremities, especially if there is injury to the descending long tracts

Clinical symptoms of CSM may include the following:

- A history of peculiar sensations in the hands, associated with weakness and lack of coordination
- Numbness, weakness, cramping, or pain in the arms or legs
- Neck pain is mentioned by only one third of patients with CSM.
- Gait disturbances
- Spasticity
- Leg weakness
- Spontaneous leg movements
- Older patients may describe leg stiffness, foot shuffling, and a fear of falling.
- Incontinence is a late manifestation

In CSM, physical examination may reveal the following:

- Weakness of the appendages in association with spasticity and fasciculations
- Sensory deficits including decreased dermatome sensation and loss of proprioception and clonus in the upper and lower extremities
- Cauda equine syndrome is a serious condition that results from very serious narrowing. This syndrome occurs when there is pressure on nerves in the lower back. Symptoms may include the following:
  - Loss of bowel or bladder function
  - Erectile dysfunction
  - Pain, weakness, or loss of feeling in one or both legs

Differential Diagnoses

The list of differential diagnoses to consider when a person presents with the above mentioned signs and symptoms is substantial. The following represent a number of them:

- Muscular pain
- Herniated disc

- Compression fracture
- Degenerative joint disease
- Infectious diseases (osteomyelitis, epidural abscess, subacute bacterial endocarditis)
- Neural compression from neoplastic disease to bone
- Seronegative spondyloarthropathies
- Leaking aortic aneurysm
- Renal colic
- Spinal stenosis
- Peripheral vascular disease
- Trauma

Essential Diagnostic and Laboratory Tests

Diagnosis of spinal stenosis is best done by obtaining a focused history, observing the patient with regard to functional activities, and attempting to replicate pain via positioning. If possible, the clinician should attempt to perform a Phalen's test which is particularly useful in making the diagnosis of spinal stenosis (Borenstein, 2001). This test attempts to reproduce symptoms of leg pain, weakness, or numbness by causing neural ischemia. The patient is asked to stand in full extension for a minute. A positive test occurs if an increase in leg symptoms is noted, followed by a rapid relief of these symptoms by having the patient bend forward with hands on the examination table and one foot on a stool. Studies that will aid in making the diagnosis include the following:

- Plain radiographs of the spine
- Magnetic resonance imaging (MRI) without contrast
- Computerized axial tomography (CAT)
- Myelogram
- Bone scan

Plain radiographs reveal advanced degenerative disease with narrowed disc spaces, osteophytes, facet joint sclerosis, and cervical instability. Magnetic resonance imaging (MRI) without contrast should be done to make the final diagnosis and facilitate treatment options. MRI is useful in detecting the extent of spinal cord compression and the effects of compression on the integrity of the cord. The MRI can also help to differentiate spinal stenosis from other possible causes of back pain such as evidence of a spinal tumor or compression fracture. Combined MRI and CAT scan may be requested in some cases. A trefoil canal seen on CAT scan is virtually pathognomonic for LSS (Alvarez & Hardy, 2002).

Management Plan

Patients with spinal stenosis have pain that progresses over an extended period of time. Education about appropriate spinal biomechanics used in activities of daily living and those positions of the spine that exacerbate back and leg pain is a key component of treatment. Other pharmacologic and nonpharmacologic strategies for the treatment of spinal stenosis include the following:

Nonpharmacologic

Several nonpharmacological strategies may be implemented to treat the pain associated with stenosis and improve functioning although there are no randomized controlled trials to demonstrate the effectiveness of some of these treatments, and others demonstrated only modest efficacy (Tadokoro, Miyamoto, Sumi, & Shimomura, 2005):

- The following changes in posture may help people with spinal stenosis by enlarging the spinal canal and decompressing neural elements:
  - Flexing the spine by leaning forward while walking tends to relieve symptoms.
  - Lying with the knees drawn up to the chest also can offer some relief.

- As appropriate, patients should be encouraged to reduce weight to achieve a body mass index that is appropriate for their given age and gender.

- Back braces can be used for short periods of time (4 to 8 weeks) and may provide support while the patient regains mobility. This approach is sometimes used with patients who have weak abdominal muscles or older patients with degeneration at several levels of the spine (Lieberman, 2004).

- Alternative treatments such as acupuncture and acupressure

- Rest followed by a gradual resumption of activity

- Consider referrals for occupational and physical therapy.

Pharmacologic

- Nonopioid analgesic agents are usually the initial choice for treating pain associated with spinal stenosis, but opioid agents may be required if patients fail to adequately respond (Beers & Berkow, 2000).

- NSAIDs are useful in decreasing inflammation, soft tissue swelling, and neuronal compression. They should be used with caution, especially in the elderly, and may be needed for an extended period of time while improvement of function continues (Papadakis & McPhee, 2006).

- The utility of epidural corticosteroid injections into facet joints is questionable, as they tend to be more effective for radicular pain associated with herniated intervertebral discs than for spinal stenosis (Borenstein, 2001). However, they may be considered as an option for pain control if medications are not fully relieving symptoms. Epidural injections may be repeated in 4 to 6 months if good response is achieved (AGS Panel on Persistent Pain in Older Persons, 2002).

Surgical

Spinal decompression by surgery may be indicated if a patient does not respond to conservative approaches or if function is severely compromised. Surgery may also be warranted when there is documentation of herniation by an imaging procedure, a consistent pain syndrome, and a consistent neurological deficit (Papadakis & McPhee, 2006). Surgical consultation is needed urgently for any patient with a large or evolving neurological deficit. The following surgical procedures have been shown to be effective in relieving pain and improving symptoms (Gelalis et al., 2005; Chang, Singer, Wu, Keller, & Atlas, 2005):

- Laminectomy

- Decompressive laminarthrectomy

- Microdiskectomy

- Laminoplasty

Patient, Family, and Staff Education

- Explain natural history and management options for spinal stenosis.

- Explain benefit of exercise and an activity program.

- Explain strategies to protect the back in daily activities.

- Educate on importance of weight reduction, if indicated.

Physician Consultation

- If symptoms and signs suggest epidural or spinal abscess, cauda equine syndrome, or new metastatic cancer (Papadakis and McPhee, 2006)

- If patient is a candidate for surgery, refer to orthopedic surgeon for joint surgery.

- Consider referral to rheumatologist if joint pain persists or response to treatment is inadequate.

SEIZURES

Definition

A seizure is a brief, paroxysmal clinical event characterized by the following:

- Loss of consciousness
- Altered state of consciousness
- Cessation of motor activity
- Abnormal motor activity, abnormal sensory perceptions
- Loss of bladder and bowel control

Each manifestation may occur alone or in combination with any or all of the others. The condition may be referred to as a seizure disorder or epilepsy when seizures are recurrent.

A seizure disorder is a manifestation of underlying brain dysfunction, not a disease entity. Therefore, any person with a seizure disorder requires careful diagnostic evaluation to determine the etiology. A specific cause can be found in 50% of both adult-onset and childhood onset seizures.

Seizures can be divided into two broad groups, according to their etiology: (a) unprovoked, idiopathic, or primary epilepsy, in which etiology or cause is unknown because no structural abnormalities of the brain can be detected, and (b) provoked, symptomatic, or secondary epilepsy, in which there is a structural or metabolic disruption of the neuronal membranes that is genetic, acquired, or environmentally induced. Seventy-five percent of seizures are idiopathic and 25% are symptomatic (Yamamoto, Olaes, & Lopez, 2004).

Epidemiology

Epilepsy and seizures affect approximately 2.5 million Americans. An estimated 10% of Americans will experience a seizure, and approximately 3% will have a diagnosis of epilepsy by age 80. The onset of epilepsy is most common during childhood and after age 65, but the condition can occur at any age (Chang & Lowenstein, 2003).

One in 100 adults is diagnosed with epilepsy. The incidence increases over the age of 65. Approximately 600,000 people over the age of 65 have a seizure disorder, and 33% over 75 years of age have had at least one seizure. This results in an estimated annual cost of $12.5 billion in medical care and accounts for 8.4 million office visits annually (Schachter, 2002, 2004).

Susceptibility to seizures is determined by a complex interplay between genetic factors and acquired brain disorders. The most likely cause of seizure disorders relates to the age at onset. Idiopathic epilepsy onset is usually between the ages of 5 and 20 years and is rarely initiated after the age of 25 years. Thus, beyond 25 years of age, generalized seizures may often come from some identifiable cause. However, in the adult population, the etiology of seizures varies remarkably. Etiology of seizures is outlined in Table 14-8.

TABLE 14-8   Etiology of Seizures in Older Adults

   I. Idiopathic
  II. Structural
    A. Degenerative disease
    B. Neoplasm
    C. Scar from birth trauma, other head trauma, anoxic damage, infection
 III. Metabolic
    A. Hypoglycemia
    B. Hyperosmolar state
    C. Hyponatremia
    D. Hypomagnesia
    E. Hypoxia
    F. Uremia
    G. Thyroid disease
    H. Nutritional deficiency
 IV. Toxin
    A. Alcohol
    B. Drug withdrawal
    C. Drug overdose
  V. Vascular
    A. Subdural hematoma
    B. Epidural hematoma
    C. Intraparenchymal hematoma
    D. Stroke
    E. Subarachnoid hemorrhage
    F. Arteriovenous malformation
 VI. Eclampsia

The most common origins of seizures are tumors, infarctions, alcohol and substance abuse or withdrawals, and acute infections. Head trauma is one of the most usual causes of epilepsy in younger adults, especially when it is associated with skull fracture or intracerebral or subdural hematoma. With severe closed head injuries, seizures occur in about 5.5% of persons (Yamamoto, Olaes, & Lopez, 2004).

In almost half (49%) of all seizures in older adults, the cause is unknown. However, by far, the most common underlying etiology in this age group is cerebrovascular. Approximately 4–14% of infarcts are associated with seizures within the first one to two weeks, and up to 10% are associated with seizures two weeks or more after the acute insult (Schachter, 2002, 2004). Other known causes of seizures in older adults include neurodegenerative diseases such as Alzheimer's dementia, trauma, tumors; and metabolic disorders such as uremia, hyperglycemia, hypoglycemia, hyponatremia, alcohol withdrawal, or infection (Velez & Selwa, 2004).

Common Presenting Signs and Symptoms

Because abnormal brain cell activity causes seizures, having a seizure can result in the sudden occurrence of any activity that is coordinated by the brain. This can include temporary confusion, complete loss of consciousness, a staring spell, or uncontrollable, jerking movements of the arms and legs. Signs and symptoms may vary depending on the type of seizure. Most people with epilepsy experience the same type of seizure, with similar symptoms, each time they have a seizure, but others may experience a wide range of types and symptoms.

Seizures are classified as either partial or generalized, based on the origin of the epileptogenic focus. Partial seizures occur when a discharge begins as a single focus in one localized area of the cortex and produces abnormalities in one area of the electroencephalogram (EEG). Generalized seizures begin bilaterally in both hemispheres of the cerebral cortex without an exciting focus and show diffuse EEG abnormalities. Seizure classification is outlined in Table 14-9.

TABLE 14-9   Seizure Classification

SEIZURE TYPE	KEY FEATURES	OTHER FEATURES
Partial seizures	*Involvement of only restricted part of the brain; may become secondarily generalized*	
Simple partial	Consciousness preserved	May be manifested by focal motor, sensory, or autonomic symptoms
Complex partial	Consciousness impaired	Above symptoms may precede, accompany, or follow other symptoms that may include involuntary laughter, screaming, bicycling motions, and sexually suggestive movements.
Generalized seizures	*Diffuse involvement of brain at onset*	
Absence	Consciousness impaired briefly; patient often unaware of attacks	May be clonic, tonic, or atonic components; autonomic components; or accompanying automatisms. Almost always begin in childhood and frequently cease by age 20.
Atypical absences	May be more gradual onset and termination than typical absence	More marked changes in tone may occur
Myoclonic	Single or multiple myoclonic jerks	
Tonic-clonic	Tonic phase: sudden loss of consciousness, with rigidity and arrest of respirations, lasting < 1 minute. Clonic phase: jerking occurs, usually for < 2–3 minutes. Flaccid coma: variable duration	May be accompanied by tongue biting, incontinence, or aspiration; commonly followed by postictal confusion variable in duration .
Status epilepticus	Repeated seizures without recovery between them; a fixed and enduring epileptic condition lasting 30 minutes	

The three subclassifications of partial seizures include: (a) simple seizures, (b) complex seizures, and (c) secondary generalized seizures. Simple partial seizures begin from a small area in the brain, usually last no longer than 10 seconds, and do not result in loss of consciousness. Complex partial seizures also begin from a small area of the brain but result in alterations in consciousness and usually cause disturbances in higher-level functions such as memory, thought processes, and complex motor behavior. These seizures vary in duration from 5 seconds up to 2 minutes. Secondary generalized seizures are partial seizures with secondary generalization. These seizures occur when simple or complex seizures spread to involve the entire cerebral cortex.

Generalized epilepsy makes up only about one third of all classified cases. They typically last from a few seconds to 5 minutes, rarely longer. The most common types of generalized seizures are: (a) tonic-clonic (grand mal), (b) myoclonic seizures, (c) absence (petit mal), and (d) atypical seizures.

Primary generalized seizures are rare in older patients and tend to occur in people with a past history of tonic-clonic seizures. Elderly persons with epilepsy nearly always have partial seizures, and complex partial seizure cases occur most often. Moreover, the clinical manifestations of complex partial seizures in this age group remain to be fully characterized. Behaviors such as confusion, disorientation, and unresponsive staring may be both subtle and quite prolonged. Some ictal behaviors in the elderly, such as orofacial automatisms, rubbing, tapping, stroking, disrobing, and wandering, may have different causes and can lead to misdiagnosis. Many people with some degree of dementia who live in long-term care settings may manifest similar behaviors from time to time, and it is not uncommon for complex partial seizures in these patients to be mistaken for features of dementia (Schachter, 2002, 2004).

Nonepileptic seizures (NES) are also a frequent problem in elderly patients. Compared with a younger control group, physiologic NES (transient ischemic attack (TIA) or stroke, movement and sleep disorders) and psychogenic NES (somatoform, anxiety, and mood disorders; reinforced behavior patterns) are equally frequent in the elderly. Unlike seizures in children that originate from temporal lobe foci, seizures in older adults tend to be from frontal or parietal lobe foci. These individuals generally present with an altered mental state, staring, blackouts, and confusion. In addition, it is not unusual for an older adult to have a simple partial seizure and present with numbness in a hand or leg (Kellinghaus, Loddenkemper, Dinner, Lachhwani, & Luders, 2004).

In older adults, the postictal state is prolonged in 14% of cases and may last even longer than 24 hours. After even a brief seizure, older patients may experience a prolonged state of confusion, temporary paralysis, or be at increased risk of falls for up to 7 days. As a result, seizures can have a significant impact on quality of life among these individuals (Schachter, 2002, 2004).

Because the possible causes of seizures are many, clinicians are advised to conduct a comprehensive seizure assessment and perform several diagnostic tests. A comprehensive seizure assessment involves collecting a detailed history from the patient and eye witnesses that includes the following:

- A description of past and present seizure events
- An exploration of risks and predisposing factors
- Past and present medical conditions and treatments

Moreover, because syncope, transient ischemic attack (TIA), transient global amnesia (TGA), or vertigo are commonly noted to mimic seizure and complicate the differential diagnosis, the length of the episode in question is particularly important information to help with the differential diagnosis.

- A seizure is believed to last approximately a minute.
- Syncope is briefer than seizure, usually lasts for less than a minute, and tends to be reproducible in the office setting.
- The TIA lasts several minutes to hours. Like TIA, TGA typically lasts for hours rather than minutes (Resnick, 2004).

A complete physical examination should be performed with a special focus on a neurological evaluation.

Differential Diagnoses

There are many conditions that may result in abnormal movements, sensations, or loss of awareness, but are not associated with an abnormal electrical discharge in the brain. These various disorders can be confused with seizures, and care must be taken to distinguish between them and actual seizure disorders. Common diagnoses that should be considered when developing a differential for persons having seizures include the following:

- Syncope
- Cardiac arrhythmias
- Stroke or transient ischemic attacks

TABLE 14-10   Differential Diagnoses of Seizure According to Adult Age
Early adulthood (18–25)
Idiopathic
Drug and alcohol withdrawal
Trauma
Middle age (25–60)
Drug and alcohol withdrawal
Trauma
Tumor
Vascular disease
Late adulthood (over 60)
Vascular disease
Tumor
Degenerative disease
Metabolic

- Pseudoseizures
- Panic attacks
- Migraines
- Narcolepsy

A detailed history and physical can usually distinguish among these various conditions. Another helpful way to generate differential diagnoses for patients who are having seizures is to consider the most likely causes of seizures according to age. Differential diagnoses according to age are outlined in Table 14-10.

Essential Diagnostic and Laboratory Tests

Laboratory evaluation should include a complete blood count and comprehensive metabolic panel. Additional tests can be used to further establish the diagnosis, including the following:

- Complete blood count
- Complete metabolic panel
- Anticonvulsant levels
- Drug and toxic screens
- Serologic testing for syphilis
- Computerized tomography
- Magnetic resonance imaging (MRI)
- Electroencephalograph (EEG)
- Repeated Holter monitoring may be necessary to establish the diagnosis of cardiac arrhythmias.

Management Plan

Goals for the management of seizures are to prevent reoccurrences, avoid adverse drug reactions, and maintain patient's safety and quality of life.

The decision to initiate treatment with medication for a seizure should be based on evidence of recurrent seizures, onset of epilepsy as status epilepticus, or a clear structural predisposition for seizures (Ramsay, Rowan, & Pryor,

2004). Medication should likely be initiated if the individual has seizures that impact quality of life.

Nonpharmacologic

- Routine patient monitoring for response to treatment regimen

- Regular monitoring of anticonvulsant levels

- CBC and complete metabolic panel as indicated

- Monitoring medication side effects and adverse drug reactions

- *Surgery*—Many academic centers are finding success with stereotactic surgery for seizures that fail conventional therapy. However, surgery is most commonly done when tests show that seizures originate in a small, well-defined area, or focus, in the temporal lobes or the frontal lobes of the cerebral cortex. Surgery is rarely an option if a patient has seizures that start in several areas of the brain or if seizures originate from a region of the brain that contains vital brain functions. Although many people continue to need some medication to help prevent seizures after surgery, most require fewer drugs at reduced dosages. Surgical risks include permanent alteration of cognitive abilities and personality (Aminoff, 2006a).

- Other treatment options for epilepsy include ketogenic diets and vagus nerve stimulation (Aminoff, 2006a).

Pharmacologic

Pharmacologic interventions are the primary management of seizure disorders, and treatment choices are generally based on seizure type, individual needs, existence of co-occurring diseases, and specific drug profiles (Velez & Selwa, 2004). However, the newest antiepileptic agents, such as gabapentin, lamotrigine, oxcarbazepine, and topiramate, are widely being recommended as first treatment options because of their more favorable side effect profiles (Ramsay, Rowan, & Pryor, 2004). With regard to drug dosing, clinicians are recommended to start low and go slow, monitoring drug response in terms of prevention of seizures. Extended-release formulations may be helpful for drug adherence.

Evaluation and treatment of seizures should be geared toward helping individuals obtain and maintain optimal quality of life through seizure elimination balanced by tolerance of the medication. Most people with epilepsy can become free of their seizures by using a single antiepileptic drug. For others, medication can make seizures less frequent and less intense. Many adults can discontinue medication after two or more years without seizures (Blanchard & Toffler, 2006).

Finding the right medication and dosage can be complex. It might take more than one drug or trying several different drugs until the right one is found. Although the initial management plan will be developed in consultation with the primary physician or neurologist, the nurse practitioner should consider the following factors when initiating or maintaining drug therapy:

- Anticonvulsant drug treatment is generally not required for a single seizure unless further attacks occur or investigations reveal some underlying untreatable pathology.

- Treatment with anticonvulsant drugs is generally not required for alcohol withdrawal seizures because they are self-limited.

- Drug dose is generally increased until seizures are controlled or unwanted side effects occur.

- Optimal dosage is based on prevention of seizure and not on reaching therapeutic drug levels.

- If seizures continue despite treatment at maximum dose, a second drug is added and the first drug is gradually withdrawn.

- A combination of two drugs may be indicated when two or more single drug regimens have been tried without success.

- Discontinue medication only when the patient is seizure free for at least 3 years.

- Dose reduction should be gradual over a period of weeks or months.
- Reinstitute previous drugs if seizures recur.
- Order a bone densitometry for older adult patients on long-term antiepileptic drug therapy to evaluate risk of osteoporosis. Treat osteopenia and osteoporosis.

In general, anticonvulsant medications include the following:

- Phenytoin (Dilantin, Phenytek)
- Carbamazepine (Carbatrol, Tegretol)
- Valproic acid (Depakene)
- Divalproex (Depakote)
- Levetiracetam (Keppra)
- Gabapentin (Neurontin)
- Phenobarbital
- Ethosuximide (Zarontin)
- Clonazepam (Klonopin)
- Primidone (Mysoline)
- Oxcarbazepine (Trileptal)
- Lamotrigine (Lamictal)
- Topiramate (Topamax)
- Felbamate (Felbatol)
- Tiagabine (Gabitril)
- Zonisamide (Zonegran)

For prolonged or cluster seizures, sedatives such as diazepam (Diastat, Valium) or lorazepam (Ativan, Lorazepam, Intensol) may be prescribed. Caution must be used when prescribing sedatives because of the potential for falls, especially in older adults. Commonly used medications for seizure management and related information are listed in Table 14-11.

TABLE 14-11   Commonly Used Medications for Seizure Management

DRUG & DOSAGES	SIDE EFFECTS	SEIZURE INDICATION	ADVANTAGES	DISADVANTAGES
Phenytoin 200–400 mg daily	Osteoporosis Rash Slowed thinking	Partial; generalized tonic-clonic	Low cost	Many side effects; drug and food and nutrient interactions
Carbamazepine 600–1200 mg two to three times daily	Osteoporosis Rash	Partial; general tonic-clonic	Minimal sedation and cognitive adverse effects	Many drug interactions; may exacerbate myoclonic seizures
Valproic acid 1500–2000 mg three times daily	Thrombocytopenia, nausea, vomiting, diarrhea, tremor	Partial; generalized tonic-clonic; absence; myoclonic	Broad spectrum efficacy	Extensive protein binding; multiple drug interactions
Gabapentin 900–1800 mg three times daily	Fatigue	Partial; generalized tonic-clonic	No hepatic metabolism; drug interaction only with antacids	Dosage modification in renal disease; weight loss, sedation, fatigue
Tiagabine 32–56 mg twice daily	Slowed thinking Fatigue	Partial; generalized tonic-clonic	None	Dosage modification in liver disease
Lamotrigine 100–500 mg twice daily	Prolonged half-life Rash	Partial; generalized tonic-clonic	Interaction with antiepileptic drugs only	Dosage modification in liver disease
Topiramate 200–400 twice daily	Renal stones Slowed thinking	Partial; generalized tonic-clonic	Interaction with antiepileptic drugs only	Weight loss; dosage modification if creatinine clearance is < 60 mL/minute

Note: Refer to manufacturer's profile of each drug for specific contraindications, precautions, and significant possible interactions.

Patient, Family, and Staff Education

Patient, family and staff will benefit from education that enables them to more confidently and competently support and care for persons with seizure disorders or epilepsy. Information that should be shared with families and staff might include the following points:

- Complications of recurrent seizures that place the person with the seizure disorder and others at risk of physical harm (e.g., falls, driving accidents)
- Life-threatening complications from epilepsy are uncommon, but do occur. People who have severe, prolonged, or continuous seizures (status epilepticus) are at increased risk of permanent brain damage and death.
- If you see someone having a seizure, call for medical help immediately and then follow these steps:
  - Gently roll the person onto one side and put something soft under his or her head.
  - Loosen tight neckwear.
  - Do not put your fingers or anything else in the person's mouth. The tongue cannot be swallowed, and you can cause harm to the person having a seizure or to yourself by trying to put something in his or her mouth.
  - Do not try to restrain the person or shake or shout at him or her. If the person is moving, remove dangerous objects from his or her path.
  - Stay with the person until medical personnel arrive. If possible, observe the person closely so that you can provide details on his or her signs and symptoms and how long the seizure lasted

After assessing a patient's capacity and interest in learning about their seizure disorder, the clinician may want to discuss the following points, especially if the patient will reside in an independent living situation:

- Maintenance of overall health by getting adequate rest, eating a balanced diet, performing regular exercise, and managing stress effectively
- Importance of medication adherence
- Avoidance of alcohol and recreational drugs
- Use of medical alert bracelets stating who to contact in an emergency and antiseizure medications
- Maintenance of a detailed seizure record
- Consider modifying activities that involve driving, swimming, and heights.
- Maintain a strong support system.
- Set reasonable goals.

Physician Consultation

Physician referrals are not necessary each time a patient with a known diagnosis of epilepsy has a seizure, as long as nurse practitioners are comfortable treating patients when seizures occur. It may be prudent to seek medical advice in the following circumstances:

- Patient's first seizure
- Seizures lasting more than five minutes
- Patient recovery from seizure is slow
- Second seizure follows immediately
- Patients with poorly controlled diabetes
- Signs of injury or illness are present.
- Seizures change in frequency and severity.
- Patient complains of a change in the way they typically feel during and after the seizures occur.
- Seizure is preceded by a sudden, severe headache or other signs and symptoms of stroke.
- Seizure occurs after medication changes.

Most persons who experience seizures do not need to be hospitalized. The following circumstances support hospital admission for persons experiencing seizures:

• Status epilepticus
• Video monitoring unit to distinguish pseudoseizures from epileptic seizures
• If surgery is contemplated

STROKE

Definition

The term *cerebrovascular disease* refers to disorders of the arterial or venous circulatory systems of the central nervous system. The term *stroke*, sometimes called a brain attack, is used when the symptoms begin abruptly, either as a result of inadequate blood flow (ischemic stroke) or hemorrhage into the brain tissue (parenchyma hemorrhage) or surrounding subarachnoid space (subarachnoid hemorrhage). Approximately 80% of strokes are ischemic in origin. Focal ischemic stroke is caused by either thrombotic or embolic occlusion of a major artery, whereas global ischemia usually results from inadequate cerebral perfusion such as that which occurs after cardiac arrest or ventricular fibrillation.

For years, strokes have been subdivided pathologically into infarcts (thrombotic or embolic) and hemorrhagic and clinical criteria between these possibilities have been emphasized. However, it is often difficult to determine on clinical grounds the pathologic basis for stroke. Major stroke subtypes include the following:

• Ischemic
  ○ Lacunar infarct
  ○ Carotid circulation obstruction
  ○ Vertebrobasilar occlusion
• Hemorrhagic stroke
  ○ Spontaneous intracranial bleed
  ○ Subarachnoid hemorrhage
  ○ Intracranial aneurysm
  ○ Arteriovenous malformations (AVMs)

Epidemiology

Stroke remains the third leading cause of death and the second most frequent cause of morbidity in developed countries. In the United States, stroke remains the third leading cause of death, despite a general decline in the incidence of stroke in the last 30 years. Since 1990, only heart disease and cancer cause more deaths annually. Every year about 700,000 Americans experience a stroke and about 160,000 of these people die. Twenty-seven percent of those die within one month, 10% of stroke survivors make complete recoveries, 10% are severely and permanently disabled, and 80% have significant deficits that affect their ability to live independently (Counihan, 2001). The cost of care for patients with stroke has been estimated at $20 billion per year. Stroke is the most common medical condition leading to medical rehabilitation services (Rodin, Saliba, & Brunmel-Smith, 2006).

Since 1990, the incidence of stroke in the United States has declined by about 1.5% annually to about 0.5 to 1.0 per thousand people, accounting for about 1 in every 15 deaths. It is believed that this steady decrease is the result of improvements in general public health and is coincident with the decline of cardiovascular deaths and better control of hypertension and other risk factors. Rates of stroke among men and women are similar, although the incidence and rate of mortality from stroke are higher in African-Americans than Caucasians (Hachinski, 2006).

Although the reasons for the decline in the incidence of stroke remain somewhat unclear, a greater understanding of the importance of controlling risk factors in stroke prevention may in part be responsible. The increasingly successful management of hypertension and the reduction in smoking habits have been major factors in reducing the incidence of stroke. In addition, the increasing public awareness of the warning symptoms of stroke as constituting a brain attack (analogous to chest pain as a warning of a "heart attack") is beginning to improve primary stroke prevention (Counihan, 2001).

Causes and Risk Factors

Cerebral ischemia may result from thrombotic or embolic occlusion of a major vessel that reduces blood flow within the involved vascular territory, or it may be a consequence of diminished systemic perfusion. Prolonged brain ischemia results in infarction characterized histologically by necrosis of neurons, glia, and endothelial cells.

Global cerebral ischemia usually results from cardiac arrest or ventricular fibrillation. Some neuronal populations are selectively vulnerable to transient global ischemia inducing so-called laminar necrosis. Pure hypoxia causes cerebral dysfunction, manifested clinically as lethargy and confusion, but rarely produces irreversible brain injury unless accompanied by other factors such as hypoglycemia. When neurons are rendered ischemic, a number of biochemical changes take place: intracellular membranes are no longer able to control ion fluxes, which leads to increased intracellular concentrations of calcium and arrest of mitochondrial function. Activation of membrane lipases further compromises membrane integrity and leads to release of excitatory neurotransmitters, which in turn may further exacerbate tissue injury. If blood is restored within 15 minutes, the effects of these events may be reversible.

Cerebral ischemia due to atherosclerosis of the cerebral vasculature accounts for two thirds of all strokes, either through embolization of plaque into distal vessels (artery-to-artery embolus) or by in situ thrombosis. Cardiogenic emboli make up the majority of the remaining third of ischemic strokes, arising most commonly as a result of atrial fibrillation. Mural thrombi, vascular vegetations, and atrial myxomas are also potential sources of emboli, as are paradoxical emboli of venous origin passing through a patent foramen ovale. Causes of cerebral ischemia and hemorrhagic strokes and causes of strokes in young adults are summarized in Tables 14-12, 14-13, and 14-14. Many factors can increase stroke risk. Risk factors for ischemic stroke are listed in Table 14-15.

TABLE 14-12   Causes of Cerebral Ischemia

Focal
- Mural abnormalities
- Atherosclerosis
- Vasculitis
- Vasospasm (migraine, subarachnoid hemorrhage)
- Compression (by tumor, aneurysm)
- Fibromuscular dysplasia/Moyamoya
- Dissection (spontaneous, traumatic)

Embolism
- Cardiogenic (atrial fibrillation, mural thrombus, myxoma, valvular vegetations)
- Artery-to-artery
- Fat
- Air
- Paradoxical

Hematologic
- Hypercoagulable state
- Sickle cell disease
- Homocystinuria
- Antiphospholipid antibodies (lupus anticoagulant, anticardiolipin antibodies)
- Protein C or protein S deficiency

Global
- Hypoperfusion
- Cardiac arrest
- Ventricular fibrillation

TABLE 14-13   Causes of Spontaneous Intracerebral Hemorrhage

Intraparenchymal Hemorrhage
- Trauma
- Hypertension
- Amyloid angiopathy
- Arteriovenous malformation
- Bleeding diathesis (anticoagulants, thrombolytics)
- Drugs (amphetamines, cocaine)

Subarachnoid Hemorrhage
- Congenital saccular aneurysm (85%)
- Unknown

Common Presenting Signs and Symptoms

Signs and symptoms of stroke are varied and relate to the mechanism of the stroke and to location of the lesion. Cerebral arterial circulation derives from four major extracerebral arteries.

TABLE 14-14   Causes of Stroke in Young Adults

General factors
- Migraine
- Arterial dissection
- Drugs (cocaine, heroin, oral contraceptives)
- Premature atherosclerosis (homocystinuria, hyperlipidemia)
- Postpartum angiopathy

Cardiac factors
- Atrial septal defect
- Patent foramen ovale
- Mitral valve prolapse
- Endocarditis

Hematologic factors
- Deficiency states (antithrombin Ill, protein S, protein C)
- Disseminated intravascular coagulation
- Thrombotic thrombocytopenic purpura inflammatory

Inflammatory factors
- Systemic lupus erythematosus
- Polyarteritis nodosa
- Neurosyphilis
- Cryoglobulinemia

Other factors
- Fibromuscular dysplasia
- Moyamoya syndrome

TABLE 14-15   Risk Factors for Ischemic Stroke

- Advanced age
- Male gender
- Diabetes
- Hypertension
- Smoking
- Family history of premature vascular disease
- Hyperlipidemia
- Atrial fibrillation
- History of transient ischemic attack (TIA)
- History of recent myocardial infarction
- Severe carotid stenosis
- History of congestive heart failure (left ventricular ejection fraction < 25%)
- Drugs (sympathomimetics, oral contraceptives, cocaine)

Paired internal carotid arteries (ICAs) bring blood from the heart along the front of the neck, and paired vertebral arteries bring blood from the heart along the back of the neck inside the spinal column. The major components of cerebral vasculature and defects that occur when these pathways are interrupted are summarized in Table 14-16. Features of major hemorrhagic stroke subtypes are outlined in Table 14-17.

Evaluation of the patient with a suspected stroke should seek to answer two questions: "What is the mechanism of the stroke?" and "Where is the lesion?" Useful elements of the history include the time of the onset of symptoms and the temporal course and progression of the symptoms. The type of activities and the presence of associated symptoms are also useful to determine, as is the presence of stroke risk factors.

The physical examination determines lesion location, as well as identifies clues to pathogenesis. Components of the physical examination that are particularly important when a person presents with a suspected stroke include the following:

- Thorough cardiovascular assessment, including measurement of blood pressure and cardiac rhythm, is essential.
- Thorough neuromuscular examination including mental status assessment, motor and sensory evaluation, assessment of cranial nerves and reflexes
- Palpation of the facial arteries may reveal reversal of flow, which indicates ICA occlusion.
- Auscultation of the neck for carotid bruits

Ophthalmoscopy can detect platelet and cholesterol emboli, as well as give information about the chronicity and severity of systemic hypertension; papilledema may accompany cerebral venous occlusion.

Transient Ischemic Attacks
Transient ischemic attacks (TIA) need to be distinguished from other paroxysmal events

TABLE 14-16   Clinical Manifestations of Ischemic Stroke

MAJOR VESSEL	AREAS SUPPLIED	DEFECTS
Anterior Circulation		
Internal carotid arteries (ICA)	Retinas, lateral and medial hemisphere surfaces	Visual impairment or ipsilateral blindness, contralateral motor/sensory disturbances
Middle cerebral artery (MCA)	Lateral portions of hemispheres; motor and sensory to face, upper extremities, and speech centers	Contralateral motor/sensory loss (face/arm > leg), dysphagia or aphasia, spatial/perceptual problems, homonymous hemianopsia
Anterior cerebral arteries (ACA)	Medial and superior surfaces; motor and sensory for lower extremities; large portions of frontal lobe	Contralateral motor/sensory loss (leg > arm), confusion & perceptual problems, personality changes
Posterior Circulation		
Vertebral artery (VA), posterior area inferior cerebral artery (PICA), basilar artery (BA), superior cerebellar artery (SCA), posterior cerebral (PCA) artery	Multiple branches supply brain stem (medulla oblongata, pons, mid brain) and cerebellum	Varied signs and symptoms depending on of brain stem involved: VA/PICA—Ipsilateral facial sensory loss, hemiataxia, nystagmus, Horner's syndrome SCA—Gait ataxia, nausea, vertigo, dysarthria BA—Quadriparesis, dysarthria, dysphagia, diplopia, somnolence, amnesia, often fatal PCA—Contralateral homonymous hemianopsia, amnesia, sensory loss

TABLE 14-17   Features of the Major Hemorrhagic Stroke Subtypes

STROKE TYPE	CLINICAL FEATURES
Spontaneous intracerebral hemorrhage	Commonly associated with hypertension or bleeding disorders and amyloid angioplasty Usually occurs suddenly and without warning, often during activity Consciousness is initially lost in 50% of patients, vomiting is frequent at onset Focal signs and symptoms follow depending on site of bleed: Basal ganglia—Severe headache, normal pupils, normal eye movements, hemiparesis, confusion and aphasia Thalamus—Moderate headache; small, poorly reactive pupils; hyperconvergent eye movements with absent vertical gaze; hemisensory > motor loss; hypersomnolence Pons—Severe headache; pupils small and reactive; horizontal gaze paresis; quadriplegia; coma Cerebellum—Severe occipital headache; normal pupils; normal eye movements; ataxia, early vomiting
Subarachnoid hemorrhage	Presents with sudden onset of worst headache of life, may rapidly lead to loss of consciousness; signs of meningeal irritation often present; etiology usually aneurysm or AVM, but 20% have no identified source
Intracranial aneurysm	Most located in the anterior circle of Willis and are typically asymptomatic until bleed occurs; 20% bleed again in the first 2 weeks
Arteriovenous malformation	Focal deficit from hematoma or bleed itself
Cerebellar hemorrhage	Sudden onset of nausea and vomiting, disequilibrium, severe occipital headache, and loss of consciousness that may terminate fatally within 48 hours

affecting the nervous system. Recognition of TIAs and proper treatment is essential in order to prevent stroke. TIAs are focal, ischemic, cerebral neurological deficits that last for less than 24 hours. Deficits usually last for a few minutes and in most cases, signs and symptoms disappear within 1 to 2 hours. Embolization is an important etiology and may explain why separate attacks affect different parts of the territory supplied by the same vessel. Cerebrovascular sources of TIA must also be considered.

About 30% of people who have a stroke have a history of TIAs. The incidence of stroke is not related to the number or duration of individual TIAs but is increased in patients with hypertension or diabetes. The risk of stroke is highest one month following a TIA and then progressively declines.

The signs and symptoms of TIAs resemble those found early in a stroke and vary markedly among patients, but tend to be consistent in a given individual. TIAs in the carotid territory may manifest with the following:

- Contralateral weakness or heaviness of the arm, leg, face, singly or in combination
- Numbness or paresthesias may occur either as the sole manifestation or in combination with motor deficits.
- Dysphagia
- Sudden blindness in one or both eyes or double vision
- A carotid bruit or cardiac abnormality may be present.

Vertebrobasilar TIAs may manifest with the following:

- Vertigo
- Ataxia
- Diplopia
- Dysarthria
- Dimness or blurring of vision
- Weakness or sensory complaints on one, both or alternating sides of the body
- Drop attacks due to bilateral leg weakness

Complications of Stroke

- Neurologic complications of stroke include stroke progression, seen in over 25% of patients.
- Seizures can occur in up to 10% of patients at some point after stroke and are more common after subarachnoid or intracerebral hemorrhage and large lesions involving the cerebral cortex.
- Increased intracranial pressure (ICP) is the most lethal poststroke complication and may be a direct effect of a hematoma or brain edema. Signs and symptoms of raised ICP include depressed level of consciousness, pupillary asymmetry, abducens nerve palsy, papilledema, and periodic breathing.
- Medical complications after stroke include cardiac arrhythmias, myocardial infarction, pulmonary embolism, pneumonia, urinary tract infection, and gastrointestinal bleeding (Zweifler, 2003)
- Review code status and intensity of care issues in patients experiencing complications following a stroke. Discuss need for transfer back to the acute hospital and/or emergency 911 services with physician when indicated.

Differential Diagnoses

The acute onset of a stroke generally distinguishes it from other brain lesions although hemorrhage into primary or metastatic tumor may manifest in a strokelike fashion. Strokes and seizures may coexist, and 10% of strokes are associated with seizures at time of onset. As a general rule, stroke rarely manifests with an alteration in consciousness unless there are other signs of brain dysfunction. The differential diagnoses for ischemic strokes are summarized as follows:

- Hypoglycemia
- Transient ischemic attacks
- Intracranial hemorrhage or other mass lesion
- Focal seizure

- Migraine
- Peripheral causes of vertigo

The differential diagnoses of hemorrhagic strokes include the following:

- Ischemic stroke
- Subarachnoid hemorrhage
- Space-occupying lesion
- Subdural or epidural hemorrhage

Essential Diagnostic and Laboratory Tests

Ancillary laboratory and other tests include the following (Aminoff, 2006b):

- Complete blood count and platelet count
- Sedimentation rate
- Glucose
- Coagulation screen
- Lipid profile
- Serologic test for syphilis
- Homocysteine
- Blood cultures if endocarditis is suspected
- ECG to help exclude a cardiac arrhythmia or recent myocardial infarction that might be the source of the emboli
- Holter monitoring if paroxysmal cardiac arrhythmia is suspected
- Examination of cerebral spinal fluid is not always necessary but may be useful if there is diagnostic uncertainty; it should be delayed until after CT.

Recommended imaging studies include the following (Aminoff, 2006b):

- CT scanning without contrast is important for excluding or confirming hemorrhage and if present, for determining the size and site of the hematoma.
- CT is superior to MRI for detecting intracranial hemorrhage of less than 48 hours' duration.

- Carotid duplex studies, MRI, and MR angiography may also be necessary.
- Diffusion-weighted MRI is more sensitive than standard MRI in detecting ischemia.
- If the patient's condition permits further intervention, cerebral angiography may reveal an aneurysm or AVM.
- Echocardiography with bubble contrast if heart disease is suspected
- Carotid duplex ultrasonography can detect significant stenosis of the internal carotid artery.

Management Plan

In most cases, getting prompt medical treatment for stroke is important. Specific treatment will depend on the type of stroke. To treat an ischemic stroke, arterial obstruction must be removed and blood flow to the brain restored.

Acute Phase Care

Persons who have sustained a massive stroke from which meaningful recovery is unlikely should receive palliative care (Aminoff, 2006b). In other cases, the goals of acute ischemic stroke management are to limit size of infarct, prevent and treat complications, and prevent recurrences. The following strategies are recommended for the management of patients during the acute phase (Meschia, 2000):

- Intravenous thrombolytic therapy with tissue plasminogen activator (t-PA) is effective in reducing neurologic deficit in selected patients without CT evidence of hemorrhage when administered within 3 hours after onset of ischemic stroke. The agent carries a 6–7% risk of intracerebral hemorrhage, but a 33% chance for functional improvement to independence at 3 months after stroke onset (Bath, 2002).
- Maintain oxygenation.
- Monitor cardiac rhythm for 48 hours.
- Control hyperglycemia.

- Prevent hyperthermia.
- Cautious lowering of BP is essential and not recommended to be attempted for the first two weeks following stroke unless systolic pressure exceeds 200 mm Hg.
- Monitor cardiac status and administer anticoagulant drugs if there is a cardiac source of embolization.
- After excluding hemorrhagic stroke by CT scan, heparin therapy (5000 units every 12 hours) may be of value in limiting or arresting further deterioration of the neurologic deficit.
- Ventilate as needed.

Subacute and Chronic Phase Care
- Deep vein thrombosis (DVT) prevention—low dose unfractionated heparin following an ischemic stroke
- Antithrombotic stockings
- Discontinue Foley catheter as soon as possible; monitor for urinary retention.
- Assessment of skin integrity; prevention of pressure ulcers. See chapter on wound care.
- Nutritional assessment; tube feeding, if indicated.
- Assessment for, and treatment of depression, a common occurrence after stroke. See chapter on psychological disorders.
- Initiate physical, occupational, and speech therapy to facilitate early mobilization and active rehabilitation. It is important that rehabilitation be provided in a coordinated and organized setting such as a skilled nursing facility or hospital-based rehabilitation unit using an interdisciplinary team approach. See chapter on rehabilitation

The prognosis for survival after cerebral infarction is better than after cerebral or subarachnoid hemorrhage. Loss of consciousness after a cerebral infarct implies a poorer prognosis than otherwise. The extent of the infarct governs the potential for rehabilitation.

Treatment for hemorrhagic strokes depends on the location and extent of the hematoma. In cerebellar hemorrhage, prompt surgical evacuation of the hematoma is appropriate and may lead to complete resolution of the clinical deficit. Untreated cerebellar hemorrhage can spontaneously deteriorate with a fatal outcome from brainstem herniation. Decompression is helpful when a superficial hematoma in cerebral white matter is causing mass effect and herniation. In noncerebellar hemorrhage, neurological management is generally conservative and supportive, either in cases of profound deficit with associated brainstem compression or more localized deficits. The treatment of underlying structural lesions or bleeding disorders depends on their nature (Aminoff, 2005, 2006b).

Transient Ischemic Attacks: Embolization from the Heart
Anticoagulations should be started immediately unless contraindicated. The fear of causing hemorrhage into an infarcted area is misplaced, because there is a far greater risk of further embolism to the cerebral circulation if treatment is withheld.

- Use IV heparin (loading dose of 5000–10,000 units of standard molecular weight heparin).
- Maintenance infusion of 1000–2000 units/hour, depending on the PTT while warfarin is introduced.
- Warfarin is more effective than aspirin in reducing the incidence of cardioembolic events, but when contraindicated, aspirin (325 mg/day) may be used in nonrheumatic atrial fibrillation.

Transient Ischemic Attacks: Embolization from the Cerebrovascular System
In presumed or angiographically verified atherosclerotic changes in the extracranial or intracranial cerebrovascular circulation, the

following antithrombotic medication can be prescribed:

- Treatment with aspirin, 325 mg by mouth daily, significantly reduces the frequency of TIA and stroke.
- Dipyridamole (Persantine) added to aspirin does not offer any advantage over aspirin alone.
- In patients intolerant of aspirin, clopidogrel (Plavix) may be used.
- There is no convincing evidence that anti-coagulant drugs are beneficial (Aminoff, 2006b).

Prevention

Management of modifiable risk factors, especially TIAs, hypertension, and cigarette smoking, has the greatest impact on prevention of first stroke. Other primary prevention strategies include the following (Hachinski, 2006):

- Oral anticoagulation with warfarin for selected high-risk patients with nonvalvular atrial fibrillation
- Carotid endarterectomy for selected patients with carotid artery stenosis greater than 60%
- Regular physical exercise
- Treatment with statin medications for patients who have coronary artery disease with or without hyperlipidemia

Routine use of antiplatelet medication has no proven role in primary stroke prevention, although aspirin is often prescribed for patients with vascular risk factors who have not yet had symptoms of either stroke or ischemic heart disease (Ingall, 2000).

The following are the major strategies for secondary stroke prevention:

- Appropriate evaluation to identify the mechanism of the initial stroke
- Carotid endarterectomy is the best prevention for secondary stroke in patients with TIA or minor stroke and ICA stenosis of > 50%.
- Surgical extracranial-intracranial arterial anastomosis is generally not helpful in TIAs or stroke associated with stenotic lesions, distal internal carotid, or proximal middle cerebral arteries.
- Oral anticoagulation with warfarin for patients with nonvalvular atrial fibrillation
- Use of various antiplatelet agents, including aspirin, clopidogrel (Plavix) and the combination of aspirin and slow-release dipyridamole (Aggrenox); these agents and the typical doses are outlined in Table 14-18.
- Reduction of risk factors may also reduce the risk of secondary stroke.

Patient, Family, and Staff Education

Patients and family members should be educated regarding both short- and long-term clinical expectations. Symptoms of post-stroke depression should be reviewed and discussed. Applicable secondary stroke preventive

TABLE 14-18 Antiplatelet Agents		
AGENT	**TYPICAL DOSE**	**COMMENTS**
Aspirin	50 to 325 mg once daily	First-line drug choice for stroke prophylaxis
Clopidogrel	75 mg once daily	Used if stroke recurs on aspirin or if patient is unable to tolerate aspirin
Aggrenox	One capsule (200 mg dipyridamole/50 mg ASA) twice daily	Combination aspirin and slow release dipyridamole

strategies should be discussed and stroke symptoms should be reviewed.

Knowing risk factors and living healthfully are the best steps a person can take to prevent a stroke. The American Heart Association (AHA) has made recommendations that may be shared with patients and their families as well as staff as a means to stay healthy by preventing the recurrence of strokes and myocardial infarction:

- *Early risk factor screening and risk estimation—* The AHA recommends that all people, beginning at age 20, undergo risk factor screening and recommends estimation of risk every five years for people age 40 or older, or for anyone with two or more risk factors.

- *Lower cholesterol and decrease saturated fat intake.* Eating less cholesterol and fat, especially saturated fat, may reduce the plaques in your arteries. If cholesterol can't be controlled through dietary changes alone, you may have to take a cholesterol-lowering medication.

- *Take B vitamins.* B complex vitamins can work together to reduce blood levels of homocysteine, thereby lowering your risk of a stroke.

- *Don't smoke.* Quitting smoking reduces your risk of stroke. Several years after quitting, a former smoker's risk of stroke is the same as that of a nonsmoker.

- *Control diabetes.* You can manage diabetes with diet, exercise, weight control, and medication. Strict control of your blood sugar may reduce damage to your brain if you do have a stroke.

- *Maintain a healthy weight.* Being overweight contributes to other risk factors for stroke. Weight loss of as little as 10 pounds may lower your blood pressure and improve your cholesterol levels.

- *Exercise regularly.* Aerobic exercise, like walking, reduces your risk of stroke in many ways. Exercise can lower your blood pressure, increase your level of HDL cholesterol, and improve the overall health of your blood vessels and heart. It also helps you lose weight and control diabetes and can reduce stress. Gradually work up to 30 minutes of activity on most, if not all, days of the week.

- *Manage stress.* Stress can cause a temporary spike in your blood pressure. It can also increase your blood's tendency to clot, which may elevate your risk of ischemic stroke. Simplifying your life, exercising, and using relaxation techniques are all approaches that you can learn to reduce stress.

- *Drink alcohol in moderation, if at all.* Alcohol can be both a risk factor and a preventive measure for stroke. Binge drinking and heavy alcohol consumption increase your risk of high blood pressure and of ischemic and hemorrhagic strokes. However, drinking small to moderate amounts of alcohol can increase your HDL cholesterol and decrease your blood's clotting tendency. Both factors can contribute to a reduced risk of ischemic stroke.

- *Don't use illicit drugs.* Many street drugs, such as cocaine, are associated with a definite risk of stroke.

Regarding advanced directives, review intensity of care issues and discuss CODE status. Often patients and families require education and counseling regarding the expected course of their recovery, treatment plan, and prognosis. Patients who have suffered significant neurological impairment and have a poor prognosis may be candidates for hospice referral.

Physician Consultation

- Consult physician for any significant neurological change in patient.
- Consult physician when transfer back to the acute hospital is needed.
- Consult physician when unable to control blood pressure adequately.

SUBDURAL HEMATOMA

Definition

Intracranial bleeding is caused by an injury to the head, often as a result of an automobile or motorcycle accident or a seemingly trivial event, such as a bump to the head. Mild head trauma is more likely to cause a hematoma in older persons.

Subdural hematomas form as venous blood collects below the dural surface. Because the bleeding is under venous pressure, the hematoma formation is relatively slow. However, the clot formation will cause pressure on the brain surface and may eventually displace brain tissue. If this expanding clot is not evacuated, it can contribute to the rise in intracranial pressure and its sequelae, including a progressive decline in consciousness, possibly resulting in death. Although these mass lesions are a direct threat to life and brain function, they are usually amenable to clinical diagnosis.

There are three types of subdural hematomas. However, regardless of type, all three require medical attention as soon as signs and symptoms are apparent or permanent brain damage may result:

- *Acute (ASH)*—This type is the most serious and potentially life threatening. It is generally caused by trauma involving an acceleration or deceleration head injury. Signs and symptoms of an acute subdural hematoma usually appear immediately. In this instance, the age of the hematoma is three days or less.

- *Chronic (CSH)*—Less severe head injuries may cause a chronic subdural hematoma. Bleeding from a chronic subdural hematoma may be much slower, and symptoms may take days, or even months, to appear. Chronic subdural hematoma is often the result of trivial head injury in older persons. One fourth to one half of these individuals do not have a history of head trauma. The chronic hematoma is classically older than

three weeks and is associated with an encapsulating membrane.

- *Subacute (SSH)*—In subacute subdural hematoma, signs and symptoms take longer to appear, generally several hours. Subacute subdural hematoma appears 4 to 21 days from maturation of acute subdural hematoma.

Epidemiology

Acute and chronic subdural hematomas occur in 1–2/100,000 Americans and both types of hematomas are more prevalent in men. The risk of developing subdural hematoma is greater for people who use *aspirin or anticoagulants daily*. Other people who are at greater risk for developing subdural hematomas include alcoholics and the very young or very old. ASH is more prevalent among people younger than 60 years of age. Those who develop CSH are generally over the age of 60 years (Aminoff, 2005).

Acute subdural hematomas are caused by high-velocity acceleration or deceleration head injury that results in tearing of the bridging veins between the cerebral cortex and the dural venous sinuses. ASH also results when there is injury to the surface of the brain that precipitates bleeding from injured cortical vessels.

Chronic subdural hematomas are often caused by trivial head injury in adults. Cerebral atrophy is common in older adults and predisposes them to subdural hematoma development. A balance between recurrent bleeding from the hematoma membrane and resorption determines the ultimate size of the hematoma (Wiederholt, 1995).

Five to 22% of people who sustain head trauma (resulting from falls, motor vehicle accidents, blunt head injury, and suspected nonaccidental trauma in infants) will develop subdural hematomas. In the community and in nursing homes head trauma may also be due to physical abuse by caregivers. However, trauma is not the only cause of subdural hematomas. Other causes include coagulopathies, blood vessel disorders such as arteriovenous malformation (AVM), or aneurysms; brain tumors; liver disease; use of blood anticoagulants and antiplatelet agents; certain autoimmune diseases; cerebral spinal fluid shunt for hydrocephalus; bleeding disorders, such as hemophilia, leukemia and sickle cell anemia; and rarely, metastatic carcinoma to the subdural space (Gottfried & Weinand, 2006).

It is estimated that 35–40% of community-dwelling adults older than 65 years of age fall annually. Incidence increases after age 75. Fall rates in hospitals and nursing homes are three times greater, with an estimated 1.5 falls per bed, annually. Ten to 25% of these falls result in serious injury (American Geriatrics Society (AGS), British Geriatrics Society, & American Academy of Orthopaedic Surgeons Panel on Falls Prevention, 2001).

Unrecognized subdural hematoma is the cause of many lawsuits brought against nursing homes. Many were the result of falls or physical abuse by staff.

Common Presenting Signs and Symptoms

A subdural hematoma can become serious because of its location and compression of vital areas. If a patient who has been conscious for several weeks or months after a head injury becomes unconscious and develops neurological symptoms, a subdural hematoma should be suspected. The focal neurological signs from clot formation can be related to the site of the clot. A Cushing response (hypertension, bradycardia) is suggestive of intracranial mass and can be a useful warning sign, particularly in the comatose patient.

Therefore it is imperative that clinicians are aware that signs and symptoms of an intracranial hematoma may occur from immediately to several weeks or longer after a blow to the head. As time progresses, pressure on the brain increases, producing the typical signs and symptoms associated with both ASH and CSH.

Although symptoms of intracranial hematoma may not be immediately apparent, the nurse practitioner should watch closely for subsequent physical, mental, and emotional changes.

In ASH the following signs and symptoms may be apparent:

• Altered level of consciousness (90%)
• Pupillary irregularity that is usually unilateral to hematoma (47–53%)
• Hemiparesis usually contralateral to hematoma (34–47%)
• Decerebrate posturing (47%)
• Papilledema (16%)
• Cranial nerve III abnormality (5%)

The following signs and symptoms may occur in persons who develop CSH:

• Impaired consciousness (53%)
• Hemiparesis (45%)
• Papilledema (24%)
• Cranial nerve III abnormality (11%)
• Hemianopsia (7%)

Differential Diagnoses

The following might be included in a differential diagnosis list if patients present with the above mentioned signs and symptoms:

• Concussion
• Cerebral contusion or laceration
• Acute epidural hemorrhage
• Acute subdural hemorrhage
• Cerebral hemorrhage
• Dementia
• Stroke
• Transient ischemic attack
• Brain tumor
• Subdural empyema
• Meningitis
• Depression

Essential Diagnostic and Laboratory Tests

Diagnosing a hematoma can be difficult. However, clinicians generally presume that the progressive loss of consciousness after a head injury is caused by a hemorrhage inside the head until proved otherwise. Those who are stable but whose status is questionable need to undergo a diagnostic study. The CT scan (with intravascular contrast if the hemoglobin is less than or equal to 9 gm/dL) is the most efficient diagnostic tool and best method to define the position and size of an ASH.

The CT scan is also the preferred method for evaluating CSH. Usually hematomas evolve from isodense to hypodense by three weeks. An MRI head scan is often necessary for hematomas that appear isodense within the brain due to the mixture of chronic hematoma with recurrent hemorrhage.

Management Plan

The goals for management of subdural hematoma are early recognition and transfer to an acute care setting for evaluation and treatment.

The inpatient setting is the appropriate one for the treatment of subdural hematomas because hematoma management often requires surgery. On the other hand, some subdural hematomas do not need to be removed because they are small and produce no signs or symptoms. However, patients who are rapidly deteriorating require immediate surgical evacuation.

If a patient is still communicative, close observation and steroids should suffice, and a CT scan should be rapidly obtained to determine treatment options. However, if surgery is required to evacuate a significant hematoma, it should be carried out as soon as possible, because delay of more than 4 hours after injury results in poorer outcome.

General medical treatment goals and intervention measures for ASH include controlling elevated intracranial pressure with osmotic and loop diuretics and hyperventilation to induce hypocapnia ($PaCO_2$ of 22–28 mm Hg). For CSH,

interventions must be aimed at maintaining adequate airway and ventilation and support of the cardiovascular system to promote normal cerebral profusion.

Surgical measures for ASH include emergent craniotomy for hematomas causing significant mass effect. If a patient with a SSH is neurologically stable, surgery may be delayed until the hematoma matures and becomes chronic at which time a burr hole drainage can be performed. However, SSH causing significant mass effect and neurological defect may require craniotomy for evacuation. In cases of CSH, burr hole drainage of the hematoma may suffice. Some surgeons will leave a catheter in the subdural space for 24 hours after the operation to facilitate drainage (Gottfried & Weinand, 2006).

Patient, Family, and Staff Education

All interested parties should be taught how to prevent or minimize the occurrence of head injuries that may lead to hematoma formation. In nursing home settings this includes interventions to prevent falls. The nurse practitioner may assist in the development and evaluation of fall prevention programs and should be vigilant in identifying fall risks and in staff education. The nurse practitioner is also legally bound to report suspected physical abuse of residents by caregivers.

Patients, families, and facility staff may also benefit from anticipatory guidance regarding coping strategies that might be effective while trying to recover from a head injury or to support someone who is recovering. Adults will experience the majority of their recovery during the first six months. Smaller improvements may occur for as long as two years after the hematoma. The following tips for patients/caregivers may help make for a smoother recovery:

- Get plenty of sleep at night, and rest during the day.
- Return to normal activities gradually, not all at once.

- Avoid activities that could result in a second head injury.
- Take only those drugs prescribed or approved by your provider.
- Refrain from alcohol consumption until fully recovered. Alcohol may hinder recovery, and can put you at risk of further injury.
- Record things that are hard to remember.
- Talk with family or close friends before making important decisions.

Physician Consultation

Consult if patients sustain any significant blow to the head in which there is a loss of consciousness or demonstration of any of the signs and symptoms listed above.

▬ WEB SITES

- National Institute of Neurologic Disorders and Stroke—www.ninds.nih.gov/disorders/multiple_sclerosis/multiple_sclerosis.htm
- National Multiple Sclerosis Society—www.nmss.org or http://www.nationalmssociety.org/Brochures-Guide%20for.asp
- National Parkinson Foundation—www.parkinson.org
- Nursing Home Care of Individuals with Multiple Sclerosis: Guidelines and Recommendations for Quality Care—www.nationalmssociety.org/PRC%20Publications.asp
- National Stroke Association—www.stroke.org

▬ REFERENCES

AGS Panel on Persistent Pain in Older Persons. (2002). The management of persistent pain in older persons. *Journal of the American Geriatric Society, 50* (Suppl. 6), 205.

Alvarez, J. A., & Hardy, R. H. (1998). Lumbar spine stenosis: A common cause of back and leg pain. *American Family Physician, 57*, 1825–1945.

American Geriatrics Society, British Geriatrics Society, & American Academy of Orthopaedic Surgeons Panel on Falls Prevention. (2001). Guideline for prevention of falls in older persons. *Journal of the American Geriatrics Society, 49*, 664–672.

Aminoff, M. J. (2005). Nervous system. In L. M. Tierney, S. T. McPhee, & M. A. Papadakis (Eds.), *Current medical diagnosis and treatment* (pp. 944–1006). New York: Lange Medical Books/McGraw-Hill.

Aminoff, M. J. (2006a). Epilepsy. In M. A. Papadakis, & S. J. McPhee (Eds.), *Current consult in medicine* (pp. 356–357). New York: Lange Medical Books/McGraw-Hill.

Aminoff, M. J. (2006b). Ischemic stroke. In M. A. Papadakis, & S. J. McPhee (Eds.), *Current consult in medicine*. New York: Lange Medical Books/McGraw-Hill.

Aminoff, M. J. (2006c). Multiple sclerosis. In M. A. Papadakis, & S. J. McPhee (Eds.), *Current consult in medicine* (pp. 655–645). New York: Lange Medical Books/McGraw-Hill.

Aminoff, M. J. (2006d). Parkinsonism. In M. A. Papadakis, & S. J. McPhee (Eds.), *Current consult in medicine* (pp. 706–708). New York: Lange Medical Books/McGraw-Hill.

Bath, P. (2002). Anticoagulants and antiplatelet agents in acute inschaemic stroke, *Lancet Neurology, 1*, 405.

Beck, R. W., Cleary, P. A., Anderson, M. M., Keltner, J. L., Shults, W. T., Kaufman, D. I. et al. (1992). A randomized, controlled trial of corticosteroids in the treatment of acute optic neuritis. The Optic Neuritis Study Group. *New England Journal of Medicine, 326*, 581.

Beers, M. H., & Berkow, R. (2000). *The Merck manual of geriatrics* (3rd ed.). New Jersey: Merck Research Laboratories.

Ben-Shlomo, Y. (1997). The epidemiology of Parkinson's disease. *Clinical Neurology, 6*, 55–68.

Blanchard, S. H., & Toffler, W. L. (2006). In M. R. Dambro (Ed.), *Griffith's 5-minute clinical consult* (pp. 1022–1023). Philadelphia: Lippincott Williams & Wilkins.

Borenstein, D. (2001). Low back and neck pain. In L. Robbins, C. S. Burkhardt, M. T. Hannan, & R. J. DeHoratius (Eds.), *Clinical care in the rheumatic diseases* (2nd ed., p. 244). Atlanta: Association of Rheumatology Health Professionals.

Bowling, A. C. (2001). *Alternative Medicine and Multiple Sclerosis*. New York: Demos.

Brex, P. A., Ciccarelli, O., O'Riordan, J. L., Sailer, M., Thompson, A. J., & Miller, D. H. (2002). A longitudinal study of abnormalities on MRI and disability from multiple sclerosis. *New England Journal of Medicine, 346*, 158–164.

Caspi, O., & Thomson, C. (1999). Parkinson's disease: "Don't become your disease." *Integrative Medicine, 2*, 37–42.

Chang, B. S., & Lowenstein, D. H. (2003). Epilepsy. *New England Journal of Medicine, 349*(13), 1257–1266.

Chang, Y., Singer, D. E., Wu, Y. A., Keller, R. B., & Atlas, S. J. (2005). The effect of surgical and non-surgical treatment on longitudinal outcomes of lumbar spinal stenosis over 10 years. *Journal of the American Geriatric Society, 53*, 785–792.

Counihan, T. J. (2001). Cerebrovascular disease. In T. E. Andreoli, C. C. J. Carpenter, R. C. Griggs, & J. Loscalzo (Eds.), *Cecil essentials of medicine* (5th ed.). Philadelphia: W.B. Saunders Company.

Fillippi, M., Bozzali, M., Rovaris, M., Gonen, O., Kesavadas, C., Ghezzi, A., et al. (2003). Evidence for widespread axonal damage at the earliest clinical stage of multiple sclerosis. *Brain, 126*, 433–437.

Gelalis, I. D., Stafilas, K. S., Korompilias, A. V., Zacharis, K. C., Beris, A. E., & Xenakis, T. A. (2005). Decompressive surgery for degenerative lumbar spinal stenosis: Long-term results. *International Orthopedics, 5*, 1–5.

Golbe, L. I. (1991). Young-onset Parkinson's disease: A clinical review. *Neurology, 41*, 168–173.

Gottfried, O. N., & Weinand, M. E. (2006). Subdural hematomas. In M. R. Dambro (Ed.), *Griffith's 5-minute clinical consult* (pp. 1068–1069). Philadelphia: Lippincott Williams & Wilkins.

Hachinski, V. (2006). Stroke: Brain attack. In M. R. Dambro (Ed.), *Griffith's 5-minute clinical consult*. Philadelphia: Lippincott Williams & Wilkins.

Hess, D. C., & Hughes, M. D. (2005a). Multiple sclerosis: When to suspect-keys to diagnosis. *Consultant, 45*, 844–852.

Hess, D. C., & Hughes, M. D. (2005b). Multiple sclerosis: New help, new hope. *Consultant, 45*, 1144–1148.

Ingall, T. J. (2000). Preventing ischemic stroke. *Stroke Prevention, 107*(6), 34–50.

Jacobs, L. D., Beck, R. W., Simon, J. H., Kinkel, R. P., Brownscheidle, C. M., Murray, T. J., et al. (2000). Intramuscular interferon beta-1a therapy initiated during a first demyelinating event in multiple sclerosis. CHAMPS Study Group. *New England Journal of Medicine, 343*, 898–904.

Kellinghaus, C., Loddenkemper, T., Dinner, D. S., Lachhwani, D., & Luders, H. O. (2004). Non-epileptic seizures of the elderly. *Neurology, 251*, 704–709.

Lieberman, D. (2004, September 29–October 3). *Non-pharmacological interventions for spinal stenosis*. Program and abstracts of the National Conference of Gerontological Nurse Practitioners 23rd Annual Meeting, Phoenix, Arizona.

Lublin, P. D., & Reingold, S. C. (1996). Defining the clinical course of multiple sclerosis: Results of an international survey. National Multiple Sclerosis Society (USA) Advisory Committee on Clinical Trials of New Agents in Multiple Sclerosis. *Neurology, 46*, 907–911.

Mayeux, R., Marder, K., Cote, L. J., Denaro, J., Hemenegildo, N., Mejia, H., et al. (1995). The frequency of idiopathic Parkinson's disease by age, ethnic group, and sex in northern Manhattan, 1988–1003. *American Journal of Epidemiology, 142*, 820–827.

Meschia, J. F. (2000). Management of acute ischemic stroke: What is the role of tPA and antithrombotic agents? [Electronic version]. *Postgraduate Medicine Online, 107*(6).

Minteer, J. F. (2006). Parkinson's disease. In M. R. Dambro (Ed.), *Griffith's 5-minute clinical consult* (pp. 806–807). Philadelphia: Lippincott Williams & Wilkins.

National Multiple Sclerosis Society Long Term Care Committee. (2003). *Nursing home care of individuals with multiple sclerosis: Guidelines and recommendations for quality care*. NY: National Multiple Sclerosis Society.

O'Riordan, J. I., Thompson, A. J., Kingsley, D. P., MacManus, D. G., Kendall, B. E., Rudge, P., et al., (1998). The prognostic value of brain MRI in clinically isolated syndromes of the CNS. A 10-year follow-up. *Brain, 121*, 495–503.

Papadakis, M. A., & McPhee, S. J. (2006). *Current consult in medicine*. New York: Lange Medical Books/McGraw-Hill.

Parkinson's Disease Study Group. (1995). An alternative medicine treatment for Parkinson's disease: Results of a multicenter clinical trial. *Journal of Alternative Complementary Medicine, 1,* 149–155.

Paterson, C., Allen, J. A., Browning, M., Barlow, G., & Ewings, P. (2005). A pilot study of therapeutic massage for people with Parkinson's disease: The added value of user involvement. *Complementary Therapeutics for Clinical Practice, 11*(3), 161–171.

Paulson, G. W. (1993). Management of the patient with newly diagnosed Parkinson's disease. *Geriatrics, 48*(2), 30–40.

PRISMS (Prevention of Relapses and Disability by Interferon Beta-1a Subcutaneously in Multiple Sclerosis) Study Group. (1998). Randomized double-blinded, placebo-controlled study of interferon beta-1a in relapsing/remitting multiple sclerosis. *Lancet, 352,* 1498–1504.

Pryse-Phillips, W., & Costello, F. (2001). The epidemiology of multiple sclerosis. In S. Cook (Ed.), *Handbook of multiple sclerosis* (pp. 15–31). New York: Marcel Dekker.

Rajput, A. H. (1992). Frequency and cause of Parkinson's disease. *Canadian Journal of Neurological Science, 19* (Suppl. 1), 103–107.

Ramsay, R. E., Rowan, A. J., & Pryor, F. M. (2004). Special considerations in treating the elderly patient with epilepsy. *Neurology, 62* (5 Suppl. 2), S24–S29.

Resnick, B. (2004). Seizures and Epilepsy in the Older Adult. *Highlights of the NCGNP 23rd Annual Convention.* Retrieved February 6, 2006, from http://www.medscape.com/seizures/view authors

Rhoades, J. (2001). Neurologic problems. In L. M. Dumphy, & J. E. Winland-Brown (Eds.), *Primary care: The art and science of advanced practice nursing.* Philadelphia: F.A. Davis Company.

Rodin, M., Saliba, D., & Brunmel-Smith, K. (2006). Guidelines: Management of stroke rehabilitation. *Journal of American Geriatric Society, 54,* 158–162.

Rollins, K. E., & Corboy, J. R. (2005). Immunotherapeutic advances in multiple sclerosis. *Applied Neurology, April* (Suppl.), 1–10.

Sadovnick, A. D., Remick, R. A., Allen, J., Swartz, E., Yee, I. M., Eisen, K., et al. (1996). Depression and multiple sclerosis. *Neurology, 46,* 628–632.

Samii, A., Nutt, J. G., & Ransom, B. R. (2004). Parkinson's disease. *Lancet, 363,* 1783.

Schachter, S. C. (2002). Management and treatment of epilepsy in the elderly. *Annals of Long-Term Care, 6*(10), 33–38.

Schachter, S. C. (2004). Epilepsy: Major advances in treatment. *Lancet Neurology, 3,* 11.

Sellebjerg, F., Frederiksen, J. L., Nielsen, P. M., & Olesen, J. (1998). Double-blind, randomized, placebo-controlled studies of oral high dose methylprednisolone in attacks of multiple sclerosis. *Neurology, 51,* 529–534.

Selma, T. P., Beizer, J. L., & Higbee, M. D. (2005). *Geriatric dosage handbook* (10th ed.). New Jersey: Lexicomp.

Smith, S. G. (2006). Multiple sclerosis. In M. R. Dambro (Ed.), *Griffith's 5-minute consult,* pp. 728–729. Philadelphia: Lippincott Williams & Wilkins.

Soldan, S. S., Berti, R., Salem, N., Secchiero, P., Flamand, L., Calabresi, P. et al. (1997). Association of human herpes virus 6 (HHV-6) with multiple sclerosis: Increased IgM response to HHV-6 early antigen and detection of serum HHV-6 DNA. *Nature Medicine, 3,* 1394–1397.

Stacy, M. (2002). Sleep disorders in Parkinson's disease. *Drugs & Aging, 1,* 733–739.

Tadokoro, K., Miyamoto, H., Sumi, M., & Shimomura, T. (2005). The prognosis of conservative treatments for lumbar spinal stenosis: Analysis of patients over 70 years of age. *Spine, 30,* 2458–2463.

Tierney, L. M., Saint, S., & Whooley, M. A. (2005). *Current essentials of medicine,* (3rd ed.). New York: Lange Medical Books/McGraw-Hill.

Velez, L., & Selwa, L. (2004). Seizure disorders in the elderly. *American Family Physician, 67,* 325–332.

Verbiest, H. (1990). Lumbar spine stenosis. In J. R. Youmans (Ed.), *Neurological surgery: A comprehensive reference guide to the diagnosis and management of neurosurgical problems* (3rd ed., pp. 2895–2855). Philadelphia: W. B. Saunders.

Wiederholt, W. C. (1995). *Neurology for non-neurologists* (3rd ed.). Philadelphia: W.B. Saunders.

Whetten-Goldstein, K., Sloan, F. A., Goldstein, L. B., & Kulas, E. D. (1998). A comprehensive assessment of the cost of multiple sclerosis in the United States. *Multiple Sclerosis, 4,* 189–425.

Yamamoto, L., Olaes, E., & Lopez, A. (2004). Challenges in seizure management: Neurologic versus cardiac emergencies. *Topics in Emergency Medicine, 3*(26), 221–224.

Zifko, U. A., Rupp, M., Schwarz, S., Zipko, H. T., & Maida, E. M. (2002). Modafinil in treatment of fatigue in multiple sclerosis. Results of an open-label study. *Journal of Neurology, 249,* 983–987.

Zweifler, R. (2003). Management of acute stroke. *Southern Medical Journal, 96,* 380–385.

▆ BIBLIOGRAPHY

American College of Emergency Physicians. (2004). Clinical policy: Critical issues in the evaluation and management of adult patients presenting to the emergency department with seizures. *Annals of Emergency Medicine, 43,* 265.

Arle, J. E., & Alterman, R. L. (1999). Parkinson's disease and parkinsonian syndromes: Surgical options in Parkinson's disease. *Medical Clinics of North America, 83,* 483–498.

Delport, E. G., Cucuzzella, A. R., Marley, J. K., Pruitt, C. M., & Fisher, J. R. (2004). Treatment of lumbar spinal stenosis with epidural steroid injections: A retrospective outcome study. *Archives of Physical Medicine and Rehabilitation, 85,* 479–484.

Deuschl, G. (2000). New treatment options for tremors. *New England Journal of Medicine, 342,* 505–507.

Kawaguchi, Y., Kanamori, M., Ishihara, H., Kikkawa, T., Matsui, H., Tsuji, H., et al. (2004). Clinical and radiographic results of expansive lumbar laminoplasty in patients with spinal stenosis. *American Journal of Bone and Joint Surgery, 86,* 1698–1703.

Krupp, L. B., Coyle, P. K., Doscher, C., Miller, A., Cross, A. H., Jandorf, L., et al. (1995). Fatigue therapy in MS: Results of a double-blind, randomized, parallel trial of amantidine, pemoline, and placebo. *Neurology, 45,* 1956–1961.

Lai, B. C., Schulzer, M., Marion, S., Teschke, K., & Tsui, J. K. (2003). The prevalence of Parkinson's disease. *Parkinsonism Related Disorders, 9,* 233–238.

Liu, B., Gao, H., & Hong, J. (2003). Parkinson's disease and exposure to infectious agents and pesticides and the occurrence of brain injuries: Role of neurotransmitters. *Environmental Health Perspectives, 111,* 1065–1073.

Marshall, F. J. (2001). Disorders of the motor system. In T. E. Andreoli, C. C. J. Carpenter, R. C. Griggs, & J. Loscalzo (Eds.), *Cecil essentials of medicine* (5th ed.). Philadelphia: W.B. Saunders Company.

Spratt, K. F., Keller, T. S., Szpalski, M., Vandeputte, K., & Gunzburg, R. (2004). A predictive model for outcome after conservative decompression surgery for lumbar spinal stenosis. *European Spine Journal, 13,* 14–21.

Strayer, A. (2005). Lumbar spine: Common pathology and interventions. *Journal of Neuroscience Nursing, 37*(4), 181–193.

Weinstein, P. R. (1993). Lumbar stenosis. In R. W. Hardy Jr. (Ed.), *Lumbar disc disease* (2nd ed., pp. 241–255). New York: Raven.

CHAPTER 15

Psychological Disorders

Valisa Saunders

GENERALIZED ANXIETY DISORDER IN THE ELDERLY

The most common types of anxiety disorders include generalized anxiety disorder (GAD), panic disorder (PD), post-traumatic stress disorder (PTSD), phobias (particularly social anxiety disorder [SAD]), and obsessive-compulsive disorder (OCD). As in other geriatric syndromes, there are few age-specific studies on anxiety, and the studies that do exist are generally of short duration. GAD is commonly seen with comorbid mental health issues such as panic disorder, social or other phobias, major depression, alcohol abuse, PTSD, or personality disorders. The most common anxiety disorder to develop, for the first time, in the older adult is GAD, and this will be the focus of this section.

Definitions

Generalized anxiety is characterized by excessive worry and anxiety that are difficult to control and cause significant distress and impairment (Ciechanowski, 2005). Chronic states of anxiety may lead to GAD, which is characterized by six months or more of chronic exaggerated worry and tension. PTSD is the re-experiencing of a very traumatic event accompanied by symptoms of increased arousal and

by avoidance of stimuli associated with the trauma. In OCD, the behaviors (compulsions) or mental acts (obsessions) are aimed at preventing or reducing distress or preventing some dreaded event or situation, but these behaviors or mental acts are not connected in a realistic way with what they are designed to neutralize or prevent, or are clearly excessive. The obsessions or compulsions cause marked distress, are time consuming, or significantly interfere with the person's normal routine or relationships. In SAD there is marked fear of social or performance situations in which embarrassment may occur (American Psychiatric Association [APA], 1994).

Epidemiology

GAD has an 8% prevalence rate among primary care patients and is the most common anxiety disorder in the primary care setting. The prevalence is 16% in healthcare settings (Jacobs, 1998). GAD has approximately a 5% lifetime occurrence rate, but most patients with GAD have other psychiatric diagnoses such as substance abuse, PTSD, OCD, depression, and phobias. Of patients with depression, 35–50% meet criteria for GAD. Twice as many women as men have GAD (Ciechanowski, 2005). Untreated GAD is associated with high utilization of medical health care (Katon et al., 1990). Early environment is considered to be as or more important than genetics in the development of GAD and is often associated with traumatic events (Kessler, Davis, & Kendler, 1997). In the elderly, anxiety secondary to a medical condition is quite common.

Common Presenting Signs and Symptoms

DSM IV Criteria for Generalized Anxiety Disorder (GAD)

- Excessive anxiety and worry (apprehensive expectation), occurring more days than not, for at least 6 months, about a number of events or activities (such as work or school performance)

- The person finds it difficult to control the worry.

- The anxiety and worry are associated with three (or more) of the following six symptoms (with at least some symptoms present for more days than not, for the past 6 months). Only one item required in children.

  o Restlessness or feeling keyed up or on edge

  o Being easily fatigued

  o Difficulty concentrating or mind going blank

  o Irritability

  o Muscle tension

  o Sleep disturbance (difficulty falling or staying asleep, or restless, unsatisfying sleep)

- The focus of the anxiety and worry is not confined to features of an Axis I disorder (e.g., the anxiety or worry is not about having a panic attack, as in panic disorder), being embarrassed in public (as in social phobia), being contaminated (as in OCD), being away from home or close relatives (as in separation anxiety disorder), gaining weight (as in anorexia nervosa), having multiple physical complaints (as in somatization disorder), or having a serious illness (as in hypochondriasis), and the anxiety and worry do not occur exclusively during PTSD.

- The anxiety, worry, or physical symptoms cause clinically significant distress or impairment in social, occupational or other important areas of functioning.

- The disturbance is not due to the direct physiological effects of a substance (e.g., a drug of abuse, a medication) or a general medical condition (e.g., hyperthyroidism) and does not occur exclusively during a mood disorder, a psychotic disorder, or a pervasive developmental disorder.

- The person is unable to relax and often suffers from insomnia, as well as often having somatic complaints, such as fatigue, trembling, muscle tension, headaches, irritability, or hot flashes. The person may have difficulty concentrating and is easily startled. People with GAD usually do not avoid situations as a result of their anxiety. They may experience only mild impairment with normal daily functioning; however, severe cases may interfere with work or school, social situations, and other daily routines.

Differential Diagnosis

- Medications and substances (see Table 15-1)
- Endocrine problems
  o Hyperthyroidism
  o Hyper- or hypoparathyroidism
  o Hypoglycemia
- Anemia
- Infection
- Respiratory disease, hypoxia
- Depression
- Cardiovascular:
  o Mitral valve prolapse syndrome
  o Arrhythmias

TABLE 15-1 Medications That Can Induce Anxiety

- Caffeine withdrawal
- Alcohol withdrawal
- Benzodiazepine withdrawal
- Sympathomimetics
  - Ephedrine
  - Beta agonists
- Digoxin
- Corticosteroids
- Psychotropic drugs
  - Antipsychotics
  - Antidepressants
  - Stimulants
- Thyroxine
- Theophylline

- Angina
- Myocardial infarction
- Heart failure
- Less commonly: carcinoid syndrome, pheochromocytoma, and electrolyte disorders

Psychiatric Conditions (Differential)
- Depression or bipolar disorder
- Social or performance anxiety disorder
- PTSD
- Somatization (Briquet's) disorder or hypochondriasis
- Alcoholism or other substance use disorders
- Psychotic disorders
- Personality disorders

Essential Diagnostic and Laboratory Tests
- CBC
- Electrolytes, including calcium, serum glucose

- TSH, T4
- Urinalysis

With Indications
- EKG if chest pain or palpitations occur
- Echocardiogram for suspected valvular pathology
- Urine or serum toxicology
- Oxygen saturation

Other Assessment
- Eliciting a thorough social history from family members may be very helpful. Elicit any past psychiatric illness, substance abuse issues, stressful situations (war, rape, etc.) or hospitalization for mental health problems or other institutionalization (prison, prison or internment camps, "sanitariums," etc.). Listen for such words as "nervous breakdown." Ask about any treatment they were aware of such as medication names. Be familiar with the names of older psychotropic drugs listed in the long-term care survey which may give clues to previous illness.
- Hamilton Anxiety Rating Scale (HARS) (Hamilton, 1959). A semistructured scale of 14 items that characterize anxiety. Each item is rated on a 5-point scale, ranging from 0 (not present) to 4 (severe). This tool is recommended more as a monitoring tool than a screening tool (APA, 2000). (See Appendix A.)
- Zung Self-Rating Anxiety Scale (SAS) (Zung, 1971). The patient answers 20 questions related to the frequency of various symptoms on a 4-point scale.
- Mini-Mental State Exam (MMSE) (see section on dementia)
- Depression assessment (see section on depression)

Management Plan
The goal is to improve the patient's quality of life by alleviating symptoms through the aggressive treatment of coexisting medical or psychiatric dis-

orders. Treatment of the anxiety itself may be through supportive or problem-focused therapy, drug therapy, or both. Eliminating an anxiety disorder; however, may not be a realistic goal.

Nonpharmacologic
- Brief supportive psychotherapy (BSP)—A study by Catalan and colleagues (1984) of patients with new episodes of GAD found that family physicians who used BSP had 3- and 6-month follow-up results similar to those who used benzodiazepines.
- Cognitive behavior therapy (CBT)—Studied in elderly primary care patients with MMSE score greater than 24 (Stanley et al., 2003)
- Consistent caregivers with consistent routines and calm behavior
- Avoid known triggers of anxiety when possible.
- Elicit successful strategies from patient and family members whenever possible.
- Develop jointly agreed-upon goals and interventions with patient and family.
- Activities
- Relaxation techniques

Pharmacologic
Antidepressants are now the mainstay of treatment (see Table 15-2). Although most antidepressants are helpful in treating GAD, they do take some time to work and short-term treatment with benzodiazepines may be warranted. If possible, it is best not to start a benzodiazepine, as most antidepressants have good antianxiety effects, fewer problematic side effects, and a high likelihood of treating comorbid psychiatric problems. All classes of antidepressants, including serotonin reuptake inhibitors (SRIs), serotonin-norepinephrine reuptake inhibitors (SNRIs), tricyclic antidepressants (TCAs), and monoamine oxidase inhibitors (MAOIs) are effective in the treatment of GAD, but may take up to 6–8 weeks to be effective. Short-term benzodiazepine use during this time may be warranted. In the frail elderly, use of the benzodiazepines with short half-life is recommended. Buspirone (Buspar) is as effective as the benzodiazepines for the treatment of GAD, but the onset of action can take several weeks (Ciechanowski, 2005). Buspar has relatively few side effects, but there can be some gastrointestinal side effects. A slower titration can generally avoid this problem.

Patients with long-standing anxiety disorders have often been taking benzodiazepines for years, if not decades. They often believe that they "must have them," because they do alleviate symptoms, patients do experience increased anxiety when withdrawn, and the drugs are habituating. However, benzodiazepines do have side effects that can be of concern, which older adults experience increasingly as they age, and the older benzodiazepines have very long half-lifes. Common adverse effects from benzodiazepines in the elderly include cognitive impairment, ataxia, falls and fractures. Abrupt withdrawal is very problematic as patients will experience rebound anxiety and may also have cardiac ischemia. Dose reductions of 10–20% per week are recommended, but may take even longer.

Once effectively treating anxiety, medications should be maintained for at least 4 to 6 months and then tapered slowly. Some patients will have symptoms recur and will need longer or indefinite treatment. Abrupt withdrawal is likely to reactivate anxiety symptoms and abrupt withdrawal of SRIs can cause serotonin syndrome. Serotonin syndrome can be induced by a number of other drugs as well, either in excess or abrupt withdrawal. The symptoms can be mild to life threatening and include tachycardia, shivering, diaphoresis, mydriasis, tremor, akathisia, altered mental status, clonus, muscular hypertonicity, and hyperthermia (Boyer & Shannon, 2005).

Pregabalin (Lyrica) is a new drug showing potential for GAD treatment and is believed to have fewer problems than the benzodiazepines.

TABLE 15-2 Medications Used to Treat Anxiety in the Elderly

BRAND NAME GENERIC NAME	INDICATIONS OTHER THAN DEPRESSION X* = OFF-LABEL WITH EVIDENCE		X = FDA-APPROVED USE			AVERAGE START AND MAX DAILY DOSE (mg)	COMMENTS
SRIs	GAD	OCD	PD	PTSD	SAD		
Celexa (citalopram)	X*	X*				10–20 40 max, once daily	Sedation, weight gain, generally dose in a.m. Same active molecule as escitalopram
Lexapro (escitalopram)	X					10 20 after 1 week, once daily	Minimal side effects; contains only the active isomer of citalopram
Luvox (fluvoxamine)		X	X*			25–50 start 50–200 after 6 wk 300 max	Used primarily in OCD
Paxil (paroxetine)	X	X	X	X	X	10–20 start 40 max, once daily	Sedating, some EPS in frail elderly. CR form only in PD and SAD
Prozac (fluoxetine)		X	X			10–20 20–40 once daily	May be activating in some patients; dose in the morning.
Zoloft (sertraline)	X*	X	X	X	X	25–50 200 max, single dose	Sedating, weight gain
SNRIs	GAD	OCD	PD	PTSD	SAD		
Cymbalta (duloxetine)	X- in major depression					20–30 mg twice daily 60 max single or divided dose	Sedating, also approved for diabetic peripheral neuropathy
Effexor (venlafaxine)	X	X*	X		X	37.5–75 300 max, divided 2–3 doses or single dose of XR form	Sedating, weight gain. Activating at higher doses. Also used in neuro pathic pain—unlabeled
Remeron (mirtazapine)	X*					7.5–15 45 max, once daily	Sedation, weight gain; activates at higher doses; monitor for agranulocytosis

Benzodiazepines—Short acting; generally preferred in geriatric patients—not covered under Medicare Part D

		DOSE RANGE	HALF-LIFE	ONSET	COMMENTS
Ativan (lorazepam)		0.5–2 mg/day	8–14 hrs	1–2 hrs	Benzodiazepines are best used for acute anxiety on a short-term basis and then tapered. They do not have strong effects on OCD or PTSD.
Xanax (alprazolam)	Xanax XR is approved for PD	0.25–1 mg/day	0–14 hrs	1 hr	
Serax (oxazepam)		10–30 mg/day	10–15 hrs	1–2 hrs	
Klonopin (clonazepam)	Klonopin is approved for PD	0.25–1 mg/day	20–50 hrs	1–2 hrs	

Other

Buspar (buspirone)	For GAD. Does not block panic attacks and is not efficacious as a primary treatment of OCD or PTSD. Is often used as an adjunct with SRIs.	Start at 5 mg twice daily, then three times daily after 2–3 days, then increase by 5 mg/day, every 2–3 days to usual range of 20–30 mg/day in 2–3 doses. Max 60 mg/day	Takes 4–6 weeks to take effect. Not habit forming. Should be tapered when discontinued

Notes: CR, controlled release; EPS, extrapyramidal symptoms; GAD, generalized anxiety disorder; OCD, obsessive-compulsive disorder; PD, panic disorder; PTSD, post-traumatic stress disorder; SAD, social anxiety disorder.

All SRI medications can have GI side effects such as nausea, diarrhea, headache, sedation, restlessness, weight gain, and sexual dysfunction. May cause hyponatremia in some. Most are approved for use in obsessive-compulsive disorder (OCD). SNRIs may cause dry mouth and sedation. SRIs should not be discontinued abruptly. Check labeling for rate of taper. Monitor electrolytes and CBC for many SRIs for agranulocytosis, neutropenia, or leukopenia.

Sources: MedLinePlus, 2006; Brody & Serby, 2004; Lantz, 2004; Schatzberg et al., 2002.

This drug is involved in regulating gamma-amino butyric acid (GABA) and a compound related to gabapentin (neurontin). Currently it has FDA approval for diabetic peripheral neuropathy, postherpetic neuralgia, and as adjunctive therapy for partial-onset seizure disorder.

In the complementary medicine arena, many promote using the extract from Kava root for treating anxiety. Pittler (2000) conducted a meta-analysis of 11 studies with a total of 645 participants on kava extract compared with placebo, and the conclusions were that it is relatively effective and safe for short-term treatment (the longest study was 24 weeks). However, long-term effects are not known, and the FDA has issued a safety alert about kava use and fatal hepatotoxicity.

Patient, Family, and Staff Education

- Advise consistency in routine, but care plan must be tailored to the individual.
- Educate that this is a medical condition, but that the medications do not "cure" the disorder, although they can alleviate uncomfortable symptoms.
- Educate that the medications may take some time to be fully effective and must be increased gradually at intervals and not stopped abruptly.
- Educate regarding side effects that may be experienced and to report them, including the increased risk of suicidal thinking and behavior.
- Teach techniques to help relaxation such as touch therapy, massage therapy, guided imagery, music therapy, and deep breathing.

Physician or Other Consultation

- Suicidal or homicidal ideation
- Psychosis
- Suspected serious comorbid psychiatric illness
- Need and cognitive ability for psychotherapy

DEMENTIA

Definition

Dementia is a progressive, acquired disorder in which intellectual abilities decline and interfere with the affected person's customary occupational, functional, and social performance. Dementia is a global term that characterizes cognitive, functional or behavioral changes. One's ability to learn, reason, make judgments, communicate and carry out daily activities decline in the disease (Roman et al., 1993). The term *dementia* does not indicate a specific diagnosis of a disease.

Dementia may be reversible or irreversible depending on the etiology. Reversible causes include metabolic disturbances, endocrine disorders, vitamin deficiencies, brain tumor, increased intracranial pressures, infections, depression, and medications. Reversible causes of dementia often present as *delirium* (discussed in another section of this chapter) but may also represent an unmasking of previously unrecognized irreversible dementia. An irreversible dementing disorder cannot be diagnosed in the presence of delirium.

Common irreversible causes of dementia include Alzheimer's dementia (AD), Lewy body dementia (LBD), vascular dementia (VAD), frontotemporal dementia (FTD), Parkinson's disease with dementia (PDD), and alcohol-related dementia (ARD). Huntington's is a more rare form of dementia that has an early onset. Other terms often used for vascular dementias include Binswanger's disease (BD), which refers to diffuse white matter disease, senile leukoencephalopathy, multi-infarct dementia (MID), and subcortical ischemic leukoencephalopathy.

Epidemiology

In the year 2000 the prevalence of AD was estimated at 4.5 million cases in the United States. This number is expected to increase to 13.2 million by 2050 (Hebert et al., 2003). Alzheimer's dementia accounts for 60–80% of the chronic irreversible dementias in older persons. In Americans older than 65 years, AD affects 6–10% of the population (Black, 2005). By age 85, the prevalence increases to nearly 50%.

Vascular dementia accounts for 10–20% of all dementia and is often mixed with AD. Most patients with AD have some signs of cerebrovascular pathology on autopsy, and one third of patients diagnosed with vascular dementia show Alzheimer's disease pathology (Black, 2005). Lewy body dementia accounts for approximately 17% of all cases going to autopsy (Serby & Almiron, 2005). Other sources cite the overall incidence of LBD at only 10–20% of all dementia (Shadlen & Larson, 2005). Some sources consider LBD to be the second leading cause of dementia. Of all the dementias, VAD and LBD have the widest variability of criteria in making a diagnosis. Criteria for LBD were first published in 1996 by the American Academy of Neurology (AAN). CADASIL (cerebral autosomal dominant arteriopathy with subcortical infarcts and leukoencephalopathy) is a rare, inherited form of multi-infarct dementia (MID). This disease can cause stroke, dementia, migrainelike headaches, and psychiatric disturbances.

Dementia occurs in Parkinson's disease (PD) in approximately one third of all cases (Lieberman et al., 1979). Of the PD patients with dementia, in an autopsy study of 422 PD patients, over 50% had AD and 14% had LBD (Libow et al., 2005). Criteria for LBD and Parkinson's disease dementia (PDD) have a great deal of overlap and have the same pathological and clinical process with slightly different presentations (Serby and Almiron, 2005). With current criteria, pure PDD can only be diagnosed on autopsy by excluding AD and DLB.

Alcohol-related dementia (ARD) has also been named as Wernicke-Korsakoff syndrome. A veteran's nursing home study in Pennsylvania found 10% of their population met criteria for ARD out of 158 patients (Oslin & Cary, 2003). These were clinical diagnoses, and patients were followed for 2 years. ARD patients stabilized with treatment.

Frontotemporal dementia may represent 16% of all dementias that go to autopsy, but this disease is often found in younger persons (Chow, 2003). FTD has several distinct clinical presentations, and consensus groups have developed diagnostic criteria for frontotemporal lobe dementia (FTLD) that more specifically relate to the neuropathology. The term *FTD* refers to the behavioral presentations of FTLD (Chow, 2003). One form of FTLD is referred to as Pick's disease and indicates specific brain pathology.

Creutzfeldt-Jakob Disease (CJD) is a rare, degenerative, fatal brain disorder with usual onset at about age 60. About 90% of persons with CJD die within 1 year (www.NINDS.NIH.GOV, 2005).

Up to 23% of older adults will manifest psychotic symptoms at some time during their life. Dementia is the most frequent cause, but some do represent past mental illness. Approximately 50% of dementia patients will have psychotic symptoms, with paranoid delusions being the most common symptom followed by visual hallucinations (Khouzam et al., 2005).

Common Presenting Signs and Symptoms

Alzheimer's Disease

DSM IV criteria to diagnose Alzheimer's dementia include multiple cognitive deficits manifested by both memory impairment (short term initially) *and* one or more of the following:

- Aphasia (loss of word-finding ability)
- Apraxia (unable to do correct motor tasks)
- Agnosia (inability to recognize familiar faces)
- Disturbance in executive functioning (paying bills, preparing meals, abstract thinking)

The hallmark feature of beginning AD is isolated short-term memory loss, and a person may not initially meet the diagnostic criteria.

Persons who score 26/30 or better on the Mini-Mental State Exam (MMSE) are considered to have minimal cognitive impairment (MCI) but often progress to AD criteria within a year.

Other signs and symptoms include:

- Deficits in orientation are often noted after some progression of short-term memory problems. More likely to get lost in unfamiliar places.
- Often loses things and may blame others for their disappearance, or puts things in inappropriate places
- Frequent repetition of same information within a short period of time.
- Difficulty performing familiar tasks requiring sequencing, such as preparing a meal, using an appliance, or planning an outing or trip
- Poor or decreased judgment such as dressing inappropriately for the weather or walking into the street without regard to oncoming traffic
- Difficulties with abstract thinking, especially in finances and numbers are often the first problems that require the family to notice problems and intervene.
- Changes in mood or behavior, including sadness, outbursts, and anger and rapid mood swings. Changes in personality may also be noted.
- Withdrawal from normal activities, staying in more often, and sleeping more
- Psychosis with hallucinations or delusions tends to be later in the disease. Hallucinations tend to be more visual than auditory, but either may be present.

Vascular Dementia
- Dementia defined by cognitive decline from a previously higher level of functioning manifested by impairment of memory and of two or more cognitive domains (orientation, attention, language, visuospatial functions, executive functions, control, and praxis [ability to perform purposeful acts]), preferably established by clinical exam and documentation of neuropsychological testing; deficits should be severe enough to interfere with activities of daily living not due to physical effects of stroke alone.
- Cerebrovascular disease (CVD), defined by the presence of focal signs on neurological examination, such as hemiparesis, lower facial weakness, Babinski's sign, sensory deficit, hemianopia, and dysarthria consistent with stroke and evidence of relevant CVD by brain imaging (CT or MRI) including multiple large vessel infarcts or a single strategically placed infarct (angular gyrus, thalamus, basal forebrain, or posterior cerebral artery [PCA] or anterior cerebral arteries [ACA] territories), as well as multiple basal ganglia and white matter lacunes, or extensive periventricular white matter lesions, or combinations thereof.

A relationship between the above two disorders, manifested or inferred by the presence of one or more of the following: (a) onset of dementia within 3 months following a recognized stroke: (b) abrupt deterioration in cognitive functions; or (c) fluctuating stepwise progression of cognitive deficits (National Institute of Neurological Disorders and Stroke–Association Internationale pour la Recherche et l'Enseignement en Neurosciences (NINDS-AIREN) Criteria-1993).

Additional features often cited in other criteria sets include the following:

- The patient is often slowed in motor function and has a more variable cognitive disturbance history.
- Symptoms may be very similar to AD: poor short-term memory and verbal memory but may have more disturbances in executive function than memory initially.
- Vascular risk factors present (Black, 2005).
- Emotional lability is common.

- Important noncognitive features include depression, apathy, and psychosis (Shadlen, 2005), including auditory and visual hallucinations and delusions (Hill & Watson, 2005).

- Presentations have considerable variation due to the number of areas of the brain that can be involved.

- CADASIL (cerebral autosomal dominant arteriopathy with subcortical infarcts and leukoencephalopathy) is an inherited form of MID. This disease can cause stroke, dementia, migrainelike headaches, and psychiatric disturbances (NINDS, 2005).

- More common in men

Lewy Body Dementia

- Rapid and fluctuating course in attention, cognition, and alertness.

- Hallucinations occur in 40% of cases (Serby & Almiron, 2005); such hallucinations are well formed and recurrent and usually visual (93%) and/or auditory (50%) (Bolla et al., 2005).

- Prominent or persistent memory impairment may not occur in the early stages but is usually evident with progression (McKeith et al., 1996).

- Visuospatial problems are worse than memory problems (Geldmacher, 2004).

- Daytime sleepiness exists despite sufficient sleep the night before.

- Daytime sleep of two or more hours before 7 p.m.

- Staring into space for long periods

- Symptoms of Parkinsonism in 60% of cases: tremor, rigidity, bradykinesia

- Recurrent falls

- Syncope

- Neuroleptic sensitivity

- Delusions

Frontotemporal Lobe Dementia (FTD or FTLD)

- Often has early onset, between ages 35–75, with mean age in sixth decade

- Rarely occurs after age 75

- Both sexes equally affected

- Familial occurrence in 20–40% of cases.

- Gradual and progressive behavioral change

- Gradual and progressive language dysfunction, with fluent and nonfluent forms

- New onset of pedophilia, kleptomania, or other antisocial behavior is common.

- Obsessive-compulsive behaviors and agitation are common (Chow, 2003).

- Early major depression may precede dementia, but it may also manifest in euphoric states.

- Attention deficits early and memory problems may be later onset.

- Apathy common—emotional blunting

- Those with language impairment will show an aphasia corresponding to the affected region of the language-dominant hemisphere (Chow, 2003).

- Those with right temporal lobe variants often show hyperorality, carbohydrate craving, antisocial behavior, and rigidity of behaviors.

- Visuospatial abilities may be well retained for some time.

- There is a strong familial factor in Pick's disease variant of FTD.

- In the later stages of the disease, parkinsonian features: bradykinesia, rigidity, and postural instability develop.

- The amyloid plaques seen in AD are not seen in FTD (Chow, 2003).

Differential Diagnosis

- Depression

- Parkinson's disease dementia

- Normal pressure hydrocephalus (NPH)

- Chronic subdural hematoma
- Cruetzfeldt-Jakob disease (CJD)—Rapidly progressing
- Hashimoto's thyroiditis
- Brain tumor
- Delirium (potentially reversible) causes:
  - Medication induced (particularly analgesics, anticholinergics, psychotropic medications, and sedative-hypnotics)
  - Alcohol-related thiamine deficiency
  - Infections
  - Hypothyroidism
  - Vitamin B_{12} deficiency
  - Electrolyte problems including hyponatremia, hypercalcemia
  - Hepatic and renal dysfunction

Essential Diagnostic and Laboratory Tests

- Complete blood count with differential
- Serum electrolytes including calcium
- Serum glucose
- BUN/creatinine
- Thyroid function tests
- Liver function tests
- Serum B_{12} level

With Indications

- Syphilis screening
- CT or MRI of head
- HIV testing
- Toxicology screen
- Digitalis level or other drug levels
- Holotranscobalamin (holo TC) (in B_{12} deficiency)
- Serum methylmalonic acid (MMA) (in B_{12} deficiency)
- Intrinsic factor antibody assay (in B_{12} deficiency)
- Serum magnesium and phosphorus

- EEG
- EKG
- Chest X-ray
- Pulmonary function tests
- Lumbar puncture

Other Assessment

- Detailed history is most important. Interview caregivers and family members to identify key behavior and functional changes.
- Cognitive testing:
  - Folstein Mini-Mental State Exam (MMSE)
  - Clock drawing test
  - Trail making part B (written or verbal)
  - Other neuropsychological tests
- Depression screening
  - Ysavage Geriatric Depression Scale, short form (GDS-15) (see Appendix C)
  - Cornell Scale for Depression in Dementia (Observational Scale—appropriate in more advanced dementia) (see Appendix D)
- Functional assessment
  - Activities of daily living (ADLs)
  - Instrumental activities of daily living (IADLs), driving abilities
- Complete physical exam with thorough sensory and neurological exams

Management Plan

It is critical to manage underlying chronic medical problems including pain, constipation, thyroid disease, nutritional deficiencies, cardiovascular disease, respiratory disease, diabetes, and renal disease to maximize function and quality of life. The plan of care should be adjusted for the individual's medical care goals, risk factors, and age. Acute changes in condition should alert the practitioner to infections or other acute events that cause chronic medical conditions to deteriorate.

Nonpharmacologic
See Table 15-3.

- Environmental issues are the primary cause of behavior symptoms in dementia.
- Most dementia patients do best with a structured schedule, minimal caregiver changes, and avoidance of excessive stimulation.
- Review target behavior documentation with facility staff/caregivers and care-planning approaches.
- Activity tailored to the individual's interests, aptitude, and physical and sensory abilities

- Ensure patient has access to their glasses and hearing aids. Remove earwax.

Pharmacologic
Cholinesterase inhibitors (ChIs) (Table 15-4) are indicated for mild to moderate dementia. Primary indication is for AD-type dementia, but many sources indicate benefit in Lewy body dementia, Parkinson's disease dementia, and vascular dementia, but not in frontotemporal dementia (Chow, 2003).

A review by Wynn and Cummings (2004) provides beneficial evidence of ChI effects on

TABLE 15-3   Nonpharmacologic Treatment of Behavioral Symptoms in Older Patients with Dementia

CLINICAL FEATURES	APPROACH	COMMENTS
Delirium	Refocus in the moment. Avoid multiple commands. Avoid excessive stimulation. Ensure safety.	Search for underlying medical cause: UTI, respiratory infection, CHF, constipation, electrolyte imbalance, or medications are common causes.
Depression	Consider referral of patient to counseling in early stage of disease. Recommend meaningful, appropriate daytime activities based on past hobby and social interests. Use pet therapy if available and appropriate to client needs.	Help family and staff understand dementia and depression is different than mental illness. Explain that there is a chemical deficiency in the brain.
Anxiety	Use calm reassurance and distraction. Underlying depression may be a factor.	One-to-one attention. Mirror desired behavior or affect.
Insomnia or sleep disorders	Decrease dietary caffeine and evening fluid intake. Increase patient activity level or exercise in daytime and avoid daytime naps. Increase exposure to bright light during the day. Keep patient dressed during daytime hours. Consider lifelong sleep patterns, warm milk or high carbohydrate snack before bedtime.	Consider underlying medical problems: sleep apnea, pain, heart failure, BPH, or urge incontinence. Long-term use of benzodiazepines causes rebound insomnia, but don't discontinue abruptly. Wean slowly.
Agitation	Eliminate or minimize environmental stresses. Simplify environment. Structured routines and socialization. Advise staff and family to seek medical advice if there is sudden onset. Distract, don't confront. Use of restraints is not recommended and may be harmful. For delusions, provide validation, not reality orientation. Consider constipation, depression, infection, and pain (CDIP).	
Wandering	Ensure safety by using wander guards to alert staff to patient leaving facility. Use visual diversions in the environment at exits and patient rooms where doors are open. Stairwell doors should have electronic keypads. Evaluating the patient's needs and potential triggers is essential to developing individualized care plans. Have identification of facility on patient with phone number to call.	Wandering isn't necessarily a problematic behavior, but becomes so when patients wander into others' rooms or out of building, posing a risk to their own safety.

TABLE 15-4   Drugs Used to Treat Dementia

BRAND NAME	GENERIC NAME	START DOSE	DAILY MAXIMAL DOSE	INDICATIONS	CLASS	MOST COMMON SIDE EFFECTS*
Aricept	Donepezil	5 mg daily	10 mg daily	Mild to moderate Alzheimer's	Cholinesterase inhibitor	GI: diarrhea, nausea and/ or vomiting may be dose related. Weight loss. CV: Bradycardia and/or heart block, syncope. Use with caution in SSS or SVT, in seizures, COPD or asthma, risk of ulcer disease or in patient with bladder outlet obstruction.
Exelon	Rivastigmine	1.5 mg twice daily	6.0 mg twice daily	Mild to moderate Alzheimer's	Cholinesterase inhibitor	GI: significant, nausea and/or vomiting, and weight loss—more frequent in women. Also diarrhea, anorexia, abdominal pain, dyspepsia, constipation, flatulence. Use caution in patients with history of PUD or NSAID use. CV: Use with caution in SSS, SVT, in seizures, COPD or asthma, risk of ulcer disease or in patient with bladder outlet obstruction. CNS: Dizziness, headache, insomnia, confusion, depression, anxiety, hallucinations.
Razadyne**	Galantamine	4 mg twice daily	12 mg twice daily	Mild to moderate Alzheimer's	Cholinesterase inhibitor	GI: diarrhea, nausea and/or vomiting may be dose related. Weight loss. Abdominal pain. CV: Bradycardia and/or heart block, syncope. Use with caution in SSS or SVT, in seizures, COPD or asthma, risk of ulcer disease or in patient with bladder outlet obstruction. CNS: dizziness, headache, depression, insomnia
Namenda	Memantine	5 mg daily	10 mg twice daily	Moderate to severe Alzheimer's	N-methyl d-aspartate receptor antagonist	GI: constipation, vomiting, weight loss CV: hypertension, cardiac failure, syncope, CVA, TIA CNS: dizziness, confusion, headache, hallucinations, pain, somnolence, fatigue, aggressive reaction, ataxia, vertigo, hypokinesia Other: cough, rash

*This is not a complete list of side effects. Check drug reference for contraindications, drug interactions, and dose titration schedules.

**Formerly Reminyl; name changed to Razadyne July 2005.

Notes: COPD, chronic obstructive pulmonary disease; CVA, cerebrovascular accident; PUD, peptic ulcer disease; SSS, sick sinus syndrome; SVT, supraventricular tachycardia; TIA, transient ischemic attack.

Source: Lacy, 2005.

behavioral symptoms including neuropsychiatric behavioral symptoms in AD, as well as depression. Patients with behavioral symptoms in vascular depression, including agitation, apathy, and emotional instability, may also benefit from ChIs (Hill & Watson, 2005). These drugs work by blocking the action of enzymes that degrade acetylcholine but do not make more acetylcholine. The goal is to slow the progression of the disease. Cognitive scores are only a crude assessment of effectiveness, and functional assessments and family and staff reports are most important.

N-methyl d-aspartate (NMDA) receptor antagonist (memantine/Namenda) (Table 15-4) is indicated for use in moderate to advanced dementia. Application for use of this drug in mild

dementia is pending with the Food and Drug Administration (FDA). This drug was studied by Reisberg and colleagues (2003) in patients with AD with a base-line MMSE score of 3–14, and that is the typical range when patients are started on treatment. Tariot et al. (2004) conducted a study of AD patients with MMSE scores of 5–14 that had been receiving stable doses of Aricept for at least 6 months with significantly better outcomes than the placebo group. Little is known about the effects of this combination of therapy earlier in the disease for patients already on cholinesterase inhibitors.

Serotonin reuptake inhibitors (SRIs) (Table 15-5) are often indicated for treatment of underlying depression in dementia. The Alzheimer's brain is deficient not only in

TABLE 15-5   Serotonin Reuptake Inhibitor (SRI) Antidepressants

GENERIC NAME	BRAND NAME	AVERAGE STARTING DOSE (mg/day)	AVERAGE TARGET DAILY DOSE AFTER 6 WKS (mg/day)	USUAL HIGHEST FINAL DAILY ACUTE DOSE (mg/day)	COMMENTS
Citalopram	Celexa	10–2	20–30	30–40 once daily	Some sedation, weight gain—generally dose in morning. Same active molecule as escitalopram
Duloxetine	Cymbalta	20 twice daily	20–30	60 single or divided dose	SNRI—Sedation, also approved for treatment of diabetic peripheral neuropathy, not approved for treatment of urinary incontinence in the United States (is in Europe)
Escitalopram	Lexapro	10	20 after 1 week	20 once daily	Minimal side effects—contains only the active isomer of citalopram
Fluoxetine	Prozac	10	20	20–40 once daily	May be activating in some patients—dose in the morning.
Fluvoxamine	Luvox	25–50	50–200	100–300	Used primarily in OCD
Mirtazapine	Remeron	7.5–15	1–30	30–45 once daily	SNRI—Sedation, weight gain. Activating at higher doses
Paroxetine	Paxil	10–20	20–30	30–40 once daily	Sedating, some EPS in frail elderly
Sertraline	Zoloft	25–50	50–100	100–200	Sedating, weight gain
Venlafaxine	Effexor	25–75	75–200	150–300	SNRI—Sedation, weight gain. Activating at higher doses

Notes: EPS, extrapyramidal symptoms; SNRI, serotonin-norepinephrine reuptake inhibitors.

All SRI medications can have GI side effects such as nausea, diarrhea, headache, sedation, restlessness, weight gain, and sexual dysfunction. May cause hyponatremia in some. Most are approved for use in obsessive-compulsive disorder (OCD). SNRIs may cause dry mouth and sedation.

Sources: MedLinePlus, 2005; Brody & Serby, 2004.

acetylcholine but in serotonin and norepinephrine as well (Bolla et al., 2005). Alzheimer's and
vascular dementia patients with anxiety or irritability may also benefit from SRIs. Significant
loss of serotonergic neurons has been demonstrated in FTD, and SRIs have been reported as

successful in the treatment of disinhibition,
depression, carbohydrate craving, and compulsive behaviors in FTD subjects (Swartz et al.,
1997).

Many other psychotropic drugs (Tables
15-6 and 15-7) have been used in an attempt to

TABLE 15-6   Treatment of Behavioral Symptoms in Older Patients with Dementia—Pharmacologic Approaches

CLINICAL FEATURES	DRUGS	COMMENTS
Delirium	Conventional antipsychotic (CHAP): haloperidol—only if patient is threat to self or others, or lorazepam in < 2 mg dose	Evaluate current drugs as possible cause. Stabilize underlying medical causes. Contraindicated in Parkinson's disease or Lewy body dementia
Psychosis	Acute: CHAP* Long term: atypical antipsychotics *	Zyprexa available IM. Risperdal IM not appropriate for acute treatment
Depression	*Without psychosis*: sertraline (Zoloft) or citalopram (Celexa), escitalopram (Lexapro), duloxetine (Cymbalta), mirtazapine (Remeron), or paroxetine (Paxil). *With psychosis*: Antidepressant and antipsychotic or ECT Prozac and Effexor may be more activating. Remeron can be activating at higher doses.	Start with lowest dose and increase slowly. Effects may take weeks to manifest adequately. Most SRI antidepressants are sedating initially. Seek previous history of depression, treatment, and possibility of bipolar disorder
Anxiety	Acute: benzodiazepine (lorazepam, consider oxazepam) Long term: buspirone, SRIs, SNRIs	*Long term use of benzodiazepines should be avoided in the elderly for all indications*
Insomnia	Acute: trazodone (Desyrel). For very short term consider a benzodiazepine such as zolpidem (Ambien) or lorazepam.	Trazodone is nonhabit forming, but sedating. Not generally used as an antidepressant in the elderly.
Sundown syndrome	Acute: trazodone; consider CHAP, atypical antipsychotic (risperidone, olanzapine, or quetiapine). Long term: Cholinesterase inhibitors or glutamate blockers (Memantine), trazodone; consider atypical antipsychotic	Consider sensory deficits. *Avoid using antipsy-chotics for behavior unless the behaviors are psychosis and distressing to the patient.*
Aggression or anger	Mild acute: trazodone Mild long term: antiseizure, SRI, trazodone, buspirone Severe acute: CHAP, atypical antipsychotic Severe long term: antiseizure drug or antipsychotic or combinations	Antiseizure drugs being used off-label include: divalproex (Depakote), carbamazepine (Tegretol), gabapentin (Neurontin), levetiracetam (Keppra), lomotrigine (Lamictyl), oxcarbazepine (Trileptal), topiramate (Topamax)

*See FDA warnings on Table V.

Notes: Prior to initiating treatment with new medication, consider whether the target behavior is caused or exacerbated by a current medication. Start with low doses and go slow. Systematic trials of single agents should be tried rather than the use of multiple agents. The practitioner is advised to ensure adequate documentation of target behaviors prior to prescribing.

Target Behaviors:

• Verbal—Yelling, screaming, swearing, threatening, criticizing, scolding, verbal sexual advances

• Physically active—Hitting, kicking, biting, spitting, throwing things, using weapons, physical sexual advances

• Physically passive—Unable to sit or lie still, increased activity, wandering or pacing, increased agitation

• Psychotic symptoms—Hallucinations, paranoia, or delusions

TABLE 15-7   Pharmacologic Treatment of Behavioral Symptoms of Older Patients with Dementia

MEDICATION	CLASS	DOSE RANGE	COMMENTS
Buspirone (Buspar)	Anxiolytic	10–60 mg/dd	Few side effects or drug interactions. Takes up to 6 weeks for full effect
Sertraline (Zoloft)	AD-SRI	25–100 mg/d	GI side effects common, initially sedating
Pareoxetine (Paxil)	AD-SRI	10–20 mg/d	Somewhat sedating, Can cause EPS.
Citalopram (Celexa)	AD-SRI	10–40 mg/d	Somnolence, insomnia
Escitalopram (Lexapro)	AD-SRI	10–20 mg/d	Can titrate to full dose in 1 week
Mirtazapine (Remeron)	AD-SNRI	7.5–45 mg/d	Monitor for agranulocytosis or neutropenia—sore throat, stomatitis; sedating, weight gain. More activating at higher doses
Trazodone (Desyrel)	AD-atypical	25–150 mg	Low cardiotoxicity, sedating, postural hypotension. Interactions
Bupropion (Wellbutrin)	AD-other (DRI)	75–225 mg/dd	Lowers seizure threshold, insomnia, irritability. Low cardiotoxicity
Venlafaxine (Effexor)	AD-SNRI	37.5–150 mg/d	May worsen psychosis or mania. Useful in severe depression
Divalproex (Depakote)	Antiseizure, mood stabilizer	250–1500 mg/dd	Monitor CBC, LFTs, serum levels. Don't need therapeutic serum levels.
Gabapentin (Neurontin)	Antiseizure	200–3600 mg/dd	Wide variation in dose needs. TID dosing.
Carbamazepine (Tegretol)	Antiseizure	100–500 mg/dd	Monitor levels, CBC for aplastic anemia
Lorazepam (Ativan)	Anxiolytic/ Benzodiazepine	1–2 mg/dd	Short acting. Available in IM. Use short term
Haloperidol (Haldol)*	Conventional Antipsychotic (CHAP)	0.5–2 mg/dd	Divided doses BID or TID. High EPS. Avoid artane or cogentin use. Not very sedating.
Risperidone (Risperdal)**	Atypical Antipsychotic	0.25–2 mg/d	Expensive. Less EPS than CHAP. Sedating. Avoid in Lewy body dementia and PD
Olanzapine (Zyprexa)**	Atypical Antipsychotic	2.5–10 mg/d in evening	Expensive. Less EPS than CHAP. Sedating. Avoid in Lewy body dementia and PD
Quetiapine (Seroquel)**	Atypical Antipsychotic	12.5–200 mg/ twice daily	More sedating, transient orthostasis. Least EPS
Aripiprazole (Abilify)**	Atypical Antipsychotic	5.0–15 mg	Very expensive. Some EPS. Avoid in Lewy body dementia and PD
Zolpidem (Ambien)	Benzodiazepine-like Sedative hypnotic	5 mg in elderly or debilitated	Regular use can lead to tolerance, depression, cognitive impairment. Should be limited to 10 days or less.

Notes: AD, antidepressant; SRI, serotonin reuptake inhibitor; SNRI, serotonin-norepinephrine reuptake inhibitor; DRI, dopamine reuptake inhibitor; dd, divided doses; PD, Parkinson's disease.

*May carry a higher risk of mortality.

**FDA has issued warning of 1.6–1.7 times the risk of death from stroke, other cardiovascular complications, and infections compared to placebo in 17 controlled trials. May also cause hyperglycemia.

It should be noted that the US FDA has not approved any agent to treat agitation, aggression, or psychosis associated with dementia. Off-label uses of psychotropic drugs are based on evidence-based literature and clinical and expert consensus guidelines.

extinguish difficult behaviors, but extreme caution should be used with these drugs. Ensure that there are no other medical causes or environmental or caregiver issues precipitating the behaviors before pursuing pharmacologic interventions. Identify target behaviors carefully, and ensure thorough documentation of such. Table 15-6 outlines approaches to the psychotropic drugs commonly used; many of which, however, are off-label uses. Table 15-7 gives more specific dose ranges and indications and some of the most problematic side effects of the individual drugs.

It should be noted that the FDA has not approved any agent to treat agitation, aggression, or psychosis associated with dementia. Off-label uses of psychotropic drugs are based on evidence-based literature and clinical and expert consensus guidelines.

Recent studies have demonstrated a significant increase in the risk of cardiovascular events with the use of atypical antipsychotics, and using conventional antipsychotics are not recommended either (Sink et al., 2005; Wang et al., 2005). The unnecessary use of antipsychotic and other psychotropic drugs is carefully scrutinized in long-term care facility surveys. They are recognized as sometimes necessary in "organic mental syndromes" (now called *delirium*, *dementia*, and *amnestic* and other cognitive disorders by the Diagnostic and Statistical Manual, 4th edition, [DSM-IV]) with associated psychotic and/or agitated behaviors which, if not caused by environmental, medical, or preventable causes, are persistent and cause the resident to present a danger to self or others, or experience psychotic symptoms resulting in distress or functional impairment.

Patients with Lewy body dementia (LBD) are particularly sensitive to antipsychotics. While they can still have adverse reactions, olanzapine and quetiapine are the preferred agents to avoid the extrapyramidal symptoms (EPS) side effects. Many LBD patients do not need or respond well to dopaminergic drugs for their parkinsonian features. If treatment is needed, levodopa-carbidopa is indicated (Geldmacher, 2004).

Stopping acetylcholinesterase inhibitors (ChIs), memantine, or other psychotropic drugs—Statistically significant cognitive and functional effects for ChIs have been established in many studies. These effects have been reported for as little as 3 months delay in symptom worsening to 2–3 years in other reports

(Schneider, 2004). However, not all individual patients have the same responses of symptoms to the drugs nor do all caregivers have the same perceptions as to the significance of the response. Therefore the decision to stop treatment with these drugs becomes a matter of helping the family articulate any concerns and the goals of continuing or discontinuing therapy. The clinician can start by asking the designated spokesperson about what benefits they feel have been achieved with the medication, their concerns, or disappointments. Give factual information, but do not insist that therapy be stopped or continued, and there will be no blame for either decision on the provider's part. Let the family know that there can be further abrupt decline in cognition and function when the drugs are stopped, but that there are legitimate reasons to halt therapy such as:

- Adverse side effects including weight loss, anorexia, nausea, and nightmares
- Inability to have medication administration monitored (in community settings)
- Lack of perceived benefit
- No significant function to preserve.
- Inability to swallow

The same principles apply to Memantine therapy or antidepressants, and in any case therapy can be reinitiated if it is determined to be necessary. Weaning from the drug is recommended, but there is not clear evidence that this is necessary.

Patient, Family, and Staff Education

- Presentation of the diagnosis
  - Elicit patient and family understanding of the problem first.
  - Present the specific findings.
  - Explain how a diagnosis is derived as appropriate (no specific tests).
  - Name the disease.

- Prognosis
  - Progression variable, but ultimately terminal
  - 2–20 years course
  - Eventual decline in memory and function including cessation of eating and drinking.
- List treatment options, including risks and benefits and medication side effects.
- Discuss advance directives.
  - Code status
  - Durable power of attorney/decision maker procedures specific to state
  - Treatment directives
    - Transfer to hospital for acute episodes
    - Do not transfer to hospital—treat in facility
    - Comfort care only
    - Tube feeding decision status if known
- Behaviors to expect—Use materials from Alzheimer's Association or locally developed, culturally sensitive materials.
- Anticipatory guidance includes family reaction to their grief over loss of "the person" as well as placement issues.
- Community resources as appropriate
- Internet resources if family has access or interest
- If behavioral symptoms in dementia warrant antipsychotic therapy, include warnings regarding increased vascular events and increased mortality (see Appendix B).

Physician Consultation

- New or unexplained focal neurological symptoms
- Suspected normal pressure hydrocephalus (NPH-rapid onset dementia, urinary incontinence, ataxia)
- Unclear diagnosis
- Violent behavior

- Very rapidly progressing dementia
- Consider psychiatry consult to assist with diagnosis and medication management.

▆ LATE-LIFE DELIRIUM

Introduction

Randomized clinical studies of delirium are very difficult to perform in patients with cognitive impairment and confounding comorbidities. Therefore, recommendations for evaluating and treating delirium are based on expert opinion and clinical observations. The pathophysiology of delirium and confusion is poorly understood because of confounding comorbidities, but it is believed that acetylcholine plays an important role in delirium. This hypothesis is derived from observations that hypoxia, hypoglycemia, and thiamine deficiencies decrease acetylcholine synthesis in the central nervous system. It is also known that Alzheimer's disease, in which there is a loss of cholinergic neurons, increases the risk of delirium due to anticholinergic medications (Francis, 2004).

Recognition of delirium, even in the presence of dementia, is important in order to not overlook potential interventions that can improve outcomes and quality of life in the elderly. Delirium may be the only early finding that heralds acute illness in demented elderly patients. Some studies have found that up to 70% of cases of delirium were not recognized, but attributed to the patient's age, dementia, or to other mental disorders (Marcantonio et al., 2002). Delirium is also often referred to as *acute confusional state*, *acute brain syndrome*, or *toxic or metabolic encephalopathy*. The term *confusion* is used to indicate a problem with thinking at normal speed, clarity, or coherence, and is associated with a reduced attention span. Confusion is a component of delirium (Francis, 2004). Although there is a high percent of underlying dementia in the elderly in long term care and hospital populations with delirium, a clear diagnosis of the dementia type cannot be made in the presence of delirium.

Definition

There are four key features that characterize delirium as defined by the American Psychiatric Association's Diagnostic and Statistical Manual, 4th edition (DSM-IV).

- Disturbance of consciousness with reduced ability to focus, sustain, or shift attention

- A change in cognition or the development of a perceptual disturbance that is not better accounted for by a preexisting, established, or evolving dementia

- The disturbance develops over a short period of time (usually hours to days) and tends to fluctuate during the course of the day.

- There is evidence from the history, physical exam, or laboratory findings that the disturbance is caused by a medical condition, substance intoxication, or medication side effect.

Additionally, there may be other features present in delirium and confusion:

- Psychomotor behavioral disturbances such as hypoactivity, hyperactivity with increased sympathetic activity, and impairment in sleep duration and architecture

- Variable emotional disturbances, including fear, depression, euphoria, or perplexity

Epidemiology

Rates of delirium in hospitalized elderly medical patients vary from 14–56% with high rates of mortality ranging from 10–60%. This disorder is underrecognized and often misdiagnosed by physicians caring for elderly hospitalized patients (Inouye, 1994). Nearly 30% of elderly medical patients in the hospital experience delirium, with the higher rates being associated with the frail elderly and surgical patients (Francis, 2004). Nearly 30% of cases of delirium are produced by drug toxicity. In a meta-analysis, the prevalence of delirium on top of an underlying dementia ranged from 22% to 89% (Fick, Agostini, & Inouye, 2002). In a study of elderly patients with femoral neck fractures who underwent surgery and who were followed for 5 years, Lundstrom and colleagues (2003) found a 69% prevalence of delirium superimposed upon dementia that developed in previously undiagnosed dementia. Only 20% of the patients without postoperative delirium developed dementia. Signs of delirium may persist for up to 12 months or even longer, particularly in those with underlying dementia.

Precipitating Risk Factors

- Polypharmacy and high-risk drugs (see Table 15-8)

- Alcohol

- Infection, including sepsis and central nervous system (CNS) infections

- Dehydration

- Immobility

- Malnutrition or nutritional/vitamin deficiencies (vitamin B_{12}, niacin, folic acid), or Wernicke's encephalopathy

- Use of bladder catheters

- Fecal impaction

- Seizures

- Pulmonary disease with metabolic disturbance

- Endocrine disease, such as thyroid, parathyroid, adrenal, or diabetes

- Hypothermia or hyperthermia

- Sensory deficits, especially with dementia

- Anesthesia

- Previous delirium

Common Presenting Signs and Symptoms

- Disturbance of consciousness and altered cognition are essential components.

- Develops over a short-time period and tends to fluctuate over the course of a day.

TABLE 15-8 Common Drugs That May Cause Delirium in the Elderly

DRUG	COMMON SIDE EFFECTS	COMMENTS
Diphenhydramine (Benadryl)	Typical anticholinergic side effects:	Also contained in OTC sleep medication: Tylenol PM
Hydroxyzine (Atarax, Vistaril)	Dry mucus membranes, blurry vision,	
Cholorpheniramine (Chlortrimeton)	constipation, urinary retention, hallucinations, confusion	Common ingredient in OTC cold preparations
Tricyclic antidepressants (TCAs) (Amitriptyline, Doxepin, Imipramine, Maprotiline, others)	Anticholinergic and some cardiotoxicity	If TCA is used: disipramine (Norpramin) or nortriptyline (Pamelor)
Trihexyphenidyl hydrochloride (Artane)	Very anticholinergic	
Benztropine (Cogentin)	Very anticholinergic	
Promethazine (Phenergan)	Anticholinergic, respiratory depression	
Cimetidine (Tagamet)	Confusion common in elderly	Renal or hepatic impairment suspected
Oxybututynin (Ditropan)	Anticholinergic side effects,	
Tolterodine (Detrol)	including hallucinations	
Parkinson's drugs:	Hallucinations common for both.	Dopaminergic agents
• Sinemet	Somnolence for Mirapex	
• Mirapex		
Benzodiazepines	CNS depressant	Not covered by Medicare part D. Need to be weaned
Reserpine	Mental depression, anxiety, psychosis	
Clonidine (catapres)	CNS depression	Should be weaned
Opiates	CNS depression	May still need to treat pain
Propoxyphene	CNS disturbances common	No more effective than Tylenol and is habituating. Beers List exclusion
Corticosteroids	Psychosis	

- Disturbance is usually caused by a medical condition, substance intoxication, or medications.
- Distractibility is often evident in conversation.
- May appear drowsy, lethargic, or even comatose in more advanced cases.
- Hypervigilance may also occur in cases of alcohol or sedative drug withdrawal, but is not always present in the elderly.
- Anxiety
- Irritability
- Problems in speech and language functions. Patient may lose the ability to speak a second language and may revert to their primary language.
- Perceptual disturbances are common, as are delusions of harm.
- Visual hallucinations are common but are sometimes thought of as "misperceptions."
- May be worse at night and better in the morning
- Altered sleep-wake cycles

Differential Diagnosis

- Metabolic disease or electrolyte disturbance
- Dehydration
- Infection
- Substance intoxication (alcohol, narcotics, many medications) or drug reaction
- Brain trauma or tumor
- Seizure
- Psychiatric illness—(depression, psychosis, bipolar mania)

- Hyperparathyroidism/hypercalcemia
- Hyperthyroidism or hypothyroidism
- Hypoglycemia or hyperglycemia
- Hypoxia
- Cardiovascular disease (bradycardia, MI, arrhythmia, uncompensated heart failure)
- Sundowning syndrome—Common in the afternoon in patients with dementia
- Frontotemporal dementia—Loss of language skills, lack of judgment, and lack of spontaneous activity may be confused with delirium.
- Lewy body dementia
- Untreated or under treated pain.
- HIV Infection with dementia

Essential Diagnostic and Laboratory Tests

- Electrolytes including calcium, magnesium, phosphorus
- Renal function tests
- CBC with differential
- Urinalysis for culture and sensitivity and toxicity screens
- Thyroid studies
- Drug levels as indicated (digoxin, dilantin, valproic acid, carbamazepine, lithium, quinidine, salicylate toxicity screens). May be toxic even if within therapeutic range in malnutrition states. Check albumin in patients taking drugs with narrow therapeutic window

As Indicated
- Erythrocyte sedimentation rate (ESR)
- HIV test
- B_{12} and folate
- Liver function—consider ammonia level if liver disease suspected.
- Arterial blood gases

- Electrocardiogram
- Head CT is often indicated, but not always needed if the patient is easily aroused, there are no focal signs of neurological damage, there is no history of trauma, or the initial evaluation uncovers a treatable cause. However, it may still be needed if the problem is not resolving or is worsening.
- Lumbar puncture—highest yield is in those suspected to have meningitis. Brain imaging should be obtained first.
- EEG to exclude seizures, some metabolic encephalopathies, or infectious encephalitides. Alcohol or sedative drug withdrawal can be identified on EEG as a distinct pattern from metabolic or seizure disorders (Francis, 2004).

Other Assessment
- Sudden decline in MMSE score may be helpful but not diagnostic.
- Specific attention tasks such as reciting five random numbers at a time, spelling words backward, serial subtraction
- Confusion Assessment Method (CAM) uses questions to determine: acute onset and fluctuating course, inattention, disorganized thinking, and altered level of consciousness (Inouye et al., 1990) (see resource list).
- Oral Trail Making Part B Test—Ask patient to say out loud alternating numbers and corresponding letters up to 13. Give example of a few pairs: 1-A, 2-B, 3-C, etc.

Management Plan

Identify problems and treat within parameters of patient goals of care. Remove or reduce offending drugs and environmental problems as able. Discuss work-up and care options with spokesperson for the patient, and review treatment directives for facility care or hospitalization if necessary. Ensure safety of patient and staff in case of violent or aggressive behavior. Avoid restraints if at all possible.

Nonpharmacologic
- Redirection without confrontation
- One-to-one or closer supervision
- Avoid overstimulation with activity or loud noise
- Give the patient something to do or something to hold with pleasant textures. Stuffed animals can be helpful for some.
- Exposure to daylight sun when possible to help with sleep-wake cycles.
- Early mobilization and range of motion
- Visual aids including glasses, magnifying lenses, and phone with large numbers
- Hearing aids, or portable amplifying devices, earwax removal
- Adequate hydration

Pharmacologic
- Discontinue or reduce offending drugs.
- Short-term lorazepam or antipsychotics may be necessary. Benzodiazepines have been associated with development of delirium itself but may be necessary in withdrawal syndromes.
- Trazodone may be helpful for sleep at night.
- B_{12}, folic acid, niacin as indicated

Patient, Family, and Staff Education
- Caregivers should be given anticipatory guidance on the significance of sudden changes in mental status or function in dementia patients or even frail elderly. The changes can represent the onset of a new medical illness, exacerbation of chronic disease, or changes in the environment. Reports of these changes by family members are often the most timely and accurate information, if caregivers in a facility are not regularly with the patient.

- Changes in room assignment in the long-term care facility or change in caregivers, routines, or light or noise levels may be precipitating factors of behavioral changes that need to be addressed.
- Remind family and staff that the patient has no control over any offending behavior, although they may respond to gentle, consistent, calm reminders. Always speak to the patient in a calm tone of voice, speak clearly, and ensure they have sensory aids available such as their glasses and hearing aids.
- Ensure clear communication about behaviors, and identify the behavior clearly before considering pharmacologic intervention. Teach family and staff that getting out of bed or wandering are not behaviors warranting restraints nor medications. Work as a team to discover the unmet needs being expressed.
- Ensure family and staff understand safety issues for the patient, which may include risk of falls, wandering, inability to operate equipment, call lights, and aspiration risks in lethargy. Avoid access to glass or sharp objects.

Physician Consultation
- Violent behavior
- Alcohol withdrawal
- Problems not resolving as anticipated
- Invasive testing indicated and requested by power of attorney for health care (EEG, lumbar puncture)
- New seizure activity suspected
- Problems not within scope of practice of the practitioner

LATE-LIFE DEPRESSION

Definition

Depression is a medical illness characterized by persistent sadness, discouragement, and loss of self-worth, but in the elderly sad mood is not a reliable symptom. The traditional definition of depression requires persistent sadness, most of the time, or anhedonia (loss of pleasure in activities one usually enjoys) for a minimum of 2 weeks. Depression is a brain disease that involves the limbic and prefrontal neuronal circuits (Brody & Serby, 2004).

Epidemiology

Late-life depression affects about 6 million elderly Americans. Up to 40% of adult patients in the community have significant depressive symptoms, but less than one half meet the criteria for major depressive disorder as defined by DSM-IV. The lifetime prevalence rate for a major depressive disorder is 7–12% for men and 20–25% for women. The overall rate in primary care settings for major depression in the elderly is 17–37% (Lebowitz et al., 1997), and these rates are highest in outpatients with chronic disease (Katon & Sullivan, 1990). In long-term care facilities, approximately 30–50% of residents have depression where multiple chronic comorbidities are common (Katz & Parmelee, 1997).

The elderly in the United States have the highest suicide rates with older white males over the age of 80 being at greatest risk. Most suicides in the elderly, but not all, have depression and have seen their primary care physician within a month of death (Katz, Kennedy, & Conwell, 2004). Psychoanalytic views of depression tie it to early trauma or loss, but only half of the cases are precipitated by such experiences. There may be environmental factors and genetic factors as well (Paulson, 2005).

Depression can occur in 20–25% of elderly stroke patients, with most cases manifesting in the first month after a stroke. In Parkinson's disease patients, 40% may have significant depressive symptoms, and up to 50% of dementia patients have depressive symptoms. In Alzheimer's disease patients, up to 20% have major depression (Lebowitz, 1997).

Common Presenting Signs and Symptoms

Major Depression

- A person must have either a depressed mood and/or:

- Loss of interest or pleasure in daily activities consistently for at least 2 weeks, which is a change from the person's normal mood or function *and* several of the following symptoms:

  ○ Weight loss or change in appetite that is involuntary

  ○ Insomnia or hypersomnia

  ○ Psychomotor agitation or retardation

  ○ Fatigue or loss of energy

  ○ Feelings of worthlessness or guilt that is inappropriate

  ○ Diminished concentration or indecisiveness

  ○ Recurrent thoughts of death (not just fear of dying), recurrent suicidal ideation without a specific plan, or a suicide attempt or a specific plan for committing suicide

- The symptoms are not as a result of bereavement or caused by substances (such as drugs, alcohol, medications) or a general medical condition.

- Major depressive disorder cannot be diagnosed if a person has a history of manic, hypomanic, or mixed episodes (e.g., a bipolar disorder) or if the depressed mood is better accounted for by schizoaffective disorder and is not superimposed on schizophrenia, a delusion, or psychotic disorder (DSM-IV-Abbreviated).

- DSM-IV criteria are not specific to the elderly. Cognitive symptoms, including behavioral symptoms secondary to dementia, may be indicative of depression.

- Late-life depression is more highly associated with cognitive impairment and medical comorbidities than family history.

- Psychotic depression may overlap with major depression and include obsessive ruminations. Patient may present with more animation than apathy. Delusions rather than hallucinations are common.

- Risk factors include female gender, history of depressive illness in first-degree relatives, prior episodes of major depression, lack of social support, substance abuse, and corticosteroid use.

Primary Mania or Bipolar Disorder (DSM-IV) Criteria

- At least 1 week of elevated, expansive, or irritable mood and 3 of the following:

  - Grandiosity
  - Decreased sleep
  - Talkativeness
  - Racing thoughts
  - Distractibility
  - Increased goal-directed activity
  - Excessive involvement in pleasurable activities with a high potential for painful consequences

Patients with mania may experience secondary psychoses related to lack of sleep, substance abuse, or prescription drugs.

Differential Diagnosis

- Bipolar disorder—All patients with depressive symptoms should be screened for bipolar disorder
- Dementia
- Anxiety disorder
- Chronic pain
- Sleep disorders related to underlying medical problems
- Thyroid disease, primarily hypothyroidism
- Hypercalcemia
- Vitamin B_{12} deficiency
- Anemia

- Malignancy
- Substance-induced mood disorder
- Complicated bereavement (elevated suicide risk)
- Seasonal affective disorder
- Dysthymia—More chronic, low-intensity mood disorder for at least 2 years' duration
- Consider abuse or neglect.

Essential Diagnostic and Laboratory Tests

- Thorough medical history and evaluation
- Psychiatric history
- Institutional history (prison, prisoner of war, relocation camps, sanitariums)
- Assess for environmental, social, and spiritual issues.
- Medication history
- Nutritional history
- The minimum data set (MDS), as routinely used, is not a sufficient screening to pick up the majority of cases of depression in a nursing home population (Snowden, Sato, & Roy-Byrne, 2003).
- Geriatric depression scale (15 item) can be used in early dementia. A score of 5 or more may be indicative of depression.
- Cornell Scale for Depression in Dementia— 19-item observational scale may be more appropriate in patients with moderate to severe dementia. A score of 12 or more may be indicative of depression.
- Baseline MMSE
- Hamilton Depression Rating Scale (see Appendix A) and Beck Depression Inventory Scale are used more frequently in research than in practice.
- Diagnosis of depression should not be based solely on scores of validated depression scales.
- Suicidal ideation screening (see Table 15-9)
- Thyroid studies

TABLE 15-9   Assessing for Risk of Suicide

- Suicidal or homicidal ideation intent or plan
- Access to means
- Lethality of plan
- Presence of psychotic symptoms, command hallucinations, or severe anxiety
- Alcohol or substance abuse
- History of previous attempts
- Family history of or recent exposure to suicide

- B_{12} and folate levels
- Electrolytes, including serum calcium
- Serum drug levels that could be contributing to cognitive changes or anorexia
- Kidney function
- Liver function
- Complete blood count
- Urinalysis
- EKG

Management Plan

Reduce symptoms and maximize function. Treatment of depression in patients with dementia often improves cognitive performance and function. Start with low doses and titrate slowly, but do increase to therapeutic range whenever possible. For minor depressive symptoms, nonpharmacological treatment may be appropriate as first-line intervention. First-line treatment for residents that meet criteria for major depression without psychosis should include antidepressant therapy. For residents with major depression with psychotic features, a combination of antidepressant and antipsychotic medications is appropriate (Snowden et al., 2003).

Nonpharmacologic

- Provide referrals to psychotherapy when appropriate. Early dementia patients may benefit from behavioral or cognitive therapy.

- Socialization activities as appropriate for the individual
- Encourage physical activity or recreation therapy.
- Music therapy
- May need environmental changes
- Bright light therapy
- Offer choices as possible
- Provide frequent follow-up early in the treatment to assess for side effects and effectiveness.
- Electroconvulsant therapy (ECT) if several medication trials fail

If no improvement in symptoms has occurred by 6–8 weeks, pharmacologic intervention should be considered.

Pharmacologic

- The Alzheimer's brain is deficient not only in acetylcholine, but serotonin and norepinephrine (Bolla et al., 2005). Depression in both Alzheimer's dementia and vascular dementia may respond to either SRI medications or ChIs (Hill & Watson, 2005). Significant loss of serotonergic neurons has been demonstrated in FTD, and SRIs have been reported as successful in the treatment of disinhibition, depression, carbohydrate craving, and compulsive behaviors in FTD subjects (Swartz, 1997). Antidepressant therapy choices are based on comorbidities, mood features, and side effect profiles of the drugs. Sedating antidepressants should be dosed in the evening and may be selected for patients with insomnia. More activating antidepressants such as Prozac and some of the SNRIs are more appropriate to give in the morning. SRIs are also helpful for patients with depression and anxiety or obsessive-compulsive disorders. Selective serotonin reuptake inhibitors (SRIs) are the current first-line choice of pharmacologic treatment in the elderly. See Table 15-10.

TABLE 15-10 Antidepressants in the Older Adult

GENERIC NAME	BRAND NAME	AVERAGE STARTING DOSE (mg/day)	AVERAGE TARGET DAILY DOSE AFTER 6 WKS (mg/day)	USUAL HIGHEST FINAL DAILY ACUTE DOSE (mg/day)	COMMENTS
SELECTIVE SEROTONIN REUPTAKE INHIBITORS (SSRIs)					
Citalopram	Celexa	10–20	20–30	30–40 once daily	Some sedation, weight gain—generally dose in morning. Same active molecule as escitalopram
Escitalopram	Lexapro	10	20 after 1 week	20 once daily	Minimal side effects contains only the active isomer of citalopram
Fluoxetine	Prozac	10	20	20–40 once daily	May be activating in some patients—dose in the morning.
Fluvoxamine	Luvox	25–50	50–200	100–300	Used primarily in OCD
Paroxetine	Paxil	10–20	20–30	30–40 once daily	Sedating, some EPS in frail elderly
Sertraline	Zoloft	25–50	50–100	100–200	Sedating, weight gain
SEROTONIN-NOREPINEPHRINE REUPTAKE INHIBITORS (SNRIs)					
Mirtazapine	Remeron	7.5–15	15–30	30–45 once daily	SNRI*—Sedation, weight gain; activates at higher doses
Duloxetine	Cymbalta	20 twice daily	20–30 mg	60 single or divided dose	SNRI—Sedation, also approved for treatment of diabetic peripheral neuropathy, not approved for treatment of urinary incontinence in the United States (is in Europe)
Venlafaxine	Effexor	25–75	75–200	150–300	SNRI—Sedation, weight gain. Activates at higher doses. Also has weak dopamine activity
OTHER					
Bupropion	Wellbutrin	50–100 daily	150	300 divided dose or XL single dose	Can cause insomnia, weight loss. Can lower seizure threshold, especially at doses >150 mg, Comes in XL formulation. Use with caution in cardiac, hepatic, or renal dysfunction.

Notes: EPS, extrapyramidal symptoms.

Note: Tricyclic antidepressants (TCAs), monoamine oxidase inhibitors (MAOIs), and psychostimulants are not first-line recommendations in the elderly. Monotherapy in patient with bipolar disorder should be avoided. See FDA warnings regarding antidepressants and suicide risks.

All SRI medications can have GI side effects: e.g., nausea, diarrhea, headache, sedation, restlessness, weight gain, and sexual dysfunction. May cause hyponatremia in some. SNRIs may cause dry mouth and sedation.

Sources: MedLinePlus, 2005; Brody & Serby, 2004.

- Serotonin-norepinephrine reuptake inhibitors (SNRIs) may also be considered, especially with psychomotor retardation. Caution must be used in patients with bipolar disorder. Activating antidepressants may drive patients into state of mania.

- Mirtazapine is generally sedating at lower doses but may be activating at higher doses.

- Trazodone may be desirable if sedation is of benefit. Cardiac side effect profile is generally safer than tricyclic antidepressants.

- Bupropion may be desirable in patients that need to lose weight. It is more activating and can cause insomnia and can lower seizure threshold.

- Tricyclic antidepressants (TCAs), monoamine oxidative inhibitors (MAOIs), and psychostimulants should be avoided in the elderly as first-line treatment.

- Reevaluate response to medications at least every 6 weeks initially for dose titrations. Some newer medications can be titrated up more quickly.

- Reevaluation should also take place at 8 and 12 weeks once pharmacologic treatment starts.

- Continue treatment for 6–9 months after remission of symptoms. Some patients relapse frequently and need indefinite treatment.

Patient, Family, and Staff Education

- Explain natural history of depression and prognosis for improvement.

- Explain benefit of socialization and physical activity.

- Educate on side effects of medications or worsening symptoms.

- Educate on importance of follow-up and allowing time for medications to work.

- Immediately report any suicide ideation.

Physician or Geropsychiatrist Consultation

- Suicidal ideation with lethal plan
- When diagnosis is unclear
- Bipolar mania
- Presence of psychosis
- Treatment failure
- Patient or family request

▬▬▬ WEB SITES

- Anxiety Disorders Association of America— www.adaa.org. Patients and providers can obtain information about resources and qualified providers in their area.

- National Anxiety Foundation—www. lexington-on-line.com/naf.html

- Screening for Mental Health, Depression and Generalized Anxiety Disorder: A Guide for Health Care Clinicians—www. mentalhealthscreening.org

- Hamilton Anxiety Rating Scale (HARS)— www.fpnotebook.com/PSY84.htm

- Zung Self Rating Anxiety Scale (Zung SAS)—www.anxietyhelp.org/information/ sas_zung.html. Questions can be answered online.

- Alzheimer's Disease and Related Disorders Association (ADRDA)—www.alz.org

- National Highway Traffic Safety Administration site has the Trail Making Part B test available—www.nhtsa.gov/people/injury/ olddrive/OlderDriversBook/pages/Trail Making.html

- National Institutes of Health, senior health page on Alzheimer's disease—www. nihseniorhealth.gov/alzheimersdisease/ toc.html

- National Institutes of Health, Alzheimer's Disease Education and Referral Center (ADEAR)—www.nia.nih.gov/alzheimers

- Geriatrics at Your Fingertips—Online resource for geriatric syndromes includes many of the tools described in text. There is also a PDA version, both free online—www.geriatricsatyourfingertips.org
- Hartford Institute of Geriatric Nursing, *Try This: Best Practices in Care for Older Adults*. This is a series of assessment tools providing knowledge of best practices for care of older adults—www.hartfordign.org/resources/education/tryThis.html
- National Institute of Neurological Disorders and Stroke (NINDS)—For more detailed references on vascular dementias (see multi-infarct dementia) and Lewy body dementia—www.ninds.nih.gov/disorders/disorder_index.htm
- National Conference of Gerontological Nurse Practitioners (NCGNP) mental health toolkit (member access only)—www.ncgnp.org
- Confusion assessment method details—www.hartfordign.org/publications/trythis/issue13.pdf
- Brain disfunction in critically ill patients, patient and family education—www. icu delirium.org/delirium
- American Psychiatric Association practice guidelines—www.psych.org
- Hartford Institute for Geriatric Nursing: Resources, assessment tools, GDS 30-item scale—www.hartfordign.org
- For 30 translations of the GDS and an online version—www.stanford.edu/~yesavage/GDS.html
- Cornell Scale for Depression in Dementia—www.emoryhealthcare.org/departments/fuqua/CornellScale.pdf
- National Institute of Mental Health: Educational materials, handouts, audiotapes, CDs, and more links—www.nimh.nih.gov/HealthInformation
- U.S. Food and Drug Administration, Center for Drug Evaluation and Research, Information About the Drugs We Regulate. Enter a search for antidepressant information. A menu of sheets for various antidepressants for family or patients are available under Tables/Tools—www.fda.gov/cder/drug/default.htm

REFERENCES

Agronin, M. (2004). The man with agitation and aggression. In P. Aupperle (Ed.), *Managing moods: Diagnosis and treatment of mood problems and behavioral issues in the elderly: Case-based medicine teaching series* (pp. 29–40). New York: McMahon Publishing Group.

Alexopoulos, G. S., et al. (1998). Treatment of agitation in older persons with dementia. The Expert Consensus Panel for agitation in dementia. *Post Graduate Medicine*. Spec. No., 1–88.

American Psychiatric Association. (1994). *Diagnostic and statistical manual of mental disorders* (4th ed.). Arlington, VA: Author.

American Psychiatric Association. (2000). *Diagnostic and statistical manual of mental disorders* (4th ed.). Arlington, VA: Author.

Black, S. E. (2005). Vascular dementia: Stroke risk and sequelae define therapeutic approaches. *Postgraduate Medicine, 117*(1), 15–16, 19–25.

Bolla, L. R., Filley, C. M., Palmer, R. M., Boyer, E., & Shannon, M. (2005). The serotonin syndrome. *New England Journal of Medicine, 352,* 1112–1120.

Boyer, E. W., & Shannon, M. (2005). The seratonin syndrome. *New England Journal of Medicine, 352*(11), 1112–1120.

Brody, D. W., & Serby, M. (2004). What you should know about adult depression. *Clinical Advisor*, September, 19–25.

California Workgroup on Guidelines for Alzheimer's Disease Management. (1998). Guidelines for Alzheimer's disease management: Final report. Los Angeles: Author.

Carlsson, C. M., Gleason, C., & Asthana, S. (2005). Alzheimer disease: Update on diagnosis and treatment. *Consultant*, January, 77–88.

Catalan, J., Gath, D., Edmonds, G., & Ennis, J. (1984). The effects of non-prescribing of anxiolytics in general practice: Controlled evaluation of psychiatric and social outcome. *British Journal of Psychiatry, 144,* 593.

Chow, T. (2003). Frontotemporal dementias: Clinical features and management. *Seminars in Clinical Neuropsychiatry, 8*(1), 58–70.

Ciechanowski, P., & Katon, W. (2005). Overview of generalized anxiety disorder. Retrieved December 6, 2006, from http://www.uptodate.com

Fick, D. M., Agostini, J. V., & Inouye, S. K. (2002). Delirium superimposed on dementia: A systematic review. *Journal of the American Geriatrics Society, 50,* 1723.

Geldmacher, D. (2004). Dementia with Lewy bodies: Diagnosis and clinical approach. *Cleveland Clinic Journal of Medicine, 71*(10), 789–800.

Hamilton, M. (1959). Hamilton anxiety rating scale. *British Journal of Medical Psychology, 32,* 50–55.

Hebert, L. E., Scherr, P. A., Bienias, J. L., Bennett, D. A., & Evans, D. A. (2003). Alzheimer disease in the US population: Prevalence estimates using the 2000 census. *Archives of Neurology, 60,* 1119–1122.

Hill, M., & Watson, L. (2005). Use of psychotropic drugs in cerebrovascular disease. *Clinical Geriatrics, 13*(9), 37–45.

Inouye, S. K. (1994). The dilemma of delirium: Clinical and research controversies regarding diagnosis and evaluation of delirium in hospitalized elderly medical patients. *American Journal of Medicine, 97*(3), 278–288.

Inouye, S., van Dyck, C., Alessi, C., Balkin, S., Siegal, A., & Horwitz, R. (1990). Clarifying confusion: The confusion assessment method. *Annals of Internal Medicine, 113*(12), 941–948.

Jacobs, D. (1998). *Depression and generalized anxiety disorder: A guide for health care clinicians.* Retrieved December 28, 2005, from http://www.mentalhealthscreening.org

Katon, W., & Sullivan, M. D. (1990). Depression and chronic medical illness. *Journal of Clinical Psychiatry, 51*(6), 3–14.

Katon, W., Von Korff, M., Lin, E., Lipscomb, P., Russo, J., Wagner, E., et al. (1990). Distressed high utilizers of medical care: DSM-III-R diagnoses and treatment needs. *General Hospital Psychiatry, 12,* 355.

Katz, I. R., Kennedy, M. D., & Conwell, Y. (2004). Prevention of suicide in older persons: Lessons and limitations of evidence-based interventions. *Annals of Long-Term Care, 12*(8), 43–48.

Katz, I. R., & Parmelee, P. A. (1997). Overview. In R. L. Rubinstein, & M. P. Lawton (Eds.), *Depression in long-term and residential care: Advances in research and treatment* (pp. 1–28). New York: Springer.

Kessler, R. C., Davis, C. G., & Kendler, K. S. (1997). Childhood adversity and adult psychiatric disorder in the US National Comorbidity Survey. *Psychological Medicine, 27,* 1101.

Khouzam, H. R., Battista, M. A., Emes, R., & Ahles, S. Psychoses in late life: Evaluation and management of disorders seen in primary care. *Geriatrics, 60*(3), 26–33.

Lacy, C. (2005). *Lexicomp drug information handbook* (13th ed.). Hudson, OH: Lexicomp.

Lantz, M. (2004). Chronic benzodiazepine treatment in the older adult: Therapeutic or problematic? *Clinical Geriatrics, 12*(5), 21–23.

Lebowitz, B. D., Person, J. L., Schneider, L. S., Reynolds, C. F., III, Alexopoulos, G. S., Bruce, M. L., et al. (1997). Diagnosis and treatment of depression in late life. Consensus statement update. *Journal of the American Medical Association, 278,* 1186.

Lehninger, F., Ravindran, V. L., & Stewart, J. T. (1998). Management strategies for problem behaviors in the patient with dementia. *Geriatrics, 53*(4), 55.

Lieberman, A., Dziatolowski, M., Kupersmith, M., Serby, M., Goodgold, A., Korein, J., et al. (1979). Dementia in Parkinson's disease. *Annals of Neurology, 6,* 355–359.

Lundstrom, M., Edlund, A., Bucht, G., Karlsson, S., & Gustafson, Y. (2003). Dementia after delirium in patients with femoral neck fractures. *Journal of the American Geriatrics Society, 51,* 1002.

Marcantonio, E., Ta, T., Duthie, E., & Resnick, N. M. (2002). Delirium severity and psychomotor types: Their relationship with outcomes after hip fracture repair. *Journal of the American Geriatric Society, 50,* 850.

McKeith, I., Galasko, D., & Kosaka, K. (1996). Consensus guidelines for the clinical and pathologic diagnosis of dementia with Lewy bodies. *Neurology*, 47(5), 1113–1124.

Moretti, R., Torre, P., Antonello, R., Cazzato, G., & Bava, A. (2003). Gabapentin for the treatment of behavioural alterations in dementia; Preliminary 15-month investigation. *Drugs in Aging*, 20(14), 1035–1040.

Oslin, D. W., & Cary, M. S. (2003). Alcohol-related dementia: Validation of diagnostic criteria, *American Journal of Geriatric Psychiatry*, 11(4), 441–447.

Osterweil, D. (2004). Alzheimer's disease in the long-term care setting—Management of behavioral disturbances with cholinesterase inhibitors. *Annals of Long-Term Care*, 12(7), 18–24.

Paulson, R. (2005). *Depression in adults: Pathophysiology, clinical manifestations, and diagnosis.* Retrieved June 25, 2005, from http://patients.uptodate.com/topic.asp?file=psychiat/6523

Pittler, M. H., & Ernst, E. (2000). Efficacy of kava extract for treating anxiety: Systematic review and meta-analysis. *Journal of Clinical Psychopharmacology*, 20(1), 84–89.

Reisberg, B., Doody, R., Stoffler, A., & Mobius, H. J. (2003). Memantine in moderate to severe Alzheimer's disease. *New England Journal of Medicine*, 348, 14.

Roman, G. C., Tatemichi, T. K., Erkinjuntti, T., Cummings, J. L., Masdeu, J. C., Garcia, J. H., et al. (1993). Vascular dementia: Diagnostic criteria for research studies. Report of the NINDS-AIREN International Workshop. *Neurology*, 43(2), 250–260.

Schatzberg, A., Kremer, C., Rodrigues, H. E., Murphy, G. M., Jr., & Mirtazapine vs. Paroxetine Study Group. (2002). Double-blind randomized comparison of mirtazapine and paroxetine in elderly depressed patients. *American Journal of Geriatric Psychiatry*, 10, 541–550.

Schneider, L. S. (2004). Commentary: AD2000: Donepezil in Alzheimer's disease. *Lancet*, 363(June), 2100–2101.

Serby, M., & Almiron, N. (2005). Dementia with Lewy bodies: An overview. *Annals of Long-Term Care*, 13(2), 20–22.

Shadlen, M. F., & Larson, E. B. (2005). *Dementia syndromes.* Retrieved June 16, 2005, from http://patients.uptodate.com/topic.asp?file=nurogen/5175

Sink, K. M., Holden, K. F., & Yaffe, K. (2005). Pharmacological treatment of neuropsychiatric symptoms of dementia: A review of the evidence. *Journal of the American Medical Association*, 293(5), 596–608.

Snowden, M., Sato, K., & Roy-Byrne, P. (2003). Assessment and treatment of nursing home residents with depression or behavioral symptoms associated with dementia: A review of the literature. *Journal of the American Geriatrics Society*, 51, 1305–1317.

Stanley, M., Hopko, D., Diefenback, G., Bourland, S., Rodriguez, H., & Wagener, P. (2003). Cognitive-behavior therapy for late-life generalized anxiety disorder in primary care: Preliminary findings. *American Journal of Geriatric Psychiatry*, 11(1), 92–96.

Sutor, B., Rummans, T. A., & Smith, G. E. (2001). Assessment and management of behavioral disturbances in nursing home patients with dementia. *Mayo Clinic Proceedings*, 76, 540–550.

Swartz, R., Miller, D. L., Lesser, I. M., Booth, R., Darby, A., Wohl, M., et al. (1997). Behavioral phenomenology in Alzheimer's disease, frontotemporal dementia, and late life depression: A retrospective analysis. *Journal of Geriatric Psychiatry Neurology*, 10, 67–74.

Tariot, P., Farlow, M., Grossber, G., Graham, S., McDonald, S., & Gergel, I. (2004). Memantine treatment in patients with moderate to severe Alzheimer disease already receiving donepezil: A randomized controlled trial. *Journal of the American Medical Association*, 291(3), 317.

Towle, M. (1997). Pharmacologic management of dementia-related aggressive behavior. *Nursing Home Medicine*, 5(10), 354.

Wang, P., Schneeweiss, S., Avorn, J., Fischer, M., Mogun, H., & Solomon, D. (2005). Risk of death in elderly users of conventional vs. atypical antipsychotic medications. *New England Journal of Medicine*, 353, 22.

Zung, W. W. K. (1971). A rating instrument for anxiety disorders. *Psychosomatics*, 12, 371–379.

■ BIBLIOGRAPHY

Alzheimer's Association. (1999). *Alzheimer's disease and related dementias.* Retrieved June 6, 2005, from http://www.alz.org

American Geriatrics Society, & American Association for Geriatric Psychiatry. (2003). Consensus statement on improving the quality of mental health care in U.S. nursing homes: Management of depression and behavioral symptoms associated with dementia. *Journal of the American Geriatrics Society, 51,* 1287–1298.

Bolla, L. R., Filley, C. M., & Palmer, R. M. (2000). Office diagnosis of the four major types of dementia. *Geriatrics, 55*(1), 34–37.

American Psychiatric Association (APA). (2003). Assessing and treating suicidal behaviors: A quick reference guide. Practice Guideline. Arlington, VA: Author.

Cole, M. (2004). Delirium in elderly patients, clinical review. *American Journal of Geriatric Psychiatry, 12*(1), 7.

Fife, A., & Schreiber, J. (2004). *Psychiatric emergencies: Agitation or aggression?* Retrieved July 2, 2005, from http://www.patients.uptodate.com/topic.asp?file=psychiat/5564

Francis, J. (2004). *Prevention and treatment of delirium and confusional states.* Retrieved June 14, 2005, from http://patients.uptodate.com/topic.asp?file=medneuro/2278

Francis, J., & Young, G. B. (2006). *Diagnosis of delirium and confusional states.* Retrieved June 14, 2005, from http://patients.uptodate.com/topic.asp?file=medneuro/2425

Ganzini, L. (2004). Depression and delirium at the end of life. *Long-Term Care Interface, 5,* 55–58.

Garavaglia, B. (2004). Unmasking the hidden problem of depression among LTC residents. *Long-Term Care Interface,* October, 43–46.

Gershenfeld, H. K., Philibert, R., & Boehm, G. (2005). Looking forward in geriatric anxiety and depression: Implications of basic science for the future. *American Journal of Geriatric Psychiatry, 13*(12), 1027–1040.

Hermida, T., & Malone, D. *Anxiety disorders.* Retrieved December 28, 2005, from http://www.clevelandclinicmeded.com/diseasemanagement/psychiatry/anxiety/anxiety.htm#definition

Hvas, A. M., & Nexo, E. (2003). Holotranscobalamin as a predictor of vitamin B_{12} status. *Clinical Chemistry and Laboratory Medicine, 41*(11), 1489–1492.

Knopman, D. S., Dekosky, S. T., Cummings, J. L., Chui, H., Corey-Bloom, J., Relkin, N., et al. (2001). Practice parameter: Diagnosis of dementia (EBR). *American Academy of Neurology, 56*(9), 1143–1153.

Marcantonio, E., Simon, S. E., Bergmann, M. A., Jones, R. N., Murphy, K. M., & Morris, J. N. (2003). Delirium symptoms in post-acute care: prevalent, persistent, and associated with poor functional recovery. *Journal of the American Geriatrics Society, 51,* 4–9.

Menza, M., Marin, H., Kaufman, K., Mark, M., & Lauritano, M. (2004). Citalopram treatment of depression in Parkinson's disease: The impact on anxiety, disability and cognition. *Journal of Neuropsychiatry and Clinical Neurosciences, 16,* 315–319.

Serby, M., & Mi, Y. (2003). There's good news about depression in the elderly. *Clinical Advisor* (September), 64–75.

Truman, B., Gordon, S., & Ely, W. (2004). Delirium: A neglected danger in the intensive care unit. *Annals of Long-Term Care, 12*(5), 18–22.

Westanmo, A., & Gayken, H. R. (2005). Duloxetine: A balanced and selective norepinephrine and serotonin-reuptake inhibitor. *American Journal of Health System Pharmacies, 62*(23), 2481–2490.

Hamilton Anxiety Rating Scale

I. Background
  A. Authored by Max Hamilton in 1959
  B. Public domain anxiety rating scale
II. Symptom Rating Scale (0 = Not Present, 4 = Disabling)
  A. Anxious mood
    1. Worries
    2. Anticipates worst
  B. Tension
    1. Startles
    2. Cries easily
    3. Restless
    4. Trembling
  C. Fears
    1. Fear of the dark
    2. Fear of strangers
    3. Fear of being alone
    4. Fear of animal
  D. Insomnia
    1. Difficulty falling asleep or staying asleep
    2. Difficulty with nightmares
  E. Intellectual
    1. Poor concentration
    2. Memory impairment
  F. Depressed mood
    1. Decreased interest in activities
    2. Anhedonia
    3. Insomnia
  G. Somatic complaints: muscular
    1. Muscle aches or pains
    2. Bruxism
  H. Somatic complaints: sensory
    1. Tinnitus
    2. Blurred vision
  I. Cardiovascular symptoms
    1. Tachycardia
    2. Palpitations
    3. Chest pain
    4. Sensation of feeling faint
  J. Respiratory symptoms
    1. Chest pressure
    2. Choking sensation
    3. Shortness of breath
  K. Gastrointestinal symptoms
    1. Dysphagia
    2. Nausea or vomiting
    3. Constipation
    4. Weight loss
    5. Abdominal fullness
  L. Genitourinary symptoms
    1. Urinary frequency or urgency
    2. Dysmenorrhea
    3. Impotence
  M. Autonomic symptoms
    1. Dry mouth
    2. Flushing
    3. Pallor
    4. Sweating
  N. Behavior at interview
    1. Fidgets
    2. Tremor
    3. Paces
III. Interpretation
  A. Above 14 symptoms are graded on scale
    1. Not present: 0
    2. Very severe symptoms: 4
  B. Criteria
    1. Mild anxiety (minimum for Anxiolytic): 18
    2. Moderate anxiety: 25
    3. Severe anxiety: 30

APPENDIX B

Behavior Drugs in the Elderly

In 2005, the FDA issued a safety announcement regarding the treatment of behavioral problems in elderly patients with dementia with atypical antipsychotics such as olanzapine (Zyprexa), aripiprazole (Abilify), risperidone (Risperdal), or quetiapine (Seroquel). Studies have shown increased deaths in the drug-treated group compared to the placebo-treated patients. The specific causes of these deaths were mostly either due to heart-related events (e.g., heart failure, sudden death) or infections (mostly pneumonia).

The atypical antipsychotics are FDA approved for the treatment of schizophrenia and bipolar mania. None of these drugs are FDA approved for the treatment of behavioral disorders in patients with dementia. This does not mean these drugs cannot be used for this purpose, but you should use caution, and the patient should be reassessed frequently if a decision is made to continue their use. All drugs have risks and benefits to be considered.

There are a number of studies of these atypical antipsychotic medications that do show they help with problem behavior symptoms in elderly patients with dementia. However, there are things that can help besides medication, and there are different classes of medications that can be helpful.

Many Alzheimer's dementia patients will have behavioral symptoms sometime during the course of their disease. It is most helpful to first try environmental adjustments and talking in a very calm voice. A regular routine with activities, attention to medical problems such as constipation, pain, and depression, may improve behavior. In some situations you may decide that the benefits of using these antipsychotics are worth the risks.

To read the complete FDA safety warning, visit www.fda.gov/cder/drug/advisory/antipsychotics.htm.

Geriatric Depression Scale (Short Form)

1. Are you basically satisfied with your life? ....yes/**NO**

2. Have you dropped many of your activities and interests? ....**YES**/no

3. Do you feel that your life is empty? ....**YES**/no

4. Do you often get bored? ....**YES**/no

5. Are you in good spirits most of the time? ....yes/**NO**

6. Are you afraid that something bad is going to happen to you?..**YES**/no

7. Do you feel happy most of the time? ....yes/**NO**

8. Do you often feel helpless? ....**YES**/no

9. Do you prefer to stay at home, rather than going out and doing new things?.................**YES**/no

10. Do you feel you have more problems with memory than most?.......................................**YES**/no

11. Do you think it is wonderful to be alive now? ....yes/**NO**

12. Do you feel pretty worthless the way you are now? ....**YES**/no

13. Do you feel full of energy? ....yes/**NO**

14. Do you feel that your situation is hopeless? ....**YES**/no

15. Do you think that most people are better off than you are? ....**YES**/no

Score _____

(count up all the bold answers that were circled)

Normal   0–3

Mildly depressed   4–7

Very depressed   8+

Cornell Scale for Depression in Dementia

NAME_____ AGE_____ SEX_____ DATE_____

WING_____ ROOM_____ PHYSICIAN_____ ASSESSOR_____

Ratings should be based on symptoms and signs occurring during the week before interview. No score should be given if symptoms result from physical disability or illness.

SCORING SYSTEM

A = Unable to evaluate   0 = Absent   1 = Mild to intermittent   2 = Severe

A	0	1	2

A. Mood-Related Signs
1. Anxiety: anxious expression, rumination, worrying
2. Sadness: sad expression, sad voice, tearfulness
3. Lack of reaction to present events
4. Irritability: annoyed, short tempered

A	0	1	2

B. Behavioral Disturbance
5. Agitation: restlessness, hand wringing, hair pulling
6. Retardation: slow movements, slow speech, slow reactions
7. Multiple physical complaints (score 0 if gastrointestinal symptoms only)
8. Loss of interest: less involved in usual activities (score only if change occurred acutely (i.e., in less than one month).

A	0	1	2

C. Physical Signs
    9. Appetite loss: eating less than usual
   10. Weight loss (score 2 if greater than 5 pounds in one month)
   11. Lack of energy: fatigues easily, unable to sustain activities

A	0	1	2

D. Cyclic Functions
   12. Diurnal variation of mood: symptoms worse in the morning
   13. Difficulty falling asleep: later than usual for this individual
   14. Multiple awakening during sleep
   15. Early morning awakening: earlier than usual for this individual

A	0	1	2

E. Ideational Disturbance
   16. Suicidal: feels life is not worth living
   17. Poor self esteem: self-blame, self-depreciation, feelings of failure
   18. Pessimism: anticipation of the worst
   19. Mood congruent delusions: delusions of poverty, illness or loss

Score _____ Score greater than 12 = probable depression

Notes/Current Medications: _____

CHAPTER 16

Respiratory Disorders

Deborah Cox

ASTHMA

Definition

Asthma is a common chronic disease of the respiratory system often underdiagnosed in the elderly (Wisnivesky, Foldes, & McGinn, 2002). Asthma is a clinical syndrome characterized by inhalation of allergens, airway inflammation/hyperresponsiveness, and eventual airway narrowing. For the elderly patient with a history of severe asthma, incomplete resolution of airflow obstruction is generally symptomatic.

Epidemiology

Asthma is a common cause for emergency room visits and hospitalization. Current evidence suggests increasing incidence of new onset asthma occurs among the elderly. Prevalence is confounded by similar diagnostic features of asthma and chronic obstructive lung disease (COPD) (Wisnivesky, Foldes, & McGinn, 2002). Men and women are equally affected. The duration and concentration of exposure to natural and manmade pollutants other than pollutants associated with occupational asthma are features of asthma that increase in the elderly. Gastroesophageal reflux disease (GERD) is also a frequent asthma trigger in the elderly. Age-related organ pathophysiology and underlying chronic disease often complicate treatment. Clinical presentation of asthma may be atypical, as symptoms of chest pain and tightness also signal coronary artery disease. The elderly tend to underreport dyspnea probably because of lessened perception of increases in airway resistance and sedentary life styles (Wisnivesky, Foldes, & McGinn, 2002). The clinical course of asthma varies with natural decline in lung function and coexisting chronic disease. The opportunity to enhance optimal functional activities and preserve quality of life begins with distinguishing the features of asthma from other obstructive airway disease. Desirable clinical outcomes rest with cautious medication management and modifications in treatment necessary to maintain symptom control.

Common Presenting Signs and Symptoms

- Episodic wheezing is frequent in asthma and less evident in COPD, although "cardiac asthma" can present as wheezing precipitated by uncompensated heart failure.

- Common allergic symptoms are nasal mucosal swelling, rhinitis, sinusitis, nasal polyps, eczema, and atopic dermatitis.

- Nocturnal symptoms are frequent in asthma, less evident in COPD. Increase in bronchoconstriction between 3 and 4 a.m. related to variations in bronchomotor tone and bronchial reactivity (circadian variations). Tachypnea and tachycardia may also occur.

- Chronic dry cough or productive cough is evident in asthma and COPD—common in the elderly.

- Lungs—Adequate inspiratory aeration, symmetry of breath sounds, wheezing, prolongation of expiratory phase and hyperinflation

- Use of accessory respiratory muscles, cyanosis, and tachycardia correlate with severity of obstruction. Status asthmaticus is persistent severe obstruction for days or hours. Airflow may be too limited to produce wheezing—a danger sign.

Differential Diagnosis

- Chronic bronchitis
- Emphysema—COPD features
- Upper airway obstruction caused by foreign body, tumor, or laryngeal edema
- Eosinophilic pneumonia
- Congestive heart failure

Essential Diagnostic and Laboratory Tests

- The diagnosis of asthma is based on a thorough history, physical examination, and pulmonary function tests. The initial goal is to distinguish between asthma with airway obstruction and COPD.

- Spirometry should be used to measure FEV1, FVC, FEV/FVC before and after administration of a short-acting bronchodilator.

- Laboratory markers: CBC may show eosinophilia; IgE may show mild elevation. Marked increase may suggest allergic bronchopulmonary aspergillosis.

- Sputum examination—eosinophilia. Presence of increased neutrophils suggests bronchial infection.

- Chest X-ray not always necessary, and may be normal in uncomplicated asthma. Useful for excluding underlying disease such as complicating infection.

- Peak expiratory handheld flow (PEF) meter establishes peak flow variability. Predicted values based on age, height, and gender are not well standardized. Inadequately controlled asthma is defined as a 20% change in PEF from morning to afternoon or from day to day. PEF values less than 200 L/min indicate severe airflow obstruction (Chestnutt & Prendergast, 2004).

- Allergy testing in the elderly has not been well documented. Skin testing to assess sensitivity to relevant environmental irritants/allergens may be useful with persistent asthma.

- Evaluation and treatment for paranasal sinus disease or GERD should be considered in patients with persistent symptoms and poor response to bronchodilators and anti-inflammatory agents.

Management Plan

The treatment goal for asthma is to minimize chronic symptoms that disrupt maintenance of normal activity and quality of life. Pharmacologic therapy is directed at symptom control, prevention of exacerbations, and medication side effects. Begin with influenza and pneumonia immunizations per CDC guidelines.

Nonpharmacologic

- Smoking cessation—smoke-free environment
- Adequate hydration and nutrition
- Frequent allergen control—dusting, eliminate perfumes, pet control
- Dental care with focus on reducing oral bacteria
- Weight loss, if needed

- Regular exercise
- If contributing factor: nonpharmacological treatment of reflux, including weight loss, avoid caffeine, elevate head of bed, stop eating prior to bed time

Pharmacologic
- Drugs to avoid or use cautiously:

  ○ Aspirin—induced asthma or "triad-asthma" involves ASA sensitivity, asthma, and nasal polyps. The syndrome can be triggered by NSAIDs. Avoid NSAIDs if polyp/sinus problems exist.

  ○ Beta-blockers—may exacerbate asthma, in oral medications or topical ophthalmic preparations. If beta-blockers are necessary, use cardioselective agents.

- Antireflux therapy often reduces or eliminates asthma symptoms. A trial of proton pump inhibitor (PPI) can be started and increased before clinical improvement is seen.

- Allergic rhinitis and asthma often coexist because of similar causes and inflammatory mediators. If allergic rhinitis occurs with uncontrolled asthma, try antihistamines, decongestants, or nasal corticosteroids. Cetirizine is a well-tolerated antihistamine—watch creatinine clearance below 35 mL/min. If irritants are controlled, treatment usually will not require decongestants.

- The approach for managing asthma in the elderly patient should avoid aggravating other medical conditions. Inhalation is the preferred method of therapy. Metered dose inhalers (MDIs) with spacers are common but sometimes difficult to manage. Improper use results in subtherapeutic effect and uncontrolled symptoms. Table 16-1 suggests basic guidelines to consider when

Table 16-1   Low-Dose Adult Asthma Therapy

Mild asthma
   B_2-agonist as needed—short acting = Albuterol 1–2 puffs every 2–6 hrs
Mild asthma persistent
   B_2-agonist as needed—short acting = Albuterol 1–2 puffs every 2–6 hrs
   Inhaled corticosteroids twice daily = Fluticasone 44 μg 1–2 puffs
Moderate asthma persistent
   B_2-agonist as needed—short acting = Albuterol 1–2 puffs every 2–6 hrs
   Inhaled corticosteroids twice daily = Fluticasone 110 μg 1–2 puffs
   plus
   B_2-agonist twice daily—long acting = Salmeterol 50 μg Blister 1 inhalation
   or
   Combination Fluticasone/Salmeterol twice daily 100/50 μg 1 inhalation
Severe asthma persistent
   B_2-agonist as needed—short acting = Albuterol 1–2 puffs every 2–6 hrs
   Inhaled corticosteroids twice daily = Fluticasone 110 μg 3 puffs
   plus
   B_2-agonist twice daily—long acting = Salmeterol 50 μg Blister 1 inhalation
   or
   Combination Fluticasone/Salmeterol twice daily 250/50 μg 1 inhalation

Notes: Leukotriene modifiers can be used as add-on therapy to reduce inhaled corticosteroid dose requirements, for moderate to severe asthma: Montelukast 10 mg at bedtime.
Methylxanthines—nocturnal relief of asthma—starting dosage 10 mg/kg/day sustained-release tablets.
The addition of *oral* corticosteroids for moderate to severe exacerbations can shorten recovery time. Short-term is preferred.
Elderly patients have a high incidence of heart disease and do not tolerate side effects of medication well.
Source: Adapted from Wisnivesky, Foldes, & McGinn, 2002.

selecting medications to achieve asthma control with minimal side effects.

- Antibiotic use should be correlating with status change and evidence of infection. Antibiotic use has no role in treatment of acute exacerbations of asthma without infection.
- Calcium and vitamin D supplement to prevent bone loss associated with steroid therapy or therapy with bisphosphonates to decrease fracture risk

Patient, Family, and Staff Education

- Explain management of asthma including use of MDI and spacer and warning signs of exacerbation.
- Explain benefit of health maintenance and exercise.
- Educate patient, caregiver, and staff to recognize early signs of respiratory distress.
- Educate staff about management of environmental pollutants that may exacerbate asthma.

Physician Consultation

- Collaborative management provides continuity of care.
- Physician consultation is advised if change from stable control.
- Pulmonology referrals for frequent exacerbations

▀▀▀ BRONCHITIS

Definition

Bronchitis is a common disorder of the lower airways. Chronic bronchitis evolves as an inflammatory process of bronchial smooth muscle and mucus linings of the airways. Smooth muscle hypertrophy and thick mucus plugging of the small airways contribute to chronic coughing. Airway inflammation becomes chronic and contributes to reactive hyperresponsiveness to irritants and eventual airflow limitation.

Acute bronchitis is an inflammation of the tracheobronchial tree typically resulting from viral infection with adenovirus or influenza.

Epidemiology

Cough is a common symptom. Three cough-associated conditions have increased over the past 20 years; asthma, GERD, and chronic obstructive pulmonary disease (COPD). Bronchitis is also a common cause of cough. Chronic bronchitis is a feature of COPD (Lie, 2000). Excessive sputum production, shortness of breath, and cough are presenting respiratory complaints of older adults in the fifth and sixth decade of life. Symptoms are often present for 10 years or more. A good history is key to diagnosis. Chronic bronchitis accounts for the majority of COPD in the United States; characteristics of chronicity include excessive secretion of bronchial mucus and productive cough for 3 or more months during 2 consecutive years. Chronic exposure to inhaled allergens and pollutants, especially cigarette smoke, impair mucociliary clearance. Loss of airway cilia contribute to acute episodes of chronic cough and eventual airflow limitations, a feature of irreversible pulmonary disease. Acute bronchitic events often follow a respiratory tract infection. Secondary bacterial infection is common following influenza and in patients with chronic lung disease. For the elderly person eventual pulmonary disability imposes a clinical course significantly impairing function and quality of life. Often the cycle and frequency of acute bronchitic exacerbations precipitate long-term care admission and loss of independence.

Common Presenting Signs and Symptoms

- Exertional dyspnea and productive mucoid cough/sputum are typical early symptoms.
- In severe disease, dyspnea may occur at rest. Individual may be overweight or present with weight loss due to anorexia.

- Chest is noisy—wheezes and rhonchi.
- Fluid retention (pedal edema), morning headaches, sleep disruption, and cyanosis may be present. Neck vein distension may be observed during expiration in the absence of heart failure.
- In advanced disease, dyspnea at rest, ruddy or cyanotic skin color, decreased heart/lung sounds, clubbing of fingertips, and pursed lip breathing. Hypoxemia and hypercarbia metabolic changes are present.
- Severe oxygen desaturation is frequently associated with obstructive sleep apnea.
- Increased exacerbations include frequent respiratory infections, cycles of coughing, fever, and sputum purulence. Underlying bacterial colonization.
- In acute bronchitis, common symptoms include cough, anorexia, malaise and headache, chest pain, and fever.

Differential Diagnosis
- Asthma
- GERD
- Chronic rhinitis
- Chronic sinusitis
- Bronchiectasis
- COPD
- Congestive heart failure

Essential Diagnostic and Laboratory Tests
- The diagnosis of bronchitis is based on a thorough history, physical exam, and radiographs. The initial goal is to rule out GERD, asthma, acute viral syndromes, upper airway chronicity (sinusitis), and possibly cough from ACE inhibitors. Features of COPD may prevail (see next section).
- Radiographic findings—Plain chest X-ray shows hyperinflation, increased anteroposterior diameter of thorax, and local radiolucencies. May see pulmonary hypertension, increased interstitial markings, or infiltrates. Diaphragm not flattened.
- Laboratory markers—Hemoglobin elevated (15–18 g/dL). WBCs increased with infection.
- Arterial blood gases—Compensated respiratory acidosis (usually not practical to obtain in long-term care settings)
- PPD current and PPD history to dismiss tuberculosis
- Pulmonary function tests if COPD is suspected
- A sputum culture is advised during acute exacerbations if resistance (nosocomial) or unusual bacterial infection is suspected, or if empiric antibiotic therapy is not resolving infection.

Management Plan
The treatment goals for chronic bronchitis are directed toward symptom relief and control of disease progression. Individualize treatment with prompt recognition and therapy during acute exacerbations. Acute bronchitis should be managed with reference to precipitating factors or exposures if chronic pulmonary disease is not an existing comorbidity.

Nonpharmacologic
- Adequate hydration, effective cough training methods, or handheld flutter device to mobilize secretions
- Graded aerobic exercise—Walking programs to prevent deterioration of functional activities
- Breathing exercises including pursed lip to slow rate of breathing and abdominal breathing to reduce accessory muscle fatigue
- Supplemental oxygen as needed
- Smoking cessation if not achieved
- Swallowing/speech evaluation to rule out GERD. Look at liquid thickness. If tube feeding, check positioning before and after eating; order or evaluate assisted feeding.

Cough may also reflect an effect of dysphagia. Avoid feeding in bed or elevate head of bed more than 30°

Pharmacologic

- *Start with bronchodilators*—Use handheld MDI with spacer or nebulizer/mask system if severe physical impairment. Match medication to severity of disease.

  ○ For quick symptom relief, a short-acting B_2-agonist may be adequate.

  ○ Combination anticholinergic and B_2-agonist bronchodilators are usually effective for moderate or less than optimal results.

  ○ An anti-inflammatory inhaled corticosteroid may be added to complement a

long-acting, B_2-agonist bronchodilator especially for nighttime symptoms.

  ○ Select drugs preferred for treating older persons. Class adverse effects for short- and long-acting B_2-agonists and inhaled corticosteroids may influence dosing selection. Table 16-2 suggests basic guidelines in a stepwise approach with first-line medications listed first.

- *Acute exacerbations*—Short duration oral steroids 5–20 mg daily for 7 days. Long-acting anticholinergic—Tiotropium (1 inhalation daily). This is a relatively new drug for long-term care setting use and may not be covered by usual plans. Side effect profile includes the following:

Table 16-2   Stepwise Escalation Therapy and Common Drugs for Chronic Bronchitis Management

Class/Drug: Anticholinergics—Ipratropium bromide
Dosage: 2–6 puffs MDI or 0.5 mg by nebulizer 4 times daily
Class effect: Do not increase with exacerbations
Add or use alone

Class/Drug: B_2-agonists—short-acting Albuterol
Dosage: 2–6 puffs MDI every 6 hrs or 2.5 mg by nebulizer 4 times daily
Class effect: Rapid onset, use half dose with known or suspected coronary disease
or
Class/Drug: B_2-agonists—long-acting Salmeterol
Dosage: 1 cap dry powder inhaler. Max: twice daily
Class effect: *Not for acute use
add
Class/Drug: Inhaled steroid—Fluticasone
Dosage: 1 puff twice daily. Start with 44 µg/puff
Class effect: Oropharyngeal thrush
or
Class/Drug: Inhaled steroid—Triamcinolone
Dosage: 2 puffs twice or three times daily or 4 puffs twice daily
Class effect: Oropharyngeal thrush
Class/Drug: Albuterol-Ipratropium
Dosage: 0.09/0.018 mg/puff, 2–3 puffs 4 times daily: 3 mg/0.5 mg by nebulizer 4 times daily.

Class/Drug: Salmeterol-Fluticasone
Dosage: 1 puff twice daily (50 µg/100, 200, or 500 µg/inhalation

---

Note: Combination inhalers are available.
Source: Chestnutt & Prendergast, 2004.

○ Evaluate the degree of renal impairment.

○ Avoid in the presence of narrow angle glaucoma.

○ Watch use with other anticholinergics.

- For cough and tenacious thick mucus—Guaifenesin 600 mg, 5–10 mL every 4 hours can provide relief. Requires adequate hydration to be effective. Maximum dosage 60 mL/day.

- For cough in combination with guaifenesin mucolytics—Benzonatate 100 mg capsules 3 times per day can provide relief during coughing cycles. Do not give with impaired gag reflex or inability to swallow capsule.

- Antibiotics for acute exacerbations—Use should be based on clinical symptoms correlating with status change and evidence of infection. Some patients may present acutely with no specific warning. Patients in long-term care facilities are vulnerable to nosocomial infections. Chest X-ray may not be conclusive. Overuse of antibiotics increases resistance. The key is early treatment of infection. Table 16-3 provides guidelines for early recognition of infection.

- Immunizations—Influenza annual immunization and pneumonia immunization if before 65 years or at 65 repeat in 5 years as indicated—depends on clinical judgment of risk factors and facility protocols. Follow CDC guidelines (see Chapter 3).

- When symptoms are controlled for 3 months, try stepwise medication reduction. Review every 1–6 months for effectiveness.

- A trial of acid proton pump inhibitors (PPI) may be prudent and worth trying if cough or increased sputum follows meals or if swallowing issues become a concern.

Patient, Family, and Staff Education

- Explain management options for bronchitis and related pulmonary disease characteristics.

- Explain benefit of exercise and respiratory hygiene programs.

- Explain benefit of hydration and balanced nutrition for weight management.

- Discuss prognosis if clinically significant disease progression.

Physician Consultation

- If chronic bronchitis is not stable or does not respond to treatment refer to the pulmonologist. Collaborate with physician if major comorbidities are present.

CHRONIC OBSTRUCTIVE PULMONARY DISEASE

Definition

The American Thoracic Society (1999) describes chronic obstructive pulmonary disease (COPD) as a disease state characterized by progressive airflow obstruction caused by chronic bronchitis or emphysema; air-flow resistance may be accompanied by hyperreactivity and may be partially reversible. Clinical findings are generally absent in the early course of the disease, but as the disease progresses into the fifth or sixth decade of life,

---

Table 16-3   Indicators of Possible Respiratory Infection

Look for at least 3 of the following symptoms:
- New or increased sputum
- Fever (> 38°C or 2° above base line)
- New or increased cough
- Pleuritic chest pain
- New or changed physical findings, shortness of breath
- Worsening mental or functional status

Source: Adapted from Chestnutt & Prendergast, 2004.

two characteristic symptom patterns tend to emerge—dyspnea and chronic cough. As COPD progresses, notable systemic consequences develop. Like asthma, COPD exacerbations occur with increased inflammation from pulmonary infection and in response to allergic and nonallergic triggers. Unlike asthmatics, COPD patients are seldom symptom free, and the disease progresses (Edmunds & Mayhew, 2000).

Epidemiology

COPD affects 14 million Americans. Two million have emphysema, and approximately 12 million suffer from chronic bronchitis (Celli, 1998). COPD ranks as the fourth leading cause of death in the United States. There is evidence of increasing mortality in women. Most middle-aged adults with severe dyspneic COPD do not survive to truly old age (Chestnutt & Prendergast, 2004). However, new treatment strategies for COPD have shown decreased symptom severity and improved survival time (Cote & Celli, 2005).

Cigarette smoking is the most significant risk factor for disease development. Respiratory changes occur with normal aging as respiratory reserve capacity adapts to annual decline of forced expiratory volume (FEV1). Approximately 30 mL in FEV1 declines annually in the normal aging individual. Smoking increases the rate of decline in FEV to approximately 45 mL per year. Occupational exposures, air pollution, and airway hyperreactivity may influence the severity of COPD and should be factors to consider in the history taking process. COPD-associated disability progresses as:

- Chronic hypoxemia
- Shorter intervals between respiratory exacerbations
- Lower extremity edema
- Weight loss
- Increasing dyspnea

Often the acute exacerbation precipitates changes in treatment plans including admission to a skilled nursing facility (SNF).

Common Presenting Signs and Symptoms

- Chronic cough with morning sputum production, considered a "first" symptom of the chronic bronchitis component of COPD. History of chronic cough 3 months out of the year or more for 2 successive years in absence of any specific disease. Sputum is initially clear mucoid but becomes thick, increasing in frequency and mucopurulent with acute exacerbations.

- Mild exertional dyspnea progresses to dyspnea at rest. Audible wheezing during prolonged expiration is a symptom of emphysema progression. Assess for rhonchi, wheezing, and hyperresonance.

- Changes in general appearance, weight loss, cyanosis, lower extremity edema. In advanced disease the anterioposterior diameter of the chest increases. The "barrel chest" accounts for apparent hyperinflation on chest X-ray.

- In advanced disease changes in respiratory patterns (use of accessory muscles of respiration and purse-lip breathing) interfere with activities of daily living (ADLs), sleep, and eating.

- Frequent respiratory infections occur seasonally or often exacerbate at night. Expiratory wheezing and decreased breath sounds occur at night; often awakenings at night occur with air hunger (paroxysmal nocturnal dyspnea).

- Vital signs and pulse oximetry values may change from baseline.

- Bacterial colonization may shift to active infection.

- Notable consequences of systemic change include jugular venous distention, ankle edema, or hepatic congestion; features of right-sided heart failure and cor pulmonale.

- Complaints of morning headache, increased irritability, or altered mental status are symptomatic of acute or chronic carbondioxide excess and alveolar hypoxia. Sleep apnea may contribute to oxygen desaturation. Be alert for delirium.

- Review current and relevant admission history and physical. Note available labs, chest X-rays, prior pulmonary function studies, immunization history (influenza, pneumonia) and tuberculosis screening results. Include some evaluation of functional abilities and exercise tolerance if feasible during the assessment. Note changes in vital signs and pulse oximetry values. Oxygen desaturation on room air or at 2 liters may support further pulmonary testing.

- The history and physical examination may not establish early COPD but does present important reference points for tracking progressive disease. It is important to consider the systemic scope of COPD and the effect of treatment modalities on the normal aging process. During physical exam look for signs of the following:

  ○ Right-sided heart failure—Peripheral edema, jugular venous distention, hepatomegaly

  ○ Pulmonary hypertension—Fatigue, cyanosis, light headedness, clubbing of digits, murmur

  ○ Cor pulmonale—Dyspnea, cough, fatigue, increased sputum production, S3 gallop, peripheral edema, jugular venous distention

Differential Diagnosis

- Acute bronchitis
- Bronchiectasis
- Asthma
- Malignancy

- Occupational interstitial lung disease
- Tuberculosis

Essential Diagnostic and Laboratory Tests

- Use radiologic tests to identify other cause of airway obstruction, infiltrates, or evidence of lung cancer. Mobile X-ray services may provide only limited value for early COPD detection. P/A and lateral chest X-ray quality and diagnostic accuracy are best if provided in a radiology department.

- Computed tomography (CT scan) is a sensitive tool in early diagnosis. CT scan specificity includes pleural thickening, mediastinal changes, diffuse infiltrates, and lung tissue emphysemetous changes.

- Laboratory tests:

  ○ CBC with differential. Screen for polycythemia that may accompany COPD. Don't forget anemia of chronic disease. Serum electrolytes, blood urea nitrogen (BUN), creatinine. On acute exacerbation, ABGs (arterial blood gases), electrolytes, glucose, creatinine, BUN, CBC to rule out infection, anemia, and check theophylline level if applicable.

  ○ Sputum cultures are not generally obtained. Research has demonstrated viral infections precede bacterial involvement in the majority of patients with exacerbations (Chestnutt & Prendergast, 2004). Culture may reveal *Streptococcus pneumoniae, Haemophilus influenza*, or *Moraxella catarrhalis* in acute exacerbations. Keep track of bacterial colonization, such as MRSA history, seasonal risk factors, and pulmonary infection trends in the facility as they are useful indicators for treatment choices. Collaborating with local care facilities and obtaining current antibiograms can provide information about influenza and pneumonia prevalence and trends in antibiotic effectiveness.

○ Pulmonary function tests (PFTs) are clearly indicated in COPD management guidelines to confirm diagnosis, determine reversibility, and support treatment protocols. Clinical values of FEV1 and change in ratio to vital capacity values are important indicators for COPD progression. Some elderly patients have difficulty performing spirometry. Other measures such as distance walked without symptoms may be more reliable.

• ECG—Obtain for baseline if not recently performed. May show sinus tachycardia. Over time chronic pulmonary hypertension can produce abnormalities.

• Obtain *alpha-globulin peak level* to rule out a genetic antiprotease deficiency. Important for patients with no smoking history.

Management Plan

Short- and long-term therapy for the elderly person with COPD is directed toward controlling symptoms, maximizing self-care, and improving health-related quality of life. Individuals with symptomatic lung disease are benefiting from structured rehabilitation programs (Cote & Celli, 2005).

Nonpharmacologic

Nonpharmacologic approaches include smoking cessation and exercise. Monitor for optimal response and individualize each treatment plan.

• Smoking cessation can minimize progressive airways damage from chronic bronchitis.

• Adequate hydration, nutrition, and regular exercise; pulmonary rehabilitation programs provide an increase in exercise endurance and a good treatment plan for patients with symptomatic lung disease.

• Therapeutic oxygen—Studies have established that long-term oxygen therapy extends survival in hypoxemic COPD, and survival is related to the number of hours of oxygen administration per day (Cote & Celli, 2005). An oxygen saturation of 88% or less should initiate long-term oxygen use.

• Involve resident in diversional activity therapy programs, and tailor living environment to maximize self-care activities.

• Provide annual dental care as periodontal disease harbors bacteria capable of bronchial seeding and lower respiratory infection.

Pharmacologic

Pharmacologic management is aimed at relieving bronchospasm, reducing secretions, managing infections, and correcting hypoxemia to improve quality of life by maximizing lung function and minimizing periods of dyspnea. Symptoms may increase and exacerbations may occur. Focus on the following key components of care:

• Review and verify compliance with current therapy.

• Monitor adequacy of current therapy.

• Increase therapy to maximize results.

• Add medications directed at presenting symptoms or precipitating cause. Be alert for signals of escalating disease: increasing oxygen demand, escalation of nebulizer treatment more often than every 4 hours, and a need for intravenous therapy.

Therapy for management of COPD usually is described as a stepwise process. Adjusting dosages, adding short-term medications, and relieving symptoms are hallmarks of current management trends. Table 16-4 outlines four levels of COPD medication management with inhaled medications. Inhaled bronchodilators are most effective in improving pulmonary function and decreasing dyspnea. For the elderly patient using handheld metered dose inhalers (MDI), use a spacer. Observation of inhalation effectiveness can ensure medication

Table 16-4 Four Levels of COPD Management with Inhaled Medications

LEVEL 1 MILD COPD SYMPTOMS

- Selective B_2-agonist MDI (Albuterol) 1–2 puffs every 2–6 hrs, as needed. Not more than 8–12 puffs every 24 hrs.
  or
- Anticholinergic MDI (Ipratropium bromide), 2–6 puffs, 4 times daily

LEVEL 2 MILD TO MODERATE CONTINUING COPD SYMPTOMS

- Long-acting B_2-agonist MDI (Salmeterol), 1 puff twice daily
  or
- Long-acting anticholinergic (Tiotropium bromide) 1 capsule daily
  or
- Anticholinergic MDI (Ipratropium bromide) 2–6 puffs every 6–8 hrs (not to be used more frequently)
  plus
- Selective B_2-agonist MDI (Albuterol) 1–4 puffs, as needed, 4 times daily (Indications are rapid relief, as needed or regular control)

Alternative choice

- Combination (Albuterol and Ipratropium bromide) MDI. 2 puffs 4 times daily (maximum 12 puffs every 24 hours)

LEVEL 3 MILD TO MODERATE COPD, SYMPTOMS INCREASING

- Add a sustained release formulation of theophylline 200–400 mg twice daily or 400–800 mg at bedtime for nocturnal bronchospasm.

LEVEL 4 SUBOPTIMAL CONTROL OR FREQUENT COPD EXACERBATIONS

- Add inhaled corticosteroid (Fluticasone) 2–4 puffs twice daily (start low dose 88 mg twice daily)

Notes: Elderly patients have a high incidence of heart disease and do not tolerate side effects of medication well. All medication should be based on patient response and relative toxicity. The table does not address severe exacerbations.
Source: Adapted from Cote & Celli, 2005.

benefit. If a patient reports a strong medication taste, the dose is concentrated in the mouth, not the lungs, and effectiveness will be decreased. Some residents may respond better to a less portable nebulizer and oral mouthpiece method of medication delivery.

- COPD maintenance
  - Bronchodilators:
    - B_2-agonists—MDI—careful dosing in patients with arrhythmias or heart disease.
    - Anticholinergics—MDI—may cause insomnia, dizziness.
    - Methylxanthines—potential for toxic side effects. Check serum levels, target range 8 to 12 µg/mL.
  - Corticosteroids—Add inhaled if bronchodilators fail to provide optimal control.
  - Other anti-inflammatory agents—Leukotriene inhibitors are useful for an asthma component of COPD. Example: Montelukast 10 mg daily. Not extensively studied in older adult populations.
  - Antibiotics—Not for prophylaxis
  - Expectorants—Guaifenesin 5–10 mL every 4 hours, as needed, for 5–7 days.

Short-term use can promote liquification of tenacious sputum.

- COPD exacerbation—acute or severe Consult with physician if IV medications are required. Maintain pulse oximetry > 91%. COPD patients prefer humidification.
  - Bronchodilators:
    - B$_2$-agonists—Increase MDI dose to 4–6 puffs every 3–4 hrs or inhalant solution unit dose every $\frac{1}{2}$–2 hrs. (Watch for side effects.)
    - Anticholinergics—Increase ipratropuim dose MDI to 6–8 puffs every 3–4 hrs or inhalant solution of ipratropuim 0.5 mg every 4 hr *and*
    - Methylxanthines—Available as IV; consult with physician.
  - Corticosteroids—Add short-term course, orally, 40–60 mg daily for 7 days, and taper over 1–2 weeks.
  - Antibiotics—The key is early treatment of infection. Clinical symptoms correlating with status change include fever, elevated WBCs, and change in sputum color (see Table 16-3). Choice of antibiotic depends on nosocomial patterns, cost, and consideration of colonization history (e.g., MRSA).
  - Sedation—Not usually recommended.
  - Expectorants—Assure adequate hydration to enhance medication effects. If severely compromised, look at daily hydration requirements and order specific fluid goals.
- Yearly influenza vaccination, if not contraindicated.

Pneumococcal vaccine should be given once and repeat in 5 years if given before age 65. Follow CDC guidelines.

Patient, Family, and Staff Education

- Explain management of the chronic symptoms of COPD and levels of change as exacerbations occur. Educate on smoking cessation.
- Explain benefit of hydration, nutrition, and exercise.
- Instruction in proper technique of inhaler and spacer use. The elderly may complain of palpitations and tachycardia with beta-adrenergic inhalers. Side effects are usually transient. Include oral care, especially rinsing after inhaled steroids to prevent oral candidiasis.
- Explain oxygen safety.
- Where appropriate, discuss end-of-life issues with resident and caregivers.

Physician Consultation

- The psychosocial and physical aspects of COPD care are interrelated. Referral and evaluation of depression is an essential quality of care measure.
- Collaborative management provides continuity of care. Physician consultation is advised in all but stable mild to moderately symptomatic patients.
- Consultation with a pulmonary specialist for frequent exacerbations and for surgical options.

▬ INFLUENZA

Definition

Influenza is an acute febrile illness, worldwide in distribution. The illness is characterized by a very abrupt onset, followed by febrile illness with moderately severe systemic symptoms and cough. Several days of respiratory symptoms often extend as a prolonged convalescence during which weakness and lack of energy are prominent features. The clinical picture may be extremely variable resulting in mild respiratory to fatal influenza and/or bacterial pneumonias.

Epidemiology

Influenza occurs in sporadic community outbreaks that begin abruptly and spread rapidly. Seasonal patterns of influenza are associated with geographical variations, often occurring in winter months and spread via social and behavioral habits. Outbreaks correspond to school reopenings or returning to work after winter holidays. Influenza is spread from person to person by droplets or by direct contact with articles contaminated with nasopharyngeal secretions. Viral shedding in a nasal secretion usually ceases within 7 days of illness onset but can be prolonged in young children and the elderly (Waldman, 1984). Epidemic disease is caused by influenza virus types A and B. Control measures are directed toward immunization with inactivated viral strains vaccine. The effectiveness of influenza immunization is evident in adult populations, varying from 50–90% depending on the closeness of vaccine strain match to the wild strain. The duration of vaccine protection is assumed to be less than 1 year. Elderly persons living in close, communal residential settings benefit from annual influenza immunization. The Centers for Medicare and Medicaid Services (CMS) now require that nursing homes offer residents influenza vaccine annually, unless it is contraindicated or refused by the patient or legal guardian (CMS, 2005). Despite immunization efforts, excess rates of hospitalization attributable to influenza virus infection are common. Secondary bacterial pneumonia is the most common pulmonary complication of influenza for elderly persons residing in long-term care settings.

Common Presenting Signs and Symptoms

- Typical onset is a sudden fever, chills or rigors, headache, malaise, diffuse muscle fatigue, and a nonproductive cough.

- Within 48 hours after onset signs of sore throat, nasal congestion, and rhinitis occur. More prominent signs of cough with greenish or blood-tinged sputum may be present. Pleuritic chest pain and dyspnea may also occur.

- Abdominal pain, nausea and vomiting can occur, contributing to dehydration and potentially deadly renal failure.

- Consider primary influenza pneumonia: usually severe and will develop 1–3 days after initial onset of influenza symptoms. It is marked by high fever, dyspnea, and cyanosis. (Chest X-ray reveals infiltrates usually in midlung fields). It is often confused with pulmonary congestion in heart failure (Waldman, 1984).

- Consider bacterial pneumonia. Usually occurs in 3–14 days after initial onset of first influenzal symptoms. It is characterized by deteriorating clinical states and a cough productive of purulent sputum (chest X-ray shows consolidation). Hypoxemia is usually less severe, and cyanosis is absent.

- Combined viral and bacterial pneumonia—There may be a 4-day interval between initial symptoms and evidence of pulmonary involvement. Watch out for "false" signs of improvement in the 4-day window period before pulmonary disease blends with the original influenza (Blinkhorn, 1998).

- Signs and symptoms in the elderly nursing home resident may be subtle. Fever may be more mild than expected, and the first sign of illness may be mental confusion.

Differential Diagnosis

The diagnosis of influenza virus infection is a clinical and epidemiologic one. The fact that influenza occurs in characteristic outbreaks during winter months may be very helpful in making a clinical diagnosis:

- Viral influenza—acute respiratory illness
- Mixed viral pneumonia and bacterial pneumonia
- "Primary" influenza viral pneumonia or secondary bacterial pneumonia

Essential Diagnostic and Laboratory Tests

- Viral cultures or rapid diagnostic tests may be performed on specimens obtained within the first 72 hours of illness. The local health department should be notified and will usually provide pertinent guidance on nasopharyngeal secretion collection and management plan. Prevention through early immunization is important. Follow CDC guidelines.

- Leukocyte counts are variable during illness, frequently low early in illness and normal or elevated later. Severe leukopenia may occur in overwhelming viral or bacterial infection, while leukocytosis with counts greater than 15,000 cells per cubic millimeter should alert suspicion that secondary bacterial infection is present.

Management Plan

The treatment goals for influenza management include early identification, cohorting, comforting and supportive measures to prevent secondary infections, and promote recovery.

Nonpharmacologic

- Infection control plan—Cohort ill patients. Close off wings and cohort staff by not switching them around units. Be vigilant

and aware of community trends, and stay connected with the local health department.

- Be sure appropriate signage is on entrance doors to educate and cue the public and family members. Enforce hand washing.

- If main dining room is used, consider keeping residents on the units until situation is resolved or under control.

- Start line listing of signs and symptoms and track to assure a resident will not be overlooked if significant change is subtle.

- Hydrate—encourage use of comfort foods such as teas, soups, and easy to chew and swallow diets.

- Bed rest is usually self-imposed due to fatigue; however, repositioning and pulmonary hygiene is important to keep secretions moving. Supply oxygen as needed and nebulizer treatments via mask with sterile saline.

Pharmacologic

- Control fever with acetaminophen or other appropriate antipyretics. If aspirin is used, be aware that marked swings in temperature, with intense sweating and chills, may exhaust the resident and cause dehydration.

- Cough management might include codeine as a dry cough suppressant. Guaifenesin, if a mucolytic is needed, requires hydration.

- Antibiotic therapy is required if bacterial pneumonia supervenes, but antibiotics prophylactically will not reduce the likelihood of bacterial pneumonia and may increase potential antibiotic-resistant bacteria. Selection of antibiotic should consider common pathogens: *Streptococcus pneumoniae*, *Staphylococcus aureus*, and *Haemophilus influenzae*.

- Amantadine or rimantadine are approved for treatment of Influenza A in adults—if given within 48 hours of onset, symptom relief is reduced by 50%. Central nervous system side effects often deter use of these medications. In the 2005–2006 influenza season these drugs were found to be ineffective against influenza A strains. Check the CDC guidelines annually to monitor further recommendations for their use. Other antiviral agents, the neuraminidase inhibitors oseltamivir and zanamivir, are available for the treatment of uncomplicated acute illness due to influenza A and B virus in patients who have been symptomatic for no more than 2 days.

- Intravenous fluids for hydration or support may be required depending on change in condition and presenting blood chemistry.

Patient, Family, and Staff Education

- Education about prevention should be ongoing. Encourage staff and family to include immunization for themselves as well as their elderly family member.

- Educate staff to be aware and report changes in resident condition immediately.

- Educate staff about the importance of health maintenance to avoid shortages of personnel during high-volume/high-risk influenza activity in the nursing home.

- Educate staff and monitor hand washing procedures before, during, and after each resident/patient contact.

Physician Consultation

Consultation with physicians, medical director, and the local health officer are essential to assure the influenza outbreak does not impact on morbidity and mortality. The resolution without unnecessary death and disability requires a team effort.

LUNG CANCER

Definition

Primary lung cancer usually presents as a malignant nodule or mass originating in the bronchial epithelium. Clinical presentation is influenced by the cell type, location of the primary tumor, and local or distant metastases. Bronchogenic cancers are classified as small cell (SCLC) and non-small cell (NSCLC), essential staging criteria for treatment protocols. Secondary lung cancers result from malignant spread to lung tissue via vascular and lymphatic networks from extra pulmonary sites. Tumor extensions are often associated with thyroid or breast cancer primary sites. Secondary lung cancers are linked with primary prostate cancers. Lung cancer diagnosis is ultimately defined by cytology and tissue type.

Epidemiology

Lung cancer is the leading cause of cancer death for American men and women. Lung cancer in women has increased by 124% over a 30-year period compared to a 10% increase for men (Rugo, 2004). Tobacco use, particularly cigarette smoking, is a major factor in the development of lung cancer. Age is also an important cancer risk factor. The aging trend in Americans has doubled cancer incidence projections from 1.3 million annual cases to 2.5 million cases by 2050 (Rugo, 2004). Strongly linked with progressive decline in compensatory mechanisms, lung cancer usually presents in older patients after the fifth decade. Associated risk factors include genetics and environmental and occupational exposure. Most lung cancers are symptomatic at the time of diagnosis and tend to surface during an abrupt functional decline. Unfortunately, detection often will occur after disease progression is beyond a treatable stage and complicated by coexisting chronic disease. Symptom management and palliative care are often the primary focus for intervention. The goals for older patients may differ from those of younger patients, for whom cure of disease and prolongation of life are of paramount concern. Although some elderly patients residing in long-term care may seek a plan for life extension, others are clearly candidates for comfort measures to maintain quality of life and a peaceful death. Patients affected by progressive disease with few curative options benefit from diligent attention to the essentials of palliative care and pain management. The overall survival rate for lung cancer is 15% (Chestnutt & Prendergast, 2004).

Common Presenting Signs and Symptoms

Periodic screening of asymptomatic non-smokers at risk for lung cancer is without demonstrated benefit.

- Anorexia, weight loss, or fatigue—Loss of strength, energy, and weight suggest distant liver metastases.

- New cough, change in chronic cough, and hemoptysis are associated with central bronchogenic tumors.

- Pain, cough, and symptoms of pleural effusion or lung abscess are associated with lesions in peripheral lung tissue.

- Dysphagia, hoarseness, or tracheal obstruction are associated with primary lung cancer. Bronchial obstruction with atelectasis may occur.

- In advanced disease, superior vena cava syndrome (obstruction with supraclavicular venous distention) disrupts cervical and paravertebral nerve function.

- Organ dysfunction impacted by the secretory effect of tumors can precipitate several paraneoplastic syndromes in 10–20% of lung cancer patients.

  ○ Digital clubbing occurs in about 20% of patients at diagnosis (Chestnutt & Prendergast, 2004).

  ○ Small-cell lung cancer patients can develop syndrome of inappropriate antidiuretic hormone secretion (SIADH).

  ○ Hypercalcemia develops in 10% of patients with squamous cell cancer.

  ○ Other syndromes include increase in ACTH, anemia, neuropathies, and hypercoagulability.

Early recognition of symptoms is important as side effects may resolve with primary tumor treatment even in noncurable states.

Differential Diagnosis

- Tuberculosis
- Pneumonia
- Sarcoidosis
- Asbestosis
- Pleural effusions
- Bronchiectasis

Essential Diagnostic and Laboratory Tests

- The diagnosis of lung cancer is initiated during assessment of symptoms suggestive of disease. A thorough history, physical examination, radiographs, laboratory tests, bronchoscopy, and tissue biopsy initiate the process of tumor location—primary or secondary, and staging for treatment and prognosis. The initial goal is differentiating malignancy from nonmalignant respiratory disease.

- Nearly all patients with lung cancer have abnormal findings on chest radiography or CT scan. Comparison with prior studies is important if a pulmonary nodule is found. Most nodules less than 3 cm are asymptomatic and carry a risk of malignancy (Chestnutt & Prendergast, 2004).

- Sputum cytology is specific for diagnosis of bronchogenic lesions but considered insensitive as a diagnostic test.

- Thoracentesis may be indicated to distinguish a cytology diagnosis from pleural effusion.
- Good diagnostic results are obtained from fine-needle aspiration/fiber-optic bronchoscopy.
- Pursuit of diagnosis if less invasive measures fail, may depend on thoracotomy.
- CBC and blood chemistries for evidence of paraneoplastic syndromes.

Management Plan

The treatment goals for lung cancer management include symptom and pain relief. For NSCLC, cure is unlikely without surgery and radiation. Chemotherapy and radiation are current treatments for SCLC. Chemotherapy is usually palliative for non-small cell carcinoma (NSCLC).

Nonpharmacologic
- Dyspnea—Supplemental oxygen via face mask or nasal cannula. A fan may provide relief.
- Hot or cold packs, massage, or physical therapy for musculoskeletal pain are adjuncts to pharmacotherapy.
- Pastoral counseling, support groups, prayer, are valuable for psychologic issues and pain management.
- Review advance directives with resident and caregivers.
- Nutrition and hydration—At end of life, have right to refuse these options. Nutrition may increase oral and airway secretions and increase the risk of choking, aspiration, and dyspnea (see chapter on end-of-life care).

Pharmacologic
- Continue medical management of coexisting chronic disease; influenza, and pneumonia immunizations.

- Pain management—Tailor to cover somatic, visceral, or neuropathic pain. Start with acetaminophen every 6 hours up to 2 g/day for elderly without liver disease. NSAIDs are an option but consider side effect profile.
- If response is inadequate, use opioid medications. Hydrocodone and codeine are typically combined with acetaminophen for mild to moderately severe pain.
- Chronic stable pain—Give sustained-release morphine (2–3 times/day), oxycodone (2–3 times/day), or transdermal fentanyl, starting dose 25 μg every 3 days (with 24–40 hours to achieve full analgesia).
- Neuropathic pain, "pins and needles"—May respond to tricyclic antidepressants or anticonvulsants (gabapentin, clonazapam, and carbamazepine). The lidocaine patch is effective for postherpetic pain and may be effective for other types of neuropathic pain.
- Nausea and vomiting—If associated with a particular opioid, substitute with a sustained-release formulation. Phenergan 12.5 mg orally or rectal suppository at 4–6 hour intervals may be effective. Watch for side effects, especially with a history of asthma.
- Constipation—A common problem. Start a prophylactic bowel regime of stool softeners (docusate) and stimulants (bisacodyl or senna).

Patient, Family, and Staff Education
- Smoking cessation
- Explain treatment options and provide referrals.
- Explain to staff the central role of family, friends, and staff in providing supportive care.
- Provide pain medications and as needed medications on time; monitor effectiveness and report pain relief failures.

- Follow-up with advance directives and do not resuscitate preference information. Assure that staff is aware of code status and hospital transport requirements.

- Educate about hospice and provide referrals.

Physician Consultation

- Collaboration with physician assures continuity of care, treatment follow-up, or referral, if feasible, to oncologist or pulmonologist.

- If patient is a candidate for surgery refer to cardiothoracic surgeon.

◼ PLEURAL EFFUSION

Definition

Pleural effusion occurs in a variety of disease states. Pleural effusions signal an abnormal change in lung physiology involving the fluid formation and fluid removal processes within the pleural space and lung tissue. Treatment goals are influenced by history, clinical presentation, risk factors, and radiographic evidence. Dyspnea is the most common symptom. Chest pain is frequently a signal for cardiac ischemia, infection (pleuritis), or trauma. Pleural effusion may present without symptoms.

Epidemiology

Pleural effusions develop in one million patients annually. Pleural effusions are generally classified as transudative or exudative. There are five common pathophysiologic causes. Transudative effusions occur in normal pleura as a result of disequilibrium in hydrostatic/oncotic pressure gradients. In patients over the age of 60, congestive heart failure (CHF) accounts for 90% of transudative effusions. Pulmonary embolism, cirrhosis, and left ventricular failure are common causes of transudative pleural effusion. Pleural diseases produce plasma exudates from increased permeability of the pleural capillary or from decreased efficiency of lymphatic fluid removal from the pleural space. Prominent causes of exudative effusions are bacterial pneumonias, viral infection, malignancy, and pulmonary embolism. Malignant pleural effusions are the most common cause of exudative effusion in patients over the age of 60 (Chestnutt & Prendergast, 2004). Infection in the pleural space (empyema) and bleeding into the pleural space (hemothorax) are also causative pathologic factors to consider during the diagnostic process. It must be appreciated that increasingly diverse subsets of elderly populations residing in assisted living and long-term care represent an important fraction of the workforce with a history of occupational and toxic waste exposures. A range of hazards such as asbestos, coal dust, cotton dust, or animal care may provide the diagnostic variable in exudative pleural disease. Family history and tuberculosis exposure are important clues. Expanding global immigration over several decades increases the probability of diagnosing an exudative parasitic pleural effusion from the common blood fluke seen in people from Mediterranean regions. Despite a full evaluation incorporating all the variables, the underlying cause for effusion in 25% of patients will not be established (Chestnutt & Prendergast, 2004).

Common Presenting Signs and Symptoms

- Dyspnea, cough, and sharp superficial rib pain aggravated during inspiration are common complaints.

- Small effusions may cause no symptoms.

- Underlying disease may cause emergent symptoms:

  ○ DVT risk (immobilizaton, recent fracture). Pulmonary embolus symptoms include tachycardia, hemoptysis, and dyspnea.

○ CHF-associated symptoms: Orthopnea, dyspnea, paroxysmal nocturnal dyspnea and pedal edema

○ Malignancy: Weight loss, anorexia, and hemoptysis

○ Pneumonia: Acute illness, productive cough, fever, chills, and night sweats

- Physical findings include dullness to percussion of lung field, diminished breath sounds over the affected side, and a pleural friction rub, auscultated in the anterior-lateral area of the lower lung field on the affected side.

- Large pleural effusions with increased intrapleural pressure may cause deviation of the trachea from the affected side and bulging of the intercostal spaces.

Differential Diagnosis

The presence of the effusion is established. The cause of the effusion may require differentiating the two main types of effusions: transudative versus exudative. An important goal is focusing on the associated symptoms and underlying illness that might produce a pleural effusion.

- CHF vs. pericardial disease
- Pneumonia/pleurisy, pulmonary embolism vs. tuberculosis
- GERD vs. gastrointestinal disease
- Rib fracture, costochondritis (Tietze's syndrome) vs. hemothorax
- Pneumonia vs. metastatic disease

Essential Diagnostic and Laboratory Tests

- The diagnosis of pleural effusion is based on a thorough history, physical examination, and radiographs. Further studies may include ultrasound and thoracentesis. The initial goal is to document the presence

and size of the effusion. The second task is determining the cause of the effusion.

- Radiographic study—Posterior/anterior and lateral chest X-ray. Chest X-ray is the typical starting point. The most common appearance of pleural effusion on chest X-ray is obliteration of the sharp angle between the diaphragm and rib cage. Appearance of an elevated hemidiaphragm suggests a subpulmonic effusion beneath the lung. Lateral decubitus views help estimate the size of the effusion. Pleural effusions may be missed on anterioposterior X-ray if taken in the supine posture as the liquid layers of the effusion gravitate posteriorly.

- Ultrasound can detect small effusions as small as 5 to 50 mL of fluid. Small pockets of fluid are identifiable markers for thoracentesis, if necessary.

- Spiral CT scan is ultrasensitive in differentiating changes in the pleura from focal masses.

- There are no specific laboratory markers for pleural effusion. Screen for underlying diseases, a practical and appropriate approach in the long-term care setting. CBC to rule out infection; comprehensive metabolic panel (CMP) for electrolytes, pre-albumin, liver profile (if clinical presentation suggests malignancy); international normalizing ratio (INR) if taking warfarin.

- Referral for thoracentesis of undiagnosed pleural effusion, if appropriate (some situations may imply further testing that is not clearly defined or desired in the overall plan of care). Note that if the cause is apparent from clinical presentation (i.e., CHF), then symptom relief and observation may be appropriate. For suspect tuberculosis with suggestive bacilli on direct microscopy, refer to local health department.

Management Plan

The treatment goals pending lab and X-ray results should focus on treating emergent symptoms or pain as they present. Emergent situations such as MI should be managed according to facility protocol.

Pneumonia and CHF are common underlying conditions precipitating pleural effusions in the elderly and may be the apparent focus for initiating the treatment plan. However, symptoms may not resolve, and diagnostic measures may require referral.

Nonpharmacologic
- Oxygen therapy
- In CHF—Pre-Lasix weight and post-Lasix weight, and electrolyte monitoring.
- Hydration—Oral 30 mL/kg in 24 hours, if on diuretic therapy
- Follow-up chest X-rays to monitor resolution of infiltrates if symptoms remain a concern.

Pharmacologic
- Pain management: Start with acetaminophen 650 mg orally or rectally 4 times/day up to 4 grams per day; or codeine with acetaminophen #3, 1–2 tabs every 4 hours. Be sure to discontinue acetaminophen if opioid-plus-acetaminophen is ordered to avoid increased dosing of acetaminophen. Another option is immediate release oral oxycodone 2.5–5 mg with acetaminophen 325 mg every 6 hours.
- Pain with dyspnea/shortness of breath— Consider morphine sulfate liquid 20 mg/mL, 0.5 mL orally every 2 hours, as needed. Be alert for fall risk.
- Pain associated with costochondritic signs— etiology could be tuberculosis. Prednisone as an anti-inflammatory agent would be contraindicated in tuberculosis. Proceed with caution if considering a short trial of prednisone. Systemic corticosteroids should be stopped immediately if final diagnosis is CHF related.
- Pain associated with undiagnosed GERD; when not currently receiving reflux/acid suppression therapy. Trial of antacid-aluminum hydroxide 10–20 mL 4 times/ day or a trial of acid proton pump inhibitor (PPI) may provide relief. Also if on a PPI consider dose increase and look at when medication is given. Often medication is not given early enough—at least 60 minutes before breakfast, or in combination with other a.m. medications. Change to hour of sleep (10 p.m.) dosing.
- CHF symptoms with interstitial edema on chest X-ray—can start and/or increase Lasix (monitor electrolytes). Lasix dosage depends on severity and renal status. A low dose 20–40 mg may be effective for a very elderly person currently on Lasix. Use sublingual nitroglycerin (0.4 mg) and aspirin 81 mg initially if chest pain suggests ischemia and refer.
- Antibiotic therapy is often part of the initial plan, especially if fever is present, and certainly should be considered if chest X-ray is suggestive of pleural infiltrates. Addition of another antibiotic may be necessary if symptoms persist.

Patient, Family, and Staff Education
- Explain disease state and diagnostic workup.
- If infection is present or suspected, cohort staff according to infection control management. (If tuberculosis is suspected, contact the local health department for instructions on isolation and transfer.)

Physician Consultation
- If symptoms are significant and laboratory data is pending, collaborate with physician on further diagnosis and treatment plan.

- Collaborate with physician in situations where renal failure, hydration, and fluid replacement become a concern.
- Refer or consult with physician if emergent condition presents.

PNEUMONIA

Definition

Pneumonia, an infection of the lower respiratory tract, is a leading cause of illness, hospitalization, and death among older people residing in nursing homes. Age and comorbidities are risk factors for pneumonia. Pneumonias begin as an acute inflammatory response involving the bronchioles and pulmonary alveoli. Infected alveoli are congested with increased cellular blood flow and exudative edemas. Cellular response mechanisms cascade from alveoli to alveoli. The alveolar macrophage, a primary cellular defense, is often depressed in the elderly. Bacteria, mycoplasmas, or viruses are potential pathogens contributing to fluid-filled lung tissues or consolidation of a lobe. Viral primary pneumonias set the stage for bacterial superinfection. *Streptococcus pneumoniae* is a frequent causative agent. Clinical symptoms include fever, cough, sputum, and pleuritic chest pain. Altered pulmonary function reduces diffusing capacity; hypoxemia and hypercapnia influence exacerbations of underlying chronic disease and altered mental status.

Epidemiology

Most segments of the general population will experience a lower respiratory tract infection. Despite improvement in diagnosis and treatment, pneumonia ranks sixth as a cause of death in the United States and is a leading cause of death in persons older than 65 years. The incidence of pneumonia among nursing home patients is 10 times that experienced by community-based elderly (Chestnutt & Prendergast, 2004).

Characteristics of pneumonia are typically classified as community acquired or hospital acquired (nosocomial). And recently classified, nursing home-acquired pneumonia (NHAP) emerged to address the skilled nursing facility. Recent statistics indicated that 28% of Medicare beneficiaries were hospitalized for pneumonia (Naughton & Mylotte, 2000). Pneumonia in the elderly is a severe clinical situation and often a diagnostic challenge in atypical situations. Comorbidity is high—80–90% of elderly patients cope with one or more illness (Yoshikawa, 2002). Chronic disease lowers physiologic defense mechanisms including alveolar macrophage activity. Aspiration is frequently a mode of bacterial entry into the lower respiratory tract (Muder, 2000). Colonization of the oropharynx with gram-negative bacilli occurs with chronic disease and disability. Seeding of bronchial structures is inevitable through inhalation, aspiration, direct spread from adjacent sites including periodontal disease, and hematogenous spread. Nursing home-acquired pneumonias comprise widely varied bacterial isolates (Yoshikawa, 2000). Specific bacterial diagnosis is difficult to achieve in most nursing home patients. Antibiotic selection is generally empiric, and the incidence of resistant organisms in long-term care facilities has fostered focused research and retrospective study (Naughton & Mylotte, 2000).

Guidelines and clinical pathway criteria address pneumonia presentations, specific and nonspecific, in an effort to determine illness severity and appropriate treatment for long-term care residents. The current principle of NHAP is early, appropriately aggressive, empirical treatment selected on the basis of the *most* likely organisms for the setting in which the pneumonia developed (Mehr et al., 2001).

Infection control plays an important role in NHAP. Prevention is a key factor—immunization and surveillance are essential measures. Inadequate application of infection control standards—infrequent hand washing—contributes to the spread of micro-organisms in the living environment of the elderly person depending on safe long-term care.

Common Presenting Signs and Symptoms

Pneumonia in the elderly may present with atypical symptoms. Pneumonia may result from the aspiration of oropharyngeal flora—usually an assortment of aerobic and anaerobic bacteria. Criteria for diagnosis may reflect "typical" or "atypical" clinical changes. Table 16-5 provides common signs and symptoms. Additional clinical manifestations may include the following:

- Common physical findings—Tachycardia (pulse greater than 100 beats per minute), tachypnea (respiratory rate greater than 25 breaths per minute), and
  - Temperature 38.1°C (100.5°F)
  - Temperature < 35.6°C (96°F)

or

  - 1.1°C (2°F) more than usual baseline

- New or worsening hypoxia. Severely hypoxic patients may appear cyanotic. Pulse oximetry may not be accurate.

- Decline in cognitive or functional status. Recent history of upper respiratory tract infection.

- Shaking chills or "rigors"—several episodes in 48-hour period
- Severe myalgia accompanied by vomiting should suggest bacteriemia (Blinkhorn, 1998).

Differential Diagnosis

- Influenza
- Pneumonitis related to fungal agents
- Tuberculosis
- Upper respiratory tract infections—adenoviruses
- Congestive heart failure
- Lung cancer
- Reactive airway disease/bronchiolitis
- Pulmonary embolism
- Atelectasis
- COPD exacerbation

Essential Diagnostic and Laboratory Tests

- The diagnosis of pneumonia is based on prompt review and response to new clinical information from nursing observation and resident status change. The initial goal is to establish bedside predictors of severity and

Table 16-5   Pneumonia Signs and Symptoms

TYPICAL PNEUMONIA SYNDROME	ATYPICAL PNEUMONIA SYNDROME
Sudden onset of fever	Fever onset more gradual
New or worsening cough	Dry cough
Purulent sputum—rusty, green	Limited secretions
Pleuritic chest pain	Headache, malaise, myalgias, sore throat, GI distress
Signs of pulmonary consolidation	Minimal signs other than crackles (rales)
Lobar infiltrate on chest X-ray*	Abnormal, often patchy chest X-ray pattern
Consider bacterial pathogens including *Streptococcus pneumoniae*	Consider mycoplasma or chlamydia, pneumoniae, or oral anerobes. Viral pneumonia may be atypical in presentation.

*Chest X-ray may be normal on day 1 and day 2; chest X-ray may show infiltrate as symptoms persist.
Source: Adapted from Hutt & Kramer, 2002; Furman, Rayner, & Tobin, 2004.

order radiographs of the chest. Infiltrates may not be present initially if dehydration is present. Infiltrates may show up 24–48 hours later after rehydration. Some providers obtain follow-up chest X-ray after treatment—residual can last 6 weeks, or more.

- Sputum gram stain and culture (optional). The organism identified on culture may not be the offending pathogen. Colonization of the oropharnyx with multiple organisms is common in long-term care patients.
- Laboratory tests:
  ○ CBC with differential
  ○ WBC count may be normal but left shift evident.
  ○ BUN, creatinine, electrolytes, glucose
  ○ Blood cultures from two different sites; 20% positivity rate. Positivity is associated with increased risk for complications (Chestnutt & Prendergast, 2004). Antibiotic therapy should not be delayed for culture results.
- Arterial blood gases or oximetry are useful in determining severity. Arterial blood gases (ABGs) not usually available in LTC setting.
- Sputum for mycobacterium tuberculosis culture and acid-fast bacilli. Isolate and contact health department if a risk factor exists.
- If in an outbreak situation, consider urine antigen for *Legionella*, or if seriously ill patients are not responding to current antibiotics. Consider notification of local health department if trend is apparent or questionable.

Management Plan

Treatment goals for pneumonia are based on a timely working diagnosis.

- Select location for treatment—LTC or hospital
- Initiate oral or parenteral antibiotics; determine when to switch from parenteral to oral, and duration of treatment.

- Assure treatment guidelines are consistent with advance directives.
- Provide comfort, and focus on reduction of infection and associated symptoms.

Nonpharmacologic
- Oxygen per cannula or mask to prevent hypoxia
- Oral care to reduce bacterial load and improve nutritional intake. Use comfort foods, high caloric if not contraindicated. Monitor hydration.
- Monitor body weight especially if anorexia is present. Low body weight is associated with death from pneumonia.
- Address deconditioning with mild to moderate activity as condition improves.
- Dementia increases pneumonia risk profile—remain alert for exacerbations of illness consistent with hygiene and functional limitations.
- Follow facility infection control guidelines if patient returns from hospital with history of MRSA-positive sputum.
- Pulmonary hygiene to mobilize secretions: suctioning, incentive spirometry, turning, coughing, deep breathing, repositioning
- Monitor pain management and provide comfort.
- Use prevention measures to avoid aspiration.

Pharmacologic
Selection of antibiotic therapy is influenced by clinical setting, potential organisms, and comorbidities. Early initiation of antibiotic therapy is an essential principle of pneumonia management. Empirical treatment is selected on the basis of the most likely organism for the setting in which the pneumonia developed. See Table 16-6.

- Prevention—Immunization for pneumonia (Pneumovax) should be up to date including for all new admissions. Influenza

Table 16-6   Empiric Antibiotic Selections for Nursing Home-Acquired Pneumonia

FLUOROQUINOLONES*	PENICILLIN RELATED*	THIRD-GENERATION CEPHALOSPORINS
First choice, if no contraindications Moxifloxacin (Avelox) 400 mg, orally daily for 7–10 days (no renal dose adjustment required) or Levofloxacin 500 mg orally daily for 7–10 days (requires renal adjustment) Monitor INR if patient is on warfarin Reduces GI flora Both are available for intravenous infusion Check data on fluoroquinolone-resistant organisms locally and regionally	First choice, or second treatment choice if suboptimal responses Amoxicillin and clavulanic acid 500 mg every 12 hrs or 250 mg every 8 hrs for 10–14 days Severe respiratory distress: 500 mg every 8 hrs (requires renal adjustment; do not use 875 mg with severe renal impairment) Diarrhea can occur Suspension available Some products contain phenylalanine	Ceftriaxone IV or IM Immediate use to avoid hospitalization or sepsis. 1 gram daily for 3 days; then switch to an oral fluoroquinolone or penicillin-related antibiotic IM: pain at injection site Prolonged use causes superinfection

Source: Current practice principles of author.

immunization is administered to all eligible residents early each fall, per CDC guidelines and CMS regulations.

- Comfort and fever management—Start with acetaminophen 650 mg 4 times daily, either tablet, suppository, or syrup. Avoid aspirin products for fever control as fever relief can cause sweating and increased loss of fluid.

- Antibiotics are often selected on the basis of organism sensitivity. Broad spectrum antibiotics are usually initiated. Oral medications are effective; however, some situations require the parenteral, intramuscular, or intravenous route to avert sepsis. Empiric choices are listed in Table 16-6. Selection of antibiotics would include facility interim box supplies, insurance approved lists, immediate availability of medication, and data on resistant organisms.

- Parenteral antibiotic options: third- or fourth-generation cephalosporins. Clindamycin or vancomycin are usually initiated

in acute care and are often reserved for methicillin-resistant staphylococcus, (MRSA).

- Hydration concerns—Oral versus intravenous. Base decisions on electrolyte monitoring, diuretic therapy, and ability to meet oral fluid requirements. Oral daily requirements are 25 mL/kg or 30 mL/kg if resident is on diuretics. Hydration orally is a team effort!

- Maintain inhalation therapy for any comorbidity and adjust accordingly. Cough management may improve with nebulizer treatments.

- Oral candidiasis—Treat with swish and swallow mycostatin suspension (4–6 mL 4 times/day) or trochees (1 dissolved slowly in mouth 4–5 times/day).

- Diarrhea—Check for *C. difficile* toxin and treat. See Chapter 12.

- Don't use benzodiazepines—they increase the risk of aspiration.

- H$_2$ blockers—Older studies suggest acid suppression in the stomach increases enteric bacterial colonization and associated risk for pneumonia (Muder, 1998).

- Watch for delirium associated with medications and comorbidities.

- GERD—For patients with aspiration risk who are on PPIs (proton pump inhibitors), look at compliance with medication dosage and schedule. Order elevated head of bed or other interventions to assure control of risk factors.

Patient, Family, and Staff Education

- Family, resident, and staff should receive education about immunization and benefits of prevention. Include education about seasonal risk during winter months and hand washing protocols.

- Explain benefit of hydration, nutrition, and exercise to family, staff, and patient.

- Educate visitors and staff on health maintenance. Post reminder signs at entrances encouraging visitors not to visit residents if sick.

- Educate infection control staff regarding line-listing for MRSA colonized residents.

Physician Consultation

- Collaborative management provides continuity of care. Physician consultation is advised in situations where a high risk of mortality occurs to assure the clinical setting and resources contribute to appropriate outcome. The need for parenteral therapy may require consultation.

- Comorbidities can mask actual pathophysiologic changes. For example, radiology reports can "suggest" pneumonia or "indicate" infiltrate "suggestive" of pneumonia or congestive heart. If little clinical history is available, the treatment plan may depend on the collaborative communication.

PULMONARY EMBOLISM

Definition

Pulmonary embolism (PE) may present as dyspnea or as severe chest pain. It is a potentially fatal complication of clot formation, usually blood, originating in the venous circulation. Pulmonary embolism is a non-ischemic cause of life-threatening chest pain. Some pulmonary emboli are associated with infarction, as a thrombus occludes the pulmonary artery or one of the branches. Most PEs occur as a result of a change in the coagulation system of the blood. Pulmonary embolism, often a missed diagnosis, can present with a variety of nonspecific symptoms. It is often clinically silent until presentation.

Epidemiology

Venous thromboembolism affects 1 in 1000 people annually. Each year in the United States, pulmonary embolism contributes to high mortality with approximately 50,000 pulmonary embolus-associated deaths. Fewer than 10% received PE specific treatment before death (Chestnutt & Prendergast, 2004). The incidence rate climbs steadily with age. Occurrence is about 3% in elderly over 85 years. Generally most PE can be linked to a "migrating" substance originating anywhere in the venous circulation or heart. Thrombus formation in calf muscles rarely embolize; however, proximal popliteal and ileofemoral venous systems tend to accumulate clots that break off and travel to the lungs. Blood as well as other migrating substances have the potential to manifest as a pulmonary embolism. Long bone fractures may release fat emboli, severe infections produce septic emboli, tumor cells release from cancers, and air from central venous catheter complications—all are associated PE risk factors in the elderly patient. Stasis and prolonged immobility or medication-induced hypercoagulability may initiate a cascade of risk potentials. An acute event, trauma, or chronic disease can be a pivotal crisis in the life of an older person, increasing the potential for clinically induced complications. Iatrogenic illness is an important factor in morbidity and mortality data. An essential course of action for the elderly person in long-term care is prevention and prophylaxis.

Common Presenting Signs and Symptoms

- Assessment of patients with or without a history of thromboembolic disease should include objective and subjective attention to complaints of pain, swelling, tenderness, and increased tissue turgor especially when presented unilaterally on an upper or lower extremity.

- Increased resistance or pain during dorsiflexion of the foot (Homan's sign) is an unreliable diagnostic test for deep vein thrombosis (DVT).

- Dyspnea, chest pain, and hemoptysis are considered typical symptoms in PE.

- Tachycardia and tachypnea, cough, diaphoresis, anxiety, and apprehension may occur in combination or as a single presentation.

- A sudden onset of dyspnea, excessively rapid breathing, and pleuritic or angina-like chest pain with sensations of syncope are prevalent in patients with massive pulmonary embolism, or an acute response in elderly patients.

- Unrecognized PE can be fatal. Immediately refer patients to their physician or emergency medical services (911) for further evaluation, diagnosis, and treatment.

Differential Diagnosis

- Pneumonia
- Myocardial infarction
- Pleural effusion
- CHF
- Pneumothorax
- Asthma
- Esophageal rupture
- Pericarditis
- Fractured rib
- Herpes zoster before rash

Essential Diagnostic and Laboratory Tests

Diagnostic tests are often combined to rule in or rule out pulmonary embolism. The PE diagnostic algorithm looks at clinical probability of a pulmonary embolism (Well et al., 1998).

- Chest X-ray
- Electrocardiogram
- Spiral computed tomography—CT scan or MRA or ultrasound scan
- Arterial blood gases
- Ventilation and perfusion scan—A common noninvasive test
- D-Dimer blood assay testing
- Pulmonary angiography—Considered the gold standard.

Management Plan

Anticoagulation is the therapy of choice to treat existing PE and to prevent new clot formation while the body degrades existing clot. Anticoagulation is usually continued for a minimum of 3 months, depending on the risk of reoccurrence or risks associated with anticoagulation therapy.

Nonpharmacologic

- Fall prevention precautions including the addition of assistance in ADLs. Patients at high risk for falls, especially if cognitively impaired, may require close activity monitoring and personal alarms. The risk-benefit approach should be discussed and documented for "frequent fallers."

- Monitor adverse anticoagulant effects. Check for bleeding, increases in bruising. Some patients may present with a scleral hemorrhage. Artificial tears may help the eye irritation.

- A dietary change after INR dosing maintenance is achieved may require follow-up INRs, especially if fortified protein drink is added.

- Laxative use or GI upset resulting in frequent loose stools can disturb bowel flora and change INR stability. Watch for *Clostridium difficile* infection in patients with recent antibiotic therapy.

- Encourage ambulation and avoid prolonged sitting. Avoid dependent edema and use antiembolic stockings—order several pairs. Most antiembolic stockings should be "thigh-high" unless body habitus creates a gartertype roll at the popliteal area. Then knee-highs are suitable.

- Medic alert bracelet or warfarin ID if receiving care from other medical providers, dentists, or podiatrist.

- Hydrate—Remind patient/resident to drink adequate fluids.

Pharmacologic
- Intravenous heparin is the usual initial therapy with no active bleeding or contraindications. Contraindications could include recent surgery or trauma, uncontrolled hypertension, or inadequate facilities to monitor anticoagulation.

- The usual treatment of choice after initial heparin therapy is a combination of low molecular weight heparin injections (Lovenox) and oral warfarin tablets (Coumadin). Lovenox is usually discontinued when the INR is between 2.0–3.0, about 7 days. Usual maximum 17 days.

- Warfarin (Coumadin) is used for long-term maintenance. Measurement frequency of the INR will be adjusted depending on the stability of the target PT-INR. Anticoagulation is always individualized and may continue for 6 months or indefinitely after pulmonary embolism.

- Maintenance of adequate anticoagulation may be disrupted by interactions with other drugs, dietary intake, and alterations in comorbid state, including dehydration.

- The addition of another medication, such as an antibiotic for a new infection, should prompt a review of the lab schedule for PT/INR and follow-up labs several days after addition of new medication. The list of medications disturbing stable INRs is extensive.

- Usual PT/INR is 2.0–3.0 for DVT and PE. If INR is elevated warfarin may be held and, if indicated, oral vitamin K, or FFP (fresh frozen plasma) may be given. This depends on facility practice guidelines. Resident may need to be transferred to acute care for treatment.

Patient, Family, and Staff Education
- Explain management and benefit of activity and exercise for PE prevention.

- Educate on importance of anticoagulant therapy monitoring, lab schedule, and medication compliance.

- Educate on safety measures, use of razor, soft toothbrush, antiembolic stockings and injury follow-up.

- Encourage and support facility fall prevention programs

Physician Consultation
- Once the emergent evaluation and treatment plan is established, physician follow-up is based on individualized risk factors, postsurgical evaluation, or surgical consultation.

- Collaborate with physician if therapeutic INR levels cannot be maintained.

- Consider referral for patients with major contraindications to anticoagulation or recurrent DVT or PE. Placement of an inferior vena cava filter may reduce incidence of recurrence of PE associated with proximal lower extremity DVT.

▌ WEB SITES

- American Lung Association—www.lungusa.org/noframes

- Global Initiative for Chronic Ostructive Lung Disease—www.goldcopd.com

- US Chronic Obstructive Pulmonary Disease Coalition—www.uscopd.com

- Current Medical Diagnosis and Treatment—www.cmdtlinks.com

- National Lung Health Education Program—www.nlhep.org

- National Association for Medical Direction of Respiratory Care—www.namdrc.org

- National Guideline Clearinghouse—www.guidelines.gov

- Centers for Disease Control and Prevention—www.cdc.gov/ncidod/diseases/flu

- National Center for Complementary and Alternative Medicine—www.nccam.nih.gov

- Oncology practice guidelines—www.cancernet.com

- Chronic Lung Disease Resource—www.cheshire-med.com/forums

- American Thoracic Society—www.thoracic.org

▌ REFERENCES

American Thoracic Society. (1999). Pulmonary rehabilitation—1999. *American Journal Respiratory Critical Care Medicine, 159*, 1666–1682.

Blinkhorn, R. J. (1998). Community-acquired pneumonia. In G. L. Baum, J. D. Crapo, B. R. Celli, & J. B. Karlinsky (Eds.), *Pulmonary diseases* (6th ed., pp. 503–530). Philadelphia: Lippincott-Raven.

Celli, B. R. (1998). Clinical aspects of chronic obstructive pulmonary disease. In G. L. Baum, J. D. Crapo, B. R. Celli, & J. B. Karlinsky (Eds.), *Textbook of pulmonary diseases* (6th ed., pp. 843–858). Philadelphia: Raven.

Chestnutt, M. S., & Prendergast, T. J. (2004). Lung. In L. M. Tierney, S. J. McPhee, & M. A. Papadakis (Eds.), *Lange 2004 current medical diagnosis and treatment* (pp. 212–305). New York: Lange.

CMS. (2005). CMS will require nursing homes to vaccinate residents against the flu. Retrieved February 5, 2006, from http://www.cms.hhs.gov/apps/media/press/release.asp?counter=1688

Cote, C. G., & Celli, B. R. (2005). New treatment strategies for COPD: Pairing the new with the tried and true. *Postgraduate Medicine, 117*(3), 27–34.

Edmunds, M. W., & Mayhew, M. S. (2000). *Pharmacology for the primary care provider* (pp. 294–309). St. Louis, MO: Mosby.

Furman, C. D., Rayner, A. V., & Tobin, E. P. (2004). Pneumonia in older residents in long-term care facilities. *American Family Physician, 70*, 1495–1500.

Hutt, E., & Kramer, A. M. (2002). Evidence-based guidelines for management of nursing home-acquired pneumonia. *Journal of Family Practice, 51*, 709–716.

Lie, D. A. (2000). Cough. In R. B. Taylor (Ed.), *The 20-minute diagnosis manual: symptoms and signs in the time-limited encounter* (pp. 149–150). Philadelphia: Lippincott Williams & Wilkins.

Mehr, D. R., Binder, E. F., Kruse, R. L., Zweig, S. C., Madsen, R., Popejoy, L., et al. (2001). Predicting mortality in nursing home residents with lower respiratory tract infection. *Journal of the American Medical Association, 286*, 2427–2436.

Muder, R. R. (1998). Pneumonia in residents of long-term care facilities: Epidemiology, etiology, management and prevention. *American Journal of Medicine, 105*, 319–330.

Muder, R. R. (2000). Approach to the problem of pneumonia in long-term care facilities. *Comprehensive Therapy, 26*, 255–262.

Naughton, B. J., & Mylotte, J. M. (2000). Treatment guideline for nursing home-acquired pneumonia based on community practice. *Journal American Geriatrics Society, 48*, 82–88.

Rugo, H. S. (2004). Cancer. In L. M. Tierney, Jr., S. J. McPhee, & M. A. Papadakis (Eds.), *2004 Lange current medical diagnosis and treatment* (pp. 1577–1599). New York: Lange/Mc Graw-Hill.

Waldman, R. H. (1984). Influenza virus. In R. H. Waldman, & R. M. Kluge (Eds.), *Infectious diseases* (pp. 485–499). New York: Medical Examination Publishing.

Well, P. S., Ginsberg, J. S., Anderson, D. R., Kearon, C., Gent, M., Turpie, A. G. G., et al. (1998). Use of a clinical model for safe management of patients with suspected pulmonary embolism. *Annals of Internal Medicine, 129*, 997–1005.

Wisnivesky, J. P., Foldes, C., & McGinn, T. G. (2002). Management of asthma in the elderly. *Annals of Long-Term Care, 10*(4), 61–68.

Yoshikawa, T. T. (2002). Antimicrobial resistance and aging: Beginning the end of the antibiotic era? *Journal of the American Geriatrics Society, 50*, 226–229.

■ BIBLIOGRAPHY

American Academy of Pediatrics—Influenza. In L. K. Pickering (Ed.), *Red Book 2003 Report of the committee on infectious diseases* (26th ed., pp. 382–390). Elk Grove Village, IL: American Academy of Pediatrics.

CHAPTER 17

Vascular Disorders

Deborah Caswell and Michelle Eslami

ABDOMINAL AORTIC ANEURYSM

Definition

An abdominal aortic aneurysm (AAA) is a dilation of the aorta anywhere along its course from below the renal arteries to the bifurcation of the iliac arteries. It is present when there is an increase in aortic diameter of 150% of normal diameter, usually considered to be greater than 3–4 cm. Aneurysms may dissect and bulge leaking blood between vessel layers and may eventually rupture.

Epidemiology

Large aneurysms are known to be associated with approximately 9000 deaths per year. The prevalence of an AAA appears to be gender specific: 5–9% in men and 1% in women. Risk factors for AAA include increasing age, male gender, family history of aneurysm, smoking history, hypertension, peripheral vascular disease, coronary artery disease, chronic obstructive pulmonary disease, and presence of other aneurysms. The strongest risk factor for rupture of an AAA is the maximal aortic diameter and rapid rate of expansion (> 1.0 cm/year). Approximately 95% of abdominal aneurysms are infrarenal.

The true cause of AAA is not known. Histologically, AAAs reveal fragmentation of the elastin layers and decreased elastin content with the aneurysm ultimately left with a thin tunica media and only a few elastin layers remaining. Atherosclerosis in the intima is typical, but the medial degenerative process for aneurysm is quite different from the typical intimal-medial thickening that occurs with an occlusive atherosclerotic process. A thick layer of thrombus is typically layered over the intimal layer of the aneurysm, which provides some protection from rupture.

Common Presenting Signs and Symptoms

- Vague abdominal pain is the most common symptom if symptoms are present.
- Patients may report feeling pulsation in the abdomen, most noticeable when supine.
- Back pain that is constant may be present, described as dull aching and not associated with movement. This occurs when the aneurysm is large enough to cause compression on the spinal cord.
- The triad of shock, pulsatile mass, and excruciating pain in the abdomen or back is highly suggestive of rupture.

- Physical examination may reveal a pulsating mass in the abdomen in the area adjacent to the umbilicus.
- A bruit may be auscultated over the aneurysm.
- Dissecting or ruptured aneurysms may present with vital sign changes associated with hypovolemia, shock, ecchymosis in the flank area, and severe pain in the abdomen or back that is sudden in onset.

Differential Diagnosis
- Urinary tract infection
- Renal obstruction
- Ruptured disc
- Diverticulitis
- Pancreatitis
- Upper gastrointestinal (UGI) hemorrhage
- Abdominal neoplasm
- Peptic ulcer perforation
- Myocardial infarction

Essential Diagnostic and Laboratory Tests
- Screening abdominal ultrasonography in asymptomatic individuals is an accurate test with 95% sensitivity and near 100% specificity. See Table 17-1 for screening recommendations.
- CT scan is more accurate and provides a more precise interpretation of the size and location of the aneurysm. CT scan is always performed prior to surgical intervention. A special CT scan with 3 mm cuts is required if considering endovascular intervention.
- MRI/MRA are comparable to CT scan, but are more expensive.
- Arteriogram is not an accurate technique to determine the presence or size of the AAA because of the presence of thrombus lining the lumen of the aorta at the aneurysmal site.

TABLE 17-1   Screening Recommendations for Abdominal Aortic Aneurysm
Initial Screening:
1. All males between the ages of 60–85
2. Women between the ages of 60 and 85 with history of cardiovascular risk factors
3. Men and women over the age of 50 with a family history of AAA
Follow-up Screening:
1. No further testing recommended if aortic diameter is less than 3.0 cm
2. Yearly screening if aortic diameter is between 3.0 and 4.0.
3. Ultrasound every 6 months if aortic diameter is between 4.0–4.5 cm
4. Referral to vascular surgeon if aortic diameter is greater than 4.5 cm
Source: Kent et al., 2004.

- Routine laboratory testing is not indicated for a patient presenting for AAA evaluation. Clinical decisions should be made on an individual basis but may include CBC with platelets, electrolytes, BUN, creatinine, fasting blood sugar, liver function tests, coagulation profile, and urinalysis.

Management Plan
The goals for management of an aortic aneurysm are early recognition and referral and aggressive management of risk factors.

Nonpharmacologic
- Order screening as indicated.
- Order serial ultrasounds to assess progression of disease.
- Screen for other risk factors and assist in modification.

Pharmacologic

Hypertension should be carefully controlled in patients in whom aneurysms are being followed.

Patient, Family, and Staff Education

- Instruct in nature, onset, and course of disease including rupture.
- Inform patient/family that routine follow-up will be necessary with repeat ultrasound or CT scans to determine the course of aneurysm progression.
- Inform patient/family/staff that sudden, severe pain in the back or abdomen (signs of rupture) requires emergency care.

Physician Consultation

All abdominal aortic aneurysms require referral to a vascular surgeon. Suspected rupture of an aneurysm is a surgical emergency, and the patient should be sent directly to the emergency room.

CAROTID DISEASE

Definition

Atherosclerotic plaque affecting the carotid arteries can reduce blood supply to the brain. The atherogenesis process begins as an inflammatory process involving the mononuclear leukocytes being recruited to the intimal layer of the vessel wall. This action initiates changes within the intimal layer allowing foam cells to form a "fatty streak" within the vessel wall. Increasing accumulation of foam cells in the intima transforms the fatty streak into a more advanced plaque. This plaque can then become stable, causing stenosis that may eventually lead to occlusion; or it may become unstable, leading to emboli and acute occlusion or infarction. Most carotid plaques occur at the bifurcation of the internal and external carotid artery within the bulb of the common carotid.

Epidemiology

Atherosclerotic vascular disease frequently affects multiple areas. Vascular risk factors for other atherosclerotic vasculapathy are identical in carotid disease. Hypertension is twice as common in patients with carotid disease than in those without it. Smoking, dyslipidemia, and diabetes are all associated with carotid artery disease. Some studies suggest that patients with asymptomatic carotid bruits are more likely to have significant carotid stenosis if they are older, are hypertensive, smoke, or have advanced peripheral vascular disease. Additionally, coronary heart disease and peripheral vascular disease are prevalent in this population.

Common Presenting Signs and Symptoms

- May present with signs of transient ischemic attack (TIA) or stroke. TIA is a brief episode of loss of brain function that can usually be localized to a specific portion of the brain supplied by a single vascular system and lasts less than 24 hours. Ischemic stroke occurs when symptoms last more than 24 hours or cause death. Signs of TIA/stroke include the following:
  - Paresthesia/weakness of one extremity (hand, arm or face most typical)
  - Hemiplegia/hemiparesis
  - Aphasia
  - Dysarthria
  - Vertigo
  - Diplopia
  - Amaurosis fugax
  - Acute confusion
  - Memory loss
  - Profound weakness
- Amaurosis fugax is a transient (< 24 hours) loss of vision in one eye or a portion of the visual field, frequently described as a curtain across a portion of the eye.

- Carotid bruit will usually be present and may be transmitted as a cardiac murmur. The bruit is found using the bell of the stethoscope listening over the area from the upper end of the thyroid cartilage to just below the angle of the jaw over the area of the carotid artery.

- Patient may be asymptomatic.

Differential Diagnosis
- Migraine headache
- Metabolic abnormalities
- Brain lesions
- Focal seizures
- Peripheral nerve disorders
- Cardiac arrhythmia
- Vertigo from labyrinthitis or Meniere's disease
- Temporal arteritis
- Optic nerve disorders

Essential Diagnostic and Laboratory Tests
- Duplex ultrasound of both carotid arteries is recommended. Duplex ultrasound is now considered the gold standard for diagnostic workup of carotid artery disease. For asymptomatic lesions of less than 75%, follow-up ultrasound should be performed at least yearly.

- Magnetic resonance angiography and CT angiography are quick, noninvasive means of ruling out alternative abnormalities during the patient workup.

- Carotid angiogram is the cornerstone for diagnosis in the workup of the patient. It is a preoperative study and should not be ordered unless the patient and the surgeon are ready to proceed promptly with surgery.

- Routine laboratory tests should include CBC, platelet count, coagulation tests, electrolytes, glucose, calcium, and sedimentation rate.

- Long-term care residents may not be candidates for surgical intervention and may not require presurgical diagnostics.

Management Plan
The goals of treatment are early detection, management of risk factors, and prevention of complications.

Nonpharmacologic
- Asymptomatic carotid stenosis less than 75% should be followed with yearly ultrasound to evaluate progression of stenosis.

- Risk factor modification: diet, exercise, smoking cessation

Pharmacologic
- Risk factor modification with lipid lowering agents, antihypertensives, beta blockers, as indicated

- Antiplatelet agents are indicated for asymptomatic carotid stenosis less than 75%.

  - ASA 81 mg daily
  - Clopidogrel 75 mg daily

Patient, Family, and Staff Education
- Teach the signs of TIA/stroke.

- If signs or symptoms develop, transfer to acute care.

- Risk factor modification for atherosclerotic disease including diet, exercise and smoking cessation

Physician Consultation
- Patients with asymptomatic carotid bruit and less than 75% stenosis on ultrasound can be followed by the primary care provider but

should be seen by a vascular surgeon to determine if further workup is indicated.

- Patients who are symptomatic or who have stenosis greater than 75% should be referred for surgical consultation, if they are candidates for surgical intervention. Research clearly shows that risk of stroke at this point is greater than risk of surgery.

DEEP VEIN THROMBOSIS

Definition

Deep venous thrombosis (DVT) refers to occlusion within the venous system. Deep venous thrombosis occurs typically in the lower extremities. Distal DVT is occlusion confined to the deep calf veins, and thrombosis at or above the popliteal vein is considered proximal DVT. A distal DVT becomes clinically important if it extends proximally, where the chance of pulmonary embolization is clinically significant.

Epidemiology

Deep vein thrombosis affects more than 2 million Americans annually and of this number, only 280,000–300,000 are objectively diagnosed. Symptoms tend to be nonspecific and the first sign of DVT may be pulmonary embolus (PE).

Deep vein thrombosis is more common in hospitalized patients with some types of conditions. Without prophylaxis, DVT occurs after approximately 20% of all major surgical procedures, and PE occurs in 1–2%. Over 50% of major orthopedic procedures are complicated by DVT and up to 30% by PE if prophylactic treatment is not implemented. Of the 31 million nonsurgical patients admitted to the hospital each year up to 16% develop DVT without prophylaxis.

Virchow's triad, developed in 1856 by Dr. Rudolf Virchow, describes the conditions that promote hypercoagulability and thrombus formation. The triad is composed of the following:

- Hypercoagulability
- Stasis
- Endothelial injury (See Table 17-2 for a detailed list of risk factors.)

Hypercoagulability of the blood results in a procoagulant state. These activities can include increases in thrombocytosis with increased adhesiveness of platelets, alterations in the coagulation cascade, and an inhibition of endogenous fibrinolytic activity. Stasis of blood in the veins, as with prolonged bed rest,

TABLE 17-2 Risk Factors for Venous Thrombosis		
ACQUIRED	**INHERITED**	**MIXED/UNKNOWN**
Age	Anticardiolipin antibody	Hyperhomocysteinemia
Previous thrombosis	syndrome	High levels of factor VIII
Immobilization	Antithrombin deficiency	APC-resistance in the absence
Major surgery	Protein C deficiency	of factor V Leiden
Orthopedic surgery	Protein S deficiency	
Malignancy	Factor V Leiden	
Oral contraceptives	Dysfibrinogenemia	
Hormone replacement	Myeloproliferative disorders	
therapy	Polycythemia vera	
	Antiphospholipid syndrome	

Source: Adapted from Rosendaal, 1999. APC=activated protein C.

allows prolonged contact of activated platelets and clotting factors, with the endothelial lining of the vein wall theoretically inducing the clotting mechanism and development of a DVT. Endothelial injury can occur from trauma, infection, venipuncture, myocardial infarction, chemical agents, or as the result of excessive dilation.

The most common site of thrombosis is the soleus muscle of the calf. About 80% of DVTs will remain isolated to the calf and usually be spontaneously lysed by the body's fibrinolytic activity or will have some degree of recannalization. The other 20% will propagate into the major deep veins such as the femoral, popliteal, or peroneal veins. Thrombi may extend into iliac and vena cava. Thrombosis propagation frequently results in formation of a "tail" of fibrin. It is this unstable tail that breaks away and becomes the life-threatening embolus.

Common Presenting Signs and Symptoms

Symptoms will vary depending on the location of the DVT, size of the thrombus, and the degree of collateral circulation that is present in the extremity.

- Many patients with DVT will be asymptomatic.

- Swelling of the affected extremity is the most common symptom identified. Swelling will usually be unilateral, will be dramatic, and rather sudden in onset. Swelling may not resolve with elevation.

- Pain may be present, made worse by standing or exercise, improved with rest and elevation. Pain may be sudden in onset and may be severe or mild.

- Patients may have a low-grade fever.

- There may be tenderness to palpation along the course of the thrombus.

- Homan's sign (pain in the calf upon dorsiflexion) is present in only 20% of patients with DVT.

- Patients with a pulmonary embolus may be asymptomatic or present with varying degrees of dyspnea, tachypnea, or chest pain. Symptoms can vary from mild to very severe with hemodynamic compromise.

Differential Diagnosis

- Cellulitis
- Lymphedema
- Muscle injury
- Ruptured Baker's cyst
- Postphlebitic syndrome

Essential Diagnostic and Laboratory Tests

- Plasma D-Dimer has almost 100% sensitivity for predicting PE, but false positives increase with age (Righini, Goehring, Bounameaux, & Perrier, 2000). It has good negative predictive value in outpatients with equivocal signs and symptoms. It does not, however, demonstrate usefulness in ruling out DVT and PE in the hospitalized patient, those with a previous thrombus, and those with comorbidities that are risk factors for DVT/PE development such as immobility, surgery, and cancer (Schrecengost et al., 2003; Wells et al., 2003).

- Hypercoagulability workup is indicated for patients who have more than one episode of DVT (PT/PTT, protein S, protein C, anticardiolipin antibody)

- Duplex ultrasound with compression is sensitive and specific for diagnosing DVT in proximal vessels. It may be inconclusive in obese patients and those with significant edema. This technique is less sensitive for detection of isolated calf vein thrombosis. Positive duplex confirms the diagnosis of DVT; negative duplex requires additional testing as calf vein thrombosis may go undetected.

- Contrast venography, though not performed as frequently, remains the gold standard in diagnostics. The finding of a constant intra-luminal filling defect on two or more views confirms the diagnosis of acute DVT. This test is seldom the first diagnostic test due to several disadvantages such as reaction to the contrast dye, renal insufficiency, and cost.

- Impedance plethysmography allows di-agnosis of DVT by impairment of venous drainage from the lower extremity.

Management Plan

The goals for management of DVT are dissolv-ing the thrombus, prevention of further clot for-mation, prevention of pulmonary emboli, and pain relief.

Nonpharmacologic
- Elevate extremity higher than heart during acute phase along with bed rest.
- Warm compresses may be helpful to reduce inflammation and control pain.
- Graduated compression stockings should be worn after acute phase to control edema. The recommended starting compression is 20–30 mmHg; for recalcitrant edema the com-pression can be increased to 30–40 mmHg.

Pharmacologic
- Heparin therapy with a bolus of 5000 to 10,000 units intravenously with infusion to keep activated partial thromboplastin time (aPTT) 1.5 to 2.5 times the control is first-line therapy. Be alert for heparin-induced thrombocytopenia.
- Low-molecular weight heparin 1.5 to 2.0 mg/kg twice daily given subcutaneously can be used instead of heparin infusion and/or as a bridge to warfarin therapy.
- In appropriate patients warfarin therapy may be utilized for treatment of DVT. Give a loading dose of 10 mg for 2 days then titrate to keep international normalizing ra-tio (INR) at desired level, usually 2.0–3.0.

Continue heparin therapy until the INR is stable. Warfarin therapy is usually contin-ued for 6–12 months with a first episode. Longer duration of therapy may be con-sidered for patients at increased risk for recurrent DVT/PE.

- In high-risk patients, other antiplatelet med-ications have been utilized such as ASA 325 mg daily alone or in combination with Clopidogrel 75 mg daily. (No scientific data is currently present to support this method; however, there are anecdotal reports.)
- Initiate any needed pain control with medication that will not interfere with anti-coagulation management such as acetomi-nophen, hydrocodone, propoxyphene, or tramadol.

Patient, Family, and Staff Education

- Cause and course of DVT should be ex-plained.
- Medication teaching specific to anticoagu-lation therapy:
  - Give medication as prescribed at the same time every day.
  - Pay attention to drug interactions with warfarin.
  - Instruct patients and caregivers upon discharge about safe use of warfarin in-cluding the following:
    - Inform any healthcare providers of warfarin use.
    - Cautious intake of any foods high in vitamin K such as organ meats, leafy green vegetables, and green tea.
    - Report any unusual bleeding or ex-cessive bruising
    - Review need and schedule for blood drawing for monitoring of INR.
- Review application and use of graduated compression stockings.

Physician Consultation

- Any new DVT
- Any DVT above the popliteal vein
- Symptoms of PE: transfer to acute care immediately.

■ PERIPHERAL ARTERIAL DISEASE

Definition

Peripheral arterial disease (PAD) is a group of diseases that result in stenosis or occlusion of the blood flow in the arteries, exclusive of the coronary and intracranial vessels. The most common cause of PAD is atherosclerosis. Atherogenesis begins as an inflammatory process involving the mononuclear leukocytes being recruited to the intimal layer of the vessel wall. This action initiates changes within the intimal layer allowing foam cells to form a "fatty streak" within the vessel wall. Increasing accumulation of foam cells in the intima transforms the fatty streak into a more advanced plaque. This plaque can then become stable (causing stenosis that may eventually lead to occlusion) or unstable (leading to emboli and acute occlusion or infarction).

Epidemiology

The prevalence of PAD is thought to be even higher than that of myocardial infarction and stroke and is estimated to affect approximately 8 to 12 million Americans. When utilizing the standard criteria of ankle-brachial index (ABI) less than 0.9, studies have found that most patients diagnosed with PAD are asymptomatic. The mortality rate for established PAD is estimated to be approximately 4% per year even in the asymptomatic patient. Patients with critical limb ischemia who have the lowest ankle-brachial index have an annual mortality of 25% (Hirsch et al., 2001). The prevalence of peripheral arterial disease is age dependent. It increased from 9% of subjects 55 to 59 years of age to 57% of patients 85 to 89 years of age

(Meijer, Hous, & Rutgers, 1998). Similarly, the prevalence of PAD (diagnosed using noninvasive tests) increased from 2.5% in subjects 40 to 59 years of age to 18.8% in subjects 70 to 79 years of age in the San Diego population study (n = 624) (Dormandy et al., 1991).

Main modifiable risk factors for PAD include the following:

- Diabetes mellitus
- Hyperlipidemia
- Hypertension
- Obesity
- Elevated homocysteine
- Smoking
- Physical inactivity

Risk factors that cannot be modified include age, male gender, and family history. Screening for atherosclerotic disease should be performed on any patient age 70 or greater or age 50 with associated risk factors of smoking or diabetes.

Common Presenting Signs and Symptoms

- Intermittent claudication is present in approximately one third of patients with PAD. Intermittent claudication is pain that begins in one or both legs with walking a certain distance, does not go away with continued walking, is relieved with 5–10 minutes of rest, and returns upon walking that same distance. Pain may be described as aching, tiredness, numbness, weakness, or cramping.
- More than 50% of patients with PAD diagnosed based on ankle brachial index (ABI) < 0.9 will not have typical claudication. These patients may have no symptoms, or they may have other types of leg pain with exercise.
- Pain may be masked in patients who have diabetic neuropathy.

- Rest pain occurs with advanced disease and affects primarily the toes and ball of the foot. Rest pain occurs when arterial compromise is so severe that circulation relies on gravity to assist with blood flow. When the patient lies down or elevates the leg, pain from ischemia results. The patient may have a history of sleeping in a chair or with affected leg on the floor to alleviate the pain. The patient may also present with swelling as well as pain because of the need to keep the extremity dependent. At this point, the compromise to the circulation is so severe that the patient is in limb threat and needs surgical evaluation. Delay may result in gangrene and/or amputation of the affected extremity. Depending on the degree of vascular compromise, the patient may be a candidate for a revascularization procedure either with bypass or angioplasty/stenting. The use of catheter-based interventions for revascularization has proven an effective treatment for even the most frail patient. Failure to intervene can result in prolonged severe pain from the ischemic extremity and may lead to emergent amputation. Some patients may not be candidates for surgical intervention, even at the late stages of vascular compromise, but it must be remembered that the pain from an ischemic extremity is excruciating and can be very difficult to alleviate.

- Nonhealing ulcers may be a presenting symptom. Severe restriction of blood flow inhibits healing and significantly compromises skin integrity. Arterial ulcers are usually on pressure points such as between toes, and over bony prominences. The patient may present with cyanosis or gangrene of toes. In this case the patient needs urgent surgical evaluation.

- Trophic changes in an extremity may be present due to chronic ischemia. These include hair loss, thin shiny skin, thickened nails, and skeletonization of the extremity.

- Diminished or absent pulses on the extremity may be present below the occlusion.

- Dependent rubor of the affected extremity appears as deep red color of the foot with dependence that blanches quickly with elevation and is slow to return (:10 seconds) when extremity is once again dependent.

- If the patient presents with symptoms that are sudden in onset suspect acute arterial occlusion. This usually involves "5 P's": pain, pallor, paresthesia, paralysis, and poikilothermia (cold). This patient must be referred for emergent vascular consult.

Differential Diagnosis

- Arthritis

- Spinal stenosis

- Peripheral neuropathy

- Venous stasis disease

- Musculoskeletal injury

Essential Diagnostic and Laboratory Tests

- All patients with PAD should be evaluated for atherosclerotic risk factors including hypertension, lipid abnormalities, and diabetes mellitus.

- Laboratory evaluation should include complete blood count, platelet count, fasting blood glucose or hemoglobin A1c, creatinine, fasting lipid profile, hypercoagulability screening, homocysteine level, and urinalysis for glycosuria and proteinuria.

- An ankle-brachial index should be performed on any patient with symptoms of peripheral vascular disease, any patient over the age of 70, and any patient age 50 or older with diabetes or smoking history. ABI < 0.90 establishes a diagnosis of PAD with a 95% sensitivity and specificity of 100%. Patients with diabetes or the elderly may have artificially elevated pressures due to calcified arteries. Instructions for performing an ABI are presented in Figure 17-1.

FIGURE 17-1   The Ankle-Brachial Reflex

How to perform ABI:

1. Patient supine for 5 minutes
2. Measure systolic pressure in both brachial arteries.
3. Apply blood pressure cuff just above malleolus on leg.
4. Obtain systolic pressure at the dorsalis pedis and posterior tibial artery.
5. Repeat on opposite leg.
6. Using highest brachial pressure, obtain ratio of leg:arm pressure.

ABI Interpretation

Above 0.90—Normal
0.71–0.90—Mild obstruction
0.41–0.70—Moderate obstruction
0.00–0.40—Severe obstruction

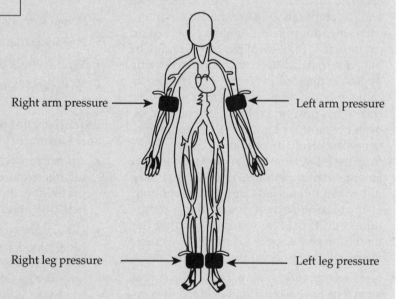

Right arm pressure ⟶   Left arm pressure

Right leg pressure ⟶   Left leg pressure

Right ABI:
Higher right ankle pressure = ___ mmHg
Higher right arm pressure   = ___ mmHg

Left ABI:
Higher left ankle pressure   = ___ mmHg
Higher left arm pressure   = ___ mmHg

Right ABI:
Higher right ankle pressure = 80 mmHg
Higher right arm pressure   = 130 mmHg

= 0.62 mmHg (see interpretation chart)

- Digit photoplethysmography or toe brachial index can be beneficial in patients with calcified vessels.
- Arterial duplex ultrasound can be performed to locate arterial lesions, but this test is not needed to diagnose PAD. It is used to address specific questions such as location and degree of stenosis, occlusion or aneurysm, measure vessel diameter, or to determine length of occlusion. It is also useful to assess patency of previous arterial grafts.
- Magnetic resonance angiography (MRA) or computerized tomographic angiography (CTA) testing is frequently used in place of diagnostic angiography for patients.
- Angiography once was the gold standard in locating the specific lesions to be addressed with surgical interventions; however, the trend is to use the less invasive MRA or CTA or to perform angiography at time of intervention in the operating room to spare the patient multiple anesthetic episodes.

Management Plan

Management of patients with PAD has two primary goals: to address the risk factors important in the progression of generalized atherosclerosis and to improve the patient's functional status. In long-term care settings the goal may be medical management and palliative care for nonsurgical candidates.

Nonpharmacologic
- Establishing a regular, formal walking program has been shown in numerous trials to be beneficial for the patient with moderate to severe PAD. Regular walking improves not only the walking distance but also the quality of life and functional capacity. A rigorous walking program has been shown to be as beneficial as a bypass procedure and more beneficial than angioplasty.
- Foot care should be made a priority including inspection every day; use of a moisturizer

every day to prevent skin cracks; keeping nails trimmed; and wearing comfortable, well-fitting shoes.
- Refer to the dietician, if indicated, for low-fat diet.
- In long-term care *carefully document physical findings and pulses* to follow disease progression or improvement.

Pharmacologic
- Pharmacologic agents have been used to improve walking distance. Pentoxifylline 400 mg three times daily was approved for treatment of claudication in 1984, but most studies do not show an increase in walking distance. Pentoxifylline improves the deformability of red cells, lowers the plasma fibrinogen concentration, and has antiplatelet effects.
- Cilostozol was approved in 1999 for treatment of claudication. Cilostozol has been shown in repeated clinical trials to improve both pain-free walking and maximal walking distance. A dose of 100 mg twice daily has the most beneficial effect. Cilostozol inhibits platelet aggregation, formation of arterial thrombi and vascular smooth muscle proliferation, and causes vasodilation. The mechanism of effect on claudication is unknown. The most common side effect is headache. *The drug should not be given to patients who have heart failure.*
- Risk factor modification should include an aggressive smoking cessation program and interventions aimed at keeping blood pressure below 130/85, HDL < 100 mg/dL, and Hb A1c < 7.0.
- Antiplatelet drug therapy should be implemented with either ASA 75–325 mg daily or clopidogrel 75 mg daily.
- If patient has nonoperable vascular disease with rest pain, recognition and treatment of the severe associated pain is essential.

Patient, Family, and Staff Education

- Educate patient and family regarding nature and course of disease.
- Reassure patient that claudication is not dangerous and that it is not dangerous to continue walking past onset of pain.
- Teach the importance of a regular, sustained walking program in appropriate patients.
- Assist patient to understand the importance of aggressive risk factor modification.
- Teach patient and staff danger signals such as development of tissue loss, rest pain, and gangrene.
- Teach medication purpose, dosage, frequency, and side effects.

Physician Consultation

Any new onset or increasing rest pain, any new or worsening ischemic ulceration, or any incidence of new or progressive gangrene is cause for urgent vascular consult as the presence of any of these symptoms indicates that the degree of vascular compromise has progressed to limb threat.

- Rest pain—New onset is cause for urgent vascular consult.
- Ischemic ulceration, new or worsening, is cause for urgent vascular consult.
- Gangrene—new or progressing—is cause for urgent vascular consult.
- ABI < 0.4.
- If patient feels quality of life is significantly impaired by arterial disease

▬▬ VENOUS INSUFFICIENCY

Definition

Venous insufficiency occurs when there is impaired return of blood flow in the venous system because of incompetence of the valves in the deep system, superficial system, or perforating veins, or with failure of the calf muscles.

Epidemiology

Venous dysfunction can manifest in many ways with varying degrees of severity, from telangectasias to ulcerations. Exact incidence is difficult to define as there are a variety of definitions used; however, it is estimated that 50% of the population over age 50 have some form of varicosity or telangectasia. Between 10% and 20% of adults will present with some degree of varicosity. About 2,000,000 people in the United States suffer from some venous ulceration as a result of chronic venous insufficiency. Risk factors for the development of varicose veins include the following:

- Age 50 years or over, peak incidence is sixth decade of life
- Hereditary
- Female gender
- Multiparty
- History of oral contraceptives
- Obesity
- History of an occupation requiring prolonged standing

Venous insufficiency results when there is failure of any or all of the parts of the venous system. These components work together to facilitate return of venous blood to the heart. The arterial flow operates as a high-pressure system with cardiac contraction forcing the blood through the arteries out to the body. Venous flow is relatively low pressure with blood being propelled primarily by external contraction of the calf muscle pump and foot action that continuously pushes against the force of gravity. Orderly flow out of the leg can only occur if the valvular system is competent. Valves prevent reversal of flow in the venous system to protect the lower extremities from the deleterious effects of continuous elevated hydrostatic pressure. Patients with a history of deep vein thrombosis will have postphlebitic syndrome and valvular incompetence.

Common Presenting Signs and Symptoms

- Complaints of dull ache, heaviness, tiredness, night cramps, swelling exacerbated by a history of prolonged standing, heat, and/or walking. Symptoms may be improved by elevation, walking, and/or compression stockings.

- May present with varying degrees of concerns about varicose veins. May present with large varicosities or ulceration.

- Edema may be present in varying degrees and may be from a variety of causes. See Table 17-3.

- Skin changes are associated with chronic venous insufficiency. These include brown staining over gaiter distribution from hemosiderin breakdown, and hair loss and dry skin from damage and scarring in the tissues due to chronic swelling.

- Progressive disease will present with the following:

  ○ Brawny edema—Chronic edema progresses to chronic changes converting the skin from a diffusely edematous state to a pigmented atrophic, tightly scarred area that gives the leg the classic inverted champagne bottle appearance.

  ○ Stasis dermatitis due to chronic inflammation in the subcutaneous tissue. The skin becomes atrophic as a result. Stasis dermatitis will present as a scaling or plaque formation much like eczema, and will present almost exclusively in the gaiter distribution.

  ○ Ulcerations may be present, most commonly at the medial malleolar region, with lateral malloelus ulcers occurring less often. Venous ulceration almost always occurs in the distal third of the extremity.

Differential Diagnosis

- Peripheral arterial disease
- Edema due to other causes such as CHF
- Lymphedema
- Osteoarthritis
- Peripheral neuritis

TABLE 17-3 Differential Diagnosis of Chronic Leg Swelling

CLINICAL FEATURE	VENOUS	LYMPHATIC	CARDIAC ORTHOSTATIC	LIPEDEMA
Consistency of swelling	Brawny, may have inverted champagne bottle appearance	Spongy	Pitting	Noncompressible (fat)
Relief by elevation	Complete	Mild	Complete, recurs quickly with dependence	Minimal
Distribution of swelling	Maximal in ankles and legs, feet spared	Diffuse, greatest distally	Diffuse, greatest distally	Maximal in ankles and legs, feet spared
Associated skin changes	Atrophic and pigmented, subcutaneous fibrosis	Hypertrophied, lichenified skin	Shiny, mild pigmentation, no trophic changes	None
Pain	Heavy ache, tight or bursting	None or heavy ache	Little or none	Dull ache, cutaneous sensitivity
Bilaterality	Occasionally, but usually unequal	Occasionally, but usually unequal	Always, but may be unequal	Always

Source: Adapted from Rutherford, 1995.

Essential Diagnostic and Laboratory Tests

- No blood tests will assist with diagnosis of venous insufficiency.

- Doppler ultrasound allows imaging of the veins and valves identifying valvular incompetence in the deep veins, superficial veins, and perforators.

- Photoplethysmography allows assessment of the degree of venous insufficiency and can separate superficial venous reflux from deep venous valvular insufficiency but does not add anything to Doppler ultrasound.

- Ankle-brachial index (ABI) to assess arterial circulation if no pulse is palpable or arterial disease is suspected.

- Magnetic resonance venography may be indicated for complicated patients or very obese patients.

Management Plan

The goals of treatment include management of pain and edema and prevention of further progression of the disorder.

- Graduated compression stockings are the mainstay of venous insufficiency treatment. Return flow is facilitated by graduated compression with the highest pressure at the ankle. For patients with mild symptoms and minimal to moderate edema use 20–30 mm Hg compression. For patients with more severe swelling/symptoms or a history of ulceration, 30–40 mm Hg or higher may be prescribed. Thromboembolic (TED) stockings are not the same as graduated compression stockings.

- Horse chestnut 300 mg twice daily has been shown to be helpful in controlling symptoms of swelling and aching. Most common side effect is headache. Do not use for patients on anticoagulation.

- Diuretics may be helpful for severe, difficult to manage edema. May use hydrochlorothiazide (HCTZ) 25 mg daily or furosemide 20–40 mg daily.

- Leg elevation with ankles higher than heart as much as possible during the day will help alleviate the discomfort associated with edema.

- Encourage walking at least 20 minutes a day to facilitate venous return by pumping action of the calf muscle.

- Encourage weight loss if indicated.

- Sclerotherapy injections will effectively treat smaller varicosities and telangectasias.

- If ulceration is present refer for wound consult. Patient will need wound treatment as well as compressive therapy. If cellulitis is present in extremity, treat with an antibiotic with gram-positive coverage.

Patient, Family, and Staff Education

- Teach the nature, course, and expected outcome of disease. Venous insufficiency is a chronic problem but can be effectively managed with conservative measures in most cases.

- Instruct on proper use of compression stockings.

- Patients with chronic venous insufficiency should avoid long periods of time standing or sitting.

- Exercise feet or walk frequently as feasible.

Physician Consultation

- Refer for surgical consultation if reflux is found in the superficial veins or perforators.

- Refer for treatment if acute deep vein thrombosis is seen with ultrasound.

- Refer for wound care consultation if stasis ulceration is present.

WEB SITES

- Medscape: Continuing education, medical news, full-text journal articles, and more—www.medscape.com
- National Library of Medicine, National Institutes of Health—www.nlm.nih.gov
- Agency for Health Care Research and Quality (AHRQ), U.S. Department of Health and Human Services—www.ahrq.gov
- Prevention of Venous Thromboembolism, from the AHRQ Evidence Report/Technology Assessment No. 43, "Making Health Care Safer: A Critical Analysis of Patient Safety Practices"—www.ahrq.gov/clinic/ptsafety/chap31a.htm
- American College of Phlebology—www.phlebology.org
- American Venous Forum—www.venous-info.com

REFERENCES

Dormandy, J., Mahir, M., Ascady, G., Balsano, F., De Leeuw, P., Blomberg, P., et al. (1991). The fate of the claudicant—A prospective study of 1969 claudicants. *European Journal of Vascular Surgery, 5,* 132–133.

Hirsch, A. T., Criqui, M. H., Treat-Jacobson, D., Regensteiner, J. G., Creager, M. A., Olin, J. W., et al. (2001). Peripheral arterial disease detection, awareness, and treatment in primary care. *Journal of the American Medical Association, 285,* 1317–1324.

Kent, K. C., Zwolak, R. M., Jaff, M. R., Hollenbeck, S. T., Thompson, R. W., Schermerhorn, M. L., et al. (2004). Screening for abdominal aortic aneurysm: A consensus statement. *Journal of Vascular Surgery, 39,* 267–269.

Meijer, W. T., Hous, A. W., & Rutgers, D. (1998). PAD in the elderly: The Rotterdam Study. *Arteriosclerosis, Thrombosis, and Vascular Biology,* 155–192.

Righini, M., Goehring, C., Bounameaux, H., & Perrier, A. (2000). Effects of age on the performance of common diagnostic tests for pulmonary embolus. *American Journal of Medicine, 109,* 357–361.

Rosendaal, F. R. (1999). Risk factors in venous thrombotic disease. Retrieved February 3, 2006, from http://www.medscape.com/viewarticle/426344?src=search

Rutherford, B. (1995). The vascular consultation. In R. Rutherford (Ed.), *The surgical approach to vascular problems.* Philadelphia: W.B. Saunders.

Schrecengost, J. E., LeGallo, R. D., Boyd, J. C., Moons, K. G. M., Goners, S. L., Rose, C. E., et al. (2003). Comparison of diagnostic accuracies in outpatient and hospitalized patients of D-Dimer testing for the evaluation of suspected pulmonary embolism. *Clinical Chemistry, 49,* 1483–1490.

Wells, P. S., Andersons, D. R., Rodger, M., Forgie, M., Kearon, C., Dreyer, J., et al. (2003). Evaluation of D-Dimer in diagnosis of suspected deep-vein thrombosis. *New England Journal of Medicine, 349,* 1227–1235.

BIBLIOGRAPHY

Abbade, L. P., & Lastoria, S. (2005). Venous ulcer: Epidemiology, physiopathology, diagnosis and treatment. *International Journal of Dermatology, 44,* 449–456.

Elliott, C. G. (2000). The diagnostic approach to deep vein thrombosis. *Seminars in Respiratory Critical Care Medicine, 21,* 511–519.

Ennis, W., & Meneses, P. (2003). Standard, appropriate and advanced care and medical-legal considerations: Part two—venous ulcerations. *Wounds, 15*(4), 107–122.

Geerts, W. H., Heit, J. A., Clagett, G. P., Pineo, G. F., Colwell, G. W., Anderson, F. A., et al. (2001). Prevention of venous thromboembolism. *Chest, 119*(Suppl.), 132S–175S.

Gey, D., Lesho, E., & Manngold, J. (2004). Management of peripheral arterial disease. *American Family Physician, 69,* 525–532.

Goldstone, J. (1998). Aneurysms of the aorta and iliac arteries. In: W. Moore (Ed.), *Vascular surgery, a comprehensive review.* Philadelphia: W.B. Saunders.

Hiatt, W. R. (2001). Medical treatment of peripheral arterial disease and claudication. *New England Journal of Medicine, 344,* 1608–1621.

McGee, S. (2001). *Evidence-based physical diagnosis.* Philadelphia: W.B. Saunders.

Morris, R., & Woodcock, J. P. (2004). Evidence-based compression: Prevention of stasis and deep vein thrombosis. *Annals of Surgery, 239,* 162–171.

Ouriel, K. (2001). Peripheral arterial disease. *Lancet, 358,* 1257–1264.

SECTION III

Special Considerations

CHAPTER 18

Wound Care

Evonne Fowler

INTRODUCTION

Patients requiring wound care are frequently managed in long-term care facilities. There are over 2.8 million patients with chronic wounds treated at a cost of billions of dollars per year in the United States. Nationally, 9.8% of nursing home residents have pressure ulcers. The prevalence of pressure ulcers in individual facilities ranges from 2.5–24%. The annual cost of treating a pressure ulcer has been quoted conservatively to range from $500 to $50,000 per ulcer with a significantly higher cost for more severe wounds (Mendez-Eastman, 2003). Nurse practitioners working in skilled nursing facilities are often involved with the management of a variety of wounds and therefore need to be knowledgeable about the evaluation, management, and documentation of wounds. Management of complex wounds often requires an interdisciplinary team approach. Members of the team usually include the physician, nurse practitioner, treatment nurse, dietician, and at times a wound care specialist, podiatrist, surgeon, and infectious disease specialist.

Clinically, chronic wounds may be associated with pressure, trauma, venous insufficiency, diabetes, vascular disease, or prolonged immobilization. The treatment of chronic wounds is variable and costly, demanding lengthy skilled nursing stays and costly supplies. Many patients are debilitated with one or more coexisting chronic medical conditions, making treatment a challenge. Healing the wound is often the expected outcome; however, in some cases pressure ulcers may not be preventable. For example, a patient who is terminally ill may develop a pressure ulcer as part of their dying process.

Some wounds may take a long time (6–9 months) to heal while other wounds may never heal. Institutionalized immobile adults with progressive advanced disease(s), who are severely compromised are considered frail patients. Often, these frail elderly patients have chronic wounds that are unlikely to heal because of their poor overall status and/or treatment priorities. Many elderly people have diseases associated with significant pain, such as arthritis, ischemia, or cancer. Immobility related to these conditions may lead to pressure ulcer development. Often those who are at risk for skin breakdown also have poor nutrition that can lead to poor muscle mass and wasting of protective subcutaneous fat adding to their risk potential. Accepting nonhealing wounds as an endpoint may be appropriate and in the best interest of many frail patients. This acknowledgment will likely avoid unrealistic expectations and allow clinicians and patients alike to focus on the effective management of symptoms control and supportive care (palliative management). The question to be asked during the initial assessment is "Should the wound be approached with the goal of healing or symptom control and comfort measures?" (Alvarez et al., 2002; Ennis, 2001).

PRESSURE ULCER QUALITY IMPROVEMENT AND RISK MANAGEMENT

In some cases, pressure ulcers may at least be partially related to "substandard care." In the year 2000, pressure ulcer prevention and healing was the fourth most common category of deficiencies reported during nursing home inspections. The Centers for Medicare and Medicaid Services (CMS) cited almost 19% of facilities for insufficient skin care—failure to assess risk, plan appropriate care, execute the plan consistently, or monitor the plan's effectiveness of care (Duncan, 2004).

It has been difficult to determine both the incidence (new cases appearing during a specified period) and the prevalence (a cross-sectional count of the number of cases at a specific point in time) because methodological limitations have prevented researchers from drawing meaningful conclusions from available data. These problems exist in data available from acute care hospitals, long-term care facilities, and home care settings (U.S. Department of Health and Human Services [DHHS], 1996). Endorsement of the staging system recommended by the National Pressure Ulcer Advisory Panel (NPUAP) would help in comparing and interpreting data. In addition a systematic assessment guide detailing the sites of the pressure ulcers should be used. Information about the type of wound, healthcare facility, diagnosis, patient's mobility, and other risk factors would be helpful in planning and allocating services to those populations at risk.

Pressure ulcers are considered a measure of quality and, in particular, considered a nursing home quality-of-care indicator (QI). Pressure ulcer prevalence is included as one of the minimum data set (MDS) quality measures and is reported for all Medicare-certified nursing homes on consumer Web sites. However, the quality indicator looks at pressure ulcer prevalence, not incidence. Therefore, it includes not only pressure ulcers that occur in the facility, but also those that occur prior to admission to the facility. This means a facility that has a wound care program and seeks to admit patients with pressure ulcers would have a high prevalence of patients with pressure ulcers. It is difficult for facility staff to show that a pressure ulcer is unavoidable when the minimum data set (MDS) from which the QIs are derived is limited in that it captures only the major risk factors for the development of pressure ulcers. It is felt by some that pressure ulcer prevalence is not an appropriate measure of quality, and the use of an additional validated scale could provide more information, such as details on sensory perception, skin moisture, and friction and shear (Vance, 2002).

According to the U.S. Department of Health and Human Services (DHHS), (1996), institutions and healthcare agencies are responsible for developing and implementing educational programs for patients, families, and caregivers. These programs should translate knowledge about pressure ulcers into effective treatment plans and should cover the entire continuum of care, from prevention through treatments that promote healing and prevent recurrence. Accurate assessment of tissue damage should be emphasized as well as principles of treatment and outcome monitoring.

Lumetra is a nonprofit quality improvement oversight corporation who has contracted with CMS to monitor nursing homes for quality indicators. Pressure ulcers are one of those indicators. The Lumetra Web site offers free materials and other resources at www.lumetra.com.

There is a lack of evidence for much of what is done to predict and treat pressure ulcers. Risk assessment is required at the time of admission and at least quarterly after admission. Federal regulators require nursing facilities to ensure that a resident who enters the facility without pressure ulcers does not develop any, unless the individual's clinical condition demonstrates that pressure ulcer development was unavoidable. A facility's care processes are the main focus of discussion when investigating quality care once pressure ulcers do occur in a facility.

Litigation regarding pressure ulcers has risen dramatically since the passage of the Omnibus Budget Reconciliation Act (OBRA) of 1987. Lawsuits related to pressure ulcers have drawn a great deal of attention due to high payouts, settlements, and jury verdicts. Although pressure ulcers are time consuming and expensive to treat, an organized and systemic approach can make the prevention and treatment of pressure ulcers an attainable goal, while reducing legal liability for the facility and staff (Weinberg, 2005). Documentation by the facility and medical staff is one key to reducing liability. This applies to a facility's full range of protocols, from instituting proper procedures, ulcer assessment, prevention, and treatment to ensuring that staff continually follow procedure and document their steps.

Photographs of wounds can be a valuable addition to a risk-management program in a nursing home. They are extremely helpful when residents are admitted from other facilities with ulcers, providing proof that the ulcer was acquired elsewhere. However, photographs taken on admission or at the time of first diagnosis, while helpful in documenting the presence and staging of these ulcers, does not reduce the facility's obligation to prevent their progression (Weinberg, 2005). In addition, clinicians need to be open when informing and discussing the presence of a pressure ulcer with family members.

PREVENTION OF PRESSURE ULCERS

The Agency for Healthcare Research and Quality (AHRQ) has identified the following basic principles for pressure ulcer prevention:

- Use a validated tool to assess risk such as the Braden Scale (see Appendix A) or Norton Scale.
- Implement a preventive plan for residents at risk focusing on avoiding friction and shear trauma to skin regions at risk, avoiding maceration from moisture, and addressing nutrition and mobility. Repositioning may also be needed for those high-risk patients.
- Inspect skin daily for high-risk residents. Skin and deep tissue damage can occur in as little as 2 hours.

In addition the 1996 American Medical Directors Association (AMDA) clinical practice guideline on pressure ulcers highlights the following responsibilities for clinicians to help prevent pressure sores:

- Identify and manage underlying medical risk factors, some of which may not be reflected in the Braden score, identify disease states, nutritional compromise, skin disorders, and drugs that affect skin, such as corticosteroids.
- Identify and treat modifiable causes of decreased alertness, incontinence, and immobility.
- Identify and manage acute changes in condition that may increase the risk of skin breakdown, such as delirium.
- Identify subacute changes that increase risk, such as weight loss or progression of dementia.

- Clarify overall condition, prognosis, and realistic goals; if appropriate to the resident's condition, discuss the option to withhold treatment with the resident or responsible party.
- Document when residents have significant risk factors for skin breakdown.

In addition, those patients with pressure ulcers or those at risk for developing pressure ulcers must be placed on a therapeutic mattress or an appropriate support surface. Examples include pressure-relieving pad, overlay for mattress with low air loss feature, and flotation bed. Pressure ulcers involving the heel regions commonly occur in patients who are bedridden, even if they are immobilized for just a few days, such as after hip surgery. Prevention and treatment of heel pressure ulcers requires off-loading. Off-loading devices are usually based on availability and include booties, boots made from a firm outer shell lined with pressure relief padding, and suspension devices that isolate the heel and transfer the weight to the lower leg, and inflatable devices made from plastic sheets that surround the heel and adjacent tissues (Stillman, 2005).

Selection of a product must be based on the patient's management plan and the evaluation of an individual's risk factors for developing a pressure ulcer. These risk factors must be monitored, and the modalities must be reevaluated as the patient's condition improves or worsens. Finally, cost and service support must be considered (Salcido, 2005).

DEFINITION OF WOUNDS AND HEALING

Wounds heal as a result of several complex physiological processes, occurring individually or in combination during the healing process (Finney, 2000). The phases of wound healing include *inflammatory, proliferative,* *and maturation*. The *inflammatory* phase is the initial reaction to the injury where cells, (platelets, neutrophils, and macrophages) migrate to the injured site. Platelets assist with the clotting and act as a chemoattractant for neutrophils, which destroy bacteria and aid in debridement. Macrophages continue the process of clean up and also secrete some growth factors essential for healing. This stage can take 4–6 days. The *proliferative phase* is the reconstructive phase where angiogenesis, granulation, and epithelialization occur and can take 4 to 24 days. During the *maturation phase* wound contraction and resurfacing of the wound occur which can take 21 days to 2 years until complete scarring occurs. Even with scarring, the skin will only regain 70–80% of its former strength, and its possible that the wound may reopen (Henkel, 2004).

Unlike normal wound healing in acute wounds, chronic nonhealing wounds have biochemical differences that delay healing such as increase in proinflammatory cytokines, decrease in mitogenic activity, increase in matrix metalloproteinases (MMP), and varied levels of growth factors and senescent cells (Schultz et al., 2003).

Wounds are classified as *partial thickness* and *full thickness* wounds. Partial thickness wounds primarily involve the epidermis and do not penetrate below the dermis (see Figure 18-1). Partial thickness wounds heal by epithelialization. In some instances, there may be pigmentary changes but no scarring. Full thickness wounds extend through the dermis into the subcutaneous tissue, fascia, or muscle; the bone may be exposed (see Figure 18-2). Full thickness wounds heal by granulation, contraction, and scar formation.

A nonhealing (chronic) wound is "a wound which has not proceeded through a timely, orderly, sequence of healing and/or fails to achieve sustained anatomic and functional integrity" (Lazarus et al., 1994). A wound is not a diagnosis in itself, but rather a manifestation

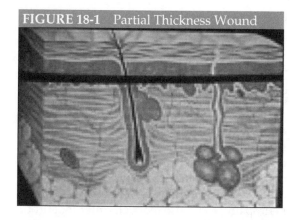

FIGURE 18-1 Partial Thickness Wound

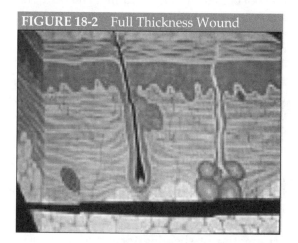

FIGURE 18-2 Full Thickness Wound

of some underlying local or systemic condition or a combination of factors that have resulted in a wound. A chronic nonhealing wound is an area of skin breakdown that is not healing at the expected rate, provided the cause has been corrected and the patient is adherent to treatment (Fowler, Krasner, & Sibbald, 2002). Chronic wounds continue to be affected by local and systemic factors. Local factors include bacterial burden, infection, trauma, edema, pressure, and moisture. Systemic factors include age, anemia, diabetes, renal and hepatic dysfunction, and nutritional status (Hess & Trent, 2004).

TYPES OF WOUNDS

The following are the most commonly seen wounds in long-term care settings:

- Skin tears
- Neuropathic foot ulcers
- Vascular ulcers (arterial and venous)
- Postoperative surgical wounds
- Radiation-related skin changes
- Pressure ulcers

SKIN TEARS

Skin tears are traumatic wounds usually seen on the extremities of older adults resulting from separation of the epidermal-dermal junction due to friction or shearing forces. Because the epidermis thins with age and is more susceptible to injury, older patients are at increased risk for skin tears. In the United States it is estimated that 1.5 million skin tears occur annually among institutionalized adults. Patients who are dependent on others for activities of daily living are at greatest risk for skin tears. The Payne-Martin Skin Tear Classification System defines skin tears by category:

- Category I—Skin tears without tissue loss
- Category II—Skin tears with partial thickness skin loss
- Category III—Skin tears with complete tissue loss (Payne & Martin, 2000)

When a skin flap is visible and can be rolled back to cover the wound, apply a gentle adherent silicone dressing and treat as a skin graft by not disturbing the wound for 4–5 days. Implementation of a protocol that includes a gentle skin cleanser, a longer-lasting barrier cream or skin sealant, thin hydrocolloid, low adhesive, and the use of extremity sleeves or long sleeve clothing can make a significant difference. When necessary, porous adhesive tapes should be used and removed with extreme caution.

NEUROPATHIC FOOT ULCERS

Neuropathic ulcers are often associated with diabetes mellitus. They are generally traumatically induced ulcers that occur in areas affected by peripheral neuropathy—most commonly the feet. They develop over regions of high pressure such as the metatarsal heads. Often the resident presents with fever, chills, and a strong odor of the wound. Residents with infected neuropathic ulcers have a much higher mortality rate than those whose ulcers are free of infection (Kiemele & Takahashi, 2004). Diabetic foot ulcers are commonly classified by a grading system. See Table 18-1 for the Wagner grading system for diabetic foot ulcers.

When an adequate vascular supply and appropriate wound care are available, wounds most likely will heal. In the complicated non-healing wound, aggressive debridement or a surgical intervention may be necessary. More inpatient hospital days are spent caring for foot-related complications in diabetics than any other diabetic problem. Off-loading of pressure on a diabetic foot ulcer is essential for wounds to heal.

Foot ulcers in a patient with diabetes can be neuropathic or ischemic. Most diabetic foot ulcers are neuropathic or have a component of neuropathy (sensory, motor, or autonomic) that renders them susceptible to wounds. The most common disabling complication in people with diabetes is decreased pain, which suppresses warning signals. Without pain as a warning, trivial injuries become a threat to limbs. Sensory nerves carry information to the brain about shape, movement, texture, warmth, coolness, or pain from special sensors in the skin and from deep in the body. Motor nerve fibers carry signals to muscles to allow motion like walking and fine finger movement. The autonomic nerve fibers are those that are not consciously controlled such as in the supply to the bladder, intestinal tract, and sexual organs. They help the heart contract, maintain blood pressure, and control sweating. Sensory neuropathy can cause burning, numbness, and tingling. Motor neuropathy can cause foot deformity, foot drop, and tripping. Muscle weakness and splaying of the foot occurs on weight bearing. The result is a convex foot with a rocker-bottom appearance. Multiple fractures go unnoticed, until bone and joint deformities become marked. This is termed a Charcot foot and is observed most commonly in people with diabetes, affecting approximately 2% of persons with diabetes (Stillman, 2005). Autonomic neuropathy is associated with heat intolerance, excessive moisture on the feet, or dry, cracked skin.

Adequate off-loading is important in treating neuropathic ulcers. Although this is ideal, it is not always practical in long-term care. Residents need to wear appropriate footwear or remain non-weightbearing. Even the slightest amount of shearing force over a neuropathic ulcer will inhibit healing. Inserts help off-load problem areas by directing pressure away from the ulcer and distributing it to the rest of the foot. Referral to a podiatrist can be helpful in managing this condition (Kiemele & Takahashi, 2004).

TABLE 18-1 Wagner Grading System for Diabetic Foot Ulcers	
Grade 0	High-risk foot, no ulcer
Grade 1	Superficial ulcer
Grade 2	Deep ulcer, no bony involvement
Grade 3	Deep ulcer, open to the bone, osteomyelitis or abscess present
Grade 4	Localized gangrene of the forefoot or toe(s)
Grade 5	Gangrene of the whole foot

VASCULAR ULCERS

Ischemic Ulcers

Ischemic ulcers are chronic wounds caused by vascular insufficiency or trauma. They are associated with other medical conditions such as atherosclerosis obliterans, inflammatory diseases, and vasospastic conditions. The incidence of ischemic ulcers is nearly 20% in people over 65 years of age. The male to female ratio is 2:1. Most elderly residents are asymptomatic (Kiemele & Takahashi, 2004).

Ischemic ulcers occur distally, have discrete borders, and are usually painful. The skin is thin, shiny, and dry. Dependent rubor is present, and elevation pallor occurs within seconds after elevating the foot. The wound base is pale, and distal pulses are not palpable. Sedentary residents who do not walk to the point of claudication may initially present with foot pain at rest or with gangrene in advanced disease. Resting foot pain is an ominous indicator that blood flow has been reduced to less than 10% of normal (Kiemele & Takahashi, 2004). See vascular chapter for assessment and management of peripheral artery disease (PAD).

Smoking cessation is paramount in managing ischemic wounds. Nicotine is a potent vasoconstrictor that not only promotes atherosclerosis but further impedes blood flow to an ischemic limb. Diabetes, hypertension, and pain need to be optimally controlled. Keeping ischemic area warm promotes vasodilation that improves arterial blood flow. Lamb's wool can be woven between the toes to keep the interdigital areas padded and to prevent ulcer formation. Care needs to be taken when sharply debriding the eschar so that no further damage is done to surrounding tissue. Gangrene should be kept dry and covered with dry gauze dressings. Use of cadexomer iodine gel may also be helpful in keeping the ulcers dry. Referral to vascular surgery for further evaluation is indicated; however, elderly patients with multiple comorbidities may not be candidates for revascularization. Lower extremity amputation may be necessary to definitively treat ischemic ulcers (Kiemele & Takahashi, 2004).

Venous Ulcers

Nearly 90% of the estimated 600,000 leg ulcers that occur annually in the United States are due to chronic venous insufficiency or a combination of arterial and venous insufficiency.

Venous leg ulcers are the most common cause of all leg ulcers and increase in frequency with advancing age (Trent, Falabella, Eaglstein, & Kirsner, 2001). The ulcer usually occurs near the medial aspect of the ankle or lower leg and is often shallow with irregular borders. The periwound skin changes (hemosiderin deposits, fibrosis, and edema) are related to chronic venous stasis. Major factors to consider with prevention and management interventions are compression, elevation, and exercise. Prior to applying compression the blood circulation to the leg must be evaluated. A palpable pulse in the dorsum of the foot means the blood pressure is at least 80 mmHg (Sibbald, 2003). A noninvasive test for the ankle-brachial index (ABI) should be done to determine the circulatory status.

Lower leg edema is a frequent condition seen with venous insufficiency and venous leg ulcers. The clinician should document the amount of swelling within the leg and around the wound. This can be done in a subjective fashion, or it can be quantified by measuring the circumference of the involved extremity. Frequently, chronic ulcers are of mixed etiology, with an ischemic or pressure component coexisting with a venous component. The exam should also evaluate the cardiac, hepatic, and pulmonary systems. An ischemic process needs to be excluded (Kiemele & Takahashi, 2004).

Often excessive fluid oozes from the pores of the skin in edematous limbs. Lower leg edema can be controlled with compression therapy. Compression therapy is the deliberate application of pressure using bandages to force fluid back into the venous and lymphatic systems. This facilitates venous return by enhancing the calf pump mechanism and valve functioning within the veins. Underlying factors causing edema or venous hypertension must be treated such as congestive heart failure, liver failure, chronic kidney disease, and cellulitis. Mechanical methods of reducing edema are safe and effective. Thirty minutes of leg elevation 3–4 times a day can be effective in reducing mild edema. For significant edema, compression wraps are necessary.

POSTOPERATIVE WOUNDS

Many patients who experience a traumatic incident necessitating a surgical procedure may develop a postoperative wound. These patients can also be compromised with multiorgan failure, massive soft tissue loss, poor tissue perfusion, insensate tissue (spinal cord injury) or a combination of all the above. Under these conditions, surgical incisions have an increased risk for dehiscence. Heavily contaminated abdominal wounds are sometimes left open to heal by secondary intention or because edema and/or poor tissue quality precludes a tension-free wound approximation (Ennis et al., 2004).

The best way to heal a wound is to close it according to surgical standards as soon as possible after injury. However, this procedure is limited to those wounds and those anatomical regions that allow both excision and adaptation of wound borders to close the wound by primary intention (wound is surgically closed).

In large surface and deep wounds in which the primary wound closure is not possible the most important issue is to dress the wound with appropriate materials to allow the following:

- Keep the wound free of infection.
- Reduce or eliminate pain.
- Reduce or eliminate all factors inhibiting natural healing (necrotic tissue).
- Replace or substitute the missing tissue as much as possible.

Several options are available for surgical management of pressure ulcers, including direct closure, skin grafting, skin flaps, and musculocutaneous flaps. Surgical management of pressure ulcers can provide skin coverage as well as soft tissue coverage (Salcido,

2005). However, for many patients, this technique may not be practicable for a variety of reasons, and the wound may be allowed to heal by second intention (wound left open) to achieve sufficient granulation, contraction, and epithelialization for spontaneous closure.

RADIATION-RELATED SKIN CHANGES

Radiation-related skin changes may create problems or ulcerations that occur during therapy, immediately after therapy, or years after the completion of therapy. The changes usually occur to the area of treatment. The most common types of skin reactions include the following:

- Erythema
- Alterations in pigmentation
- Hair loss
- Flaking or peeling (dry desquamation)
- Ulceration (moist desquamation)
- Loss of perspiration or sebaceous excretion
- Changes in superficial blood vessels
- Edema and scarring (Smith et al., 2004)

Most radiation related lesions are superficial. The Oncology Nursing Society (ONS) has adopted the following classification system for skin reaction:

- 0—Normal skin within the radiation field
- 1—Faint or dull erythema, follicular reactions
- 2—Bright erythema
- 3—Dry desquamation
- 4—Small to moderate wet desquamation
- 5—Confluent moist desquamation
- 6—Ulceration, hemorrhage, or necrosis

The treatment of radiation-induced skin reactions is similar to the treatment of skin tears. The skin within the radiation field must be considered high risk for potential breakdown and needs to be kept clean, soft, and supple. If the patient experiences burning or itching, a topical hydrogel or steroid cream can be applied.

PRESSURE ULCERS

Stages of Pressure Ulcers

Pressure ulcers are defined as an injury to the skin and muscle that is caused by constant pressure that develops when the skin and underlying structures are deprived of oxygen and other nutrients necessary for cell growth and proliferation (Agency for Healthcare Research and Quality [AHRQ]). Pressure ulcer development occurs in four stages (National Pressure Ulcer Advisory Panel [NPUAD], 1995). Intact dark discolored heel blisters are staged as "unable to determine" (UTD). See Table 18-2 for staging of pressure ulcers. Currently, the definition of a Stage I ulcer is being reconsidered.

The NPUAP has developed a Pressure Ulcer Scale for Healing known as "PUSH," which rates the size, exudate, and tissue appearance. There are 15 items for a total score ranging from 13–65. The score is plotted on a continuum. This tool is available at www.npuap.org.

Wound Care Assessment and Tools

Assessment of pressure ulcer status is perhaps the most useful method in evaluation of pressure ulcer healing. All clinical practice guidelines for treatment of pressure ulcers view assessment as the starting point in preparing to treat or manage a person with a pressure ulcer (Bergstrom, Bennett, & Carlson, 1994). The nurse practitioner needs to be familiar with assessing and accurately describing the wound. Assessment of the wound characteristics should include the following:

- Stage and depth
- Size
- Location
- Wound bed and necrotic tissue
- Exudate
- Granulation tissue
- Epithelialization
- Undermining and tunneling

PATIENT ASSESSMENT

Optimal wound care for patients with nonhealing wounds requires a holistic and systematic approach. The nurse practitioner should include the following in the assessment:

- Wound etiology
- Complete history and physical
- Contributing factors and comorbidities affecting wound healing, including underlying ischemia
- Dietary evaluation—For serum albumin < 3.5, weight < 80% ideal, 5% weight loss in 30 days, < 75% intake at most meals, body mass index < 20%, 10% weight loss

TABLE 18-2	National Pressure Ulcer Advisory Panel Staging for Wounds
Stage I	Nonblanchable erythema of intact skin; the heralding lesion of skin ulceration. Discoloration of skin, warmth, or hardness also may be indicators.
Stage II	Partial thickness skin loss involving epidermis and/or dermis. The ulcer is superficial and presents clinically as an abrasion, blister, or shallow crater.
Stage III	Full thickness skin loss involving damage or necrosis of subcutaneous tissue that may extend down to, but not through, underlying fascia. The ulcer presents clinically as a deep crater with or without undermining of adjacent tissue.
Stage IV	Full thickness skin loss with extensive destruction, tissue necrosis, or damage to muscle, bone, or supporting structure (e.g., tendon, joint capsule).

in 180 days. There is no evidence that providing vitamin and mineral supplements including vitamins A and E, zinc, or arginine will accelerate wound healing in pressure ulcers. These supplements should be provided to those who are deficient or at high risk for deficiency according to the recommended daily allowances (Grey, 2003a; Grey, 2003b; Grey & Whitney, 2003).

- Environmental and social factors influencing wound healing

- Pain

- Family and caregiver support

- Patient's motivation to comply with the medical treatment plan

- Patient's mobility and functional status

See Table 18-3 for lab values affecting delayed wound healing.

Careful review of the holistic assessment is often sufficient to make a diagnosis of the wound etiology. However, many wounds look alike, and to avoid misdiagnosis it is useful to differentiate the most common types of wounds.

▬ MANAGEMENT OF WOUND

Successful wound healing depends on an accurate management plan. Management begins

TABLE 18-3   Lab Values Indicative of Increased Risk for Delayed Wound Healing

Serum transferrin < 170 mg/dL
Prealbumin < 16 mg/dL
Serum albumin < 3.5 mg/dL with normal hydration status
Hemoglobin < 12 g/dL
Hematocrit < 33%
Serum cholesterol < 160 mg/dL
Total lymphocyte count < 1800/mm
Serum osmolality >295 mOsm/L
BUN/Creatinine > 10:1

Source: Bergstrom et al., 1994.

with understanding the physical findings; addressing the causative, local, and systemic factors; evaluating the laboratory values and diagnostic tests; assessing nutritional needs; and selecting appropriate management modalities.

Because of the many issues involved, it is difficult to create simple policies and procedures to cover all treatment options. Each facility should use clinical practice guidelines to develop step-by-step details for managing pressure ulcers, allowing flexibility for clinicians. Several organizations have published detailed guidelines on managing pressure ulcers such as AHCPR and AMDA. These guidelines discuss currently accepted principles of treatment that include the following components:

- Relieve pressure.

- Debride necrotic tissue.

- Treat infection.

- Keep the wound moist to promote granulation.

- Protect the surrounding skin.

- Manage the patient's overall condition.

- Track wound-healing progress accurately.

▬ WOUND BED PREPARATION AND TIME

Wound bed preparation and TIME is a new way of thinking that integrates proven concepts to build a platform for the treatment of chronic wounds. It organizes currently approved medical standards, practices, and products into a holistic approach that can be used to evaluate and remove barriers to the wound-healing process. The major barriers to wound closure are nonviable tissue, inflammation or infection, moisture imbalance, and nonadvancing or undermined wound edge. The system is known as TIME (Smith et al., 2004):

- T—Tissue
- I—Inflammation/infection
- M—Moisture imbalance
- E—Edge of wound

See Figure 18-3 for time system of managing wounds.

Tissue (T)

Evaluation of tissue of a wound will help in determining the direction of care. Questions should be asked such as does the wound need debridement of necrotic tissue? Does the wound appear inflamed or infected? What is the status of the periwound skin? Assessing the status of the wound can be done by classifying the wound both by depth (partial or full thickness) and color (red, yellow, black). The RYB (red, yellow, black) color classification describes the wound in terms of the surface appearance (Cuzzell, 1988). See Table 18-4. Wounds need to be free of non-viable tissue to heal. A wound with a red base usually indicates granulation tissue (red). Necrotic tissue may appear yellow and fibrinous (slough) or when the tissue is dried out and it forms a thick black or brown leathery texture (eschar). See Figure 18-4 for red, yellow, and black wounds.

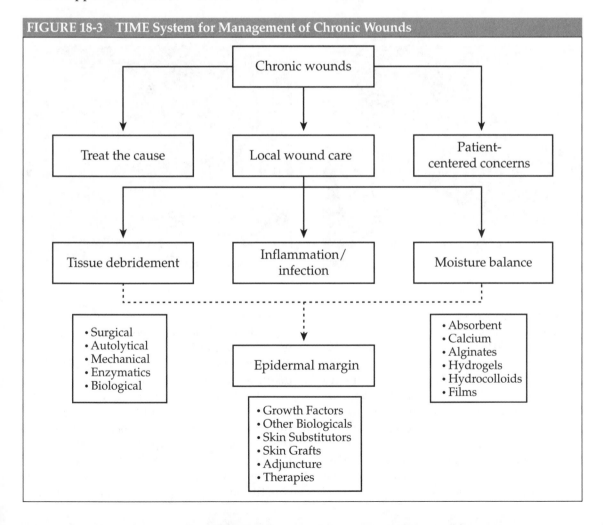

FIGURE 18-3   TIME System for Management of Chronic Wounds

TABLE 18-4   RYB Color Classification of Wounds

R: Red wounds may vary from pale pink to a beefy red with the color indicating the presence and depth of granulation tissue. Red wounds can be in the inflammatory or proliferative phase of wound healing. There is a need to cover a red wound for protection and to keep it moist. Both protection from trauma and a moist wound bed enhance wound healing.

Y: Yellow wounds vary in color from pale ivory to various shades of yellow, green, and brown. The yellow/green/brown color indicates the presence of slough (dead but moist tissue). Yellow wounds actively generate wound fluid and need to be debrided to remove the slough and reduce the bacterial load.

B: Black wounds are covered with tissue that is black, brown, or tan. The color indicates the presence of dead tissue that is dehydrated to various degrees. Often black wounds are referred to as being covered with eschar, a thick, hard leathery appearing material. When eschar is covering a wound, the depth cannot be accurately assessed until the eschar is removed. In most cases, eschar provides an excellent medium for bacterial proliferation and needs to be removed to prevent infection and promote wound healing. In diabetics with inadequate blood supply, dry eschar is kept intact until a thorough vascular exam has been completed.

The amount of necrotic tissue (yellow or black) is documented by percentage such as: 50% red, 25% yellow, 25% black.

FIGURE 18-4 (A)   RYB Wounds

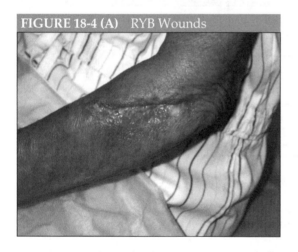

FIGURE 18-4 (B)   RYB Wounds

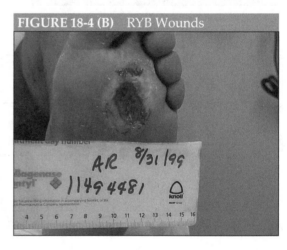

The appearance of the wound is documented by percentage of color seen within the wound (e.g., 50% red, 25% yellow, and 25% black). This type of documentation allows the progress or deterioration of the wound to be tracked through time. The surface appearance of most wounds is a combination of colors (mixed). In these wounds, care is planned to remove the necrotic tissue first. When dry eschar or gangrene is present, assess the vascular circulation near the location of the wound prior to debridement.

All wounds need to be cleansed; some wounds need debridement. Cleansing with water or saline is usually sufficient. Wound cleansers with surfactants are available when debris is tenacious or embedded in the wound.

Debridement is the removal of necrotic or contaminated tissue and foreign material in the wound. Necrotic tissue is a physical barrier to healing and supports bacterial growth. Bacterial colonies can produce damaging proteases, which can break down important constituents of the extracellular matrix and

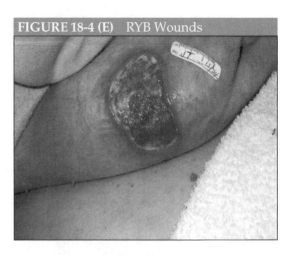

FIGURE 18-4 (E)   RYB Wounds

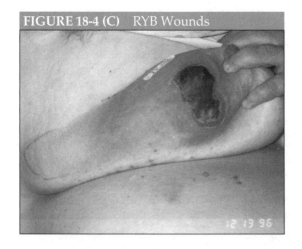

FIGURE 18-4 (C)   RYB Wounds

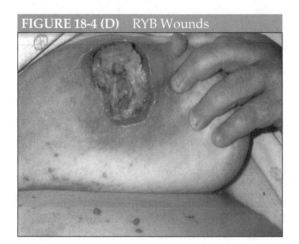

FIGURE 18-4 (D)   RYB Wounds

inhibit the formation of granulation tissue (Sibbald et al., 2003). Debridement can be accomplished using several different methods as follows:

- Sharp
- Autolytic
- Enzymatic
- Mechanical
- Biosurgical (maggot therapy)

See Table 18-5 for methods for wound debridement.

Usually a combination of methods works best. Sharp debridement for excessive or adherent necrotic tissue followed by enzymatic agents and/or covered with an occlusive dressing (autolytic) is effective. Autolytic debridement is a process that occurs naturally when occlusive dressings maintain a moist wound bed. These dressings provide an optimal environment for autolytic debridement because they contain the body's own phagocytic cells at the wound surface to liquefy necrotic tissue. This method of debridement can produce a significant amount of wound fluid. When occlusive dressings are used, they should be left in place 2–3 days and changed only if leakage, dislodgement, or signs of infection are present. If necrotic tissue is still present, continue sharp debridement with each dressing change. Using this combination of debridement methods, a red granular bed should be seen in approximately 2–3 weeks.

The most common form of mechanical debridement is the application of wet to dry dressings. Wet to dry dressings are nonselective and cause mechanical separation of necrotic tissue from the wound bed when the dressing is removed. This can cause significant pain and damage to newly formed tissue and should be the last choice, if not

TABLE 18-5	Debridement Methods for Wounds		
METHOD	DESCRIPTION	ADVANTAGES	DISADVANTAGES
Instrument/sharp	Devitalized tissue is removed using a scalpel or scissors.	Rapid, effective, and selective if performed by a skilled professional	Facilities and qualified healthcare professionals may not be readily available; may cause bleeding and pain.
Mechanical	Wet or moist dressings are applied, then removed when dry.	Easy to perform; supplies/facilities are readily available.	Slow; nonselective; may be painful and cause maceration of surrounding skin
Chemical	Debriding agent (enzyme) is applied over necrotic tissue.	Easy to perform; selective when used appropriately	Slow; prescription required; may irritate surrounding skin or cause pain or allergic reactions
Autolytic	Moisture-retentive dressing is applied, retaining endogenous enzymes.	Easy to perform; selective; painless	Slow; not indicated when risk of infection is high
Biosurgical (maggot therapy)	Sterile maggots are inserted into the wound and covered with a dressing to contain them in the wound. The maggots release collagenase and may also destroy pyogenic bacteria. The action of maggots is restricted to selective removal of necrotic tissue.	Selective; painless	Mental anguish for patient/family. Need to order maggots. No data from controlled studies.

Source: Fowler & van Rijswijk, 1995.

eliminated all together from debridement options.

When the wound is red with granulation tissue and still slow to heal, the use of enzymatic or autolytic debridement techniques can be used as an extended "maintenance" phase of debridement. This occlusive dressing represents more selective debridement, is much less painful for the patient, and is very helpful in maintaining appropriate moisture in the wound.

Inflammation and Infection (I)

Patients predisposed to pressure ulcers are at higher risk of morbidity and mortality. Infection is the most common major complication of pressure ulcers. The offending pathologic organisms in pressure ulcers can be anaerobic or aerobic. Aerobic pathogens commonly are

present in all pressure ulcers. Anaerobes tend to be present more often in larger wounds, stage 3 and above. The most common organisms isolated from pressure ulcers are *Proteus mirabilis,* group D streptococci, *Escherichia coli, Staphylococcus* species, *Pseudomonas* species and *Corynebacterium* organisms. These wounds do not need to be cultured routinely unless systemic signs of infection are present (Salcido, 2005). Research studies have shown that wounds that do not heal often have a high bacterial burden. Depending on the host's resistance and the number and virulence of the organism, bacteria may continue to proliferate and progress to an increased state (critical colonization) and on to a local or systemic infection. See Figure 18-5 for colonization versus infection.

Proliferating bacteria can form microcolonies that attach to the wound bed and secrete a

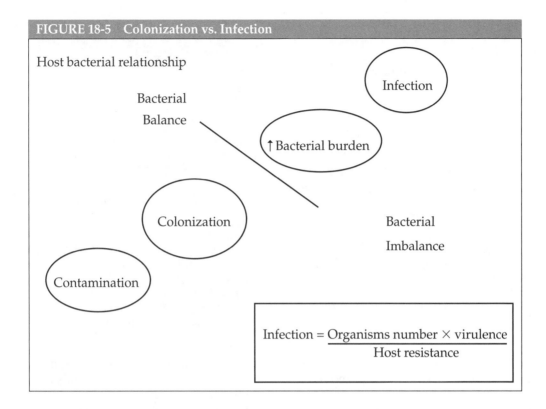

FIGURE 18-5   Colonization vs. Infection

Host bacterial relationship

Bacterial
Balance

↑ Bacterial burden

Infection

Colonization

Bacterial

Imbalance

Contamination

$$\text{Infection} = \frac{\text{Organisms number} \times \text{virulence}}{\text{Host resistance}}$$

biofilm that protects the organisms. These bacterial colonies undergo several changes and express different genes, which can alter the organism's sensitivity to antimicrobial agents (Cherry, Harding, & Ryan, 2001; Schultz et al., 2003).

An increased bacterial burden can exist with subtle or unrecognized signs before frank infection is noted (Cutting & White, 2005). Signs of increased bacterial burden include the following:

- A wound that fails to heal despite treating the cause and appropriate local wound care
- Increased clear exudates may be present before frank pus forms.
- Increased devitalized tissue or increased bright red friable and exuberant (jellylike) granulation tissue with pungent odor or boggy periwound skin

- Elevated blood glucose levels despite adequate diabetic control
- Overt signs of infection including pain, swelling, warmth, and erythema

Fever, confusion, leukocytosis, increased pulse, and hypertension may be seen in systemic infection. See Table 18-6 for signs and symptoms of infection.

Osteomyelitis may be associated with fever, malaise, chronic fatigue, and limited range of motion of an affected extremity and a nonhealing wound or a chronic draining wound overlying a bone or joint. Plain radiographs, CT scans, radionuclide bone scans, and MRIs have a role in the workup of osteomyelitis. Osteomyelitis is treated with appropriate systemic antibiotics. Most findings indicate that antibiotic treatment for osteomyelitis should last 6–8 weeks (Salcido, 2005). The goal is to provide a wound bed that is

TABLE 18-6   Signs and Symptoms of Infection of Wounds

LOCAL	SYSTEMIC
Erythema	Fever
Induration	Leukocytosis
Purulent drainage	Confusion
Malodorous drainage	Increased pulse
Crepitus	Hypertension

Other signs of infection may include:

- Nonhealing that can be a sign of increased bacterial burden
- Devitalized loose yellow debris and even areas of necrosis in the base of the ulcer
- Increased or bright red granulation tissue that is often friable and exuberant
- Bridging of nonviable epidermis (or nonadvancing epidermal margin)
- Increased exudate
- Exudate that becomes purulent instead of serous
- Pungent odor
- Macerated and boggy surrounding skin

TABLE 18-7   Taking a Swab Culture of a Wound

Before taking the specimen for swab culture:

- Cleanse the wound well with water or saline.
- Remove excess necrotic tissue.
- Compress the edges to elicit new drainage.

Use the end of a sterile cotton tipped applicator stick on a 1 cm area of the open wound. Swab for 5 seconds (Levine, et al.). Apply sufficient pressure to cause tissue fluid to be expressed.

- Do not swab exudates, pus, eschar, or necrotic tissue.
- Break off the swab tip in a sterile tube containing transport media.
- Label specimen with pertinent information including but not limited to:
  - Wound location
  - Antibiotics received
  - Suspected cause
- Send specimen immediately to the lab.

conducive to wound healing. Surgical debridement may be necessary for nonvitalized tissue (Stillman, 2005).

Clinicians must decide when to perform a bacterial culture and what type of culture to perform. See Table 18-7 for taking a swab culture. Quantitative biopsy is considered the "gold standard" but often unavailable, requires a skilled practitioner, causes pain in sensate soft tissue, and is expensive. Swab culture determines the number of bacteria per unit area in the underlying wound bed after the surface has been cleaned and enough pressure is applied to the swab to obtain tissue fluid (Gilchrist, 1997). Procedures should be performed selectively and used in conjunction with clinical signs of local or deep tissue infection to decide if topical or systemic antimicrobial treatment is appropriate. If the patient demonstrates signs and symptoms of infection as outlined above, obtain both aerobic and anaerobic cultures, especially in wounds with undermining and tunneling. Consider culturing a wound if there is no improvement and all factors have

been optimized. Sending a specimen for gram stain gives quick results while awaiting the final culture report.

When superficial signs of infection are present, topical antimicrobials can be used initially. The general principles for using topical antimicrobials include the following (Sibbald, 2003):

- Do not use agents that are used systemically because of the ability to breed resistant organisms (e.g., topical gentamicin or tobramycin).
- Do not use agents that are common allergens (e.g., neomycin, gentamycin, amikacin, bacitracin, lanolin).
- Do not use agents that have high cellular toxicity in healable wounds (e.g., povidone iodine, chlorhexidine, hydrogen peroxide).
- Reevaluate every few weeks and make changes as required.

Topical antiseptic products can be effective antimicrobial agents. Antiseptics target bacteria at the cell membrane, cytoplasmic organelle, and nucleic acid levels. The toxicity of antiseptic agents may vary and may depend on the delivery system for the concentration used. The longer the wound has been present, the broader spectrum the antimicrobial agent must be used. Newer agents such as silver dressings, cadexomer iodine, and topical antibiotic creams or ointments can address surface bacterial balance, maintain moisture, and facilitate debridement. Antimicrobials can be used in selected cases of critical colonization or infection. Table 18-8 lists commonly used topical antimicrobials.

When a large bacterial wound contamination is suspected or confirmed, a 2-week course of topical antimicrobial may benefit by reducing the bacterial load within the wound (Rodeheaver, 1997). Oral antibiotic therapy is *not* recommended when bacteria, sepsis,

cellulitis, or osteomyelitis is present (Stotts & Hunt, 1997) and generally requires systemic antibiotics. The choice of antibiotics depends on the organism involved, the antimicrobial sensitivities, previous antibiotic use, the duration of the wound, and host resistance.

Moisture Imbalance (M)

Nonhealing wounds frequently produce a substantial amount of exudates. Several studies have demonstrated biochemical differences between the exudate component of acute and chronic wounds. Chronic wound exudates slow down or block the proliferation of cells such as keratinocytes, fibroblasts, and endothelial cells that are all important to wound repair. The exudates contain a number of

TABLE 18-8   Commonly Used Antimicrobials

AGENT	VEHICLE	STAPH. AUREUS	STREPTO- COCCUS	PSEUDO- MONAS	COMMENTS
†Cadexomer Iodine (Iodosorb)	Yellow-brown powder/ paste/ointment	MRSA ✓	✓	✓	Releases iodine slowly, less toxic to granulating tissue Broad spectrum, including virus and fungus
Gentamicin sulphate cream/ointment	Alcohol cream base or petrolateum ointment	✓	✓	✓	Good broad spectrum vs gram negatives
†Metronidazole gel/cream	Wax—glycerin cream and carbogel 940/ propylene glycol gel				Good anaerobe coverage and wound deodorizer
†Mupuricin 2% cream/ointment	Propylene glycol ointment	MRSA ✓	✓		Good choice for MRSA Excellent topical penetration
†Polymyxin B sulphate—Gramacidin	Cream	MRSA ✓	✓	✓	Broad spectrum Low cost Ointment contains bacitracin, a new sensitizer
Polymyxin B sulphate—Bacitracin zinc—neomycin*	Ointment	✓	✓	✓	Neomycin is a potent sensitizer and may cross-react, in 40% of cases, to aminoglycosides
†Silver sulfadiazine	Water-miscible cream	MRSA ✓	✓	✓	Do not use in sulfa-sensitive individuals
†Silver (ionized)	Absorbent bilayered sheet, burn dressing, alginate, foam and other forms	MRSA ✓	✓	✓	Ionized silver is activated with sterile water. Saline will precipitate the silver chloride

MRSA   methicillin-resistant *Staphylococcus aureus*
*   Contains common sensitizer
†   Preferred products

matrix metalloproteinases and serine proteases that can break down or damage essential extracellular matrix materials. Essential growth factors are also inhibited by macromolecules that are found in chronic wound exudates. Managing the amount of fluid produced can minimize the detrimental effects of the wound exudates (Schultz et al., 2003).

Edge of Wound (E)

The failure of the epidermal margin or wound edge to migrate across the wound bed prevents healing. The wound may be undermined or tunneled under the wound edge, and the biochemical environment of the wound bed may be hostile for migrating epithelial tissue. At the cellular level, the lack of epidermal migration is due to nonresponsive wound cells and abnormalities in protease activity that degrade the extracellular matrix while it is

being formed (Cook, Davies, Harding, & Tomas, 2000). Consideration of the use of growth factors, biological dressings, skin substitutes, skin grafts, negative pressure, or other adjunctive therapies may enhance the healing cycle.

When the wound is clean of slough and necrotic material and/or the infection has subsided, healing should occur. Wound healing is indicated by the development of granulation tissue and a decrease in wound volume and surface area (Stotts & Hunt, 1997). If there is no progress toward healing, an overall comprehensive reassessment of the patient's health status and the wound is necessary. Adequate tissue perfusion is essential; correction of abnormalities or adjustment of co-medications for other conditions, poor nutrition, or lifestyle may be factors in nonhealing. A change in the plan of care is indicated in these cases, and adjunctive therapy may be considered. See Figure 18-6 for a wound care decision guide.

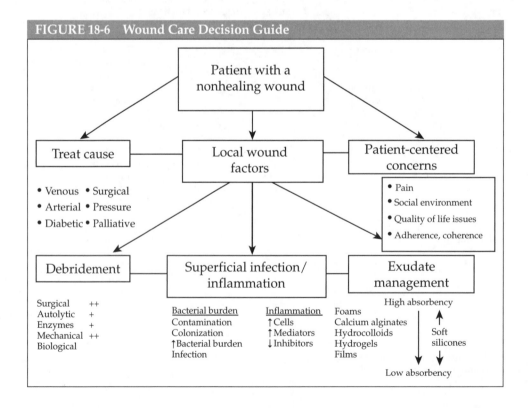

FIGURE 18-6   Wound Care Decision Guide

SELECTING A DRESSING

Although saline wet to moist gauze has been a popular dressing choice for most wounds, research has developed more efficient dressing types both for healing and frequency of applications (Ovington, 2001). Studies show that the best environment is developed by a dressing that provides an appropriate degree of occlusion or blocks the passage of air (Haimowitz & Margolis, 1997; Kerstein, 1995). Clinical studies have shown that compared to conventional gauze, moist moisture-retentive dressings will reduce time to healing, the rate of wound infection, patient pain, and the cost of care (Wyatt, McGowan, & Najarian, 1990; Nemeth, Eaglstein, Taylor, Peerson, & Falanga, 1991).

A variety of wound dressings are available. Understanding the various dressings is pivotal to selecting the one most appropriate for a specific situation. In selecting a dressing, consider the following:

- The dressing's absorptive capacity
- Hydrating ability
- Adhesiveness
- The dressing's ability to conform to the wound

The clinician's challenge is to use a dressing that maintains an adequate degree of fluid within the wound without being too wet and causing maceration of the periwound and skin. In addition, to maximize efficiencies and healing consider the cost, ease of use, visits and labor required, and the frequency of dressing changes. A comprehensive listing of wound care products is available through *Kestrel Wound Product Sourcebook* and can be found online at www.woundsource.com. If the patient is to be discharged home with wound care needed, an assessment of the home environment and caregiver situation must be factored into the approach to achieve positive outcomes (Ovington, 2001).

When a wound is moist with minimal drainage, a dressing with little to no absorptive capacity is needed (e.g., transparent film). For wounds that exude a moderate amount of drainage, a thin foam or hydrocolloid might be used. When the wound is dry, a dressing that is hydrating such as an amorphous hydrogel or hydrogel sheet can be used. For heavily draining wounds, alginates and foams are the dressing of choice. See Figure 18-7 for exudate management.

Adjunctive Therapy

Advanced technologies are useful only if the wound bed has been optimally prepared. If all of these factors have been optimized and

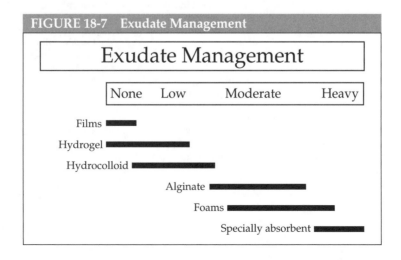

FIGURE 18-7   Exudate Management

healing has not occurred in a reasonable period of time (8–12 weeks), biological agents may be considered. A number of adjunctive therapies are evolving. Adjunctive therapies that have a current evidence base include transepidermal nerve stimulation (TENS), electrical stimulation, and therapeutic ultrasound for pressure ulcers. See Table 18-9 for advanced technologies.

Other technologies, although interesting to clinicians, require further research. Advanced technologies include skin substitutes, growth factors, and vacuum-assisted closure (V.A.C.) for pressure ulcers. The V.A.C. uses negative pressure in a closed-dressing system and is indicated for large highly exudative wounds. Negative pressure wound therapy assists in evacuation of wound fluid, stimulation of granulation tissue formation, and reduction of bacterial colonization. The continual influx of third-space fluids through the wound, into the foam, and through the tubing to the collection canister encourages a moist, clean wound, an important factor in the development of granulation tissue, epithelialization, and sustained viability of growth factors and cytokines (Mendez-Eastman, 2003).

TABLE 18-9	Advanced Technologies		
TECHNOLOGY	**DESCRIPTION**	**APPROVED INDICATIONS**	**COMMENTS**
Apligraf	Bilayered human skin equivalent (living fibroblasts and epidermal cells with a stratum corneum), on a bovine Type I collagen matrix	Resistant venous leg ulcers* Refractory diabetic neuropathic foot ulcers*	Expensive, with variable reimbursement Requires careful patient selection and optimal care Greatest benefit for patients with wounds of more than 1-year duration 5-day shelf life
Dermagraft	Viable dermal fibroblasts on a vicryl mesh (human skin equivalent)	Diabetic neuropathic foot ulcers Fistulas (pending approval)	Expensive with variable reimbursement Requires careful patient selection and optimal care 6-month shelf life (in a –40° freezer)
Oasis	Freeze-dried submucosa of porcine small intestine	Broad range of acute and nonhealing wounds (except third-degree burns)	Use selectively for patients whose wounds are refractory to appropriate wound care Relatively easy to use Relatively inexpensive Usually reimbursed Primarily anecdotal evidence only at this time
Regranex	Recombinant PDGF in a hydrogel	Full-thickness diabetic neuropathic foot ulcers with adequate blood supply and no infection*	Because infection may not be clinically apparent, this limitation reduces effectiveness. Product was approved as a drug with variable reimbursement (not reimbursed by Medicare).
V.A.C.	Negative pressure in a closed-dressing system	Highly exudative wounds	Removes excess interstitial fluid, reducing frequency of dressing changes May be used to treat multiple wound sites simultaneously. May expedite patient transfer to a lower-cost setting

TABLE 18-9   Advanced Technologies (*Continued*)

TECHNOLOGY	DESCRIPTION	APPROVED INDICATIONS	COMMENTS
Hyaluronic acid (Hyalofill)	Ester of hyaluronic acid	Hard-to-heal wounds (often with chronic inflammation)	Easy to use Relatively inexpensive Wounds need to be in bacterial balance for optimal effectiveness
Electrical stimulation (e-stim)	High-voltage electrical stimulation	Pressure ulcers	May be effective in nonhealing wounds*
Ultrasound	Mechanical vibration	Pressure ulcers	May be effective in nonhealing wounds*
Hyperbaric oxygen (HBO) therapy	Systemic delivery of oxygen to patients placed in chambers at 2–3 times atmospheric pressure, while breathing 100% oxygen	Select problem wounds: necrotizing soft tissue infections, gas gangrene, refractory osteomyelitis, thermal burns, radiation tissue damage, compromised skin grafts and flaps	Expensive Requires specialized training and equipment Some controlled studies have shown benefit. Availability and expense limit everyday use.

* Shown to be effective in randomized controlled trials.
PDGF, platelet-derived growth factor; V.A.C., vacuum-assisted closure therapy; ADLs, activities of daily living.

WEB SITES

- *Advances in Wound Care*—www.woundcare journal.com
- *Journal of Wound, Ostomy, and Continence Nursing*—www.jwocnonline.com
- *Ostomy/Wound Care*—www.journalofwound care.com
- *American Journal of Infection Control*—www.apic.org
- *Kestrel Wound Product Sourcebook*—www.woundsource.com
- *Podiatry Today*—www.podiatrytoday.com
- *Mayo Clinic Proceedings*, "Pressure Ulcers: Prevention and Management," 1995, Vol. 70, Issue 8, pp. 789–799—http://www.mayoclinicproceedings.com/Abstract.asp?AID=3983&Abst=Abstract&UID=
- *Wounds Compendium of Clinical Research and Practice*—www.woundsearch.com

REFERENCES

Alvarez, O., Meehan, M., Ennis, W., Thomas, D. R., Ferris, F. D., Kennedy, K. L., et al. (2002). Chronic wound: Palliative management for the frail population. *Wounds: A compendium of Clinical Research and Practice, 14*(8, Suppl.), 8S–12S.

Bergstrom, N., Bennett, M. A., & Carlson, C. E. (1994). *Treatment of pressure ulcers. Clinical practice guidelines No. 15* (AHCRP Publication No. 95–0652). Rockville, MD: U.S. Department of Health and Human Services, Public Health Service, Agency for Health Care Policy and Research.

Cherry, G. W., Harding, K. G., & Ryan, T. J. (Eds.). (2001). *Wound bed preparation*. International Congress and Symposium Series 250. Oxford, UK: Royal Society of Medicine Press, Ltd.

Cook, H., Davies, K. L., Harding, K. G., & Tomas, D. W. (2000). Defective extracellular matrix reorganization by chronic fibroblasts is associated with alterations in TIMP-1, TEMP-2 and MMP-2 activity. *Journal of Investigative Dermatology, 115,* 225–233.

Cutting, K. F., & White, R. J. (2005). Criteria for identifying wound infection—revisited. *Ostomy/ Wound Management, 51*(1), 28–34.

Cuzzell, J. (1988). The new RYB color code. *American Journal of Nursing, 10,* 1342–1346.

Finney, J. L., Jones, H., & Margolis, D. J. (2000). *Management of wounds: Wound repair, growth factors, and engineered tissue* (Number 9 in a monograph series). Hauppauge, NY: Curative Health Services, Inc.

Fowler, E., Krasner, D., & Sibbald, G. (2002). *Healing environments for chronic wound care: Optimizing local wound management as a component of holistic interdisciplinary patient care. Treatment of chronic wounds* (Number 11 in a series). Hauppauge, NY: Curative Health Services, Inc.

Fowler, E., & van Rijswijk, L. (1995). Using wound debridement to help achieve the goals of care. *Ostomy Wound Management, 41*(7A Suppl), 23S–35S.

Gilchrist, B. (1997). Infection and culturing. In D. Krasner, & D. Kane (Eds.). *Chronic wound care: A clinical source book for healthcare professionals* (2nd ed., pp. 109–114). Wayne, PA: Health Management Publications, Inc.

Grey, M., & Whitney, J. (2003). Does vitamin C supplementation promote pressure ulcer healing? *Journal of Wound, Ostomy and Continence Nursing, 30*(5), 245–249.

Grey, M. (2003a). Does oral supplementation with vitamins A or E promote healing of chronic wounds? *Journal of Wound, Ostomy and Continence Nursing, 30*(6), 290–294.

Grey, M. (2003b). Does oral zinc supplementation promote healing of chronic wounds? *Journal of Wound, Ostomy and Continence Nursing, 30*(6), 295–299.

Haimowitz, J., & Margolis, D. (1997). Moist wound healing. In D. Krasner, & D. Kane (Eds.). *Chronic wound care: A clinical source book for healthcare professionals* (2nd ed., pp. 49–56). Wayne, PA: Health Management Publications, Inc.

Hess, C. T., & Trent, J. T. (2004). Incorporating laboratory values in chronic wound management. *Advances in Skin and Wound Care, 17*(7), 387–388.

Kerstein, M. (1995). Moist wound healing: The clinical perspective. *Ostomy and Wound Management, 41*(7A), 37S–45S.

Kiemele, L., & Takahashi, P. (2004). Practical wound management in long-term care. *Annals of Long-Term Care, 12*(10), 25–32.

Lazarus, G. S., Cooper, D. M., Knighton, D. R., Margolis, D. J., Pecoraro, R. E., Rodeheaver, G., et al. (1994). Definitions and guidelines for assessment of wounds and evaluation of healing. *Archives of Dermatology, 130,* 489–493.

Mendez-Eastman, S. (2003). *Determining the appropriateness of negative pressure wound therapy for pressure ulcers.* Proceedings from the 2003 National V.A.C. Education Conference: Vol. 50(4A), 13–16.

National Pressure Ulcer Advisory Panel. (1995). Consensus statement. *Advances in Wound Care, 8,* 11–24.

Nemeth, A. J., Eaglstein, W. H., Taylor, J. R., Peerson, L., & Falagna, V. (1991). Faster healing and less pain in skin biopsy sites treated with an occlusive dressing. *Archives of Dermatology, 127,* 1679–1683.

Ovington, L. (2001). Hanging wet-to-dry dressings out to dry. *Home Healthcare Nurse, 8*(19), 477–483.

Payne, R., & Martin, M. (2000). Defining and classifying skin tears: Need for a common language. *Ostomy/Wound Management, 39*(5), 16–20, 22–24, 26.

Rodeheaver, G. T. (1997). Wound cleansing, wound irrigation, wound disinfection. In D. Krasner, & D. Kane (Eds.). *Chronic wound care: A clinical source book for healthcare professionals* (2nd ed., pp. 97–107). Wayne, PA: Health Management Publications, Inc.

Salcido, R. (2005). *Pressure ulcers and wound care.* Retrieved October 16, 2006, from http://www.emedicine.com/pmr/topic179.htm

Schultz, G., Sibbald, R. G., Falanga, V., Ayello, E. A., Dowsett, C., Harding, K., et al. (2003). Wound bed preparation: A systematic approach to wound management. *Wound Repair and Regeneration, 11,* 1–28.

Sibbald, R. G. (2003). Topical antimicrobials. *Ostomy/ Wound Management, 49*(Suppl. 5A), 3S–33S.

Smith, S. (2003). *The clinician's notebook. 1*(3).

Stillman, R. (2005). *Wound care.* Retrieved October 16, 2006, from http://www.emedicine.com/med/topic2754.htm

Stotts, N., & Hunt, T. (1997). Managing bacterial colonization and infection. *Clinics in Geriatric Medicine, 13,* 565–573.

Trent, J., Falabella, A., Eaglstein, W., & Kirsner, R. (2001). Venous ulcers: Pathophysiology and treatment options, parts 1 & 2. *Ostomy Wound Management, 51*(5), 38–54.

Vance, J. (2002). No easy answers to LTC conundrums: Pressure ulcer controversies. *Caring for the Ages, 3*(5), 24–27.

Weinberg, A., & Levine, J. (2005). Clinical areas of liability: Risk management concerns in long-term care. *Annals of Long-Term Care, 13,* 26–32.

Wyatt, D., McGowan, D., & Najarian, M. (1990). Comparison of a hydrocolloid dressing and silver sulfadiazine cream in the outpatient management of second-degree burns. *Journal of Trauma, 30,* 857–865.

BIBLIOGRAPHY

Ankrom, M. A., Bennett, R. G., Sprigle, S., Langemo, D., Black, J. M., Berlowitz, D. R., et al. (2005). Pressure-related deep tissue injury under intact skin and the current pressure ulcer staging systems. *Advances in Skin & Wound Care, 18*(1), 35–42.

Baranoski, S., & Avello, E. (2004). *Wound care essentials: Practice principles.* Philadelphia: Lippincott, Williams & Wilkins.

Bryant, R. A. (2000). *Acute & chronic wounds: Nursing management* (2nd ed.). St. Louis, MO: Mosby.

Falanga, V. (2001). *Cutaneous wound healing.* London: Taylor & Francis.

Falanga, V., & Eaglstein, W. (1995). *Leg and foot ulcers: A clinician's guide.* Vincent Falanga and William Eaglstein. London: Martin Dunitz.

Hess, C. T. (2002). *Clinical guide to wound care* (4th ed.). Philadelphia: Lippincott Williams & Wilkins.

Irion, G. (2002). *Comprehensive wound management.* Clifton Park, NY: Delmar Learning.

Kloth, L., & McCulloch, J. (2001). *Wound healing: Alternatives in management (Contemporary perspectives in rehabilitation)* (3rd ed.). Philadelphia: F.A. Davis.

Krasner, D., Rodeheaver, G., & Sibbald, G. R. (2001). *Chronic wound care: A clinical source book for healthcare professionals* (3rd ed.). Malvern, PA: HMP Communications, Inc.

MacLean, D. S. (2003). Preventing and managing pressure sores. *Caring for the Ages, 4*(3), 34–37.

Maklebust, J., & Sieggreen, M. (2002). *Pressure ulcers: Guidelines for prevention and management* (3rd ed.). Philadelphia: Lippincott, Williams & Wilkins.

Morison, M., Ovington, L., & Wilkie, K. (2004). *Chronic wound care: A problem learning approach.* St. Louis, MO: Mosby.

Myers, B. A. (2003). *Wound management: Principles and practice.* Upper Saddle River, NJ: Prentice-Hall.

Ovington, L. G. (1999). Dressings and adjunctive therapies: AHCPR guidelines revisited. *Ostomy/Wound Management, 45*(Suppl. 1A), 94S–106S.

Rovee, D. T., & Maibach, H. I. (2003). *The epidermis in wound healing.* Boca Raton, FL: CRC Press.

Sibbald, R. G., Williamson, D., Orsted, H. L., Campbell, K., Keast, D., Krasner, D., et al. (2000). Preparing the wound bed—debridement, bacterial balance and moisture balance. *Ostomy/Wound Management, 46,* 14–35.

Smith & Nephew, Inc. (2004). *Wound bed preparation and time: A practical guide.* Largo, FL: Author.

Stotts, N. A., Barbour, S., Slaughter, R., & Wipke-Tevis, D. (1993). Wound care practices in the United States. *Ostomy/Wound Management, 39*(3), 53–55, 59–62.

Sussman, C., & Bates-Jensen, B. (2001). *Wound care: A collaborative practice manual for physical therapists and nurses* (2nd ed.). Philadelphia: Lippincott, Williams & Wilkins.

APPENDIX A

Braden Scale

BRADEN SCALE FOR PREDICTING PRESSURE SORE RISK

Patient's Name _____ Evaluator's Name_____ Date of Assessment

SENSORY PERCEPTION ability to respond meaning- fully to pressure-related discomfort	**1. Completely Limited** Unresponsive (does not moan, flinch, or grasp) to painful stimuli, due to diminished level of con-sciousness or sedation. OR limited ability to feel pain over most of body	**2. Very Limited** Responds only to painful stimuli. Cannot communicate discomfort except by moaning or restlessness OR has a sensory impairment which limits the ability to feel pain or discomfort over ½ of body.	**3. Slightly Limited** Responds to verbal com- mands, but cannot always communicate discomfort or the need to be turned. OR has some sensory impairment which limits ability to feel pain or discomfort in 1 or 2 extremities.	**4. No Impairment** Responds to verbal commands. Has no sensory deficit which would limit ability to feel or voice pain or discomfort..
MOISTURE degree to which skin is exposed to moisture	**1. Constantly Moist** Skin is kept moist almost constantly by perspiration, urine, etc. Dampness is detected every time patient is moved or turned.	**2. Very Moist** Skin is often, but not always moist. Linen must be changed at least once a shift.	**3. Occasionally Moist:** Skin is occasionally moist, requiring an extra linen change approximately once a day.	**4. Rarely Moist** Skin is usually dry, linen only requires changing at routine intervals.
ACTIVITY degree of physical activity	**1. Bedfast** Confined to bed.	**2. Chairfast** Ability to walk severely limited or non-existent. Cannot bear own weight and/or must be assisted into chair or wheelchair.	**3. Walks Occasionally** Walks occasionally during day, but for very short distances, with or without assistance. Spends majority of each shift in bed or chair	**4. Walks Frequently** Walks outside room at least twice a day and inside room at least once every two hours during waking hours
MOBILITY ability to change and control body position	**1. Completely Immobile** Does not make even slight changes in body or extremity position without assistance	**2. Very Limited** Makes occasional slight changes in body or extremity position but unable to make frequent or significant changes independently.	**3. Slightly Limited** Makes frequent though slight changes in body or extremity position independently.	**4. No Limitation** Makes major and frequent changes in position without assistance.
NUTRITION usual food intake pattern	**1. Very Poor** Never eats a complete meal. Rarely eats more than ⅓ of any food offered. Eats 2 servings or less of protein (meat or dairy products) per day. Takes fluids poorly. Does not take a liquid dietary supplement OR is NPO and/or maintained on clear liquids or IV's for more than 5 days.	**2. Probably Inadequate** Rarely eats a complete meal and generally eats only about ½ of any food offered. Protein intake includes only 3 servings of meat or dairy products per day. Occasionally will take a dietary supplement. OR receives less than optimum amount of liquid diet or tube feeding	**3. Adequate** Eats over half of most meals. Eats a total of 4 servings of protein (meat, dairy products per day. Occasionally will refuse a meal, but will usually take a supplement when offered OR is on a tube feeding or TPN regimen which probably meets most of nutritional needs	**4. Excellent** Eats most of every meal. Never refuses a meal. Usually eats a total of 4 or more servings of meat and dairy products. Occasionally eats between meals. Does not require supplementation.
FRICTION & SHEAR	**1. Problem** Requires moderate to maximum assistance in moving. Complete lifting without sliding against sheets is impossible. Frequently slides down in bed or chair, requiring frequent repositioning with maximum assistance. Spasticity, contractures or agitation leads to almost constant friction	**2. Potential Problem** Moves feebly or requires minimum assistance. During a move skin probably slides to some extent against sheets, chair, restraints or other devices. Maintains relatively good position in chair or bed most of the time but occasionally slides down.	**3. No Apparent Problem** Moves in bed and in chair independently and has sufficient muscle strength to lift up completely during move. Maintains good position in bed or chair.	

Total Score

CHAPTER 19

Nutrition

Mary Jacob and Barbara White

Nutrition plays an integral part in the prevention and management of chronic and acute illnesses, the correction of impaired function, and the rehabilitation of the individual. Institutionalized individuals are at greater risk for malnutrition associated with nutritional deficiencies than are community-dwelling individuals. These deficiencies increase the incidence of infection and affect both quality and length of life. In nursing homes the prevalence of weight loss, tube feeding, and dehydration are also reportable quality indicators. It is crucial, therefore, that the nurse practitioner initiates early evaluation of residents' nutritional status so that appropriate management plans can be developed.

Some common nutrition-related problems encountered in nursing home patients include the following:

- Anorexia of aging, associated with decreased physical activity and metabolic changes that affect satiation, enjoyment, and feeding drive (Morley, 1997)

- Dehydration

- Malnutrition (nutrient deficiencies, excesses, or imbalances)

- Failure to thrive associated with infections, pressure sores, slow wound healing, or the stress of surgical procedures

- Anorexia tardive resulting from a previous history or disposition to anorexia nervosa or developed as a new strategy to maintain personal control or gain needed attention

- Nutritional problems associated with chronic diseases (e.g., hypertension, diabetes mellitus, dyslipidemia, thyroid disorders, cancer, and/or diseases of other organ systems)

- Food and drug interactions

- Terminal illness

Epidemiology

DiMaria-Ghalili & Amella (2005) estimated that 20–60% of older adults in home care and 40–60% of hospitalized older adults are malnourished or at risk for the problem. In long-term care they estimate the prevalence to be as high as 40–85%. Protein-energy malnutrition can occur with a variety of acute and chronic illnesses including infections, cancer, chronic obstructive pulmonary disease, congestive heart failure, malabsorption, hyperthyroidism, hyperparathyroidism, and diseases that increase the level of circulating cytokines such as acquired immunodeficiency syndrome and rheumatoid arthritis (Thomas, Kamel, & Morley, 2004). Malnutrition leads to medical complications, longer hospital stays, and increased cost of care. Risk factors for the development of nutritional problems, in addition to disease states, include the following:

- Functional limitations that affect the ability to eat
- Dental, chewing, and swallowing problems
- Diminished sense of taste and smell related to age, illness, or medications
- Food intolerances
- Unmet cultural or ethnic food preferences
- Restrictive diets
- History of excessive alcohol intake
- Fatigue
- Pain
- Dyspnea
- Constipation or fecal impaction
- Dehydration
- Polypharmacy
- Cognitive impairment and wandering
- Depression and delirium

Nutritional Assessment

Federal regulations as well as the American Medical Directors Association (AMDA) guidelines for altered nutritional status recommend nutritional evaluation of all residents within 14 days of admission to the nursing home.

Baseline Data
Admission *baseline data* should include a minimum of the following:

- Height, weight, and calculation of body mass index (BMI), with measurements taken standing or, recumbent and calculated as (weight in lbs/height in inches squared) × 704

- Resident preferences for foods, portion size, and meal timings
- Percentage of food eaten and/or food groups consumed per meal
- Risk factors for altered nutritional status

Triggers that should alert the clinician to the need for medical nutrition management to correct nutritional deficiencies include (Thomas, Ashmen, Morley, Evans, & Council for Nutritional Strategies in Long Term Care, 2000):

- Involuntary 5% weight loss in 30 days or less
- Involuntary 7.5% weight loss in 90 days or less
- Involuntary 10% weight loss in 180 days or less
- BMI $\leq$ 19–21
- Resident leaves $\geq$ 25% of food uneaten at two thirds of meals (based on 2000 kcal/ day) over 7 days

Specific Assessments
Implementation of any nutrition intervention plan must be preceded by nutritional assessment that may include clinical, dietary, anthropometric, and biochemical evaluations. The effectiveness of the intervention is monitored by continuous reassessment. See summary in Table 19-1.

Medical History History of recent weight loss per patient, family, or medical records; restrictive therapeutic diets; acute or chronic medical or surgical conditions

Psychosocial History History of delirium, dementia, depression; response to loss, environmental change

Medication Review With attention to polypharmacy and potential drug-drug and food-drug interactions that may affect appetite or ability to eat. Many drugs potentiate weight loss (Morley, 1997) by the following mechanisms:

TABLE 19-1 Summary of a Comprehensive Nutrition Assessment	
NATURE OF THE INFORMATION	
Dietary assessment	Current and past food intake using 24-hour diet recall of food Record of food frequency or direct observation Special culturally defined dietary preferences Food allergies, meal patterns Dietary/nutrient/herbal supplements Dietary restrictions related to chronic diseases Quality and quantity of foods consumed Medications—prescription and over-the-counter, amount, frequency, polypharmacy
Medical history	Chronic diseases—presence and duration GI factors, dental and oral health Sensory and psychological factors
Biochemical assessment	**Protein status** Visceral proteins: • Serum albumin • Serum transferrin • Transthyretin (prealbumin) • Retinol-binding protein **Microcytic anemia** Serum iron, serum ferritin, transferrin receptor Total iron-binding capacity (TIBC) Hemoglobin, hematocrit, RBC count Mean corpuscular volume (MCV), Mean corpuscular hemoglobin concentration (MCHC) Mean corpuscular hemoglobin (MCH) **Macrocytic (megaloblastic) anemia** Serum, RBC, folic acid, and cobalamin concentrations Homocysteine **Cardiovascular disease** Total cholesterol, low-density lipoprotein High-density lipoprotein, triglycerides C-reactive protein, homocysteine **Immunocompetence** Complete blood cell count (CBC) Total lymphocyte count (TLC) Differential white cell count **Hydration status** Serum electrolytes (e.g., sodium, potassium) Serum osmolality

- Decreasing appetite
  - Cardiac drugs: digoxin, amiodarone, procainamide, quinidine, spironolactone
  - Gastrointestinal drugs: cimetidine, interferon
  - Psychiatric drugs: phenothiazines, butyrophenones, lithium, amitriptyline, imipramine, fluoxetine, and other selective serotonin reuptake inhibitors (SSRIs)
  - Anti-infective drugs: most antibiotics, metronidazole, griseofulvin
  - Nutrient supplements: iron sulfate, potassium salts, excessive vitamin D
  - Antineoplastics

○ Antirheumatic drugs: NSAIDs, colchicines, penicillamine

○ Pulmonary drugs, such as theophylline

- Causing malabsorption (e.g., laxative, cholestyramine, methotrexate, colchicines, neomycin, ganglionic blockers)

- Increasing metabolism (e.g., theophylline, excessive doses of thyroid hormone)

Dietary Assessment In consultation with the dietician order calorie/nutrient evaluations.

Physical Examination

- Review anthropometric measures including height, weight, and body mass index.

- Assess integument including skin texture, temperature, turgor; evidence of loss of subcutaneous fat or muscle wasting; presence of poor healing wounds; and edema.

- Complete an oral examination including lips, tongue, teeth, gums, mucosa, saliva production and management, chewing and swallowing abilities, cranial nerves (gag reflex (IX, X), tongue movement and strength (XI), facial sensation and movement (V, VII), and olfaction and taste (I, VII) as needed.

- Assess vision (cranial nerves II, III, IV, VI) and hearing (VIII).

- Assess functional abilities, including the ability to sit upright for meals, upper extremity range of motion, grasp, and strength.

- Perform a gastrointestinal evaluation including abdominal distention, bowel sounds, tenderness, organ enlargement, and rectal examination for impaction and sphincter control.

- Perform a neurological examination for mental status, memory, and mood.

- For specific evaluations for dysphagia, refer to the speech-language pathologist.

- Take measurements of body composition, in consultation with the registered dietician.

Essential Diagnostic and Laboratory Tests

Baseline Biochemical Tests

Baseline laboratory data should be established for all patients, against which changes can be evaluated. These may be omitted or limited if the patient's advance directive or condition (e.g., terminal care) warrants it (AMDA, 2001). Recommended tests and abnormal values include the following:

- Serum albumin (< 3.5 mg/dL)

- Serum prealbumin (transthyretin) (< 15 mg/dL)

- Serum cholesterol (< 160 mg/dL)

- Complete blood count or hemoglobin (< 12 g/dL)

- Serum transferrin (< 180 mg/dL)

Measurements of components in blood are classified into nonspecific or nutrient-specific markers and immunological indicators of nutritional status. The nonspecific indicators are serum transport proteins such as albumin, transthyretin (thyroxine-binding prealbumin) and transferrin.

- *Serum albumin* values are easily obtained and so it is commonly used in clinical practice to detect severe malnutrition. It is a nonspecific marker because it is affected by factors other than protein-energy malnutrition (PEM). Serum albumin plays an important role in the maintenance of osmotic pressure and plasma volume, and therefore intravascular fluid changes can influence serum albumin levels. Usually hypoalbuminemia (< 2.8 g/100 dL) is accompanied by generalized edema. Serum albumin is *altered* in the presence of the following:

○ Liver and renal disease

○ Trauma

○ Surgery

○ Burns

○ Inflammation

Thus it becomes difficult to differentiate between the effects of protein-energy malnutrition and disease in chronically ill patients. The long half-life of albumin (14–20 days) tends to decrease its sensitivity to short-term changes in protein status. Decreased serum albumin (< 3.5 g/dL) is a risk factor for mortality in institutionalized individuals (Sullivan & Walls, 1995).

- *Serum prealbumin (transthyretin)* provides the earliest laboratory indication of protein-energy malnutrition and an early indication of recovery. It has the highest ratio of essential to nonessential amino acids of any body protein and is an excellent marker of protein synthesis. It has a half-life of 2 days and returns to normal after depletion in 14 days. Prealbumin is not affected by hydration state and is less affected by liver disease than serum albumin. *Transient declines* in prealbumin are seen in the following:

  ○ Postsurgically
  ○ With inflammation
  ○ With decreased levels of zinc

Levels may rise with acute alcohol intoxication and with medications, including prednisone and progestational agents (Beck & Rosenthal, 2002). The Prealbumin in Nutritional Care Consensus Group (Bernstein et al., 1995) recommended referral to a dietician for values less than 15 mg/dL and initiation of nutritional support for values less than 11 mg/dL, or values that fail to rise 4.0 mg/dL in 8 days with treatment.

- *Serum transferrin*, the iron transport protein, is a visceral protein with a relatively shorter half-life (8–9 days) than albumin. Changes in protein status result in a faster response in transferrin than in albumin. In an iron deficiency, transferrin values are elevated and the reverse is true in cases of PEM. This limits the usefulness of serum transferrin as an indicator of malnutrition if chronic PEM coexists with an iron deficiency.

- *Hemoglobin, hematocrit, mean corpuscular hemoglobin (MCH), and mean corpuscular volume (MCV)* are useful indicators that distinguish between microcytic and macrocytic anemia, which are common occurrences among institutionalized persons. Iron, folic acid, and vitamin B_{12} are often low in institutionalized individuals due to poor dietary intake, physiological changes, and concurrent effects of illness.

- *Total lymphocyte count (TLC), a differential white blood cell count, and delayed cutaneous hypersensitivity or delayed hypersensitivity reactivity (DHR)* tests are ordered to assess immunocompetence. The TLC indicates the functional capacity of T and B immune cells while the DHR measures cell-mediated immunity. The immune response is depressed in older adults due to factors that include infections, illness, PEM, nutrient deficiencies, and physical and/or emotional stress.

- The fat-soluble *vitamin D and calcium* are nutrients of concern among long-term care residents. Lack of exposure to sunlight, lactose intolerance, physiological changes in the aging skin and intestine, drug interactions, and functional changes in the liver and kidney contribute to vitamin D deficiency. Decreased absorption of calcium with advancing age, hypochlorhydria, low vitamin D status, and the use of antacids lead to calcium deficiency resulting in osteopenia and osteoporosis.

- Additional tests to consider include the following:

  ○ Thyroid stimulating hormone (TSH): Hyper- and hypothyroidism
  ○ C-reactive protein: Inflammation, excess cytokines
  ○ Blood urea nitrogen, creatinine: Dehydration, renal failure
  ○ Electrolytes: Specific imbalances

Additional Assessment Tools

The most commonly used evaluation tools are the Prognostic Nutrition Index, Subjective Global Assessment, and Mini Nutritional Assessment. Each of these protocols includes a series of specific tests that evaluate dietary intake, body composition, energy expenditure, and laboratory tests for specific components (such as enzymes, proteins, vitamins, electrolytes, and other minerals) in blood and urine that relate to nutritional status and clinical symptoms (Lysen, 1997). The types of assessment conducted depend on the health status of the person. Generally, not all measurements can be taken in one person, and therefore the dietitian will select the most feasible and meaningful ones.

The Prognostic Nutritional Index (PNI) is used to assess risk of complications, sepsis, and death in postoperative patients and is calculated as a percentage using serum albumin, serum transferrin, triceps skinfold, and DHR (Busby, Mullen, Mathews, Hobbs, & Rosato, 1995). The index identifies patients who will benefit from nutrition support although it does not identify specific nutrient deficiencies. See Table 19-2.

The Subjective Global Assessment of nutritional status is a bedside tool that evaluates history of weight change, dietary intake, gastrointestinal symptoms, functional impairment, muscle wasting, fat loss, and edema. Scoring rates the patient as well nourished, mildly/moderately undernourished, or severely malnourished. The tool can be accessed at several Internet sites.

The Mini Nutritional Assessment (MNA) uses anthropometric measures (weight, height, weight loss), general assessment (lifestyle, medication, mobility), dietary assessment (number of meals, food and fluid intake, autonomy of feeding), and subjective assessment (self-perception of health and nutrition) to evaluate nutritional status (Gibson, 2005). The Mini Nutritional Assessment has been validated in long-term care (Thomas, Kamel, & Morley, 2004). It, too, can be accessed on the Internet.

▬▬ MANAGEMENT PLAN

Nutrition support for patients/residents is warranted for those:

- Who cannot eat
- Who refuse to eat enough
- Whose increased caloric and/or protein needs cannot be met by their usual diets
- Who should not eat due to certain gastrointestinal pathologies
- For whom the benefits of improved nutrition are greater than the treatment risks
- Without an advance directive restricting nutritional support in terminal conditions

Conditions of particular concern in the nursing home include, but are not limited to, protein-energy malnutrition (PEM), undernutrition, dehydration, pressure ulcers, and chronic disease states.

Protein-Energy Malnutrition

Protein-energy malnutrition (PEM) is a complex entity that is made up of marasmus and kwashiorkor. Marasmus is defined as a primary chronic *calorie deficiency* involving many

---

TABLE 19-2   Calculation of the Prognostic Nutritional Index

$$PNI (\%) = 158 - (16.6 \times ALB) - (0.78 \times TSF) - (0.2 \times TFN) - (5.8 \times DHR)$$

Where:

ALB = serum albumin (g/dL), TSF = triceps skinfold (mm), TFN = serum transferrin (g/dL), DHR = delayed hypersensitivity reactivity (grade of reactivity to any of the three antigens (mumps, streptokinase-streptodornase, *Candida*), all graded: 0 = nonreactive, 1 = < 5 mm, 2 = > 5 mm).

Score: Low risk (< 40%), intermediate risk (40–50%), high risk (> 50%).

specific nutrients as well. Individuals adapt and use body energy stores while sparing lean body mass. Their basal metabolism is decreased to conserve energy. Hormones regulating energy are also affected. Insulin is decreased and glucagon is increased. The latter promotes fatty acid release from adipose tissue and production of ketone bodies. Glucocorticoids are required to release amino acids from the muscle for gluconeogenesis. However, the adaptation associated with starvation prevents this increase, and there is a decrease in glucocorticoids leading to the preservation of muscle. There is also decreased synthesis of tri-iodothyronine resulting in a lowering of the basal metabolic rate. In the long term these individuals utilize most of their body fat due to starvation and they appear emaciated.

In contrast, kwashiorkor is a *protein deficiency* with accompanying hypoalbuminemia (< 2.8 g/dL). It is an acute response and is referred to as hypoalbuminemic stress syndrome. These patients do not adapt to stressful situations, and therefore, both stored fat and muscle protein are used for energy. There is depression of the immune response with increased risk of infection and failure in wound healing.

Marasmus and kwashiorkor can occur separately or in combination. In the latter instance it is referred to as *protein-calorie malnutrition*. In reality there is no clear-cut demarcation of these two conditions, and usually the symptoms include those associated with both calorie and protein deficiencies.

Kwashiorkor can develop very rapidly, and marasmus is the result of a slow gradual process of wasting that goes through stages of underweight followed by mild, moderate, and severe cachexia. The hypermetabolic state in kwashiorkor requires aggressive feeding but marasmus needs a gradual refeeding protocol to avoid any complications of the refeeding syndrome (Shils, Shike, Ross, Caballero, & Cousins, 2006; Skipper, 1998).

The diagnosis of PEM is difficult in older adults because in most instances it may be secondary to an underlying illness such as cancer, cardiovascular disease, or a gastrointestinal disorder. It becomes a challenge to differentiate the underlying disease from malnutrition and to separate their effects on patient outcome. In seriously ill patients, the clinician needs to make a sound clinical judgment prioritizing treatment of the medical problem versus nutritional interventions.

Nonpharmacologic Interventions

Oral Nutrition Therapy

The thrust of any intervention is to correct the underlying cause of malnutrition as soon as it is diagnosed. If the gut is functional, nutrition support for involuntary weight loss must be decided on the basis of other related factors that affect food consumption. The focus of the nutrition plan is to increase energy intake by creating an environment that enhances food intake. The facility should provide culturally acceptable meals, adequate in energy and protein, that incorporate individual preferences. The adequacy of nutrients consumed by mouth and the ability and willingness of the patient to eat are determined before resorting to alternative methods such as enteral or parenteral nutrition.

- The following are the energy and protein requirements recommended for involuntary weight loss:
  - ○ Kilocalories = 30–35 kcal/kg/day
  - ○ Protein = 1.5 g/kg/day.
  - ○ Fat intake estimated at 30% of the total kilocalories
  - ○ Fluid intake at 1 L/1000 kcal
  - ○ In the case of protein energy malnutrition it is important to provide a calorie to nitrogen ratio ranging from 150:1 to 200:1 for optimum utilization of the protein within the total kilocalorie requirement.

- Diets ranging from clear liquid diets, full-liquid diets, mechanically altered diets, soft diets, and regular diets can be ordered to accommodate the specific needs of the patient.

  ○ The American Dietetics Association (2005) supports the concept of using less restricted diets made up of regular foods rather than an energy-controlled diet for frail older adults. Restrictive diets limiting particular foods may be low in calories and unpalatable. A liberalized diet improves compliance and the general well-being of patients.

  ○ In contrast, a rationale presented by the Society of Critical Care Medicine states that standard nutritional regimens can result in overfeeding of many critically ill patients leading to adverse consequences. They recommend providing a caloric intake of 20 kcal/g for patients with normal body mass index instead of the common strategy of giving a caloric intake of 25 kcal/g (Mazuski, 2004). The higher caloric intake should be restricted to critically ill patients with severe pre-existing malnutrition.

  ○ Diet modifications in the amounts of carbohydrate, fat, cholesterol, sodium, calcium, and other nutrients for specific chronic diseases must be assessed on the basis of risks versus benefits. A restrictive nutrition intervention may not be conducive for a nursing home resident who has a poor appetite and involuntary weight loss. The clinician should strive for a balanced approach between medical nutrition requirements and quality of life needs. Decisions to modify a therapeutic diet to meet these needs should be clearly documented in the medical record.

  ○ Snacks and high-calorie, high-protein, nutrient-rich oral supplements can be used to improve body weight and energy intake.

Oral medical nutrition therapy may include nutritional supplements. These can be tailored to any necessary fluid restriction by ordering a formula in concentrations of 1–2 kcal/mL. Supplements should be given at least one hour before a meal. Consistency of intake is required for effective weight gain. Summarizing evidence for the management of nutritional deficiencies with oral therapies in long-term care residents, Thomas et al. (2004) suggest:

- Give liquid supplements as the fluid for oral medication administration.
- Nutrient-dense supplements are hyperosmolar and may cause diarrhea.
- Order lactose-free formulas for lactose intolerant residents.
- Order fiber-rich formulas for constipation.
- Limit carbohydrates for patients with pulmonary disease.
- Order increased branched chain amino acids for liver disease.
- Decrease protein in renal disease.
- Use elemental formulas with free amino acids and monosaccharides for residents with malabsorption syndromes.

Finally, do not disregard exercise as a treatment for weight loss in selected elderly residents. Sarcopenia may be a contributing factor to weight loss in some individuals, due to reduced physical activity. With medical clearance, a resident may be referred to a kinesiologist or physical therapist for resistance exercise training, which has demonstrated effectiveness for nursing home residents to enhance not only weight but also strength, functional capacity, bone health, and protein retention.

Dehydration
Dehydration is a common problem among older adults in institutional settings. Normal fluid homeostasis is defined as the correct proportion of fluid to the major electrolytes

(sodium and potassium) in the intracellular and extracellular compartments of the body. There are three types of dehydration: hypertonic, isotonic, and hypotonic.

- *Hypertonic* dehydration or hypernatremic dehydration occurs when water losses are greater than sodium losses, such as occurs with fever or the use of laxatives or diuretics.

- *Isotonic* dehydration is present when equal amounts of water and sodium are lost as in the case of vomiting, diarrhea, and other forms of GI fluid losses.

- *Hypotonic* dehydration or hyponatremic dehydration is the excessive loss of sodium relative to water, as seen in glucocorticoid deficiency, hypothyroidism, and syndrome of inappropriate antidiuretic hormone secretion (SIADH) (Niedert & Dorner, 2004).

Inadequate consumption of water is the major cause of dehydration among the elderly. The thirst sensation and total body water decrease with aging. Environmental factors and medications also contribute to dehydration. Management of dehydration requires both water and sodium replacement.

To prevent dehydration among nursing home residents, care is taken to increase fluid intake to equal the water requirement of 1.5 L/day. Older adults must be encouraged to drink more often rather than large quantities at one time. The facility must also provide access to water for those with poor mobility. Residents with difficulties swallowing or with dysphagia can be offered flavored gelatin. Low-osmolality drinks such as broth, sports drinks, and water or high-osmolality drinks such as fruit juices and sugared drinks are additional choices to ensure adequate fluid intake. Despite all efforts, if sufficient fluid intake cannot be achieved, subcutaneous infusion (hypodermoclysis) has been used with some success.

Enteral/Parenteral Nutrition

Nutrition support in the form of enteral or parenteral feeding is used as a last alternative when older adults are unable to meet their nutritional requirements orally. The decision to provide nonoral nutrition is based on the functional capacity of the GI tract, the long-term outcome, and quality-of-life issues for the patient. The major types of nutrition support are enteral feeding via a functional gastrointestinal tract and parenteral feeding via the intravenous route in the presence of a nonfunctioning GI tract (Matarese & Gottschlich, 2003).

Enteral Nutrition

Enteral nutrition can be delivered by orogastric, nasogastric, or nasointestinal (nasoduodenal, nasojejunal) routes. Nasoenteric tubes should only be used for short term therapy (< 30 days). Feeding tubes can also be surgically placed as percutaneous endoscopic gastrostomy (PEG) or percutaneous endoscopic jejunostomy (PEJ) tubes. These tubes can be used for longer periods of time. Jejunal tubes should be selected for patients with recurrent tube-feeding aspiration (ASPEN, 1998).

The administration of enteral tube feedings can be continuous (usually tolerated the best) or by intermittent/bolus delivery over 30–60 minutes several times per day. The method of administration is based on the patient's medical condition, GI function, and feeding route. Continuous feeding is required when the tube is in the small bowel. Slower initial rate of delivery, with gradual advance to desired level, may minimize intolerance and refeeding syndrome.

Types of enteral feeding formulas (see Table 19-3) include the following:

- *Polymeric formulas* made up of intact nutrients providing 1–2 kcal/ml. These are further classified into, blenderized (1 kcal/ml) food products, milk-based products, hypercaloric (1.5–2.0 kcal/ml) lactose-free products, and normocaloric (1 kcal/ml) lactose-free

TABLE 19-3 Composition of Enteral Nutrition Solutions

	kcal/mL	PROTEIN g/L (% kcal)	FAT g/L (% kcal)	CHO g/L (% kcal)	FIBER g/L	mOsm/kg	WATER %	VOL. TO MEET RDA
Elemental/ hydrolyzed protein (e.g., Criticare HN)	1.5	38 (14)	5.3 (4.5)	220 (81.5)		650	83	1890
Fiber (e.g., Ensure with Fiber)	1.1	37.2 (14.1)	37.2 (30.5)	162 (55)	14.4	480	82.9	1420
Polymeric formulas, general purpose (e.g., Ensure)	1.06	37.2 (14.1)	25.8 (22)	169 (63.9)		555	84.5	1887
Disease-specific (e.g., Pulmocare)	1.5	62.6 (16.7)	93.3 (55.1)	105.7 (28.2)		475	78.5	947
Renal disease (e.g., Suplena)	2.0	30.0 (6)	95.6 (43.0)	255.2 (51.0)		600	71.2	947
Blenderized (e.g., Compleat Modified)	1.07	43.0 (16)	37 (31)	140 (53)	4.4	300	83.7	1500

	COMPONENTS PER SERVING (1 TBSP)							
	kcal	FAT						
Modular formula (e.g., MCT oil)	115	14						

Provides fat as a single nutrient to alter the nutrient composition of commercial formulas or food; may also provide electrolytes and increase renal or osmotic load.

	COMPONENTS PER SERVING (1 PACKET)							
	kcal	PRO	CHO	ARGININE g				
Resource Arginaid	35	4.5	4.0	4.5				

products. The normocaloric lactose-free products are isotonic, hypertonic, high nitrogen, or fiber containing. Fiber-containing formulas have low osmolality, and the fibers are derived from natural food sources or soy polysaccharide.

- *Elemental formulas* are lactose free and contain partially or fully hydrolyzed nutrients with 1–1.3 kcal/ml. These are unpalatable and usually hyperosmolar.
- *Modular formulas* have 2.8–4.0 kcal/ml and contain single macronutrients (glucose polymers, lipids, proteins).

- *Specialty formulas* are formulated for specific diseases such as diabetes, renal failure, and pulmonary or liver diseases. These formulas may need supplementation with vitamins or minerals.

Parenteral Nutrition

Parenteral nutrition is used when the function of the GI tract is impaired or the nature of the illness prevents access to it. Nutrients are delivered directly into the bloodstream through a catheter tip placed in the superior vena cava. Total parenteral nutrition (TPN) is delivered through large central veins, while peripheral parenteral nutrition (PPN) is delivered through smaller peripheral veins. Placement must be confirmed with chest X-ray. Modes of delivery can be continuous (24 hours/day) or cyclic at a fixed rate over 8–16 hours (ASPEN). Slower initial rate of delivery with gradual advance to ordered level may minimize intolerance and refeeding syndrome.

The TPN solutions contain all essential nutrients. Carbohydrates are delivered as dextrose, protein as amino acids, and lipids as an emulsion of essential fatty acids. The solutions used for parenteral nutrition are referred to as two in one (dextrose + protein) or three in one (dextrose + protein + lipids). See Table 19-4.

Delivery of solution through a peripheral vein requires a reduction in osmolarity

TABLE 19-4 Composition of Parenteral Solutions

	20% LIPID EMULSIONS	
	INTRALIPID 20%	**LIPOSYN II 20%**
kcal/mL	2	2
Fat content (g/100 mL)		
Safflower oil	—	10
Sunflower oil	20	10
Fatty acids (%)		
Linoleic acid	50	65.8
Oleic acid	26	17.7
Palmitic acid	10	6.6
Stearic acid	3.5	3.4
Linolenic acid	9	4.2
mOsm/L	260	258

	AMINO ACID SOLUTIONS		
	AMINOSYN II **FREAMINE III** **(10% SOLUTIONS)**		**HEPATAMINE** **(8% SOLUTION)**
Nitrogen (g/100 mL)	1.53	1.53	1.2
Essential amino acids (mg/100 mL)			
Isoleucine	660	690	900
Leucine	1000	910	1100
Lysine	1050	730	610
Methionine	172	530	100
Phenylalanine	298	560	100
Threonine	400	400	450
Tryptophan	200	150	66
Valine	500	660	840
Nonessential amino acids (mg/100 mL)			
Alanine	993	710	770
Arginine	1018	950	600
Proline	722	1120	800
Serine	530	590	500
Taurine	—	—	—
Histidine	300	280	240
Tyrosine	270	—	—

(Continued)

TABLE 19-4   Composition of Parenteral Solutions (*Continued*)

AMINO ACID SOLUTIONS

	AMINOSYN II	FREAMINE III (10% SOLUTIONS)	HEPATAMINE (8% SOLUTION)
Glycine	500	1400	900
Cysteine	—	< 20	< 20
Glutamic acid	738	—	—
Aspartic acid	700		
Electrolytes (mEq/L)			
Sodium	45.3	10	10
Chloride	—	< 3	< 3
Acetate	71.8	89	62
Phosphate (mmol/L)	—	10	—
mOsm/L	873	950	768–785
pH	5–6.5	6–7	6–7

PARENTERAL NUTRITION DAILY REQUIREMENTS

CALORIES	PROTEIN	FAT	FLUID	ELECTROLYTE VITAMIN MINERAL TRACE ELEMENT
25–30 kcal/kg	0.8–2.0 g/kg, 1.2–2.0 g/kg (catabolic). Start with 0.6 g/kg and increase to 1–1.2 g/kg (hepatic encephalopathy). Start with 0.6 g/kg if protein restriction is appropriate and then increase based on clinical condition (renal failure not on dialysis); 1.0–1.2g/kg (renal failure on dialysis); peritoneal dialysis may need more protein	< 30% of total kcals	30 mL/kg	TPN RDA

ENTERAL NUTRITION DAILY REQUIREMENTS

CALORIES	PROTEIN	FAT	FLUID	ELECTROLYTE VITAMIN MINERAL TRACE ELEMENT
25–30 kcal/kg	0.8–2.0 g/kg; 1.2–2.0 g/kg (catabolic). Start with 0.6 g/kg and increase to 1–1.2 g/kg (hepatic encephalopathy). Start with 0.6 g/kg and increase according to clinical condition (renal failure not on dialysis); 1.0–1.2 g/kg (renal failure on dialysis)		30 mL/kg	

limited to 900 mOsm/L. The low osmolarity is necessary to prevent inflammation of the vein (thrombophlebitis). Provision of adequate fat is not possible with this low osmolarity. A high volume of fluid is also required to provide adequate calories in PPN. These considerations prevent PPN being used to sustain long-term energy requirements. Furthermore, the catheter must be replaced frequently. It is, therefore, recommended for patients who do not require more than 10–14 days of support.

The composition of parenteral nutrition solutions is the following:

- Dextrose provides 3.4 kcal/g in concentrations of 5–70%.
- Amino acids provide 4.0 kcal/g in concentrations of 3–15%.
- Lipids provide 9.0 kcal/g in concentrations of 10%, 20%, or 30%.
- Minerals, vitamins, trace elements, and electrolytes have to be added daily to parenteral nutrition solutions based on the clinical status, renal function, nutritional status, and patient's medications.
- Fluid intake must be monitored carefully in patients receiving parenteral nutrition.

Refeeding Syndrome

In the severely debilitated and malnourished patient, refeeding syndrome may occur when nutrition rich in carbohydrates is introduced too quickly into the diet. This stimulates insulin release and draws potassium, magnesium, and phosphorus intracellularly. Resulting electrolyte imbalances can potentiate cardiac problems, sodium and water retention, and death from respiratory or cardiac failure (Niedert & Dorner, 2004). The syndrome can be avoided with slow introduction of feedings and supplemental electrolytes as needed.

Transitional Feedings

The ultimate goal of any nutrition care plan is to get the patient on an oral feeding modality using the GI tract. A period of adjustment is required when one form of nutrition support is changed to another as, for example, when parenteral feeding is discontinued and the patient is placed on oral or tube feeding. It is important to ensure that throughout the transition period the patient obtains adequate nutrient intake to meet nutritional requirements. The patient has to be monitored carefully to determine tolerance to oral intake, swallowing ability, and GI function. Changes must be introduced gradually to prevent complications such as osmotic diarrhea or problems associated with swallowing. Generally, a low fat, lactose-free diet, low in other simple carbohydrates is recommended initially (Lysen, 1997; Skipper, 1998).

Pharmacologic Interventions

Medications may improve appetite in some individuals. As with all drugs provided to the older adult, attention must be paid to the risk of adverse drug reactions. The following drugs may be helpful in stimulating appetite:

- Vitamins, trace elements, and mineral supplements
- Antidepressants: Mirtazepine (Remeron); other selective serotonin reuptake inhibitors (SSRI) such as fluoxetine (Prozac), sertraline (Zoloft), paroxetine (Paxil); or tricyclic antidepressants (many anticholinergic effects).
- Megesterol acetate (Megace): A synthetic progestin derivative that has been demonstrated to decrease cytokine excess that affects food intake, albumin synthesis, and nitrogen retention (Morley & Thomas, 2004). It is given in larger doses than for cancer patients (800 mg/day in a 40 mg/mL suspension) for 3 months. Side effects may include hyperglycemia, adrenal suppression, impotence, and deep vein thrombosis (do not prescribe for bedridden patients).
- Dronabinol (Marinol) (Schedule III): A synthetic cannabis derivative (tetrahydrocannabinol) with antiemetic, antispasmodic, and analgesic effects. Initial dose is 2.5 mg before the dinner meal. If well tolerated, add 2.5 mg before lunch 2 weeks later. Side effects may include mood disturbances, delirium, drowsiness, tachycardia, hypotension (Morley & Thomas, 2004).

- Anabolic agents: Testosterone and the anabolic steroids nandrolone and oxandrolone may also be effective agents to stimulate appetite and treat sarcopenia. Limited research, however, is available on their effectiveness in long-term care settings (Morley & Thomas, 2004).

PRESSURE ULCERS

Poor nutritional status is a risk factor for the occurrence of pressure ulcers. The prevalence of undernutrition is about 40–85% in long-term care institutions (Niedert & Dorner, 2004). Severe PEM affects tissue repair, the inflammatory reaction, and immune function. The characteristics of skin are altered by advancing age and dehydration; it loses elasticity and moisture. The skin response to temperature, pain, and pressure is decreased.

Pressure ulcers occur over bony prominences and are classified into four stages according to degree of tissue damage. The major risk factors for developing pressure ulcers are: impaired mobility, end-stage renal disease, malnutrition, and being comatose.

- Stage 1 is characterized by an observable pressure-related change of the intact skin. The alterations are: skin temperature (warm or cool), tissue consistency (firm or boggy), sensation of pain and itching.

- Stage 2 is characterized by partial-thickness skin loss involving the epidermis and/or the dermis. The ulcer is superficial and looks like an abrasion, a blister, or a shallow crater.

- Stage 3 is characterized by full-thickness skin loss that involves damage or necrosis of subcutaneous tissue that may extend down to the underlying fascia. The ulcer is seen as a deep crater, with or without undermining of surrounding tissue.

- Stage 4 is characterized by full-thickness skin loss with extensive destruction, tissue necrosis, or damage to muscle, bone, or supporting structures.

Langkamp-Henken, Hudgens, Stechmiller, & Herrlinger-Garcia (2005) used the Mini Nutritional Assessment (MNA), the Mini Nutritional Assessment Screening Form, and the standard nutritional assessment indicators on nursing home patients with pressure ulcers to determine if there was any association among the scores obtained with these three methods. The MNA showed good correlations with the standard indicators, and the researchers concluded that using visceral proteins to screen and assess nutritional status of elderly men with pressure ulcers did not provide any advantage.

The guidelines for daily nutritional support of elderly subjects with pressure ulcers are as follows:

- Energy: 30–35 kcal/kg body weight
- Protein: 1.2–1.5 g protein/kg body weight
- Fluid: Minimum of 1500 mL or 30 mL/kg body weight
- Vitamin A: Daily dietary source is recommended
- Vitamin C: Daily supplement of 500–1000 mg may be beneficial if a patient is deficient in vitamin C or has stage 3 or 4 pressure ulcer
- Zinc: 50 mg/day is often recommended for older adults with poor intake or weight loss who have stage 3 or 4 pressure ulcer. Long-term supplementation is discouraged.

No specific recommendations are given for glutamine and arginine.

CARDIOVASCULAR DISEASE

Diagnosis of risk of heart disease is based, in part, on the lipid profile that includes total cholesterol and two classes of plasma lipoproteins—LDL cholesterol and HDL cholesterol. The National Cholesterol Education Program

TABLE 19-5	Components of the TLC* Diet
Fats:	Limit to 25–35% of total calories
	Saturated fat: Less than 7% of total calories
	Limited trans fatty acids
	Polyunsaturated fat: Up to 10% of total calories
	Monounsaturated fat: Up to 20% of total calories
	Cholesterol: Less than 200 mg/day
Carbohydrate:	50–60% of total calories
	Mostly complex carbohydrates derived from whole grains
	Fruits
	Vegetables
Fiber:	20–30 grams/day
Protein:	Approximately 15% of total calories
Total calories:	To maintain body weight or reduce to desired goal

*Therapeutic lifestyle change

Adult Treatment Panel III (ATP III) guidelines (2001) are used for assessment. The ATP III treatment focuses on lowering LDL and recommends therapeutic lifestyle changes (TLC) that are mainly dietary (Table 19-5). Addition of plant stanol/sterols (2 g/day) and viscous (soluble) fiber (10–25 g/day) enhance LDL-C lowering. Inclusion of foods fortified or rich in folate reduces the risk associated with homocysteine excess. Physical activity is emphasized as part of the TLC.

HYPERTENSION

Medical nutrition therapy is individualized because of the variation in the causes and severity of hypertension in the elderly. Weight loss (if the individual is overweight) is a major strategy that lowers blood pressure. Initiating physical activity especially if the individual is sedentary, reducing alcohol intake, and decreasing sodium intake (2400 mg) with a concurrent increase in calcium, magnesium, and potassium intakes are lifestyle changes recommended in the 7th report of

the Joint Committee on Prevention, Detection, Evaluation, and Treatment of High Blood Pressure (USDHHS, 2004). The Dietary Approaches to Stop Hypertension (DASH) diet incorporates most of the changes outlined. It is a diet high in fruits, vegetables, and low-fat dairy products that has been shown to lower blood pressure. Drug therapy is indicated when the lifestyle modifications are ineffective (see Chapter 6).

DIABETES

The goals for medical nutrition therapy for older adults is to provide adequate kilocalories and essential nutrients based on individual needs so that plasma glucose levels are maintained within the acceptable range. This dietary modification is made to effectively manage any other coexisting illnesses. The daily diet composition is the following:

- Carbohydrate and monounsaturated fat together = 60–70% of total energy needs
- Dietary fiber = 15–20 g
- Saturated fat = < 10% of total kilocalories
- Polyunsaturated fat = 10% of total kilocalories
- Cholesterol = < 300 mg
- Protein = 15–20% of total kilocalories.

Alcohol must be consumed with food to prevent hypoglycemia and is limited to one drink daily for women and 2 drinks for men as is the case for the general public. A daily multivitamin tablet is recommended especially if caloric intake is reduced. In general, nursing home residents are underweight and a change in body weight is a reasonably reliable indicator of poor nutritional status. Therefore, if weight changes of 10% of body weight occurs in less than 6 months, an evaluation must be made to rule out diet-related causes.

The focus in diabetes management is on total carbohydrate rather than the source (starch versus sugar) or type (high- or low-glycemic index foods) of carbohydrate. Restriction of sucrose or sucrose-containing foods is not necessary as long as they are included in the total carbohydrate count. When changes in fiber intake are made, if individuals are not ambulatory, it is important to monitor fluid intake to prevent dehydration. Lowering protein intake to 0.8 g/kg is recommended if there is renal involvement. Medical nutrition therapy is individualized factoring in the patient's likes, dislikes, and lifestyle. Consistency and timing of meals is important if insulin dosage is not adjusted before meals.

WEB SITES

- Journal of Enteral and Parenteral Nutrition—http://jpen.aspenjournals.org
- Medical Algorithm Project—http://www.medal.org

REFERENCES

American Dietetics Association. (2005). Position of the American Dietetics Association: Liberalization of the diet prescription improves quality of life for older adults in long term care. *Journal of the American Dietetics Association, 105*(12), 1955–1965.

A.S.P.E.N. Board of Directors and The Clinical Guidelines Task Force. (January/February, 2002). Guidelines for the use of parenteral and enteral nutrition in adult and pediatric patients. *Journal of Enteral and Parenteral Nutrition, 26*(1, Suppl.).

Beck, F. K., & Rosenthal, T. C. (2002). Prealbumin: A marker for nutritional evaluation. *American Family Physician, 65*, 1575–1578. Retrieved January 23, 2006, from http://www.aafp.org/afp/20020415/1575.html

Bernstein, L., Bachman, T. E., Meguid, M., Ament, M., Baumgartner, T., Kinosian, B., et al. (1995). Prealbumin in Nutrition Consensus Group: Measurement of visceral protein status in assessing protein and energy malnutrition standard of care. *Nutrition, 11*, 169–171.

Busby, G. P., Mullen, J. L., Mathews, D. C., Hobbs, C. L., & Rosato, E. F. (1995). Prognostic nutritional index in gastrointestinal surgery. *American Journal of Surgery, 139*, 160–167.

DiMaria-Ghalili, R. A., & Amella, E. (2005). Nutrition in older adults: Intervention and assessment can help curb the growing threat of malnutrition. *American Journal of Nursing, 105*(3), 40–50.

Gibson, R. S. (2005). *Principles of nutritional assessment* (2nd ed.). New York: Oxford University Press.

Langkamp-Henken, B., Hudgens, J., Stechmiller, J. K., & Herrlinger-Garcia, K. A. (2005). Mini nutritional assessment and screening scores are associated with nutritional indicators in elderly people with pressure ulcers. *Journal of the American Dietetics Association, 105*, 1590–1596.

Lysen, L. K. (1997). *Quick reference to clinical dietetics*. Gaithersburg, MD: Aspen.

Matarese, L. E., & Gottschlich, M. M. (2003). *Contemporary nutrition support practice: A clinical guide* (2nd ed.). Philadelphia: Saunders.

Mazuski, J. E. (2004). Rationale for underfeeding the critically ill patient. *Critical Connections, 3*, 8.

Morley, J. E. (1997). Anorexia of aging: Physiologic and pathologic. *American Journal of Clinical Nutrition, 66*, 760–773. Retrieved January 26, 2006, from http://www.ajcn.org/cgi/reprint/66/4/760

Morley, J. E., & Thomas, D. R. (2004). Update: Guidelines for the use of orexigenic drugs in long-term care. *Annals of Long-Term Care, 12*(Suppl.)

Niedert, K. C., & Dorner, B. (Eds.). (2004). *Nutrition care of the older adult: A handbook for dietetic professionals working throughout the continuum of care*. (2nd ed.). Chicago: American Dietetic Association.

Niedert, K. C., & Dorner, B. (2004). Rationale for underfeeding of the critically ill. *Critical Connections, 4*(6). Retrieved January 29, 2006, from http://www.sccm.org/publications/critical_connections/2004_06dec/rationale.asp

Shils, M. E., Shike, M., Ross, A. C., Caballero, B., & Cousins, R. J. (2006). *Modern nutrition in health and disease* (10th ed.). Philadelphia: Lippincott, Williams & Wilkins.

Skipper, A. (Ed.). (1998). *Dietitian's handbook of enteral and parenteral nutrition* (2nd ed.). Gaithersburg, MD: Aspen.

Sullivan, D. H., & Walls, R. C. (1995). The risk of life-threatening complications in a select population of geriatric patients: The impact of nutritional status. *Journal of the American College of Nutrition, 14,* 29–36.

Thomas, D. R., Kamel, H. K., & Morley, J. E. (2004). Nutritional deficiencies in long-term care, part II: Management of protein energy malnutrition and dehydration. *Annals of Long-Term Care, 12*(Suppl.)

BIBLIOGRAPHY

Detsky, A. S., McLaughlin, J. R., Baker, J. P., Johnston, N., Whitaker, S., Mendelson, R. A., et al. (1987). What is subjective global assessment of nutritional status. *Journal of Parenteral and Enteral Nutrition, 11,* 8–13.

CHAPTER 20

Rehabilitation

Aquilina Saw and Deborah Truax

PRINCIPLES OF REHABILITATION

Introduction

Over the past three decades, the nursing home has emerged as an important site for rehabilitation, especially for the geriatric population. This metamorphosis is the result of converging social, political, and economic forces, including the following:

- The increasing age and frailty of the population

- Legislative incentives, such as Medicare, the prospective payment system of hospital reimbursement (PPS), and Medicaid

- Expansion and "medicalization" of the nursing home industry

- Recognition of the central role of rehabilitation in the care of the elderly (Joseph & Wanlass, 1993)

Unlike outpatient and home rehabilitation, nursing homes provide for the resident's medical and personal care needs 24 hours a day. The best nursing home-based geriatric rehabilitation programs include comprehensive interdisciplinary assessment and treatment planning (Joseph & Wanlass, 1993).

The American Geriatrics Society (AGS) defines rehabilitation as the maintenance and restoration of physical and psychological health necessary for independent living and functional independence. For some individuals, declining mobility leads to loss of independence. Progress in medicine and surgery has made it possible for acutely or chronically ill elderly patients to survive longer periods of time, but all too often the price of survival is a physical disability. The importance of rehabilitation programs that have the potential to restore function, prolong independence, and improve quality of life following injury or illness is readily apparent in the geriatric population. Rehabilitation services should be available in all settings in which older persons receive care including hospitals, nursing homes, outpatient clinics and home care programs. In addition, utilization review of rehabilitation services is needed to ensure that effective and necessary services are provided in an efficient manner (AGS, 1999).

Medicare Coverage

The 65-years and older population is growing, with the "oldest old" group, persons at or over the age of 85 years, being the fastest growing segment of the United States. The incidence and prevalence of disease and chronic conditions increase with advancing age. The geriatric patient can present with a complex set of issues and associated disability (Stewart, Phillips, Bodeneheier, & Cifu, 2004). Medicare coverage for hospital care is used by 20% of beneficiaries each year and continues to be the single most expensive component of the Medicare benefit. However, rehabilitative services provided to patients after acute care hospital stays are the fastest growing component. Medicare payments to skilled nursing facilities for postacute care rose from $2.5 billion to $11.7 billion between 1990 and 1996, and the charges for ancillary therapy and medications accounted for more than half of these expenditures (Frampton, 2005).

A nursing home receives payment for rehabilitation therapies either through Medicare Part A or Medicare Part B. Medicare Part A is used for nursing home stays that require short-term rehabilitation following an acute care hospitalization (three days or longer) or within 30 days of a previous nursing home stay using a prospective payment methodology. Medicare Part A covers up to 100 days of skilled nursing care only if the following occurs:

- Admission to a nursing home is within 30 days of hospitalization for care that is a continuation of treatment received during the hospital stay.

- Skilled rehabilitation services are required 5 days a week.

- It is only practical to provide therapy on an inpatient basis.

- Continual improvement is documented.

Medicare Part B may cover short-term skilled rehabilitation services—speech, physical, or occupational therapy—2–3 times a week for residents who are not eligible for coverage under Part A. However, coverage continues only as long as significant improvement is shown.

The Interdisciplinary Team

Interdisciplinary assessment benefits the geriatric population in several ways. Geriatric assessments, which include functional as well as traditional medical evaluations, provide improved clinical care by targeting planned interventions. The ability to reliably test persons over time supports research that in turn supports care models that are optimal for older adults.

Studies have shown that improved outcomes for patients receiving rehabilitation in the nursing home setting were associated with the following conditions:

- An on-site rehabilitation program with an interdisciplinary team

- Increased physician or nurse practitioner involvement and the presence of a teaching program

- Intensity of physical therapy and physical therapy hours available at the institution (Joseph & Wanlass, 1993)

An interdisciplinary approach focuses on patient and team goals, regular and effective communication, coordination, and integration of care. Regular team communication is necessary to discuss patient goals and outcomes and to adjust the program accordingly (Stewart et al., 2004). Nurse practitioners and physicians should work closely with experienced rehabilitation therapists in setting realistic and individualized goals for their patients. The goals should be compatible with the patient's preferences and socioeconomic environment, and should be directed toward maximum functional outcomes realistic for that patient (Kane, 2003).

Often patients admitted to a skilled nursing facility for rehabilitation have a variety of concerns that need to be addressed, including health, psychosocial, and financial issues.

Rehabilitative or restorative care for older persons with complex needs is therefore optimally provided by an interdisciplinary approach, which may involve physical, speech, occupational, and recreational therapists; physicians; social workers; and nurse practitioners. Physiatrists can be very helpful in developing appropriate and optimal rehabilitation plans for patients with complicated needs.

It is helpful to have regular team conferences to discuss the patient's progress. Members of the team include the physician, nurse practitioner, physical therapist, occupational therapist, speech therapist, nursing, and social services. The physician or the nurse practitioner can serve as the coordinator and team leader during the meeting. Patients are reviewed for weekly progress or lack of progress over the past week. Relevant information from each discipline is presented, both to ensure proper utilization and discuss problems and issues that affect patient care, progress, or outcomes. Barriers preventing a patient from making progress with their rehabilitation goals should be identified and documented. Examples of barriers may be cognitive impairment, significant pulmonary or cardiac disease, a poorly motivated patient, or severity of the underlying condition for which the patient is receiving therapy. Modification of therapy programs and the development of new goals may have to be accomplished in the presence of barriers.

Effects of Aging on Rehabilitation

The most common conditions in the elderly that require rehabilitation include arthritis and musculoskeletal problems, stroke, hip fracture, amputations, falls, and medical deconditioning and frailty (Frampton, 2005). It is important for the nurse practitioner to understand the important age-related challenges in rehabilitation caused by the high prevalence of multiple comorbid conditions seen in the elderly population. Changes in the physiologic processes accompanying aging render elderly persons more susceptible to acute and chronic illnesses and prolong recovery from these illnesses. However, declining functional status and disability is not an inevitable consequence of aging.

To optimally rehabilitate the older patient, the clinician must consider the normal physiologic changes of aging and their effects on functional status. The gradual decline of health and increased incidence of injury and diseases experienced by older individuals can be partially attributed to the gradual loss of physiologic reserves. Throughout youth and early adulthood, individuals have reserve physiologic capacities and system redundancies that enable them to adapt to physical challenges and injury without loss in functional abilities. With aging, there is a loss in this reserve capacity and redundancy. Changes in muscle tissue, articular cartilage, intervertebral disks, tendons, ligaments, and joint capsules result in increased susceptibility to injury from repetitive use or trauma. Age-related alterations in bone dramatically increase the risk of fracture with age (Voight, 2001).

Coexisting pathologic processes can exacerbate the effects of other conditions and result in greater functional limitations and disability. Rehabilitation programs must take into consideration the whole person with multiple system involvement. Chronic conditions occur more frequently with age, accumulating as people live longer. Some of the chronic conditions often experienced by older adults include the following:

- Cardiovascular disease and hypertension
- Diabetes
- Obesity
- Chronic obstructive pulmonary disease and asthma
- Parkinson's disease
- Alzheimer's disease and other dementias

- Osteoarthritis and rheumatoid arthritis
- Sensory disorders including visual and auditory disorders

Communication is essential in rehabilitation, specifically improving any sensory impairment, including vision and hearing. *Hearing loss* has a major contribution to communication and quality-of-life issues. Hearing loss can result in withdrawal, poor self-concept, depression, frustration, cognitive impairment, isolation, loneliness, and compromised physical mobility. People who use hearing aids are more likely than others to report improvements in their physical, emotional, and social comfort (Muche, 2005). This possibility for improved function emphasizes the need for hearing evaluations and treatment to help the patient make the maximal gains possible during rehabilitation.

With aging, the gradual deterioration of sensory modalities, including *vision,* can interfere with one's daily activities. If any change in vision is noted or if the patient reports a functional deficit, follow-up with an ophthalmologist is warranted for evaluation.

The *prevention of falls and treatment of osteoporosis* can improve the patient's health and longevity. Older patients who report a fall (or recurrent falls) that is not clearly the result of an accidental trip or slip should be carefully evaluated, even if the falls have not resulted in serious physical injury. A jointly developed set of recommendations for assessing people who fall has been issued by the American Geriatrics Society, the British Geriatrics Society, and the American Academy of Orthopaedic Surgeons (2001). A thorough fall evaluation consists of a detailed history, physical examination, gait and balance assessment, and in certain instances, selected laboratory studies (Kane et al., 2004). See Table 20-1 for recommendations for falls assessment.

Malnutrition affects a patient's functional status and global medical condition. A complete nutritional assessment may be warranted based on the patient's weight, body mass index (BMI), skipped or poor intake of meals, or low serum albumin level. See the chapter on nutrition.

Depression is common in the older population if a functional loss of mobility and an

---

TABLE 20-1   Recommendations for Fall Assessment

1. All older people should be asked about falls in the prior year.
2. Those with a single prior fall should have a "get-up-and-go" test or its equivalent. Those who pass and have no history of falling need nothing further.
3. Those with two or more falls should be given a full fall assessment.
4. Fall assessment consists of the following:

   - History of fall circumstances, medications, acute or chronic medical problems, and mobility levels
   - Examination of vision, gait and balance, lower extremity joint function
   - Basic neurological examination (mental status, muscle strength, lower extremity peripheral nerves, proprioception, reflexes, tests of cortical extrapyramidal, and cerebellar function)
   - Basic cardiovascular assessment (heart rate and rhythm, postural pulse and blood pressure, and possible carotid sinus stimulation test)

Source: American Geriatrics Society, British Geriatrics Society, & American Academy of Orthopaedic Surgeons, 2001.

inability to perform activities of daily living (ADLs) predominate. Persistent depression is associated with a poor outcome in rehabilitation. Since safe, effective treatment exists, persons who fail to make anticipated progress in rehabilitation should be evaluated for depression (Joseph & Wanlass, 1993).

Cognitive impairment such as *delirium* and *dementia* can affect the patient's rehabilitation goals and outcomes. It is imperative to identify and correct the cause of delirium. Factors commonly associated with this syndrome include anticholinergic medications, hypoxia, infection, and urinary retention (Perez, 1994). The treatment of dementia involves improving the patient's quality of life and maximizing functional performance by focusing on cognition, mood, and behavior. See the chapter on psychological disorders for the treatment of depression and dementia.

A driver's evaluation for an appropriate elderly candidate is an underutilized part of rehabilitation that has a considerable impact on society. Clinicians should be aware of and follow state guidelines regarding the reporting of potentially impaired drivers. Regulations vary from state to state. State-mandated tests of visual acuity are associated with lower rates of fatal accidents. In 1996, the California DMV implemented a requirement that physicians must report patients with moderate to severe Alzheimer's disease, and the DMV revokes that patient's license without additional testing. Patients with mild dementia are required to undergo repeat examination to demonstrate their driving abilities (Muche, 2005).

Functional Assessment

The goal of rehabilitation is to restore function and prevent further disability. Careful assessment of the patient's function, the setting of realistic goals, and prevention of secondary disabilities and complications of immobility are repeated measures of functional abilities

that are relevant to the patient's environment, and adapting the environment to the patient's abilities are all essential elements of the rehabilitation process (Kane et al., 2004).

Principles of rehabilitation practice emphasize a holistic assessment of medical condition, functional impairments, handicaps, societal constraints, and utility of adaptive equipment. This comprehensive approach has been shown to improve outcomes in geriatric patients (Stewart et al., 2004). A patient's functional status is usually evaluated by the following professionals:

- The medical team, usually consisting of the physician and nurse practitioner as key members of the rehabilitation team. The medical team is responsible for prescribing interventions that have been objectively defined, meaningful goals and measurable outcomes, and determining which methods of rehabilitation are appropriate. Most patients require some type of physical therapy. Because functional disabilities are so closely intertwined with medical problems the medical team should play a central role in the patient's rehabilitation.

- Occupational and speech therapy may also be indicated depending on the patient's diagnosis and specific needs.

- Physical and occupational therapists can be extremely valuable in assessing, treating, motivating, and monitoring patients whose mobility is impaired.

- Physical therapists generally attend to the relief of pain, muscle strength and endurance, joint range of motion, and gait using a variety of treatment modalities and therapeutic exercises.

- Occupational therapists focus on activities of daily living (ADLs) such as grooming, dressing, eating, and hygiene.

- Even when mobility and function remain impaired, occupational therapists can make life easier for these patients by performing environmental assessments and recommending modifications and assistive devices that will improve the patient's ability to function independently.

- Speech therapists are helpful in assessing and implementing rehabilitation for disorders of communication and swallowing (Kane, 2003).

- Evaluation by a physiatrist can be helpful in evaluating the complex needs of older patients.

Outcome Measures and Tools

In order to assess the effectiveness of rehabilitation, functional outcomes must be measured. There are several measures of disability and ability that are widely used both as clinical assessment tools and in geriatric research. The gold standard for documenting functional progress during inpatient rehabilitation is the Functional Independence Measure (FIM) (see the appendix at the end of this book). The FIM instrument has been tested for adults, including the elderly. The FIM measures disability, and its scores correlate with the level of assistance that is required for basic functions. The FIM is an 18-item assessment of daily living that looks at a seven-level continuum from completely independent to most dependent. The two major domains are motor function and cognition, and the focus is on activities related to independent living. The FIM score can be used to determine a rehabilitation efficiency ratio or the change in FIM score over the length of stay. A score of 18 is completely dependent, and a score of 126 is completely independent (Stewart et al., 2004).

The Katz index of independence in activities of daily living (ADLs) is a widely used scale in the field of geriatrics. It measures ADLs but does not include measures of mobility such as walking or stair climbing. The Katz index can be self-administered by the patient or a caregiver rather than by the clinician. It is not very sensitive to change, however. The Barthel Index is widely used as well and is an ordinal scale of 10 self-care and mobility items (see the appendix at the end of this book). A score of 0 is completely dependent, and a score of 100 is completely independent. It is not very sensitive to changes (Stewart et al., 2004).

In the timed Get Up and Go test, a patient is asked to rise from an armchair, walk 10 feet, turn around, walk back to the chair, and sit down again. The score is the time in seconds it takes to complete these tasks. It predicts whether a patient can walk safely alone outside (Stewart et al., 2004).

The Mini Mental State Examination (MMSE) contains questions on orientation, attention, and other cognitive functions. It is a brief screening tool that allows quantification of cognition over time. It is important to screen separately for both dementia and depression. The Geriatric Depression Scale-Short Form has been validated in persons over the age of 55 years. It is a brief (15-item) questionnaire with yes-no answers that the patient can self-administer (Stewart et al., 2004).

Discharge Planning

Discharge planning should begin at the time of admission. It is based on the patient's wishes, anticipated functional outcome, and psychosocial history, which includes the patient's premorbid personality, lifestyle, coping skills, family relationships, and financial resources. Discharge planning can be hindered if a patient or family member either denies or has difficulty accepting the existence of a disability or has impaired coping skills. A family conference is often helpful in these situations. The key team members involved with the patient's care meet with the patient, family members, and/or caregiver and have a thorough discussion of the progress or lack of progress of the patient and identify reasons for lack of progress or extent of disability. This allows the family to have a better acceptance and develop a realistic discharge plan that is most suitable and safe for the patient.

Therefore, early and ongoing patient and family education is an important part of the patient's stay at the skilled nursing facility. Lack of communication with the patient and family can affect the discharge process. Often a referral to social services at the facility can assist this process and provide patients and families with the necessary resources for discharge.

Typically, patients being discharged from the skilled nursing facility to the community after a course of rehabilitation will need a referral for home or outpatient therapy. Appropriate equipment for home use should be ordered. Necessary follow-up appointments with any specialists (e.g., orthopedic surgeon or the primary care provider who will be assuming care of the patient) should be made and communicated to the patient and family. Discharge instructions including medication review should be done by the nursing staff with the patient and/or family prior to discharge home. A dictated discharge summary by the nurse practitioner or physician at the skilled nursing facility should be completed in order to provide the clinicians in the outpatient setting with pertinent information regarding the patient's stay. This will ensure proper and necessary follow-up care after the patient is discharged home.

STROKE REHABILITATION

Stroke is the acute onset of a focal neurological deficit that lasts for more than 48–72 hours. The impact stroke has on society is very significant, affecting more than 700,000 people annually, of which one third will die, leaving two thirds of the survivors requiring rehabilitation. It is the third leading cause of death in industrialized nations and is second only to head trauma as the leading cause of neurogenic disability.

The incidence of stroke increases with age and ranges from 3/10,000 in the third and fourth decades of life, to 300/10,000 in the seventh and eighth decades of life (Lorish, 1993). In the United States, the incidence is decreasing, but with the increasing proportion of elderly people in the general population, the absolute number of strokes remains high, as is the socioeconomic and healthcare impact on society.

The decreased mortality after stroke leaves over 2 million survivors with multifactorial disabling consequences such as neurologic and functional deficits.

In the NHLB1 Framingham Stroke Study, it was found that 71% of stroke victims had impaired vocational capacity 7 years poststroke; 31% remained dependent in ADL; 20% needed help with mobility, and 16% were institutionalized.

Definition

Stroke rehabilitation is defined as the process by which the handicap and disability resulting from stroke are minimized through the coordinated use of medical, educational, social, and vocational measures in retraining the stroke victim to maximum potential within physiologic and environmental limitation (Zorowitz, 2000). It basically teaches patients new ways to do basic tasks such as ADLs, getting around at home or in the community safely, speaking and communicating, as well as eating strategies. The goals are to help the patients become as independent as possible and to attain the best possible quality of life.

Stroke rehabilitation requires a multidisciplinary team approach. The team members in an acute comprehensive stroke center usually consists of a physician, a nurse (at times, a specialized rehabilitation nurse), physical therapist (PT), occupational therapist (OT), speech therapist (ST), psychologist, social worker (SW), recreational therapist (RT), and in some centers, a kinesiotherapist (KT). In the skilled nursing facility, the team includes a physician/nurse practitioner, physical therapy (PT), occupational therapy (OT), speech therapy (ST), and social worker (SW).

Review of literature showed an equal number of studies to support and dispute the benefits of stroke rehabilitation, the latter especially in light of the spontaneous recovery that occurs after stroke. However, overall, the studies suggest that rehabilitation enhances functional impairment beyond that which can be expected with spontaneous neurologic recovery (Lorish, 1993), but the selection of patients does play a role.

Motor Recovery Poststroke

In 1951, a neurologist, T. E. Twitchell, published the results of his study, long considered a classic, on the motor recovery following stroke involving 121 patients. He noted that there was a remarkable uniformity in the recovery of different cases. Understanding the stages of motor recovery is helpful to the clinician, not only in the initial selection of patients that can benefit from rehabilitation, but also, in the subsequent review of the patients, aligning their progress or lack of progress with the different stages of recovery. It is also beneficial in setting goals as well as in the discharge planning. The stages of motor recovery poststroke are as follows:

- Immediately after onset of stroke, there is a decrease or loss of voluntary movement in the involved limbs and a loss of deep tendon reflexes (DTRs).

- Within 48 hours, the DTRs increase on the affected side, and may require from 3–29 days to develop.

- Within a short period, tone is increased in the wrist and finger flexors, ankle plantar flexors, the upper extremity (UE) adductors and flexors, the lower extremity (LE) adductors and extensors, progressing to developing clonus in 1–38 days.

- In 1–30 days, spasticity appears and the development of the classic hemiplegic posture is noted.

- In the UE, the shoulder is adducted (close to the body) and internally rotated, the elbow is flexed, the forearm pronated, and the wrist and fingers are flexed.

- In the LE, the hip is adducted and extended, the knee is extended, the ankle is plantar flexed, and the foot inverted.

- Recovery of movement is noted from 6–23 days, occurring proximally first in both the UE and LE, so that you see it in the shoulder and in the hip initially. The patient may show shoulder shrugs or a slight to moderate hip flexion usually manifested by a withdrawal response of the leg when given a painful stimulus. The recovering movement occurs in patterns or synergy, of which there are two types, flexor and extensor synergies. For example, attempt at flexion of the shoulder may also result in elbow flexion, forearm pronation, and even wrist and finger flexion, all in varying degrees.

- Although both types of synergy occur in the UE and LE, the flexor synergy predominates in the UE, and the extensor synergy predominates in the LE.

- With continued recovery, spasticity decreases and more volitional or isolated movements occur. The process of recovery is continuous but can stop at any stage and at times may overlap.

One simple bedside test that can help predict potential for gait is asking the patient to do a simple straight leg raise (SLR). If the patient is able to raise the involved lower limb as in doing an SLR, even if it is only a few degrees off the bed, the potential for gait is encouraging as this maneuver puts the involved leg in the higher stage of the recovery process. In doing an SLR maneuver, the patient is demonstrating a volitional, isolated hip flexion and knee extension and not a patterned movement. Therefore that leg is at a higher stage of the recovery process. As most patients are more concerned about being able to walk, this simple bedside test can be very encouraging.

Selection of Patients for Rehabilitation

Neutral predictors on rehabilitation outcome include the following:

- Age
- Sex
- Side of brain affected

Positive predictors on rehabilitation outcome include the following:

- Strong family support
- Good financial resources
- Early referral to rehabilitation
- High educational and socioeconomic level
- Rehabilitation in a comprehensive stroke center

Negative predictors on rehabilitation outcome include the following:

- Long period of coma at onset
- Persistent bowel and bladder incontinence longer than 3 weeks
- Early bowel incontinence
- Severe cognitive and perceptual deficits
- Large or deep lesion on CT scan
- Global aphasia
- Severe neglect or denial
- Severe sensory deficits despite motor return
- Disturbance in verticality
- Persistent poor balance
- Bilaterality of lesions
- Previous CVA
- Persistence of flaccidity longer than 3 weeks in the affected limbs
- Significant comorbid issues (diabetes, cardiac, or musculoskeletal)

Types of Stroke Rehabilitation Programs

Comprehensive Stroke Center

Stroke rehabilitation can be, and traditionally has been, conducted in a hospital-based inpatient rehabilitation unit. There are freestanding comprehensive rehabilitation centers also in the community that provide intensive stroke rehabilitation. Patients admitted to this program are typically medically stable, both from stroke and comorbid medical issues. An initial evaluation by a physician, such as a neurologist or a physiatrist, usually reveals that the patient is suitable for an inpatient, more intensive therapy program with reasonable to good rehabilitation potentials for functional gains. Patients are generally seen by PT, OT, and ST twice a day for a total of at least 3 hours of therapy a day. A rehabilitation nurse sees to it that there is follow through of the lessons learned in therapy during the off-therapy hours. A psychologist, social worker, and recreation therapist (in some centers) also are involved as part of the multidisciplinary team approach.

Skilled Nursing Facility

More stroke patients now receive their rehabilitation in a skilled nursing facility than in any other setting. In 1995, more than 30% of the Medicare patients discharged from the acute care hospital for a stroke received rehabilitation exclusively in a skilled nursing facility. Another 15% had rehabilitation in a skilled nursing facility in combination with an inpatient rehabilitation or home health agency (Kramer & Coleman, 1999).

Typically, these patients are transferred to the skilled nursing facility because initial evaluation at the acute hospital revealed a lower functional level, or significant comorbid medical issues, that render them unable to participate in the 3 hours/day therapy in a hospital-based inpatient program. Most of the patients are elderly with low endurance. In the skilled nursing facility, therapies consist of

TABLE 20-2   Characteristics of Patients with Stroke on Admission to Skilled Nursing Facilities

CHARACTERISTICS	PERCENTAGE
Demographics	
Age (years)	
65–74	22
75–84	47
85+	31
Female	66
Education (< 12 years)	33
Social supports	
Marital status	34
Able and willing caregiver	53
Community residence	89
Comorbidities	
Diabetes	18
Pressure ulcer	13
Fluid and electrolyte problem	9
Dyspnea	14
Seven or > medications	6
Urinary incontinence	69
Cognitive and psychological status	
Always confused	16
Depression	30
Mini Mental Status Exam score < 18	66
Coma	3

Source: Kramer et al., 1997.

PT, OT, and ST occurring generally once a day for 5–6 days a week. Adequacy of nursing staff at each facility has an impact on the carryover of the learned tasks during the off-therapy hours. See Table 20-2.

Outpatient Therapy Program
Often patients enrolled in this program are those with minimal neurologic deficits noted on initial evaluation and are more functional, yet could benefit still from therapy to fine-tune their motor or coordination skills or their ADLs. Some patients that complete their hospital-based inpatient program or have their rehabilitation at a skilled nursing facility and are then discharged home could continue their therapies on an outpatient basis as well

on a less intensive level. Treatment sessions are usually 2–3 times a week, with follow-up usually by a physiatrist. Speech therapy is often one of those areas where patients need a longer time frame to maximize their potentials. These referrals are made prior to their discharge from either the inpatient hospital or the skilled nursing facility with a referral also to the physiatrist for follow-up of the patient's progress usually in 3 weeks after discharge.

Home-Based Rehabilitation Program
This is usually best suited for those patients with transportation problems or those who require treatment by only one of the therapy services. Although this allows flexibility for patients to tailor the program to their own schedules, and also gives them the opportunity to practice the skills they have learned in their own home, the downside to this program is that patients sometimes are not as motivated to perform as when they are on an outside unit. Another disadvantage is that there is no access to specialized equipment. For those purely Medicare patients, lack of transportation is not a valid reason for home-based therapy anymore. Patients must meet Medicare's requirement for "home-bound" status to be eligible for the program.

Components of Stroke Rehabilitation
Early Intervention
Stroke rehabilitation should begin as soon as the patient is neurologically stable. This helps prevent complications of limb contractures, skin compromise from inactivity, deep vein thrombosis (DVT), pulmonary complications, stretched bladder, and aspiration. It also stimulates the patients and thereby minimizes emotional and intellectual regression and depression.

- Position the patient in bed with pillow between the axilla and the body on the involved UE to prevent adduction contracture of the shoulder which will render hygienic care difficult especially in the presence of spasticity.

- Avoid lying on the affected side to decrease edema of the hand and contracture of the limb.

- Frequent change of position, preferably every 2 hours

- Avoid elevating the head of the bed unless other medical issues indicate it, because this promotes hip and knee flexion contracture and may cause shearing forces in the sacral area leading to pressure sores.

- Patients should be positioned in bed so that most of the activities occur on the uninvolved side, especially in the presence of neglect. As neglect decreases or patient develops compensatory training, the bedside table can be moved to the affected side.

- Avoid IV lines on the affected limb.

- Encourage early involvement of the family members or caregiver.

- Personal devices such as dentures, hearing aids, and eyeglasses should be worn daily. Sometimes patients may encounter denture fitting problems poststroke and this contributes to feeding difficulties. This should be resolved as soon as feasible to prevent compromising the patient's nutritional status.

Rehabilitation in the Skilled Nursing Facility

Patients are referred to PT, OT, and ST for initial evaluation and institution of therapy within the patient's tolerance. Each therapy service may begin the training at bedside initially, but attempts to get the patient to the treatment areas are encouraged as soon as tolerated by the patient.

Physical therapy addresses the following areas:

- Bed mobility training includes rolling from side to side and getting up from a supine to sitting position.

- Standing activities begin with sit-to-stand and progress to transfer training to a bedside chair or to a wheelchair.

- Mat activities include working on increasing trunk balance for sitting and standing purposes. Many stroke patients have disturbances in verticality, and working in front of a mirror is helpful. Balance activity is preparatory work for ambulation.

- Passive range of motion (PROM) and active assistive range of motion (AAROM) exercises to the affected limbs and strengthening exercises to the uninvolved limbs are also part of the mat activities. Coordination and endurance exercises are also an important part of therapy.

- Early wheelchair mobility training provides the patient with a mode of ambulation, crucial to the patient's sense of independence, provided that the patient has no significant cognitive/neglect problems and can do the activity safely using the uninvolved upper and lower extremities (UE/LE). A dropped seat (hemi) wheelchair is generally used for stroke patients.

- Ambulation is a goal for most stroke patients, and studies have shown that many patients are able to walk in varying degrees. For ambulation to be successful, the patient must be able to follow verbal or nonverbal instructions, preferably a 3-step command, and maintain standing balance without significant contracture of the involved leg, and have adequate return of volitional control on the involved side to support the hip and knee. The return of good (G) strength in one particular muscle is especially important—the hip extensor. Therefore the detection of early return of this muscle is encouraging.

- Ambulation may begin using the parallel bars, with patients learning weight shifting, maintaining neutral balance, and later on progressing to walking with an assistive aid such as a hemiwalker, hemicane, or front wheel walker, depending on what is available in the involved upper limb that can be used for support. Oftentimes, the PT provides physical assistance in varying degrees, diminishing as the patient progresses. As gait training progresses, the patient is eventually trained in safety on stairs and ramps. It is ideal to check the patient's safety in walking on different surfaces, such as thick carpet, grass, and gravel.

- Oftentimes, a custom molded ankle foot orthosis (AFO) is prescribed to assist ambulation by providing stability to the knee and ankle. Patients can be considered for an AFO if they have good hip strength and fair to good knee strength. There are many types of orthoses available, including off-the-shelf types that in some cases, may suit some selective patients. For the most part, a custom-molded AFO is preferred, and most often, an articulating AFO is used as it gives patients a better gait as well as better assist in stair climbing. It is important to provide the orthotist with clinical information such as the strength of the involved leg, presence/absence of clonus, contractures of the heelcord, and severity of sensory deficits as these factors may affect the orthotic prescription.

- Equipment and home evaluation are services provided by the PT. Equipment may include wheelchair, walkers, canes (large-based quad cane) and ramps for access to home. A dropped seat or hemiwheelchair is most often recommended for easier propulsion as are detachable desk arms and swinging detachable leg rests for easier transfer. A one-arm drive wheelchair is usually not necessary.

- A seat cushion for the wheelchair is needed especially if the patient has limited mobility and anticipates spending a significant amount of time in the wheelchair. Usually, a 3-inch, high-density foam cushion is sufficient unless skin compromise warrants a custom cushion.

- A home evaluation is another helpful assessment to the patient and his family in preparation for discharge. It is important to check out potential barriers at home that may render the patient unsafe and at risk for injury. Sometimes home modifications may be recommended. A PT can obtain basic information from the family about the home environment early on so that potential problems can be resolved ahead before discharge, especially if a home visit is not possible.

- The strategies used by the PT in stroke rehabilitation focus for the most part on functional activities, in addition to the various combination of range-of-motion exercises, strengthening, mobilization, and compensatory techniques generally considered the conventional strategies. There is another group of strategies that were quite popular in the past, the neurophysiological techniques (Bobath/neuromuscular developmental technique [NDT], Brunstrom, proprioceptive neuromuscular facilitation [PNF], etc.), that use therapeutic exercises incorporated with neuromuscular reeducation. There are studies that compared the two groups of strategies and found that patients did better with the conventional strategy when the focus was on function. Still, there is selective sensory stimulation such as tapping or stroking a particular muscle in an attempt to generate a contraction while practicing a particular motor task and this has been shown to have some merit still. Other therapists may use a functional electrical stimulator (FES) as part of muscle reeducation. However, these are not commonly seen in the skilled nursing facility. Sometimes, the PT will work together with the OT and engage patients in games to promote coordination.

Occupational Therapy

- Address ADLs that include feeding, dressing upper and lower body, hygiene, grooming, and toileting. These activities can be done bimanually if the patient has some return on the involved limb, and if none, the OT teaches patients how to do the tasks with one hand, oftentimes with the use of adaptive aids.

- Include passive range of motion (PROM) and active assistive range of motion (AAROM) exercises of the UE, manually or with equipment such as shoulder wheel or skateboard. Remember that the most common cause of a painful shoulder in a hemiplegic patient is tightness caused by inadequate ranging.

- Teach patients self-ROM exercises of the involved limb that the patient can do during off-therapy hours and even at home, as well as compensatory strategies especially in the presence of neglect or visual field defect, while doing the ADL.

- Assess and provide adaptive aids such as eating utensils, rocker knife, suction cups/plates, button hooks, Velcro closure for clothing, sock aids, and reachers.

- Recommend toileting aids such as raised toilet seat, commode, shower aids (tub bench and flexible shower hose), and grab bars.

- Provide edema control measures such as compression glove, pneumatic compression, foam wedge, and Coban wrap.

- Assess for a wrist-hand orthosis (WHO) if indicated to prevent contracture secondary to abnormal flexor posturing or to decrease tone in a spastic hand. There are many prefabricated orthoses available, but they can be custom molded as well.

- Assess and provide other adaptive aids such as a forearm trough for the wheelchair to support the involved upper limb especially if there is subluxation of the shoulder. If the patient has poor trunk balance, a lapboard may be used for support of the UE; it also helps the trunkal balance.

- To sling or not to sling! Some say that slings may contribute to the flexor synergy and contractures. The consensus is that a sling should be worn only when the arm cannot be supported by other means, especially during gait. Note that the presence of increased tone or spasticity in the involved UE may help keep the shoulder in place and a sling will not be necessary.

- In selective patients, a kitchen evaluation can be done by the OT to determine safety of patient in meal preparation at home, as well as to determine the need for modifications and to teach the patient compensatory techniques to minimize energy expenditure while doing kitchen tasks.

Speech and Language Therapies

- Focus on speech and language retrieval poststroke, develop alternative means of communication, evaluate and work on swallowing problems, as well as help patients with cognitive issues, such as problem solving, and social skills needed to cope with the consequences of stroke.

- Dysphagia affects more than 33% of stroke survivors (Veis & Logemann, 1985) and potentially impacts the nutritional state of the patient, with a ripple effect impacting on the patient's strength, and therefore, their ability to participate in other therapies. It is imperative that patients be seen by an ST early. Noninvasive imaging techniques are used by the ST to study the swallowing patterns of the stroke survivors and identify the exact source of the problem.

- Swallowing disorders could be due to a variety of causes such as a delayed or absent swallow reflex, vocal cord paresis, oral apraxia, sensory deficits, lingual/labial/buccal weakness, so that the patient is unable to manipulate food with the tongue, or the inability to detect food remaining lodged or pocketed in the cheeks after swallowing. Patients may drool, or have a wet voice, abnormal cough, choking while eating or drinking, or nasal regurgitation. They may also show cognitive impairment and emotional lability.

- Some patients may require nasogastric tube (NGT) feeding for a period of time, and the ST works closely with the nursing staff, OT, and family members/caregiver regarding feeding precautions and the risk of aspiration.

- Percutaneous endoscopic gastrostomy (PEG) placement should be considered in patients with persistent dysphagia for long-term nutritional support. There is currently no evidence-based data to indicate when to convert from NGT to PEG feeding. PEG placement is better tolerated and safer for long-term nutritional support than is NGT feeding. The invasive nature of PEG placement and the sometimes rapid recovery of oral feeding, however, argue for temporary use of NGT feeding after stroke (Iizuka & Reding, 2005).

- The ST helps patients with dysphagia by devising strategies to overcome or minimize the problem, and this can be by simply changing body position or improving the posture during eating. Additionally, the texture of foods can be modified for easier swallowing; for example, thin liquids which are often a cause of choking, can be thickened. Teaching patients to take small bites and chew slowly are also helpful strategies.

- About one quarter of stroke survivors have some form of language impairment, including the ability to speak, read, write, and understand both spoken and written language. The patient may have expressive aphasia if the damage is to the dominant side of the brain, called Broca's aphasia. If the damage is to the rear of the brain, the patient will have receptive aphasia also known as Wernicke's aphasia.

- Speech and language therapists use special therapeutic techniques to help patients with aphasia. Short-term therapy helps improve comprehension. Other techniques include having the patient repeat the therapist's words, drills on following directions, reading and writing exercises, developing prompts or cues to help the patient recall specific words, and developing strategies such as sign language or alphabet or symbol boards to circumvent the language disability. Nowadays, computers are being used to improve communication. The ST also works with the patient on improving their short-term memory, their ability to process thoughts, and their awareness of their deficits.

- Similar to motor recovery, there is also a spontaneous recovery of language deficits poststroke; this usually occurs in the first 3 months and may continue up to 6 months in some instances. Out of eight group efficacy studies of language therapy, five studies found in their outcome a significant improvement in those who were treated versus those who were untreated or treated late (Orange & Keriesz, 1998).

Interdisciplinary team meetings are usually held weekly. Team members gather to share the weekly clinical and functional condition of the patient. Generally, the nurse reports on the vital signs, nutritional status, any weight change, feeding issues, skin integrity, bowel and bladder program, as well as any interaction that they have had with family members. The clinician gives an update on the overall clinical condition of the patient, the status of comorbid problems, any change in treatment plans, as well as the discharge plans. The various therapists report on the patient's progress or lack of progress, citing possible reasons for the latter, setting new goals based on the changes, and recommending changes in the therapy plans if needed. The social worker reports on the information gathered from the patient or family and potential discharge plans as well as pertinent background information on family dynamics that may affect discharge plans. The clinician documents the input from the team members and makes recommendations for continuation of therapies or preparations for discharge if there has been no consistent progress or if the patient has made the maximum gains from therapies.

Other Issues in Stroke Rehabilitation

Nutrition

Nutrition is an important aspect of a patient's care poststroke. The goal is to estimate the patient's nutritional needs, identify imbalances (especially important in elderly patients who have comorbidities such as hypertension, diabetes mellitus, and chronic kidney disease). Some nutritional considerations include anthropometric measures such as patient's weight, height, and skinfold; patient's dietary history; as well as lab work to include serum protein, albumin, triglycerides, cholesterol, LDL, serum transferring, glucose, electrolytes, BUN, creatinine, liver function, creatinine clearance, and total lymphocyte count.

Skin Care and Pressure Ulcers

It is important to be aware of the areas prone to develop skin compromise when the patient is supine, side lying, semireclined, or sitting up in the wheelchair. The presence of pressure ulcers can affect the patient's participation in therapy, their self-image, and their length of hospital stay, as well as the discharge plan. Whether the cause is extrinsic (pressure, friction, shear forces, or moisture) or intrinsic (anemia, spasticity, diabetes, malnutrition, contractures, edema, or obesity), the key is prevention. Therefore, hydration, nutrition, and incontinence care are important preventive measures. Heel protectors, frequent positioning change, air mattress,

seating cushions, and teaching pressure relief are specific measures to prevent extrinsic cause of pressure ulcers. See the chapter on wound care for specific treatment measures for the different stages of pressure ulcers.

Bladder Dysfunction

Bladder dysfunction occurs in 49–60% of stroke patients after 1 week, 29–42% after 4 weeks, 29% after 12 weeks, 14–15% after 6–12 months (Wade & Hewer, 1981; Borrie, Campbell, Caradoc-Davies, & Speers, 1986; Linsenmeyer & Zorowitz, 1992). Urinary dysfunction may be associated with mental status change such as confusion, communication problems, significant motor deficits with impaired mobility, drugs (diuretics, calcium channel blocker, sedatives), as well as urinary tract infections.

- Areflexic or flaccid bladder with retention is very common poststroke, especially initially. It may require in and out (I & O) catheterization, and usually resolves in 1–2 weeks. For this problem of retention, offer urinal or bedpan every 2 hours, and avoid Foley catheter as it can lead to urinary tract infection (UTI).

- Urinary incontinence may be secondary to overflow or spasticity with hyper-reflexic detrussor resulting in uninhibited contraction with complete or incomplete emptying. Discourage Foley catheter, check postvoid residual (PVR), offer urinal every 2 hours, and consider the I & O catheter program. A bedside commode or bathroom privileges may be appropriate for those with better ability to transfer and who have improved sitting and standing balance. A urology referral may at times be indicated for further studies. In a study of 38 male stroke survivors by Nitti, Adler, and Combs (1996), 82% were found to have detrussor hyperreflexia. Subsequent urodynamic studies showed 63% of male stroke survivors had outlet obstruction.

Bowel Incontinence

- Poor prognostic indicator if persistent and usually indicates bilateral cerebral involvement.
- Often due to constipation or immobility.
- Management consists of hydration, bowel care with stool softeners, and stool stimulants; allow the use of commode or bathroom privileges if balance permits.

As an outcome predictor, Barer (1989) stated "Outcome was so much better in those who remained dry that it seems possible that recovery of continence may promote morale and self-esteem which could actually hasten overall recovery."

Cognitive and Perceptual Deficits

Cognitive and perceptual deficits differ somewhat between left hemiplegic and right hemiplegic patients. Typically, left hemiplegic patients present with visuomotor perceptual dysfunction, left neglect, and loss of visual memory. Because most of these patients maintain their verbal fluency, their deficits are not readily noticed, unless severe, until they get to therapies where especially the left neglect becomes very obvious. These patients are usually impulsive, have poor insight and judgment, and safety is always a significant issue. There is poor carryover of tasks as is their potential for learning from their mistakes or watching others perform the task. Patients with significant left neglect are unsafe to walk, even with motor return, or operate a wheelchair, do kitchen activities, and they need supervision. Those with depth perception deficit may have difficulty finding the hole of the dress or shirt sleeve and putting the arm through it, or have trouble pouring a cup of coffee safely, not aware that the cup is full.

In the right hemiplegic patient, cognitive deficits can be manifested by reduced vocabulary and auditory retention. They are better able to learn from their mistakes and learning

by observing others perform the task. In both situations (right and left hemispheres), the OT and the ST collaborate using different management strategies such as basic visual scanning, size-estimation training, somatosensory awareness, visuoperceptual organization, using visually demonstrated stage by stage instructions, imitation techniques, and limiting words. In a comprehensive acute stroke center, it is not uncommon to have a neuropsychologist as team member available for consultation and follow-up for those patients with significant cognitive problems poststroke. A specific cognitive retraining program is generally available in these facilities; such a program can also be done on an outpatient basis.

Poststroke Depression

Poststroke depression (PSD) has a detrimental effect in the recovery because it causes fatigue, lack of hope, and decreased motivation for rehabilitation. The rate of PSD varies markedly, ranging from 25% to 79% (Gordon & Hibbard, 1997), for a variety of reasons such as differences in research approaches as well as inconsistent research findings. PSD has no hemispheric preference. It is more prevalent from 6 months to 2 years (Astrom, Adolfsson, & Asplund, 1993), 31% at 3 months, 16% at 12 months, 19% at 24 months, 34% at 36 months. Controversy exists as to whether PSD is a separate type of depression syndrome specific to poststroke patients or whether it is similar to any other depression among chronically ill patients, as some studies showed similar prevalence rate (Burvill et al, 1997)

A group of Swedish stroke survivors were followed for 3 months with detailed psychiatric evaluation. Predictors of immediate depression included left anterior lesion location, aphasia, and living alone premorbidly. Three months poststroke, dependency in ADL was the most important predictor of PSD, and at 1 year and onward, poor social contacts outside the family are more important in determining who are the candidates for chronic depression (Rigler, 1999).

Treatment:

- Less than 5% of patients were treated with medications.
- There is a high degree of spontaneous recovery within 6–10 weeks.
- Agents used included antidepressants such as tricyclics (SSRIs). Stimulant medications were also used such as dextroamphetamine or methylphenidate, but such use lacks large-scale randomized clinical trials.
- Cognitive behavioral treatment concurrent with medications
- Family/caregiver involvement in the counseling sessions

Vocational Rehabilitation

- In a study by Angeleri and colleagues (1993) of 180 stroke survivors with mean age of 65.29 with age-matched controls, less than 21% returned to work, not always to the same job, and most were under 65 years of age.
- Prerequisites for successful return to work include neuropsychiatric evaluation, ability to drive, work capacity evaluation, as well as a workplace evaluation.
- For those with the potential to return to work, a vocational counselor can be helpful in discovery of options. Some patients can benefit from a referral to the state vocational rehabilitation program for retraining.

A driving evaluation poststroke requires physical and mental abilities to operate a vehicle with or without adaptive modifications in the vehicle. A referral to the driver's education program, either through the DMV or community-based independent program, can be made to assess the physical and cognitive abilities of selective patients to drive safely. Those with significant motor deficits or with neglect and perceptual deficits and poor balance should not be referred.

Successful rehabilitation is contingent upon many factors, but the stability of the patient's underlying medical conditions is probably the most important. A patient's motivation is also an important factor. Some specific possible sequelae of stroke that may affect the patient and impact on the rehabilitation course include the development of significant spasticity that may require the use of medications (Lioresal, Dantrolene, Diazepam, or Tizanidine); interventions such as phenol blocks, or Botox; or even surgical treatment such as release of contractures. Complex regional pain syndrome type 1 (CRPS) may also occur poststroke affecting the involved UE. Brachial plexus injury of the involved UE is another complication and is usually due to traction injury especially in the presence of dense hemiplegia. Or the patient may have had a fall at the onset of stroke with an undetected stretch injury to the plexus. An index of suspicion is raised when one sees movement in the distal limb such as wrist and hand and a much weaker proximal arm with significant atrophy, contrary to the usual proximal-to-distal recovery pattern poststroke. An EMG test is useful to confirm the peripheral nerve injury.

Follow-Up

At the time of discharge, review the patient's future appointments and order follow-up appointments with the primary care provider and specialists such as the physiatrist in 3–4 weeks especially if the patient is continuing an outpatient therapy program. Even if the patient is not in an outpatient physical therapy (PT) program, a follow-up postdischarge is important to see if there is continuing progress or if there is regression of functional gains made earlier, as well as evaluation for any further need for equipment to help the patient at home or in the community.

REHABILITATION OF THE LOWER EXTREMITY AMPUTEE IN THE SKILLED NURSING FACILITY

Introduction

Review of several large studies on lower extremity amputations revealed that 82–93% of the amputations occurred in individuals between 59–61 years of age. Most of these were due to disease from arteriosclerosis obliterans (ASO), small vessel disease from diabetes, thromboangiitis obliterans (TAO, Buerger's disease), or thromboembolism (Kay & Newman, 1978; Esquenazi, Vacaranukunkit, & Torres, 1984). Malignancy constituted 2–2.5%; congenital causes were at 0.3%; and trauma was at 7–15%. An epidemiologic study by Dillingham (1999) of traumatic amputees showed a decline in the incidence due to improved safety standards in the workplace, even though when they occurred, especially when the amputation involved the upper extremity, the impact on vocation was significant and long lasting.

Dysvascular amputations are frequently done in the lower extremities (LE) and often due to gangrene, nonhealing ulcers, or severe claudication pain from peripheral arterial disease (PAD). At least 50% of these patients are diabetics. Medical care costs $500 million, just in this diabetic population alone, not including the cost of rehabilitation (Bild et al., 1989). See Table 20-3.

TABLE 20-4 Average Energy Consumption Increase at Different Levels of LE Amputation	
LEVEL OF LE AMPUTATION	METABOLIC ENERGY INCREASE (ENERGY EXP/UNIT DISTANCE) PERCENTAGE
Transmetatarsal	10–20
Syme's	0–30
Transtibial (below knee)	40–50
Transfemoral (above knee)	90–100
Bilateral transtibial	60–100

Source: Esquenazi, 1991.

The viability of the soft tissues will determine the most distal level of amputation that is possible, and often this is done at the time of surgery when the surgeon checks the skin bleeding. The more muscles and joints that are removed (i.e., the higher the level of amputation), the greater is the energy cost of walking and therefore, the greater is the impact on the patient's function. See Table 20-4.

From the table above, it becomes imperative that a clinician takes this increased cost of energy consumption into consideration when evaluating a new amputee for a prosthesis and factors this into the overall medical health of the patient, especially in the geriatric patient who constitute a larger percentage of the amputee population.

Preprosthetic Rehabilitation

Ideally, this process begins before surgery, especially since most of the dysvascular amputees have had a long history of decreased activity and mobility due to claudication pain, recurrent ulcers, multiple surgeries such as revascularization, or due to underlying medical illness. Deconditioning occurs invariably in these patients, and complications can occur such as decreased cardiopulmonary fitness, muscle weakness, or even joint contractures,

TABLE 20-3 Levels of Amputation	
	PERCENTAGE
Transfemoral (above knee)	37
Through knee	2
Transtibial (below knee)	48
Syme's and partial foot	8
UE amputations (all levels)	5

Source: Esquenazi, 1991.

especially of the hips and knees from pro-longed sitting. Often, initiation of a rehabilitation program does not occur till after surgery. Therefore, it is even more important that a preprosthetic rehabilitation program begin as soon as possible after surgery.

In many centers, especially freestanding amputee rehabilitation centers, a potential candidate for amputation is evaluated by a rehabilitation team before surgery for a general assessment of the patient's activities of daily living (ADLs), joint mobility, muscle strength, endurance, and ambulation skills. If there is sufficient time prior to surgery, the patient can be enrolled in physical therapy to improve the areas where limitations were noted in the assessment. The patient is given information regarding postoperative care and the subsequent rehabilitation program, as well as information on phantom phenomenon and implications of fall occurrences. The patient may also be shown different samples of prostheses or even given the opportunity to interact with a successful amputee for support and reassurance. Some patients and their families may even require psychological support due to depression from prolonged illness or fear of limb loss and its impact on lifestyle, body image perception, and self-worth.

Edema control is achieved in many different ways:

- Use of a rigid dressing immediately postoperatively with a training prosthesis (pylon) attached to the end of the cast to allow early training in standing and walking. This method also helps decrease phantom sensation and pain. The rigid dressing can also be a removable one with the cast changed periodically to accommodate residual limb (stump) shrinkage (Buergess, 1969). This procedure requires resources of the medical center and expertise of the staff.

- Use of a semirigid dressing such as the Unna dressing, which is lighter, less bulky and more flexible, allows a transtibial amputee to flex the knee through a limited range. The disadvantage is that a prosthetic component cannot be attached to the dressing and therefore no early weight bearing can occur.

- Soft dressings are most commonly used and consist of layers of gauze pad. An elastic bandaging program using Ace Wrap is eventually begun before or after suture removal, depending on the healing of the surgical wound.

- Education of the patient and the family in the proper wrapping technique is crucial because poor technique leads to skin problems, localized pockets of edema, and a poorly shaped stump. The goal of wrapping is to have a conical or cylindrical shaped residual limb as it is easier to fit with a prosthesis. Rewrapping every 3–4 hours is necessary because body movement changes the position and the tension of the bandage. Some patients are unable to learn the technique due to hand problems or from poor vision and may have to use alternate ways of shrinkage.

- A Jobst compression pump can also be used for limb shrinkage as well as the residual limb shrinkers, especially in a transfemoral amputation where Ace wrapping is not recommended as the wrap cannot be secured properly.

Amputee Rehabilitation

Rehabilitation for a patient who has undergone an amputation begins immediately after surgery and continues when a patient is transferred to an inpatient rehabilitation center or to a skilled nursing facility. Early intervention by the medical and nursing staff along with the rehabilitation team are very important. Surgical wound care, proper positioning in bed, pain control, adequate nutrition to promote wound healing, skin care of areas that are at risk for breakdown, early participation in ADL, and fall prevention, especially if there is phantom sensation, are all important areas that need ongoing assessment and management. The use of a pillow under the hip and knee is not recommended because it leads to flexion contractures and can potentially affect the eventual prosthetic fitting.

The physical therapy program consists of the following:

- Bed mobility skills training
- Instruct and monitor proper bed positioning as well as encourage proning for 30 minutes 2–3 times a day, if tolerated, to help decrease hip flexion tightness.
- Teach and monitor proper care of the residual limb by the patient/family to obtain optimal limb shrinkage and shaping and desensitization techniques of the residual limb.
- Include transfer training to all surfaces such as to bed, commode, tub, and floor.
- Teach wheelchair use to allow early mobility—most patients will be using a wheelchair for a period of time after amputation.
- Teach pressure relief techniques.
- Teach range-of-motion (ROM) exercises of all joints to prevent contractures.
- Use strengthening exercises of the upper and lower limb muscles especially those that are important in crutch walking or in using a walker.
- Teach upper body (trunk) strengthening exercises, which are important in transfer activity, mobility, and prosthetic training later on.
- Educate the patient about the phantom limb phenomenon. Reinforce fall precautions especially after discharge to home. Often, patients forget that they have lost a limb when they get up at night to go to the bathroom, leading to a fall. This can be prevented by placing a chair barrier to the side of the bed the patient usually gets up from.

- Include gait training with an assistive device, either axillary crutches or walker, without a prosthesis.
- Endurance exercises to increase cardiopulmonary fitness
- Equipment evaluation is needed for a safe discharge to home. At times, a home evaluation may be needed.
- If there is expectation that the new amputee will need a wheelchair indefinitely, then a wheelchair with an offset or more posterior wheelbase may be necessary, especially if the patient is a transfemoral or bilateral transtibial amputee. Because of the loss of forward weight after amputation, the patient's center of gravity when seated is shifted posteriorly and inferiorly, about two inches more than normal. Therefore, the wheelchair base should accommodate this shift or the patient may tip backwards when going up inclines or ramps. Either a custom wheelchair or the use of rear wheel adapters can be prescribed. In a patient with a unilateral amputation who is actively using a prosthesis but needs a wheelchair for distances, this wheelchair modification is not as crucial although antitip casters are recommended in the wheelchair and for that matter, in all wheelchairs for added safety against tipping.

The occupational therapy program consists of the following:

- ADL evaluation and training especially in dressing, bathroom activities and hygiene
- Can work in conjunction with PT in trunk balance training and coordination
- Equipment evaluation for the bathroom as needed
- Homemaking evaluation or safety in kitchen activities at the wheelchair level or using crutches or walker.

The Phantom Limb

All amputees experience phantom limb phenomenon. Up to 70% of amputees report phantom pain in the first few months after amputation (Esquenazi, 1993). Most often, the sensation or the pain decreases or disappears over time so that it does not interfere with the use of the prosthesis. It "telescopes" into the residual limb. A small number of patients may continue to experience it intermittently and when it becomes chronic it is not as amenable to treatment, unless a local cause is responsible, such as a neuroma that can be excised or an improper socket fit that can be revised. Other treatment options available for the phantom pain include desensitization techniques, use of a TENS unit, medications such as gabapentin (Neurontin), and nerve blocks. It has been noted that patients with a high anxiety level or who are under stress experience a heightened and more frequent occurrence of phantom pain. In this instance, supportive therapy and reassurance can be helpful. The pain can also be exacerbated by the progression of the underlying vascular disease. Residual limb pain is often difficult to treat and at times results in increased disability for the amputees (Sherman et al., 1985).

Prosthetic Training

Most patients who are in the skilled nursing facility for the preprosthetic rehabilitation program are discharged to their home when they have reached a level of competence in ambulation with an assistive device and there is satisfactory wound healing. They are given follow-up appointments with the surgeon and/or the rehabilitation team where the determination is made when the patient is ready for evaluation by the prosthetist for the first fitting of the prosthesis. The prosthetic training is generally done in an outpatient rehabilitation center. Patients are generally not readmitted to the skilled nursing facility for this part of the training program. Inpatient rehabilitation for amputees is underutilized even though it can improve long-term outcomes (Dillingham, 1999).

The physical therapist works very closely with the prosthetist throughout the training program. Any gait deviation attributable to the prosthetic device can be closely monitored and corrected; close observation of the integrity of the residual limb can also be done. Patients are instructed in the proper donning and doffing of the prosthesis. They are also educated on the care of the prosthesis, inspecting for cracks or missing rivets in the socket, and in the hygienic care of the socket and the stump socks and liners. The program also consists of transfer training to all surfaces, including floor transfer, or teaching how to fall safely, and gait training on different surfaces, as well as on stairs and ramps. In the first year postamputation, the residual limb continues to shrink, so it is not unusual for the patient to require different thicknesses of stump socks, initially, and eventually to require socket changes till the stump volume stabilizes.

Prosthetic Devices

A full discussion on the many varieties of prosthetic devices for lower extremity (LE) amputation is beyond the scope of this chapter. In general, partial foot amputation requires custom-molded shoes with inserts. A transtibial amputee needs a prosthetic foot, an ankle unit, a socket, suspension system, and liners (soft liners to decrease pressure on the residual limb). A transfemoral amputee needs in addition to the above, a knee joint. These are the devices in general. The specific prosthetic device and components that are issued to the patient for his or her level of amputation depends on the patient's needs, taking into consideration his or her overall medical health and activity level, lifestyle, work requirement, and leisure interests. Each general component of a prosthetic limb has numerous options and designs that can be tailored to the need of the patient so that the final prosthesis that is issued is one that the patient can wear comfortably and safely.

Conclusion

Amputation of a limb results in a dramatic change to the patient's life, and the greater the loss, the greater the impact on the patient's functional capabilities. New technologies continue to deliver more sophisticated products, lighter materials, better suspension systems, and more options in the many components. These new technologies allow all ages of amputees, but especially the geriatric population, to resume not just the ability to ambulate, but to have a prosthesis that can do many functions of the original limb. Rehabilitation of an amputee is a team approach that can make a difference in the patient's quality of life. Control of risk factors such as smoking, hypertension, elevated cholesterol, and diabetes are important ongoing goals for the patient and will help decrease morbidity and mortality risks.

REHABILITATION OF ACUTE LOW BACK PAIN IN THE SKILLED NURSING FACILITY

Acute low back pain (LBP) usually runs a benign course with as many as 90% of the patients returning to work within 3 months. Recurrences may occur later, with some patients progressing to have functional limitations. Patients are usually seen either by the primary care physician for the duration of the problem or referred to a specialist such as a physiatrist, or a spine surgeon if the symptoms are more complex. Most of the patients are treated on an outpatient basis, and this seems to be an adequate and effective approach in most instances. Bed rest for no more than 2 days is usually recommended with gradual increase in activities after that. A randomized

clinical trial published in the *New England Journal of Medicine* showed that the outcomes were the same in patients treated with 2 days versus 7 days of bed rest (Deyo, Cherkin, & Conrad, 1991). Mild to moderate analgesics and anti-inflammatory agents are usually also prescribed.

Occasionally, patients present with an acute nonsurgical LBP of such severity as to render home or outpatient care not feasible. In these instances, a short stay in a skilled nursing facility is recommended, primarily for pharmacologic therapy to control pain using a variety of regimens, which may include muscle relaxants, narcotics, and NSAIDs. See the chapter on musculoskeletal care for treatment of low back pain.

In the skilled nursing facility, physical therapy is also instituted for modalities, mobility training, and a limited flexibility exercise program as the pain control improves. The goals of therapy in the skilled nursing facility are to help decrease pain and muscle spasm and improve patient's ADLs (especially mobility to a point where the patient can be discharged to home and participate in an outpatient comprehensive back program).

- Modalities usually include superficial heat (hydrocollator packs), usually applied for 20 minutes over the affected areas 2–3 times a day. Cold packs may also be used and applied for 15 minutes, 2–3 times a day as well. Both modalities provide relief of muscle spasm that usually accompanies acute LBP. Cold packs are usually preferred in the first 48 hours after onset to decrease the muscle inflammatory response. However, some patients are not tolerant of the cold packs. Superficial heat can be used and has the additional benefit of providing general relaxation to the patient which is desirable in this setting. Both superficial heat and the cold packs are usually limited to the first 2–4 weeks after an injury resulting in acute LBP.

- Ultrasound, a deep heat modality, may at times be used on the tight paralumbar muscles prior to a stretching program. This is especially applicable in those patients with a chronic back problem, now with an acute exacerbation. Often, these patients present with chronic tightness of their low back muscles as well as hamstrings and hip flexors. It is important to remember the restrictions related to the use of ultrasound, such as a suspicion of an underlying malignancy, the presence of a skin condition over the affected area, or in the presence of an osteoporotic spine.

- Transcutaneous electrical stimulation (TENS) has been used for short-term therapy to decrease pain and relieve localized muscle spasm, and some patients have reported good results. However, it has not been shown to be of significant value in the long-term treatment of LBP.

- Some skilled nursing facilities have massage therapists on staff who can provide light or friction-type massage to the affected areas. This can usually follow the application of superficial heat. Massage therapy can be helpful in further decreasing the muscle spasm as well as provide general relaxation, which is a highly desirable goal in treating LBP. When there are myofascial trigger points involved that are contributing to the pain, friction massage or acupressure of the trigger points are helpful to release the tight myofascial bands. This is an adjunctive option to the traditional approach to myofascial trigger points.

- Mobility training is an important therapy program provided by the physical therapist. The patient is trained in bed mobility and transfer activities and is progressed to ambulation with an assistive device, usually a front-wheeled walker. Emphasis is placed on maintaining the neutral or balanced spine position at all times. The use of a mirror can be a helpful tool. Generally, as

the patient's pain control improves with the medications, participation in therapy increases, with improved effort.

- The use of a lumbosacral orthosis (corset) of any kind in patients with LBP is controversial (Walsh & Schwartz, 1990). Some patients find comfort in the use of a simple abdominal binder, especially during the early mobilization period. But any long-term use is to be discouraged. Studies showed that long-term use of an orthosis for LBP can contribute to weakness of the abdominal muscles; studies also showed that there was no substantial decrease in the intradiscal pressure from its use. However, an orthosis is indicated in patients with osteoporotic compression fractures and LBP.

- An elderly patient or a younger homemaker may require ADL evaluation and retraining in OT to make sure that proper body mechanics are utilized while doing the ADLs as well as the kitchen or housekeeping tasks. Instructions in activity modifications, energy conservation techniques and ergonomics at home or at work are also useful learning tools for the patient to take home and observe to decrease the stress on the lower back, the incidence of reinjury, and for a safe transition to home.

- When reasonable pain control is achieved, the patient is usually discharged home to continue a home program of modified activities and graduated back exercises. A referral to a community outpatient comprehensive back program is recommended. Many centers have an established Back School where patients attend for several sessions to learn about the normal spine and its biomechanics; the abnormal spine and what contributes to its pathology, what can be done about it, and the different options for treatment; information about the importance of good body mechanics at home and at work; and demonstrate understanding of such information. Additionally, some patients may be candidates for continued outpatient physical therapy for modalities.

- The exercises for a healthy back consist of *stretching* the lower back muscle and major lower extremity muscles to improve flexibility; *strengthening* of the core muscles that support the spine such as the abdominals and the spinal extensor muscles; *relaxation* exercises for help in controlling pain and relieving stress; and *aerobic* conditioning exercise to improve overall fitness and endurance as well as help in weight reduction if obesity is identified as a risk factor for LBP. There are different techniques used by the therapist to stretch and strengthen the key muscles to a healthy back. A common denominator to these exercises is the ability of the patient to learn and maintain a neutral spine position so that the exercises can be done in as pain-free range as possible. Stretching and strengthening of the lower extremity muscles are also very important for a healthy back as tightness in the hip flexors, and the hamstring muscles for example, changes the body posture and shifts the natural standing balance, which inevitably leads to LBP. Other leg muscles such as the quadriceps and the gastrocnemius are also important to stretch and strengthen, especially if the patient is to depend upon the leg muscles to provide the lifting power and spare the spine. Remember that in any exercise activity, the underlying back pathology and the general medical health of the patient are to be considered before recommending a specific program for the patient.

- Some patients admitted to the skilled nursing facility for an acute exacerbation of a chronic LBP condition may actually be appropriate candidates for the pain management program that is available in both hospital and freestanding centers. A referral should be considered after discussion with the patient. These programs utilize a multidisciplinary team approach that may include physicians of various specialties such as internal medicine, rehabilitation medicine, psychiatry, anesthesia, addiction medicine, as well as allied health personnel such as the psychologist, nutritionist, clinical social worker, pharmacist, and physical therapist. It is important to identify the patients that may benefit from such referrals before they are discharged home. It is also important to identify secondary issues that the patients may have, such as a pending workman's compensation claim, a pending litigation related to an accident, the presence of depression, family stressors, or even underlying psychiatric problems, because all these issues tend to provide a negative impetus towards earlier resolution of the pain, unless they are either treated for the problem or brought to the table for an open discussion and goal setting.

- A chiropractic approach to treatment of patients with LBP has long been a subject of debate. Many patients with spine pain seek chiropractic treatment first or solely for pain relief. Some patients report good results. Others report exacerbation of their pain. Many clinicians have long been wary of recommending it or commenting on its role when asked by their patients. Some of this probably stems from lack of understanding of the full spectrum of the field. This is changing. The new Agency for Healthcare Research and Quality (AHRQ) (Bigos et al., 1994) and the Clinical Standards Advisory Group (1994), acknowledge the potential benefit of a limited course of spinal manipulation in patients with acute LBP. More studies are still needed to identify the specific group of patients most likely to derive benefit (Koes, Assendelft, van der Heijiden, & Bouter, 1996).

Rehabilitation of LBP is very well documented in numerous articles and texts, with many protocols sharing commonalities in approach. A key point that cannot be emphasized enough is patient education. Teaching the patient ways to prevent further injury and low back strain, at home, at work, or during leisure activities, and helping the patient to maintain a level of overall physical fitness that is within tolerance in order to increase and maintain the strength and endurance of the back and lower extremity muscles, is at the core of all these different programs.

TOTAL JOINT ARTHROPLASTY OF HIP AND KNEE

Hip and knee arthroplasty are increasingly common procedures being performed in the elderly population. Replacement of damaged cartilage surfaces with artificial bearing materials has enabled surgeons to dramatically improve function and relieve pain in many patients (Voight, 2001). Early postoperative rehabilitation after total joint replacement focuses on the following:

• Restoring mobility, strength, and flexibility
• Reducing pain
• Preventing deep vein thrombosis (DVT)
• Teaching adherence to range of motion or its restrictions and weight-bearing precautions
• Ordering appropriate equipment
• Patient and family education
• Aligning home resources

Since the 1980s, with the introduction of diagnosis-related groups (DRG)-based Medicare payments to acute care hospitals, the length of stay for joint replacements has been reduced dramatically. This reduction has been accomplished through earlier mobilization of patients, streamlining care, discharging patients who are at a lower functional level, and transferring them to skilled nursing facilities to continue their rehabilitation. When patients are discharged from the skilled nursing facility to the community, they may receive continued rehabilitation services in the home or the outpatient clinic. Should the patient remain at the facility for long-term care, they may either receive continued rehabilitation under Medicare Part B or from the restorative nursing program.

Hip and knee arthroplasty procedures have the highest risk of mortality of all types of joint arthroplasty due to the increased incidence of postoperative thromboembolic events. Without anticoagulation therapy, high-risk orthopedic patients have a 40–70% chance of developing DVT. Nearly 20% will develop pulmonary emboli (PE), with approximately 1–5% being fatal (Clagett, Anderson, & Heit, 1995). Several risk factors are identified for the development of DVT:

• Age greater than 40 years
• Malignant disease
• Major trauma
• Immobility
• Obesity
• Hemostatic disorders
• Pregnancy
• Varicose veins
• Estrogen use (Voight, 2001)

Some form of prophylaxis is indicated for all patients undergoing surgery for total joint replacement (TKA, THA), and surgery for hip fracture repair. This includes the postoperative administration of various drug regimens of warfarin (maintaining the international normalized ratio [INR] between 2.0 and 3.0) or low-molecular weight heparin (e.g., enoxaparin). Adjunct therapies such as antiembolic compression stockings and intermittent external compression devices can also be used. Mobilization of the patient in the early postoperative period has been shown to reduce circulatory stasis and prevent complications (Planes, Vochelle, & Darmon, 1996).

The goal of pain management in total joint replacement is to maximize the patient's tolerance of activity while maintaining alertness. There is a wide variety of analgesia ranging from oral anti-inflammatory drugs to long-acting narcotics.

TOTAL KNEE REPLACEMENT

Knee osteoarthritis is a common, disabling condition with the rates estimated at 2/1000 per year. Total knee arthroplasty (TKA) for arthritis has emerged as one of the most common and successful procedures in the United States (Brander & Fitzgerald Mullarkey, 2002). In TKA both the femoral and tibial sides of the joint are replaced using either a long or short stem, most commonly fixated with cement. The goal is to provide a long-lasting artificial joint that relieves pain and improves function, while minimizing or avoiding surgical complications. It is indicated for disabling knee pain from advanced articular disease when conservative management has failed. A carefully thought out surgical decision considers the patient's level of pain, degree of radiographic changes, extent of potential complications, and a risk-benefit analysis of the procedure (Fitzgerald Mullarkey & Brander, 2002).

The goals of rehabilitation following TKA include the following:

- To obtain and maintain full recovery of knee range of motion
- To develop knee and hip muscle strength
- To obtain functional independence

Most often patients may begin ambulation with an assistive device (walker) as soon as postoperative day 1. If the bone is extremely osteoporotic, a delay in full weight bearing may be indicated. The progression of weight bearing is based solely on the surgeon's discretion. Restoration of range of motion as quickly as possible in order to prevent adhesions and joint contracture is critical to successful outcome in TKA (Voight, 2001). The use of continuous passive motion (CPM) machines in the early postoperative days remains controversial. Many studies have suggested that CPM allows for greater early knee flexion, decreased knee pain, fewer inpatient rehabilitation days, and decreased need for manipulation. Achieving early knee flexion facilitates independence. A minimum of 90° of knee flexion is typically required for daily activities (Fitzgerald Mullarkey & Brander, 2002).

Patients are seen by the PT for modalities such as ice packs for local pain relief as well as to decrease edema that is often present postoperatively. The PT program consists of transfer training, range-of-motion exercises to the affected knee within pain tolerance, and progressive ambulation and gait training usually with a front wheel walker. Before discharge, patients are also trained in stair climbing and walking on uneven surfaces.

Some patients may need to be seen by the OT for training in lower extremity dressing using adaptive aids and safety in bathing and toileting. This is especially true for those elderly patients with limited functional independence premorbidily.

Patient and family education is a key part of rehabilitation. Orthopedic precautions and a home exercise program are taught and emphasized during the skilled nursing facility stay. Concerns such as return to work and resumption of driving, hobbies, and sport activities are addressed. Typically, patients remain off work for 3–6 weeks after surgery, depending on the degree of physical activity required at the job. The orthopedic surgeon will instruct the patient when it is advisable to return to work and resumption of hobbies and sport activities. Resumption of driving may occur as soon as three weeks after surgery if the patient exhibits good leg control, infrequent use of narcotics, and if their overall rate of recovery is good (Fitzgerald Mullarkey & Brander, 2002).

TOTAL HIP REPLACEMENT

Hip osteoarthritis rates are estimated at .5/1000 per year (Brander & Fitzgerald Mullarkey, 2002). Total hip arthroplasty (THA) for arthritis is performed frequently in the United States. Indications for hip arthroplasty include incapacitating pain from conditions such as osteoarthritis, rheumatoid arthritis, osteonecrosis (avascular necrosis), fractures, failed previous reconstruction, and tumors. Patients commonly undergo THA after conservative measures such as activity modifications, medications for pain or inflammation that have failed to provide relief from arthritis symptoms, and patients exhibit a progressive decline in mobility and increased dependence on adaptive aids for ambulation.

THA involves surgically removing the arthritic parts of the joint, replacing the ball and socket part of the joint with artificial components made from metal alloys, and placing a high-performance bearing surface between the metal parts. Most commonly, the bearing surface is made from a very durable polyethylene plastic, but other materials including ceramics, plastics, or metals have been used. Most often cement or methylmethacrylate is used for fixation of the components. The use of cement allows early weight bearing. Hemiarthroplasty is another procedure performed for hip disease often postfracture. This procedure requires that acetabular cartilage is intact and that the joint pathology is limited to the femoral side of the hip joint.

The surgical goals of total hip arthroplasty include the following:

- Relief of persistent pain

- Improvement in mobility, function, and independence

- Improvement in quality of life

- Minimizing or avoiding surgical complications (Brander & Fitzgerald Mullarkey, 2002)

Weight-bearing restrictions after THA are not standardized and are typically prescribed based on the postoperative instructions of the surgeon. The type of implant, quality of fixation, degree of bone integrity, presence of a trochanteric osteotomy or femoral fracture, and strength of periarticular soft tissue structures can influence weight-bearing restrictions.

Commonly, patients after THA with cemented femoral stems are prescribed partial weight bearing (PWB), usually defined as allowing pressure of about 70% of body weight, or full weight bearing (FWB). In hip revisions, restricted weight bearing is often prescribed, either PWB or touch down (TDWB), which allows pressure of 10–15% of body weight (Brander & Fitzgerald Mullarkey, 2002).

The focus of the patient's PT program is on safe transfer activity and progression of ambulation with assistive devices while strictly adhering to the hip precautions. As in TKA procedures, patients are seen early for modalities such as ice packs for pain control and decreased edema as well as early ambulation.

Occupational therapy focuses on lower extremity dressing, bathing, and toileting, while adhering to hip precautions. OT may issue adaptive devices.

The rate of prosthetic hip dislocation in the postoperative phase while in the rehabilitation setting was found to be 2.1% in a retrospective study of 337 patients who underwent unilateral total joint replacement (Brander & Fitzgerald Mullarkey, 2002). Range-of-motion (ROM) restrictions are prescribed postoperatively to prevent dislocation of the prosthetic femoral head. These precautions include the following:

- No adduction (crossing over) of operative leg past the midline of the body

- No internal rotation of the hip

- No forward flexion of the trunk past 90° of the hip

Adaptive equipment and assistive devices such as elevated toilet seats and reachers are issued to help patients maintain the precautions while performing functional tasks. Hip abductor splints/pillows are commonly used to keep the legs in abduction during bed rest and when turning in bed. These hip precautions are usually followed for at least 6 weeks after surgery when hip abductors and flexors have achieved good strength. Patients and families should be instructed on hip precautions and provided written information.

▄▄▄▄ HIP FRACTURE

Hip fractures occur in approximately 80 per 100,000 persons each year. Incidence of hip fracture increases with age (Gallagher, Melton, Riggs, & Bergtrath, 1980). The mortality rate in the year after hip fracture can be as high as 30%, and as many as one third of hip fracture patients remain in a nursing home (Kane et al., 2004). Factors that contribute to increased morbidity and mortality after hip fracture include increasing age, male gender, concomitant morbidity, cognitive deficits, premorbid institutionalization, and limited premorbid function (Cifu, 1995). Incidence of hip fracture is 2–3 times greater in whites than in nonwhites, primarily because of the high rate of osteoporosis in whites. In older persons, more than 90% of hip fractures result from trauma or torsion associated with a fall (Madore, 2006).

The hip joint is composed of the head of the femur and the acetabulum of the pelvis. This articulation has a loose joint capsule and is surrounded by large, strong muscles. The construction of this stable joint allows for the wide range of motion required for normal daily activities such as walking, sitting, and squatting (Kaplan & Gilbert, 2002). Fractures of the proximal femur are classified as *femoral neck, intertrochanteric,* and *subtrochanteric* types. *Femoral neck fractures* account for approximately one half of hip fractures in the elderly,

are intracapsular, and are graded based upon their degree of displacement. They are most commonly caused by falls or near falls in the older adult (Kyle, Gustiol, & Premer, 1979). Because the blood supply to the femoral head is distally based, there is substantial risk of nonunion and avascular necrosis. Impacted and nondisplaced fractures are generally repaired by internal fixation, whereas displaced fractures are repaired either by reduction and internal fixation or hemiarthroplasty. Total hip replacement can be appropriate for patients with substantial hip arthritis before the fracture. *Intertrochanteric fractures* comprise the remaining 50% of hip fractures. They are commonly caused by significant trauma (falls and motor vehicle accidents) and occur more often in males and the vigorous elderly. They are usually categorized as either stable or unstable, and all are treated with open reduction and internal fixation. Fractures of the *subtrochanteric region* of the femur are caused by falls and motor vehicle accidents. They occur in approximately 5% of fractures in the elderly. The subtrochanteric region is also a common site of pathologic fractures from neoplastic diseases (Cifu, 1995).

The elderly patient with a hip fracture should be regarded as having a condition that is surgically urgent. Medical problems should be stabilized, and the patient should generally go to the operating room within 24 hours of the injury. In rare circumstances, especially for severely demented nonambulatory patients, or in those who have medical problems with severe risk of perioperative morbidity and mortality, a nonoperative approach may be appropriate (Ackermann, 1998).

The diagnosis of hip fracture is often straightforward, particularly when the bone fragments are displaced. The fractured leg is usually held in external rotation and the leg might be shortened if the fracture is displaced. Radiographs should be ordered on any elderly patient who complains of hip pain following a fall. Nondisplaced femoral neck fractures and fractures of just the acetabulum might not be visible on plain films and may require bone scanning, magnetic resonance imaging (MRI), or computed tomography (CT). Occasionally, hip fracture is missed for days or weeks, and a history of a fall might be absent (Ackermann, 1998).

Prevention and management of complications following surgery for hip fractures is important. Early and aggressive rehabilitation, avoidance of sedatives, and prevention of deep vein thrombosis (DVT) and pulmonary embolism is essential. All patients without contraindications should receive therapeutic doses of warfarin, or low-molecular weight heparin (e.g., enoxaparin) to reduce risk of DVT and pulmonary embolism. The optimal length of anticoagulation necessary after hip fracture surgery is unknown, but most surgeons recommend 2 to 4 weeks or until reasonable mobility is regained. Common conditions that complicate a patient's recovery following surgery to repair a hip fracture include the following:

- Fever is common in the first few days following surgery; consider sources such as lungs, urine, skin, abdomen, and wound. Appropriate tests should be ordered.

- Urinary tract infection is the most common bacterial infection in patients postoperative and is usually related to use of urethral catheters. Catheters should be removed as soon as possible after surgery.

- Gastrointestinal complications include nausea, vomiting, fecal impaction, diarrhea, abdominal pain, gastritis, and diverticulitis.

- With the use of antibiotic prophylaxis prior to surgery, the rate of superficial wound infections are low and deep wound infections are rare.

- Delirium is seen in up to 50% of patients hospitalized for hip fracture and usually occurs on postoperative days 1–5. It is associated with an increase in hospital mortality, length of stay, and institutionalization, and it requires immediate medical evaluation (Berggren, Gustafson, & Eriksson, 1987).

- Pressure ulcers are associated with a marked increase in length of stay and mortality. Pressure ulcers have been reported to occur in 13–66% of hip fracture patients (Russin & Russin, 1981). Aggressive mobilization is the most effective preventive method.

- Parenteral fluid replacement generally is needed for only 24–48 hours following surgery. A common electrolyte abnormality seen in patients is hyponatremia. Causes include diuretics, thyroid disease, and heart, liver, renal and adrenal disease. The most common reason is excessive antidiuretic hormone effect (Ackermann, 1998).

Orthopedic complications may include fracture nonunion, joint or prothesis infection, leg length discrepancy, heterotopic ossification, and prosthetic or internal fixation device loosening (Cifu, 1995).

The degree of immobility and disability caused by a hip fracture depends on several factors, including coexisting medical conditions, patient motivation, the nature of the fracture, and the techniques of management. Many older patients with hip fracture already have impaired mobility, and there is a high incidence of medical illnesses that necessitate treatment at the same time of hip fracture. Patients with these underlying conditions and those with dementia are at especially high risk for poor functional recovery (Kane et al., 2004).

Rehabilitative efforts should begin as soon as possible, either the first postoperative day or when medically feasible in nonoperative cases. Weight-bearing restrictions and instructions are prescribed by the orthopedic surgeon. The primary goals of a rehabilitation program after hip fracture is to reduce disability, maximize function, and allow the person to return to their prior activity level.

There is limited research available to clearly identify the most appropriate rehabilitation setting that is most effective. Overall, when medically and socially feasible, home-based rehabilitation has been demonstrated to be more cost-effective than nursing home or rehabilitation unit-based services. One study done by Binder et al. (2004) randomly assigned 90 hip fracture patients who had just completed the standard course of acute therapy to one of two groups. One group received six months of supervised physical therapy and exercise training, while the other group received instructions and brief training in exercises to be performed at home for six months. Participants who received supervised rehabilitation therapy that included resistance training improved on functional, strength, balance, mobility, and quality-of-life measures significantly more than those who received a prescribed, home-based regimen. Skilled nursing facilities generally provide 1–1.5 hours/day of therapy for 5 days/week and 24 hours/day nursing availability. Patients who are medically stable but too debilitated to participate in more intensive therapy programs and who cannot be treated safely at home should be considered for skilled nursing facility admission for rehabilitation services. Many patients return to the community; however, many others fail to progress, usually because of severe comorbidities, leading to placement in long-term custodial care facilities.

Areas of assessment unique to elderly hip fracture patients are for the clinician to have an understanding of the major acute and chronic medical issues. This can assist in determining the degree of physiologic reserve remaining, which is a major factor in designing more specific strategies and precautions for the rehabilitation program. It also helps to focus the medical management of the individual, which is essential for successful participation.

All postoperative hip fracture patients should have physical and occupational therapy initiated on admission to the skilled nursing facility. PT consists of mobilization of the patient out of their bed and to a chair, performing chair level exercises including quadriceps exercises and ankle pumps. The rehabilitation program exercises should progress to bed-to-chair mobility using a standing pivot transfer, wheelchair skills, pregait (sit to stand), and gait using parallel bars to walker. Occupational therapy consists of ADL training and continued performance of range-of-motion, strengthening, and conditioning exercises. Advanced skills in transfers (tub, car), mobility (stairs), and ADLs are instituted by days 6–10 postop, and equipment is procured (e.g., raised toilet sear, bathtub bench, bathroom grab bars, walker and/or wheelchair, long-handled dressing and ADL devices). Outpatient or home health therapy (usually physical therapy only) is typically utilized for 2–8 weeks after discharge to assist with the transition to the home and to advance mobility skills and endurance.

◼ DECONDITIONING

The process of aging is a challenge for individuals in unique and varied ways. Well-documented physiologic changes occur with each passing decade starting at age 20. The responses to these changes depend on uncontrollable genetic factors and avoidable risk factors specific to lifestyle choices (Vorhies & Riley, 1993).

It is important to understand the effects of deconditioning relative to both physiologic and functional losses. Physiologic losses are usually identified by a thorough medical examination that focuses on changes in organ systems. Functional losses are identified by assessing an individual's performance in activities of daily living. Early intervention of deconditioning is critical, especially for sedentary older adults, frail elderly, and older adults with neurologic, cardiac, or orthopedic impairments.

Deconditioning has historically been defined as the physiologic changes occurring with prolonged bed rest or inactivity. The types of changes depends on prior fitness level and the degree of superimposed inactivity. Prolonged bed rest can be caused by a variety of reasons, including acute hospitalization or chronic disability. It is known that a chronic sedentary lifestyle can also lead to deconditioning.

Therapists view deconditioning in functional terms. Significant organ changes that are the most debilitating are experienced in the cardiopulmonary and musculoskeletal systems. When evaluating changes such as reduced aerobic capacity, muscular weakness, and limited joint mobility, it is important to know something about the prior functional performance of the individual. Physiologic changes following a period of inactivity or low activity include the following:

- Cardiovascular changes associated with aging, disease, and inactivity
- Musculoskeletal deconditioning results in a decrease in strength, flexibility, and muscular endurance.
- Muscular endurance is the ability to contract a muscle or group of muscles for multiple repetitions.
- Muscular flexibility relates to functional range of motion available to each joint. (Vorhies & Riley, 1993)

These functional changes can usually be improved with a program of progressive low-level exercises with focus on increasing endurance using an ergometer for both upper and lower extremities. In addition to the usual ADLs, the OT may at times engage patients in game activities to improve balance and coordination. Additionally, those patients that will return home may benefit from energy conservation and work-simplification techniques such as homemaking activities and hobbies. The duration of exercise needed is highly individual and dependent on the person's previous activity level, severity of illness, and length of stay.

WEB SITES

- American Academy of Physical Medicine and Rehabilitation—www.aapmr.org
- Department of Physical Medicine and Rehabilitation—www.hopkinsmedicine.org
- American Geriatric Society—www.americangeriatrics.org

REFERENCES

Ackermann, R. (1998). Elderly patients with hip fracture. *Journal of the American Board of Family Practice, 11*(5), 366–377.

American Geriatrics Society, British Geriatrics Society, American Academy of Orthopaedic Surgeons. (2001). Panel on Falls Prevention: Guidelines for the prevention of falls in older persons. *Journal of the American Geriatrics Society, 49,* 664–672.

Angeleri, F., Angeleri, V. A., Foschi, N., Giaquinto, S., & Nolfe, G. (1993). The influence of depression, social activity and family status in functional outcome after stroke. *Stroke, 24*(10), 1478–1483.

Astrom, M., Adolfsson, R., & Asplund, K. (1993). Major depression in stroke patients: A 3-year longitudinal study. *Stroke, 24:*976–982.

Barer, D. H. (1989). Continence after stroke: Useful predictors or goals of therapy? *Age and Ageing, 18,* 183–191.

Berggren, D., Gustafson, Y., & Eriksson, B. (1987). Postoperative confusion after anesthesia in elderly patients with femoral neck fractures. *Anesthesia and Analgesia, 66,* 497–504.

Bigos, S. et al. (1994). Acute low back pain problems in adults (AHCPR Publication No. 95-0642). Rockville, MD: US Department of Health and Human Services, Public Health Service, Agency for Healthcare Policy & Research.

Bild, D. E., Selby, J. V., Sinnock, P., Browner, W. S., Braveman, P., & Showstack, J. A. (1989). Lower-extremity amputation in people with diabetes:

Epidemiology and prevention. *Diabetic Care, 12*(1), 24–31.

Borrie, M. J., Campbell, A. J., Caradoc-Davies, T. H., & Speers, G. F. S. (1986). Urinary incontinence after stroke: A prospective study. *Age and Ageing, 15*, 177–181.

Brander, V., & Fitzgerald Mullarkey, C. (2002). Rehabilitation after total hip replacement for osteoarthritis. *Physical Medicine and Rehabilitation, 16*(3), 415–429.

Cifu, D. X. (1995). Rehabilitation of fractures of the hip. *Physical Medicine. Rehabilitation: State of the Art Review, 9*, 125–139.

Clagett, G. P., Anderson, F. A., & Heit, J. (1995). Prevention of venous thromboembolism. *Chest, 108*(Suppl.), 312S–334S.

Deyo, R. A., Cherkin, D., & Conrad, D. (1991). Cost, controversy, crisis: Low back pain and the health of the public. *Annual Review of Public Health, 12*, 141–156.

Dillingham, T. (August, 1999). Amputee rehabilitation can improve results. *Biomechanics.*

Muche, J. (2005). *Geriatric rehabilitation.* Retrieved June 26, 2005, from http://www.emedicine.com/pmr/topic164.htm

Esquenazi, A., Vacaranukunkit, T., Torres, M. et al. (1984). Characteristics of a current lower extremity amputee population: Review of 918 cases. *Archives of Physical Medicine and Rehabilitation, 65*, 623.

Esquenazi, A. (Ed.). (1994). Prosthetics. *Physical Medicine & Rehabilitation: State of the Art Reviews, 8*, 1.

Fitzgerald Mullarkey, C., & Brander, V. (2002). Rehabilitation after total knee replacement for osteoarthritis. *Physical Medicine and Rehabilitation, 16*(3), 431–443.

Frampton, K. (2005). Rehabilitation services in long-term care. *Caring for the Ages, 6*(6).

Gallagher, J. C., Melton, L. J., Riggs, B. C., & Bergtrath, E. (1980). Epidemiology of fractures of the proximal femur. *Clinical Orthopedics, 150*, 163–167.

Gordon, W. A., & Hibbard, M. R. (1997). Post-stroke depression: An examination of the literature. *Archives of Physical Medicine and Rehabilitation, 78*(6), 658–663.

Iizuka, M., & Reding, M. (2005). Use of percutaneous endoscopic gastrostomy feeding tubes and functional recovery in stroke rehabilitation: A case-matched controlled study. *Archives of Physical Medicine and Rehabilitation, 86*, 1049–1052.

Joseph, C., & Wanlass, W. (1993). Rehabilitation in the nursing home. *Geriatric Rehabilitation, 9*(4), 859–871.

Kane, R., Ouslander, J., & Abrass, I. (2004). *Essentials of clinical geriatrics* (5th ed., pp. 219–244, 271–275). New York: McGraw-Hill Medical Publishing Division.

Kaplan, R., & Gilbert, A. (2002). Rehabilitation after pelvic and hip fractures. *Physical Medicine & Rehabilitation, 16*(3), 389–398.

Kay, H. W., & Newman, J. D. (1978). Relative incidence of new amputation: Statistical comparison of new amputations. *Orthopedic Prosthetics, 29*, 3.

Koes, B. W., Assendelft, W. J., van der Heijiden, G. J., & Bouter, L. M. (1996). Spinal manipulation for low back pain: An updated systematic review of randomized clinical trials. *Spine, 21*, 2860–2871.

Kramer, A., & Coleman, E. (1999). Stroke rehabilitation in nursing homes. *Clinics in Geriatric Medicine, 15*(4).

Kyle, R. F., Gustiol, R. B., & Premer, R. F. (1979). Analysis of 622 interochanteric hip fractures: A retrospective study. *Journal of Bone and Joint Surgery, 61A*, 216–221.

Linsenmeyer, T. A., & Zorowitz, R. D. (1992). Urodynamic findings of patients with urinary incontinence following cerebrovascular accident. *Neurologic Rehabilitation, 2*(2), 23–26.

Lorish, T. (1993). Stroke rehabilitation. *Clinics in Geriatric Medicine, 9*(4), 705–716.

Madore, G. R. (2006). *Hip fractures.* Retrieved October 26, 2006, from http://www.emedicine.com/emerg/topic198.htm

Nitti, V. W., Adler, H., & Combs, A. J. (1996). The role of urodynamics in the evaluation of voiding dysfunction in men after cerebrovascular accident. *Journal of Urology, 155*(1), 263–266.

Orange, J. B., & Keriesz, A. (1998). Efficacy of language therapy for aphasia. *Physical Medicine & Rehabilitation: State of the Art Reviews, 12*(3).

Perez, E. D. (1994). Physicians take more active role in patient care. *Geriatrics, 49,* 31–37.

Planes, A., Vochelle, N., & Darmon, J. (1996). Risk of deep venous thrombosis after hospital discharge in patients having undergone total hip replacement: Double blind randomized comparison of enoxaparin versus placebo. *Lancet, 348,* 224–228.

Rigler, S. (1999). Management of post-stroke depression in older people. *Stroke, Clinics in Geriatric Medicine, 15*(4).

Russin, L. A., & Russin, M. A. (1981). Hip fracture: A review of 1,166 cases in a community hospital setting. *Orthopedics, 4,* 23–24.

Stewart, D., Phillips, E., Bodeneheier, C., & Cifu, D. (2004). Geriatric rehabilitation. Physiatric approach to the older adult. *Archives of Physical Medicine, 85*(Suppl. 3), S7–S11.

Veis, S. L., & Logemenn, J. A. (1985). Swallowing disorders in persons with cerebrovascular accident. *Archives of Physical Medicine and Rehabilitation, 66*(6), 372–375.

Voight, C. (2001). Rehabilitation considerations with the geriatric patient. In W. E. Prentice & M. L. Voight (Eds.), *Techniques in musculoskeletal rehabilitation* (pp. 679–694). New York: McGraw-Hill Medical Publishing Division.

Vorhies, D., & Riley, B. (1993). Deconditioning. *Clinics in Geriatric Medicine, 9*(4), 745–763.

Wade, D. T., & Hewer, R. L. (1981). Outlook after an acute stroke: Urinary incontinence and loss of consciousness compared in 532 patients. *Quarterly Journal of Medicine, 56*(221), 601–608.

Walsh, N. E., & Schwartz, R. K. (1990). The influence of prophylactic orthosis on abdominal strength and low back injury in the work place. *Annals of Physical Medicine and Rehabilitation, 69,* 245–250.

Zorowitz, R. (June, 2000). Stroke rehabilitation update. Physical Medicine & Rehabilitation Symposium presentation.

BIBLIOGRAPHY

Andersen, T. P. (1990). Rehabilitation of patients with completed stroke. In F. J. Kottke & J. F. Lehman (Eds.), *Krusen's handbook of physical medicine & rehabilitation.* Philadelphia: W.B. Saunders Co.

Burvill, P., Johnson, G. A., Jamrozik, K. D., Anderson, C., & Stewart-Wynne, E. (1997) Risk factors for post stroke depression. *International Journal of Geriatric Psychology, 12,* 219–226.

Mooney, V., Saal, J. A., & Saal, J. S. (1996). Evaluation and treatment of low back pain. *Clinical Symposia, 48*(4), 1–32.

Evans, J., & Carlin, P. (1991). Surgical approach to amputation. *Physical Medicine & Rehabilitation Clinics of North America, 2*(2), 263–277.

Garrison, S. J., Rolak, L. A., Dodaro, R. R., & O'Callaghan, M. (1988). Rehabilitation of the stroke patient. In J. A. DeLisa (Ed.), *Rehabilitation medicine: Principles & practice.* Philadelphia: JB Lippincott.

Goldberg, G. (1991). Stroke rehabilitation. *Physical Medicine & Rehabilitation Clinics of North America, 2*(3).

Jette, D., Warren, R., & Wirtalla, C. (2005). Validity of functional independence staging in patients receiving rehabilitation in skilled nursing facilities. *Archives of Physical Medicine, 86,* 1093–1102.

Kramer, A. M., Steiner, J. F., Schlenker, R. E., Eilertsen, T. B., Hrincevich, C. A., & Tropea, D. A., et al. (1997). Outcomes and costs after hip fracture and stroke: A comparison of rehabilitation settings. *Journal of the American Medical Association, 277,* 396–404.

Klaber Moffett, J. A., Chase, S. M., Portek, I., & Ennis, J. R. (1986). A controlled prospective study to evaluate the effectiveness of a back school in the relief of chronic low back pain. *Spine, 11*(2), 120–122.

Mossman, P. L., & Sharpless, J. W. (1982). *Mossman's problem-oriented approach to stroke rehabilitation* (2nd ed.). Springfield, IL: Charles C. Thomas.

Nachemson, A. C. (1992). Newest knowledge of low back pain: A critical look. *Clinical Orthopedics, 279,* 8–20.

Patel, A., & Ogle, A. (2000). Diagnosis and management of acute low back pain. *American Family Physician, 61*(6), 1779–1786.

Stern, P. H. (1991). The epidemiology of amputation. *Physical Medicine & Rehabilitation Clinics of North America, 2*(2).

Sawner, K. A., & La Vigne, J. M. (1992). *Brunstrom's movement therapy in hemiplegia: A neurophysiological approach* (2nd ed.). Philadelphia: JP Lippincott.

Torres, M., & Esquenazi, A. (1991). Bilateral lower limb amputee rehabilitation. A retrospective review. *Western Journal of Medicine, 154*(5), 583–586.

Twitchell, T. E. (1951). The restoration of motor function following hemiplegia in man. *Brain, 74,* 443–480.

Veteran's Health Administration, U.S. Department of Defense. (2003). *VA/DoD Clinical practice guideline for the management of stroke rehabilitation in the primary care setting.* Retrieved October 26, 2006, from http://www.guideline.gov/summary/summary.aspx?doc_id=3846

Veis, S. L., & Logemann, J. A. (1984). *Incidence and nature of swallowing disorders in CVA patients.* Paper presented at a meeting of the American Speech-Language and Hearing Association, Washington, DC.

Zukerman, J. D., Cifu, D. X., & Means, K. M. (1993). In J. D. Zukermman (Ed.), *Comprehensive care of orthopedic injuries in the elderly* (pp. 23–111). Baltimore: Urban and Schwarzenberg.

CHAPTER 21

Podiatry

Guy Danon

INTRODUCTION

The senior population in America is growing at an extraordinary rate. In 2000, 13% of the population was over 65. It is estimated that by 2020 those over 65 will reach 20%. The consequence of an aging society translates to an ever-growing number of geriatric disorders.

Foot problems arise secondary to systemic illness or may begin as a primary condition. In either case, podiatric patients are seen far more frequently in the geriatric population than in any other age group. A few of the more common geriatric pathologies are arthritis (58%), hypertension (45%), heart disease (21%), orthopedic disability (19%), and diabetes (12%) (Novielli et al., 2003). A reduction in immunocompetence correlating with advancing age is a significant problem for the elderly yet remains an enigmatic process for the treating healthcare provider.

ESTABLISHING A FOOT CARE REGIMEN

Foot pathology occurs frequently during long stays in skilled nursing facilities. As geriatric, diabetic, and disabled patients become more dependent on medical staff, facilities are under greater pressure to prevent lower extremity infection, pedal ulcerations, vascular embarrassment, and traumatic injuries to the foot and ankle.

Disabilities due to compromised neuromotor function, cognitive deterioration, physical rigidity, and foot deformity can result in injuries that force patients into extended periods of dependency or permanent bed rest.

The physician and nurse practitioner are the first-line medical team and should perform the initial foot examination and evaluation at the time of admission. Establishing a baseline of the patient's condition upon admission is vital. Prompt referral to the podiatrist for abnormalities or suspected pathology is essential. The podiatrist can help to coordinate the care and treatment of serious lower extremity conditions. In addition, the podiatrist can help protect both the providers and the facility from a legal standpoint, as there is growing pressure to prevent lower extremity injuries, infections, and ulcers from occurring. For example; on admission to the skilled nursing facility, documentation of the following are recommended:

- Lower extremity skin characteristics
- The quality of pedal pulses

- History of systemic and vascular risk factors
- Differential diagnosis

This data can be very important if there is a lack of improvement or worsening in the patient's pedal ulcerations following the initial treatment plan.

Podiatric examination should include the following:

- Chief complaint or chief problem for non-verbal patients
- Secondary and tertiary complaints or problems
- Past medical and surgical history
- Family history
- Social history
- History of the chief complaint to include nature, location, duration, onset, course, aggravating and relieving methodology, and prior treatment success or failure
- Lower extremity photographs, if indicated
- Clinical observations
- Medical history and physical including any laboratory or imaging studies
- Current list of medications
- Current or prior tobacco, alcohol, and caffeine use and any illicit drug use
- Prior podiatric diagnoses
- Responses to prior podiatric treatments

In addition, bedside testing should be provided for those patients too incapacitated to go outside the facilities. Transfer back to the acute hospital and emergency services may be needed for severe life- or limb-threatening conditions.

▉ MEDICARE AND HEALTHCARE COVERAGE

Healthcare insurance plans and individual facilities vary on how often a podiatrist should visit a patient in the skilled nursing facility. Medicare has established guidelines to allow routine services for "at-risk" individuals. These include patients with one or more systemic conditions along with a specific associated peripheral complication including clinically significant circulatory embarrassment or any of the following:

- Clinically significant circulatory embarrassment
- Clinically significant diminished or absent neurological sensations
- Patients undergoing active treatment for immunocompromised states such as oral corticosteroid therapy, chemotherapy, or HIV
- Patients undergoing active anticoagulant therapy such as heparin or coumadin

These services include trimming, cutting, clipping, or debridement of long dystrophic nails and cutting or removal of corns and calluses. These may be performed no more frequently than every 60 days. In addition, the podiatrist may seek to establish preventative check-ups by making more frequent rounds to high-risk patients.

▉ DIABETIC FOOT CARE, PREVENTION, AND EDUCATION

According to the American Diabetic Association there are 20.8 million people with diabetes in the United States. One third of these individuals are undiagnosed and unaware they have the disease. An estimated 15% of diabetics will develop a pedal ulcer in the course of their lifetime. This is significant because pedal ulcerations that are not treated early can quickly progress to lower limb infection. This situation may continue to quickly deteriorate in the form of a mixed gram, anaerobic, necrotizing, systemic, and/or bony infection. In these cases, surgical intervention, including amputation, is often necessary. There is a 40% survival rate for an amputation below the knee (BKA) or above the knee (AKA) at 5 years (Leonard, Farooqu, & Meyers, 2004). Diabetes is the number one cause of nontraumatic amputation.

As a result of commonalities in immunodeficiency, there exist many common links in pathology shared between the elderly and patients with diabetes. Initial care for diabetic and elderly patients must be delivered with prevention in mind. Educational materials offered by the American Diabetes Foundation should be made available to patients and their families. Nondiabetic, neuropathic, angiopathic, and immunopathic patients may also benefit from these materials. Elderly and diabetic patients should be encouraged to take an active role in their own foot care whenever possible.

Nurse practitioners and physicians caring for patients with diabetes and neuropathy should consider ordering custom molded shoes when necessary. These shoes best protect against skin breakdown and pedal ulcerations. Frequent examinations of the feet, checking for trauma, hyperkeratosis, erythema, suspicious nevi, nail problems, or malodor should be performed by the medical team. If the patient is discharged from the skilled nursing facility to the community, the

patient or family should be instructed to set their hot water regulators to no hotter than 90° to prevent scalding injuries. Extreme cold skin contact in northern climates may also unknowingly result in similar cold burn traumas.

THE NAIL AND AGING

The nail is a hardened, keratinized extension of the epidermis; the underside forming from the stratum germinativum, the free surface comes from the stratum lucidium, the thin cuticular fold overlapping the lunula representing the stratum corneum. See Figure 21-1 for nail structures. The nail serves to provide support for the toe pad and improve sensation in the tips of the fingers and toes. The nail also maintains the shape of the tip of the toes allowing them to make contact with the ground while resisting deformity at the end of the toes. Equal toe purchase by the toes decreases the severity of weight over the metatarsals in gait allowing for improved function without trauma to the metatarsal heads. Although the majority of the toenail's function remains prehensile in

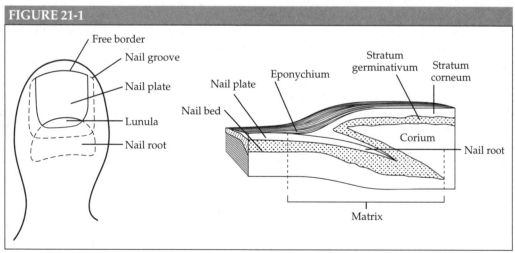

FIGURE 21-1

Source: Banks, A. S., Downey, M. S., Martin, D. E., & Miller, S. J. (2004). *McGlamry's forefoot surgery*. Philadelphia, PA: Lippincott Williams & Wilkins.

TABLE 21-1	Nail Pathology Definitions
Onychomycosis	Thickening and deformity of the nail plate. Infection whose etiology is typically a fungi, candidiasis, or nondermatolytic mold.
Onychogryphosis	Ram's horn nails most frequently associated with onychomycosis or other source of nail dystrophy
Onychoptosis	Absence of a toenail possibly as a result of autoavulsion. Commonly seen in diabetics.
Onychotrophia	Atrophic appearance of the toenail and adjacent tissue due to vascular issues, nutritional problems, or diabetes
Onychia	Inflammatory changes associated with the nail and its subungual structures
Paronychia	Inflammatory changes in subungual soft tissues with greater involvement of the posterior wall than with onychia
Onycauxis	Thickening of toenail brought on by repetitive trauma, decreased nutrition, or infection
Onycholysis	Separation between the nail bed and the nail starting at the free edge of the nail and progressing proximally. Common causes include trauma, psoriasis, onycauxis, or onychomycosis.
Onychophemia	Subungual hemorrhage commonly seen in trauma and diabetes
Onychophosis	Presence of a corn under the nail plate originating from an increase of pressure under the nail plate
Leukonychia	White streaks or spots in the nail plate
Onychia punctate	Pitting in the nail plate typically seen in psoriasis
Kilonychia	Spoon-shaped nail associated with iron deficiency
Pterigium	Hypertrophy of the eponychium related most often to arterial insufficiency

humans, this structure lends itself to many different pathologies. See Table 21-1 for nail pathologies and definitions.

The elderly population is subject to a wide array of toenail disorders. Toenail problems may present with thickened dystrophy of the nail plate leading to pressure erosions of the nail bed. According to Helfland (2003), toenails can become hypertrophied and discolored as a result of advancing age, repetitive microtrauma, previous pedal trauma, dietary deficiencies, drug reactions, skin diseases, metabolic diseases, peripheral vascular disease, or degenerative diseases. Infection is thought to occur through direct extension from the skin to the nail matrix, bed, and surrounding nail tissues. Variables affecting mycotic progression include exposure time, susceptibility to infecting organisms, poor hygiene, socioeconomic status, age and underlying systemic disease. This contagious condition begins superficially in the skin but may become entrenched deeply into the structures of the nail, making eradication a difficult process.

THE IMMUNE SYSTEM AND AGING

As the aging process proceeds, the protective mechanisms of the body become compromised, subsequently opening the door to more virulent forms of bacteria, viruses, fungi, and parasites. With the immune system in a suppressed state, there is a tendency for reduced response towards infection. As a result, the classic signs of infection (calor, dolor, rubor, tumor), may not be so classically demonstrated in the compromised patient. Delayed or missed diagnosis may ensue, leading to delayed or inappropriate care. In addition, nosocomial infection continues to grow as the result of unnecessary antibiotics leading to the development of more resistant strains of bacteria such as vancomycin-resistant enterococci (VRE).

PODIATRIC DERMATOLOGY

When assessing skin pathology, Shiraldi-Deck (2003) states the best approach to diagnosing a lesion is to organize the information into the following three categories:

- A skin component with visible, descriptive, and clinicopathologic alterations
- The applicable clinical manifestations of a disease
- The anatomical site

When evaluating open areas of the skin, the nurse practitioner should be familiar with the National Pressure Ulcer Advisory Panel (NPUAP) classification system. (See Chapter 18, on wound care.) The nurse practitioner can then assess the lesion to determine the appropriate treatment as indicated by the level of depth, necrosis, and any infection if present.

Palpation is of paramount importance when evaluating the consistency of a lesion and its level of penetration on or under the surface of the skin. In circumstances when palpation might lead to contamination of a wound or manipulation of a metastatic lesion, one should use a great deal of discretion. Palpation also serves to determine if a lesion is tender, fluctuant, nodular, rubbery, immobile, or deeply anchored.

CT scan, MRI, angiogram, and cultures may assist in differentiation of a lesion, but the gold standard for identification of a suspicious lesion is the biopsy. Though not as effective as an excisional biopsy, punch biopsies have gained acceptance in obtaining histologic information about abhorrent skin lesions.

See Tables 21-2 and 21-3 for a list of primary lesions and descriptive terms for skin lesions.

VASCULAR INSUFFICIENCY

Elderly or potentially vascular-incompetent individuals should be routinely screened for a number of different pathologic skin disorders.

TABLE 21-2 Primary Lesions

Bullae	Large blisters. Free fluid within cavities. Example: Pemphigus
Macule	Flat lesion with change of color. Greater than 1 cm. Example: Freckle, flat nevi
Nodule	Solid, elevated, 0.5 cm into the dermis Example: Wart
Papule	Small < 0.5 cm elevated, raised, or indurated solid lesion. Example: nevi
Patch	A macule with surface changes. Example: Allergic contact dermatitis
Plaque	Elevated lesion > 0.5 cm Example: Psoriasis
Pustule	A cavity filled with pus Example: Impetigo
Scale	Dried out bit of excess horny material Example: Tinea
Tumor	Elevated, larger than 1 cm, solid Example: Basal cell carcinoma
Vesicle	Small blisters, free fluid within cavities. Example: Herpes zoster
Wheel	Lesion resulting from a leakage of fluid from blood vessels Example: Immune-mediated allergen such as an insect bite

TABLE 21-3 Other Descriptive Terms for Skin Lesions

Keratosis	Circumscribed overgrowth of horny layer
Excoriation	Scratch marks
Induration	Dermal thickening resulting in skin that is thicker and firmer than usual
Lichenification	Exaggerated skin markings
Vegetation	A cauliflower appearance
Verrucous	Wartlike
Violaceous	Somewhat violet in color

The nurse practitioner should evaluate the overall fragility of the skin. How thin, how shiny, how friable is the skin? Note if there is a loss in skin tone, skin elasticity, a decrease in hair growth, or formation of telangiectasias. These findings are normal phenomenon in aging skin, and by themselves do not represent a serious health problem. By contrast, cold toes, digital cyanosis, slow capillary fill time, dependent pedal rubor, and spontaneous pallor in the limbs when elevated above the heart are signs and symptoms of a serious vascular disorder such as Buerger's disease, peripheral artery disease (PAD), or arteriosclerosis obliterans.

Treatment should be aimed at patient education, which include positive reinforcement to reduce or eliminate tobacco use, closely monitoring the underlying systemic condition, addressing nutritional problems, and enhancing circulation through daily lower extremity exercise known as Buerger's exercises.

See Figures 21-2 and 21-3 for gangrene of the foot.

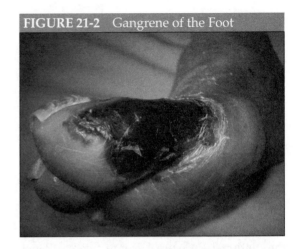

FIGURE 21-2   Gangrene of the Foot

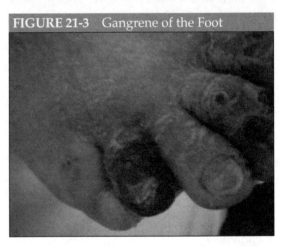

FIGURE 21-3   Gangrene of the Foot

SKIN CANCER

At first sign of a skin lesion the nurse practitioner should establish an initial documented record including photographs and all relevant lab tests. In addition a detailed notation of the lesion's size and characteristics should be recorded (width × length × depth). Commonly used methodology for analyzing melanoma is known as the ABCDs of skin cancer:

- Asymmetry—One half does not match the other half of the lesion.
- Border—The edges are irregular, ragged, notched, or blurred.
- Color—The color is not the same all over and may have patches of brown, black, blue, red or white.
- Diameter that is larger than 6 mm or noticeably growing larger

Frequent reevaluation of a lesion is necessary to record the rate of change. A timescale factoring change in growth, depth, height, color, texture, margins, quality, or quantity of discharge, and degree of patient discomfort may ultimately prove beneficial in selecting the appropriate differential diagnoses and treatment plan.

Pedal malignancies have historically proven to be a rare occurrence. Nonmalignant neoplasms are seen with some frequency in the foot. Neuroma and verruca are just two commonly observed examples in the skilled nursing facility setting. Less common are malignant tumors occurring in the foot and ankle. Nurse practitioners and other providers caring for patients in the skilled nursing facility setting need to be familiar with the characteristics and varying appearances of malignant melanoma, basal cell carcinoma, squamous cell carcinoma, actinic keratosis, and Kaposi's sarcoma. Knowing what to look for in these skin cancers followed by timely referral to the appropriate physician, podiatrist, or oncologist can be a life saving event.

In interviewing a patient, the history and physical must be extensive and complete. A malignancy in the foot may appear as a primary lesion or alternatively present as the result of a distant metastatic cancer such as a renal cell carcinoma or asymptomatic lung tumor. For this reason, it is essential to derive as much information as possible during the course of the history and physical. Palpation is very important when determining the characteristics associated with consistency and texture of the neoplasia. Palpation will determine characteristics of the lesion that will give clues as to its origin. For example, blanching on palpation may indicate vascular origin. Other palpable characteristics may include fluctuance, dermatome pain patterns, nodular aspects, cyctic aspects, hardness, sponginess, immobility, deep attachment, free floating, and so on. However, discretion is advised in circumstances where palpation might lead to disruption of a friable metastatic lesion.

DIAGNOSTIC CONSIDERATIONS

Malignant tumors arising from the dermis or subcutaneous facial layers have been observed to arise slowly or rapidly, and be isolated or in several areas of the body all growing simultaneously. Any newly discovered growth necessitates a biopsy, especially if onset and course appear to be rapid. Suspicious lesions should undergo a full thickness biopsy into the underlying subcutaneous tissue with a 1- to 2-mm border. The appearance of tense or ulcerated epidermis overlying a dermal or subdermal growth is indicative of rapid growth. This is significant as the epidermis has not had time to adequately expand.

ESSENTIAL TESTS

Blood tests, urine tests, radiographs, CT scan, MRI, ultrasonography, angiography, and cultures may assist in differentiation of a lesion. The gold standard for identification is the biopsy. Though not as effective as an excisional biopsy, the punch biopsy has gained acceptance in obtaining histological information from abhorrent skin and subcutaneous lesions. Clinical labs will frequently stage the tumor upon receiving the biopsy.

MALIGNANT MELANOMA

Melanoma is the most common foot malignancy and is more likely to be misdiagnosed than melanoma located elsewhere on the body. See Figure 21-4 for melanoma of the foot. Melanoma accounts for 75% of all deaths involving skin cancer. Incidence increases with age predominantly affecting sun-exposed skin of fair-skinned individuals. Melanoma is a form of skin cancer that involves the malignancy of the pigment-producing cells of the skin derived

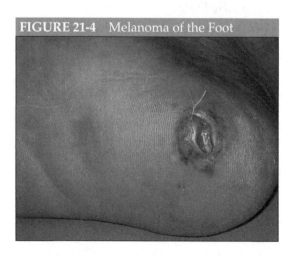

FIGURE 21-4 Melanoma of the Foot

TABLE 21-4	Clark's Staging for Melanoma
• Level I	All tumor cells above basement membrane (in situ)
• Level II	Tumor extends to papillary dermis.
• Level III	Tumor extends to interface between papillary and reticular dermis.
• Level IV	Tumor extends between bundles of collagen of reticular dermis.
• Level V	Tumor invasion of subcutaneous tissue (87% metastases)

from the neural crest cells. Incidence increases with age, predominantly affecting sun-exposed skin of fair complected individuals; however, melanoma can arise on areas of the body receiving no sun exposure. Melanoma on the bottom of the foot has been observed more commonly in persons of black or Asian ancestry. This form of cancer is particularly insidious and deadly if not caught early. See Table 21-4 for Clark's staging of malignant melanoma.

Prognostic Data

The 5-year survival rate is 52% for patients with a primary melanoma in the foot or ankle compared to 84% for patients with a melanoma of the thigh or calf (Walsh et al.). Melanomas can be found anywhere on the foot including under the toenail, where it has a disproportionately high rate of mortality. It is thought the lower survival rate in the foot is attributed to a delay by the patient bringing the condition to the attention of a healthcare professional. Frequently, incorrect diagnosis by the initial practitioner leads to a delay in definitive care.

Tumor thickness is also a prognostic indicator of long-term survival. A sudden change in color or size of an existing nevus, recent onset of pruritis, bleeding, or ulceration of a mole may indicate the presence of malignant transformation in a suspicious lesion. Risk factors may be similar to other skin cancers, such as history of skin cancer, numerous moles on the body, and having fair skin.

Once malignant melanoma has been diagnosed, the two most significant means of determining prognostic information will be the thickness of the tumor and whether or not metastasis has occurred.

BASAL CELL CARCINOMA

Basal cell carcinoma (BCC) is the most common sun-induced tumor of light complected individuals. It usually occurs in areas of chronic skin exposure and may present with chronic lymphedematous legs. In a survey conducted by the American College of Foot Surgeons (Cole & Dalauro, 1990) basal cell carcinoma was the third most common cancer of the foot. It is slow growing and rarely metastasizes. BCC most commonly occurs in adult individuals especially in elderly persons. BCC is believed to emanate from the pluripotential cells within the basal layer of the epidermis or follicular structures. These cells form during life and may develop into hair, sebaceous glands, and apocrine glands. Tumors start in the epidermis and occasionally arise from the outer root sheath of a hair follicle.

SQUAMOUS CELL CARCINOMA

Squamous cell carcinoma (SCC) is a malignancy of the keratinocyte. Cutaneous SCC is the second most common form of skin cancer and frequently arises on the sun-exposed skin of middle-aged and elderly individuals. It is one of the most common skin cancers known to arise from overexposure to the sun within solar keratoses. This form of skin carcinoma may develop from a scar or point of irritation in the lower extremity. Lesions present as ulcers with raised edges or hyperkeratotic nodules.

KAPOSI'S SARCOMA

Kaposi's sarcoma (KS) is a form of angiosarcoma classically observed in older men of Jewish or Mediterranean descent. KS was first described in 1872 by Mortiz Kaposi. An increased incidence in KS was observed during the 1960s in patients taking immunosuppressant medication. Kaposi's sarcoma later became identified as the primary sequela of patients afflicted with AIDS. Studies from the mid 1980s showed KS to be far more prevalent in homosexual AIDS patients than within groups of AIDS-infected IV drug abusers or those patients taking immunosuppressant medication; this lead researchers to believe sexual transmission may play a key role in the development of this form of cancer (Friedman-Kein & Ostreicher, 1984; Gelman & Broder, 1987). This form of cancer has various initial presentations including flat, violaceous patches, plaques, or nodules. They may also appear as translucent, keratotic, cutaneous, or hornlike lesions. Rarely do they appear as pustular lesions.

INFECTIOUS DISEASE IN GERIATRICS

Elderly individuals experience alterations in B-cells and T-cells, diminished control of regulatory immune and fever mechanisms, loss of protection by cell mediated and humoral immunity, decreased responses to immunogens and vaccines, and an increased presence of autoantibodies (Abramson, 1993). This deterioration in specific and nonspecific host defenses may facilitate colonization by micro-organisms such as bacterium, fungi, parasites, and viruses.

COMMON PODIATRIC CONDITIONS SEEN IN LONG-TERM CARE

The following sections address common podiatric conditions frequently encountered in elderly patients. In some cases the nurse practitioner may initiate treatment and refer to podiatry. Clinical guidelines presented include athlete's foot, onychomycosis, inflammation and infection in the toenail unit, polyneuropathy, pressure-induced hyperkeratosis in the neuropathic foot, and plantar neurotrophic ulcer.

The purpose of this section is to provide information that will assist the clinician in gathering data with regards to skin pathology of the foot. Clinical descriptions of pathology will be presented in order to reach a working differential diagnosis. Diagnostic tests will be presented in order to help determine a definitive diagnosis. Treatment and management plans for these various disorders, including preventative, nonpharmaceutical, and pharmaceutical treatment plans, will be discussed.

ATHLETE'S FOOT

Definition

Athlete's foot is an infection of the skin by any number of superficial fungal organisms within the foot. The most common of these organisms are dermatophytes. Dermatophytes are classified into three groups of *keratinophylic filamentous* organisms:

- *Trychophyton*
- *Mycosporum*
- *Epidermophyton*

In addition, these fungal infections can be complicated by the presence of saprophytes, yeast, or bacteria.

Epidemiology

Athlete's foot or *tinea pedis* (TP) affects both sexes and is thought to be more common in adults than in children. The environment of the foot, namely moist, warm, and usually enclosed, predisposes the foot to this type of infection. This humid environment predisposes the foot to various forms of fungal and yeast infections.

Common Presenting Signs and Symptoms

- *Tinea pedis* can present in a "moccasin" like pattern on one foot, but is more commonly observed bilaterally. *Tricophyton rubrum* is most commonly responsible for this condition and manifests clinically as a "moccasin" pattern presenting with thickened scales on the sole, generally stopping at the dorsal/plantar skin margins naming itself by pattern of infection. This type of TP is usually a chronic condition and is very difficult to completely eradicate. It frequently settles into the nail structures as a result of direct extension. (See onychomycosis section.)

- The *bullous* type presents with vesicles or pustules more commonly on one foot than bilateral. Pustules are usually seen in the arch of the foot. Presentation may be acute, subacute, or a chronic infection.

- The most common form of TP manifests as an interdigital infection. It usually presents in the form of whitish macerated skin observed equally in one or both feet. There is frequently a foul musty odor that accompanies this type of TP especially when there is a bacterial coinfection present. *Trychophyton metagrophytes* is usually the fungal species causing this infection. It is quite common and arises from between the toes where moist and macerated tissue can provide a very hospitable environment. The presentation of the lesions are usually observed in moist, soggy skin with scaly vesicular eruptions and fissures. This infection is prominently observed in skin between the fourth and fifth toes and under the toes in the plantar sulcus. This form of TP can rapidly morph into intertriginous mixed bacterial infection involving *Staphylococcus aureus, Proteus, Pseudomonas,* or *Corynebacterium minutissimus.* See Figure 21-5.

- Generally speaking symptomatic athlete's foot is probably the result of a mixed infection that may include *Candida,* gram-positive and gram-negative bacteria, and sporophytic fungi.

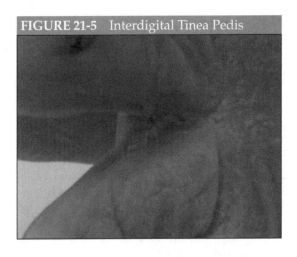

FIGURE 21-5   Interdigital Tinea Pedis

Differential Diagnosis

- Erythrasma
- *Candida albicans*
- *Staphylococcus* infection

Essential Diagnostic and Laboratory Tests

- Definitive diagnosis can be determined through use of a Wood's lamp. (Erythrasma shows up as coral red fluorescence under this blue lamp.)

- Definitive tests include KOH preparation (use epidermal scraping from active borders of the lesion).

- Histological exam (look for presence of septate and branched hyphae).

- Wound cultures and gram stain may be indicated in conjunction with X-rays to rule out gas formation or osteomyelitis.

Management Plan

Nonpharmacologic

- Regular daily or twice daily change to dry cotton socks. The patient should routinely alternate shoes to allow them to dry out between wearings to reduce the incidence of maceration between toes.

- Prevention of recurrence can be accomplished by avoiding excessive moisturizing skin cream between the toes, drying interdigital areas thoroughly after baths, and regular podiatric consults.

Pharmacologic
- For mild infection use sparse application of antifungal gel to interdigital areas and creams to plantar areas daily or twice daily for two weeks until symptoms have resolved. Clotrimazole 1%, Naftifine 1%, Loprox gel 0.77%, and Econazole nitrate 1% are examples of antifungals. Reevaluate in 2 weeks, after treatment complete.

- Treatment for moderate infection may be similar to treatment for mild infection except that results should prove more effective using sparse application of Econazole 1%. This is due to Econazole's broad spectrum of coverage against dermatophytes, some gram-positive bacteria and *Candida.*

- For severe infection, topical antifungals alone will not resolve the infection. At this stage of presentation, usually massive tissue breakdown is involved including the high probability of bacterial coinfection. If a webspace infection has been diagnosed via an interdigital portal of entry, it is important to measure the size, depth, and evaluate the area for sinus tracts. Wound cultures and gram stain may be indicated in conjunction with X-rays to rule out gas formation or osteomyelitis.

- Incision and drainage of the infected webspaces may be indicated. The addition of antibiotics or oral antifungals such as griseofulvin 375 mg twice daily for 4–8 weeks or Fluconazole 6 mg/kg first day, then 3 mg/kg thereafter for 4 weeks. Always obtain liver function tests prior to initiating oral antifungals and repeat at regular intervals especially when there is concern of hepatic compromise.

- Management is directed toward allowing air to circulate interdigitally using Lamb's wool

or cotton in between the toes. Topical drying agents such as povidone iodine, gentian violet, or carbolfuchsin paint will promote drying.

- Tepid water and domeboro soaks followed by towel drying may also help to dry and eradicate fungi. Do not use this treatment where open lesions have been identified, as maceration of these tissues may facilitate the spread of bacteria to deeper fascial planes.

Patient, Family, and Staff Education
- Encourage use of proper foot wear. Discard old shoes.
- Use foot covers especially in high-trafficked areas such as bathing areas.
- Explain importance of alternating shoes; periodically disinfect shoes, and wash feet on a regular basis.
- Report any new problems involving the feet to the nurse practitioner or physician.

ONYCHOMYCHOSIS

Definition
Onychomychosis is a common fungus infection of the nails causing thickening, roughness, and splitting.

Epidemiology
Onychomychosis is thought to originate from chronic skin infection or trauma allowing invasion of the nail matrix by such organisms as *Tinea rubrum, Tinea metagrophytes, Epidermophyton floccosum,* and *Candida albicans.* Infection is thought to occur through direct extension of the skin to the nail matrix, nail bed, and surrounding nail tissues. Increased exposure of the toenails to chronic TP infection increases the propensity for spread to contagious nail tissues. Variables affecting mycotic progression are exposure times to infected skin, susceptibility to infecting organisms, hygienic aptitude, socioeconomic status, age, and underlying systemic disease. This contagious condition is

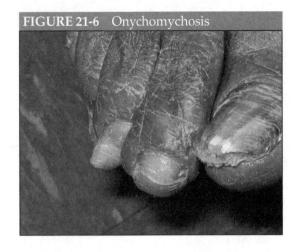

FIGURE 21-6   Onychomychosis

found invested deeply into the structures of the nail including the nail plate, nail bed, and nail matrix. See Figure 21-6.

Common Presenting Signs and Symptoms

Onychomychosis is a common nail disorder that can be clinically identified by some or all of the following:

- Marked discoloration, brittleness, crumbling of the nail plate
- Hypertrophy of the nail plate
- Subungual debris
- Lost of nail luster
- Surrounding soft tissue onychia or paronychia
- Vertical or horizontal ridges
- Ram's horn nail appearance
- Foul musty odor
- Separation of the nail from the nail bed

Differential Diagnosis

- Psoriasis
- Eczema
- Trauma
- Lichen planus
- Yellow nail syndrome

Essential Diagnosis and Laboratory Tests

Identification of the infecting organism is essential to providing management for this disorder. The following tests assist in the diagnosis of the invading *fungus* but do not rule out coinfection by *yeast, molds, or bacteria.*

- Culture
- Periodic acid Schiff stain
- KOH

Management Plan

Nonpharmacologic

- Successful management should always include mechanical debridement of the toenails.

- Reducing the amount of moisture that comes directly into contact with the skin and toenails includes the use of cotton socks, leather shoes, and frequent exposure of feet to open air. Use moisturizing creams judiciously.

- Daily application of talcum powders and rotation of shoes to allow 48 hours for shoes to dry out can also help to maintain a dry environment within the shoe.

Pharmacologic

- To date there has been no cure found for onychomychosis. Treatment results will vary with a high rate of recurrence.

- **Topical:** Currently only Ciclopirox 8% lacquer is FDA approved for the treatment of onychomychosis. It requires daily application and weekly removal by a nail file. A minimum of 48 weeks is needed to achieve fungal eradication. Results will vary depending of the severity of infection. Extremely deformed and dystrophic toenails may not return to original thickness, shape, and luster.

- **Oral:** Oral antifungals such as Terbinifine and Itraconazole have been proved relatively safe and more reliably effective than topicals. They may be preferred when treating more severe infection where the nail appears to have little chance of recovery with topical treatment alone. Terbinifine is given in a dose of 250 mg/daily for 90 days. It may be taken with or without food. Terbinifine has very limited activity against *Candida.* Itraconazole is given twice daily for the first 7 days, followed by a 21-day washout period every month for 6 months. Monitoring of ALT and AST should be done initially and every 4 to 6 weeks of treatment in both oral antifungals. If levels reach two times normal, treatment should be discontinued. Patients should be screened for prior liver disorders and allergies prior to initiating treatment.

- **Combination therapy:** Though not as heavily researched, the merits of using both oral and topical treatments together appear to be showing promising results. Demonstrably improved results have been observed in several studies when the two routes of administration are combined (Olaffson, Sigurgeirsson, & Brarn, 2003).

- **Matrixectomy:** When antifungals are contraindicated or impractical, destruction of the nail matrix may be the preferred means to prevent further growth of a pathological nail. Matrixectomy is essentially the destruction of the nail root by way of surgery or chemical cauterization. This means of nail therapy is generally considered as a last resort treatment and is contraindicated in patients with peripheral vascular disease.

Patient, Family, and Staff Education

- Follow education as outlined in the section on athlete's foot.

- Educate on importance of routine nail inspection.

▬ INFLAMMATION AND INFECTION IN THE TOENAIL UNIT (PARONYCHIA)

Definition

When an inflammatory process takes place in the nail bed and adjacent soft tissues it is usually the result of repetitive microtrauma or less frequently frank trauma to the nail and adjacent tissues. This condition involves erythema, pain, and swelling. Paronychia generally carries with it a greater involvement of the posterior nail wall and presence of purulent material compares to eponychia.

Epidemiology

Trauma to the surrounding soft tissue structures of the nail unit is generally thought to be the primary reason for initiating an ingrown nail. Trauma is defined simply as an injury. Although frank trauma to the toenail structures causes inflammation and infection, it is much more common to have inflammation arise from repetitive microtrauma to the adjacent soft tissues. Thickness and involution of the nail plate forced against the inside of a shoe or an adjacent toe is a microscopic insult that becomes significant with frequent repetition. See Figure 21-7 for infected toenail.

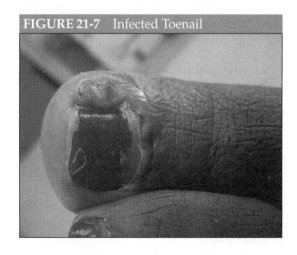

FIGURE 21-7 Infected Toenail

Common Presenting Signs and Symptoms

- Nail deformity

- Adjacent nail tissues are painful, red, swollen, and warm

- Discharge or drainage emanating from periungual soft tissue

- Presence of nail spicules left by improper cutting of nails

Differential Diagnosis

- Trauma

- Psoriasis

- Felon

- Herpetic witlow

Essential Diagnostic and Laboratory Tests

The accumulation of bacteria within tissues can be analyzed by laboratory studies and tissue biopsy. This method is one means of distinguishing between inflammation and infection and is considered the gold standard for discerning between the two. When soft tissue bacterial load reaches roughly 10^5/gm of tissue, a transformation from inflammation to infection takes place within the tissues. Though bacteriology is an important analytical tool for diagnosing infection, it is far too impractical for diagnosis of a common paronychia. Rather, diagnosis should rely on clinical determination via the appearance of purulent matter and the degree of pain, warmth, swelling, and erythema to the local tissue.

Management Plan

Nonpharmacologic

Management is usually directed towards incision and drainage of the abscess and debridement of the offending portion of the nail and its matrix.

Pharmacologic

- Antibiotics may be used in the event of cellulitis associated with paronychia, but the patient should be carefully monitored when there is potential renal impairment, drug interaction issues, or fear of allergic reaction.

- Upon obtaining wound cultures and sensitivities, treat with the most broad spectrum, least toxic, and cost-effective antibiotic. Examples include Cephalexin, Levofloxacin, and Azithromycin.

Patient, Family, and Staff Education

- Avoid footwear with pointed toes or a narrow toe box.

- Shoes should fit properly, allowing one quarter to one half inch from the tip of the longest toe to the front of the shoe.

- Report any signs of infection to the nurse practitioner or physician.

DISTAL DIABETIC POLYNEUROPATHY

Definition

Polyneuropathy is a collective sensory and motor neuropathy, most often symmetric and segmental involving autonomic neurons. It is seen frequently in older diabetic patients.

Epidemiology

Pedal lesions and callosities more commonly develop into limb-threatening illnesses in diabetic patients than with most other neuropathic disorders. Diabetes is a condition that inflicts metabolic and endocrine disturbances that interfere with wound healing and compromise the immune system. Moreover, the renal system is adversely affected as a result of hyperglycemic-induced damage to renal blood vessels. This accounts for the high incidence of end-stage renal disease observed in diabetics. If plasma glucose remains high, damage to the kidneys gradually occurs, limiting classes of antibiotics that will be effective to fight infection. Therefore, uncontrolled diabetics are at greater risk of losing a limb than are other neuropaths because the body is affected on a multiple systemic level over extended periods of chronic, overt hyperglycemia.

A number of studies have evaluated measurement of glycosylated proteins, primarily HA1c and serum fructosamine. Both glycosylated proteins are used as screening tools for diabetes. Test characteristics are compared with fasting plasma glucose to obtain a more complete picture of the patient's glucose control. Good glycemic control is important as most tissue damage occurs during fluctuation of plasma glucose.

The effects on the nerves in a poorly controlled diabetic typically result in morphological and functional changes to those nerves. These changes may also include microvascular disease leading to nephropathy, retinopathy, and distal diabetic polyneuropathy. These problems are compounded by slower recovery rates associated with the elderly population.

Common Presenting Signs and Symptoms

- Typical onset of symptoms begins in the form of tingling, loss of sensation, paresthesias, burning, or pain.
- Progression to end-stage often results in complete pedal and distal lower limb anesthesia including loss of motor ability.
- The term *diabetic distal polyneuropathy* reflects the involvement of the feet, calves, and later the hands in a "stocking and glove distribution."

Differential Diagnosis

- Arsenic intoxication
- Chronic alcoholism
- Carcinoma of the lung
- Arteriosclerosis obliterans

Essential Diagnostic and Laboratory Tests

Evaluation of a patient for neuropathy can be accomplished by use of the following instruments. Positive findings can be seen in some or all of the following methods when testing for diabetic neuropathy:

- Tuning fork: A (+) result indicates a decrease in normal time-length standards or indicates loss of sensitivity to the turning fork.
- Pinwheel: A (+) result indicates a compromised ability to discern sharp noxious stimuli.
- Calipers: A (+) result differentiates the ability of the patient to discern two individual points within the upper limit of normal.
- Cotton ball: A (+) result indicates reduced ability to feel light touch on the skin.
- Neurological hammer: A (+) result indicates relative hyper- or hyporeflexia in deep tendon reflexes.
- The Semmes-Weinstein monofilament 5.07 wire (10 gm equivalent): A (+) result indicates that the minimum sensory protective pressure threshold is not met over the specific area of skin where the test is conducted. This area is vulnerable to injury without sensory stimuli reaching the conscious level.
- Nerve conduction studies
- Gait analysis and lower extremity muscle function, strength, and range of motion tests

Management Plan
Nonpharmacologic

- Prevent skin breakdown in the lower extremity through special custom molded shoes, debridement of callosities, and encouraging the patient to exercise to maintain mobility of the joints as much as possible.
- Protect the joint of the lower extremity by evaluating joint limitation problems and consulting physical therapy.

- Anodyne therapy: An FDA-approved device that delivers non-chromatic infrared light energy (MIRE) for use as a heating method in conjunction with physical therapy.

Pharmacologic
- Tricyclic antidepressants
- Pregabalin/duloxetine
- Capsaicin cream
- Xylocain patches 5%
- Antiseizure medications such as gabapentin
- NSAIDs
- Narcotics
- Nerve block

Patient, Family, and Staff Education
- Explain the importance of good glycemic control to prevent complications of diabetes.
- Explain the importance of foot hygiene and protective supportive shoes that will prevent skin breakdown.
- Educate on the importance of inspection of the feet for signs of trauma or infection.
- Notify the provider for any changes such as erythema or skin breakdown.

PRESSURE-INDUCED HYPERKERATOSIS

Definition
Pressure-induced hyperkeratosis is the thickening of the stratum corneum brought on by focal, direct, or sheer pressure.

Epidemiology
Calluses are the skin's adaptation to frequent, low-intensity friction. They form through increased cell cohesion, reduced shedding, and a thickening of the outer epidermal layer of dead skin. The resulting indurated areas generally form over bony prominences and have accentuated normal skin lines throughout. Calluses are usually not painful and in fact can benefit athletes as the hardened skin protects areas subjected to repeated pressures.

Pressure imparted on the human foot varies from person to person, but over time, structural breakdown invariably affects the shape of the foot. Change in the shape may vary from a mild sag in the longitudinal arch of the foot to the most severe of neuropathological deformities such as in Charcot foot. See Figure 21-8.

Nearly everyone develops a pressure corn or callus in their lifetime. Hyperkeratosis may form temporarily as a result of poor fitting shoes or permanently from a severe alteration in the mechanics of gait. See Table 21-5 for disorders affecting the biomechanics of gait.

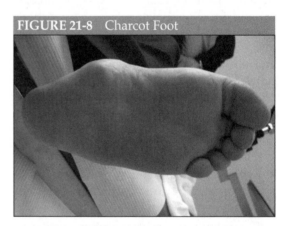

FIGURE 21-8   Charcot Foot

TABLE 21-5   Disorders Affecting Biomechanics of Gait

Ataxia: Tumor, multiple sclerosis, Wernicke's encephalopathy, alcoholic cerebellar, superior vermis

Chorea: Huntington's chorea, Fahr's syndrome

Hemiplegic: Stroke

Myopathic: Muscular dystrophy

Neuropathic: Diabetes, peroneal nerve injury

Parkinsonian: Parkinson's disease

Spastic diplegic: Cerebral palsy

Steppage gait: Posterior tibial tendon dysfunction

Major causes resulting in the formation of calluses include poor fitting shoes, pedal deformities, torsional hip and leg abnormalities, joint contractures, limb length discrepancy, ankle and forefoot equines, anomalous muscle function and tendon imbalance, bony pathology, gait abnormalities, and skin pathologies.

Common Presenting Signs and Symptoms

- Hyperkeratosis runs the gamut from a simple corn or callus to the most severely debilitating and exquisitely painful multiple lesion presentation as is observed in Unna-Thost disease.
- Clinical recognition of signs and symptoms such as verrucae bleed upon debridement from multiple punctate.

Differential Diagnosis

- Verruca planus/vulgaris
- Dyskeratosis congenita
- Reiter's syndrome
- Punctate keratoderma
- Unna-Thost syndrome

Essential Diagnostic and Laboratory Tests

Biopsy is the gold standard.

Management Plan

Nonpharmacologic

- Routine debridement is essential to reduce the potential for necrosis of the lesion.
- Functional or accommodative shoe insert to accommodate lesion
- Surgical excision of the lesion and underlying bone
- Cauterization of the lesion
- Cryotherapy
- Laser excision

Pharmacologic

- Daily application of keratylitic creams such as Keralac 50% or 40% to lesions. Over-the-counter (OTC) products are available in weaker strength formulations.
- Silver nitrate (not recommended for diabetics or patients with peripheral vascular disease).
- Monocloroacetic acid
- 5-florouracil

Patient, Staff, and Family Education

- Explain importance of properly fitting shoes.
- Explain importance of appropriate bathing and drying of feet.

PLANTAR NEUROTROPHIC ULCER

Definition

A neurotrophic ulcer can be defined as a breakdown in the skin from repetitive microtrauma that goes undetected due to sensory deprivation. The elderly are more predisposed to plantar ulcers due to progressive deterioration of sensory and motor function. Progressive and ischemic changes are typically observed in nondiabetic patients suffering from cerebrovascular accident, chronic subdural hematoma, posterior column degenerations, pernicious anemia, Parkinson's disease, neoplasms, and senile dementia. These disorders all place the elderly at increased risk for developing neuropathic decubiti.

Epidemiology

Foot lesions and callosities more commonly develop into life-threatening illnesses in diabetic patients than with other neuropathic disorders. In addition to the loss in protective sensory threshold induced by some other pathologies, diabetics also need to overcome metabolic and endocrine disturbances that alter wound healing and interfere with the immune system. Additionally, the fluctuation in plasma blood glucose affects the body on a multi-system level.

The renal system is especially prone to this type of effect. Hyperglycemia caused by diabetes damages blood vessels in the kidneys. If plasma glucose remains high, this damage gradually reduces the function of the kidneys. This accounts for the high incidence of end-stage renal disease observed in diabetics.

Diabetics are at greater risk of foot lesions progressing to limb-threatening infections and gangrene, because in addition to all above mentioned diabetic complications there is also the potential problem of the endocrine disorder itself causing a flux in blood sugar affecting the body on a multiple system level.

Pedal trauma is frequently initiated from a pressure point on the sole of the foot or in between the toes. A typical callus will develop as the result of shear forces (friction) acting upon a point on the surface of the skin. The epidermis will respond by forming a horny growth (callus) at the point on the skin in response to the deforming forces imparted on the skin by one's weight or means of ambulation. The focal pressure increases inversely to the size of the surface area undergoing such friction. As the callus thickens, the situation progresses and peak pressures result in a loss of oxygen tension (PO_2) within local capillary beds feeding adjacent skin. The patient may not feel discomfort due to neuropathy and fail to off-load resulting in necrosis of the skin just beneath the callus. The neurotropic decubitus ulcer ensues.

See wound care section for management of wounds.

Common Presenting Signs and Symptoms

- Deformity of the toes or feet
- Loss of mobility within the joints of the foot, ankle, or leg
- Erythematous areas associated with bony protuberance of the foot

- Hyperkeratosis on the soles, toes, or between the toes
- Skin erosions or fissures
- Maceration between the toes
- Insensate foot
- Absent pedal pulses
- History of prior ulcerations

Differential Diagnosis

- Basal cell carcinoma
- *Zoster gangrenosum*
- Angiosarcoma
- Squamous cell carcinoma
- Verruca planus/vulgaris

Essential Diagnostic and Laboratory Tests

- Biopsy
- Wound culture and sensitivities
- Imaging studies to assess the source of friction

Management Plan

Nonpharmacologic

- Management of preulcerous and stage 1 ulcers is geared toward eliminating the source of pressure such as reducing retro-calcaneal pressure with a heel protector or a heel-lift, or smooth-suspension boot to reduce friction.
- Address contractures and immobility in lower limbs.
- Lamb's wool between the toes or a film dressing such as Tegaderm to reduce friction.
- Management for stage 2 ulcers and above requires an interdisciplinary team approach. See wound care chapter for management of wounds.

Pharmacologic

See chapter on wound care.

Patient, Family, and Staff Education

- Educate on the importance of daily inspection of feet in high-risk patients.
- Notify the provider of any erosive skin changes.

WEB SITES

- American Diabetic Association—www.diabetes.org
- Merck Manual of Geriatrics—www.merck.com/mrkshared/mmg/home.jsp

REFERENCES

Abramson, C. (1993). Infection and the older patient. *Clinics in Podiatry Medicine and Surgery, 10,* 249–269.

Cole, D. R., & Dalauro, T. M. (1990). *Neoplasms of the foot and leg.* Baltimore, MD: Williams and Wilkins.

Friedman-Kein, A., & Ostreicher, R. (1984). Overview of classical and epidemic Kaposi's sarcoma. In A. Friedman-Kien, & L. Laubenstein (Eds.), *AIDS: The epidemic of Kaposi's sarcoma and opportunistic infections* (pp. 23–34). New York: Masson.

Gelman, E., & Broder, S. (1987). Kaposi's sarcoma in the setting of the AIDS pandemic. In S. Broder (Ed.), *AIDS: Modern concepts and therapeutic challenges* (pp. 219–232). New York: Marcel Dekker.

Helfland, A. E. (2003). Podiatric assessment of the geriatric patient. *Clinics in Podiatry Medicine and Surgery, 20,* 407–429.

Leonard, D. R., Farooqu, M. H., & Meyers, S. (2004). Restoration of sensation, reduced pain, and improved balance in subjects with diabetic peripheral neuropathy: A double-blind, randomized placebo-controlled study with monochromatic near-infrared treatment. *Diabetes Care, 27*(1), 168–172.

Olaffson, J. H., Sigurgeirsson, B., & Brarn, R. (2003). Combination therapy for onychomycosis. *British Journal of Dermatology, 149*(Suppl. 65), 15–18.

Shiraldi-Deck, F. G. (2003). Podiatric assessment of the geriatric patient. *Clinics in Podiatry Medicine and Surgery, 20,* 453–467.

BIBLIOGRAPHY

Arndt, K. A. (1991). *Manual of dermatologic therapeutics* (5th ed.). New York: Little Brown.

Beaulieu, M. D. (1994). Screening for diabetes mellitus in the non-pregnant adult. In Canadian Task Force on the Periodic Health Examination (Eds.), *Canadian guide to clinical prevention health care* (pp. 602–609). Ottawa: Health Canada.

Berlin, S. (1980). A review of 2729 lesions of the foot. *Journal of the American Podiatry Medicine Association, 70,* 318–324.

Brooks, K. E., & Bender, J. F. (1996). Tinea pedia. *Clinics in Podiatry Medicine and Surgery, 13,* 20–36.

Davidson, M. B. (1998). *Diabetes mellitus: Diagnosis and treatment* (4th ed.). Philadelphia: W.B. Saunders.

Hess, S. D. (2006). *Squamous cell carcinoma.* Retrieved November 2, 2006, from http://www.emedicine.com/derm/topic401.htm

Joseph, W. (2003). *Handbook of lower infections* (2nd ed.). St. Louis, MO: Churchill Livingstone.

Kochman, A. B., Carnegie, D. H., & Burke, T. J. (2002). Symptomatic reversal of peripheral neuropathy in patients with diabetes. *Journal of the American Podiatry Medicine Association, 92*(3), 125–130.

Lee, D., & Dauphinée, D. M. (2005). Morphological and functional changes in the diabetic peripheral nerve. *Journal of the American Podiatric Medicine Association, 95,* 433–437.

Mooser, G., Pillekamp, H., & Peter, R. U. (March, 1998). Suppurative acrodermatitis continua of Hallopeau. A differential diagnosis of paronychia. *Deutsche medizinische Wochenschrift, 123*(13), 386–390.

National Institute on Aging, U.S. National Institutes of Health. (2005). *Foot care for older people.* Bethesda, MD: Author. Retrieved November 2, 2006, from http://www.niapublications.org/agepages/footcare.asp

Ramsey, M. L. (2006). *Basal cell carcinoma.* Retrieved November 2, 2006, from http://www.emedicine.com/derm/topic47.htm

Warner, I. (2003). Nursing and long-term care concerns of the foot. *Clinics in Podiatry Medicine and Surgery, 20,* 407–429.

Zendrick, M. R., Young, M. P., Daley, R. J., & Light, T. R. (1982). Metastatic tumors of the foot: Case report and literature review. *Clinical Orthopaedics and Related Research, 170,* 219–225.

CHAPTER 22

Pain Management

Pegi Black

A challenging task in long-term care is pain management. The goal is to find an optimal balance between pain relief and maintaining function with the least side effects. This chapter is divided into two sections. The first is an overview of pain including the incidence, definitions by types, classifications, barriers, consequences, and a process to diagnosis and treat. The second section is a systematic approach to the primary types of pain: acute, chronic, cancer, rehabilitative, and pain at end of life. All of the information is based on the American Medical Directors Association (AMDA), American Geriatrics Society (AGS), Agency for Health Care, Policy, and Research (AHCPR) Acute and Cancer Pain Practice Guidelines, and American Pain Society (APS) recommendation for pain management. It is not expected to be an exhaustive review of pain but a guide in the management of this most common and challenging symptom impacting practitioners in long-term care. Given this rapidly growing field, the reader is strongly encouraged to obtain other resources that are devoted entirely to pain. (See reference list.)

EPIDEMIOLOGY, PREVALENCE, AND INCIDENCE

Pain is a dominant problem in caring for the elderly and continues to be severely undertreated. It is not a normal part of aging although research shows that after age 60 the incidence of pain doubles and increases with each decade (American Geriatrics Society, 2002). This is a result of many conditions, such as gout, fibromyalgia, neuropathies, along with bone and joint disorders that occur in individuals over the age of 65. In the long-term care setting it is estimated that 45% to 80% of the population has significant pain affecting their quality of life (Helm & Gibson, 1999). Attitudes toward pain, cognitive impairment, physiologic changes, and end-of-life issues all add to the specific needs in managing pain in the elderly.

DEFINITION

According to the International Association for the Study of Pain (IASP) the definition is an unpleasant sensory and emotional experience associated with actual or potential tissue damage or described in terms of such damage. However a definition most applicable to clinical practice proposed by McCaffery (1999) describes pain as: "Whatever the experiencing person says it is, existing whenever he/she says it does." Based on that, the patient's self-report of pain is the single most reliable indicator (Griffie, McKinnon, Berry, & Heidrich, 2002; Jacox, et al., 1994).

Pain is complex with physical, psychological, and social components that can be affected by one's spiritual and cultural belief system. In the long-term care setting, five basic types of pain are identified: acute, chronic, cancer, rehabilitative, and pain at end of life.

- *Acute pain*—Relatively brief in duration, usually an episode that lasts brief seconds to about 6 months or less. It is based on a recognized cause of pain, and as healing takes place it diminishes.
- *Chronic pain*—Experience that continues for a prolonged period of time which may or may not be associated with a recognizable disease process. It is based on a body's physiological and behavioral adaptation over time.
- *Cancer pain*—Originating from the tumor itself (e.g., chemical inflammation, mechanical pressure on nerves), remote effects of the tumor, diagnostic procedures, treatments, or pain unrelated to malignancy (Eisenber, Borsook, & LeBell, 1996).
- *Rehabilitative pain*—Convalescent pain that presents as mild to moderate pain at rest or as moderate to severe incident pain lasting approximately two weeks to two months following surgery or trauma. Pain can have a negative impact on physical therapy, thus affecting function and quality of life (Adult Pain, 2001).
- *Pain at end of life*—Pain or suffering hours to days before life ends. This process is the result of a variety of causes and requires careful assessment and management.

Classifications

To further clarify pain it is divided into sources or etiology of pain. This includes nociceptive (somatic and visceral), neuropathic (nerve), and psychologic or idiopathic.

Nociceptive Pain

Nociceptive pain is generated from tissue damage. Intact neurons from somatic (cutaneous) or visceral (gut) structures transmit electrical signals along functioning nerves and pain is experienced (Griffie et al., 2002). Somatic structures include bone, joints, muscles, skin, and connective tissue. Visceral tissue arises mainly from thoracic, abdominal, and pelvic organs.

Neuropathic Pain

Neuropathic pain is caused by either direct damage to or dysfunction of nerves rather than activation of nociceptors. However neuropathic pain frequently coexists with nociceptive pain. It is the most disturbing and complex pain occurring anywhere in the peripheral or central nervous system (Galer & Dworkin, 2002).

Psychologic or Idiopathic Pain

Psychologic or idiopathic pain is based on the patient's perception and is fundamental to how well it is tolerated. Symptoms and associated distress are to be taken seriously. Treatment begins with a full investigation of cause along with supportive care and/or pharmacotherapy for anxiety, depression, or other psychological disorders that may be experienced. Most often this diagnosis is based on exclusion and will require an outside referral.

◼ BARRIERS TO THE RECOGNITION OF PAIN

Pain is poorly identified in the long-term care setting. In an effort to achieve effective pain management one must be aware of the common misconceptions and barriers. See Table 22-1.

TABLE 22-1   Barriers to Pain Management in Long-Term Care

Patient and Family Barriers

- Elderly may not show typical signs and symptoms of pain

- May be cognitively impaired or have sensory impairments or difficulties with language or speech

- Racial, ethnic, and gender biases in both patients and staff

- Fear of medication side effects

- Concerns of addiction

- Belief that pain is part of aging

- Fear of being labeled "a bad patient"

Healthcare Professional Barriers

- Lack of education regarding pain assessment and management

- Concern over regulatory scrutiny

- Fears of opioid side effects

- Assumption that pain is a normal part of aging that can not be managed

- Coexisting illness and multiple medications limiting reporting or masking responses to pain making assessment difficult

- Reluctance to refer to access pain specialist

Healthcare System Barriers

- Insufficient numbers of qualified staff

- High turnover of staff

- Inadequate communication among interdisciplinary team members

- Insufficient time by staff to fully assess patients given high staff/patient ratios

- Limited drug formulary

Source: Adapted from American Medical Directors Association, 2003; Hanks-Bell, Halvey, & Paice, 2004.

CONSEQUENCES OF PAIN

Depression, anxiety, isolation, sleep disturbance, malnutrition, and impaired functional status are frequent occurrences of untreated or undertreated pain in the elderly (McCaffery, 1999). In the long-term care setting, pain and depression has been found to have a significant relationship that negatively impacts quality of life (Parmelee, Katz, & Lawton, 1991). For instance, patients may be treated with a psychotropic medication for behavioral issues when the real problem is unrecognized pain. Since 1999 the issue of appropriate pain management has been a standard of care evaluated by the Joint Commission on Accreditation of Healthcare Organizations (JCAHO). Failure to comply with JCAHO standards in the assessment and treatment of pain can lead to the loss of accreditation of an institution (JCAHO & National Pharmaceutical Council [NPC], 2001). It is important for nurse practitioners not to overlook the many facets to pain and how it can negatively impact the elderly in long-term care.

PROCESS TO DIAGNOSIS AND TREATMENT

Assessment

Pain is a symptom not a diagnosis and assessing elderly in long-term care creates special challenges for the entire healthcare team. Pain is multidimensional and requires a comprehensive, holistic, and systematic assessment that is fundamental to an appropriate plan of care. Many patients can have more than one type of pain, and it is important to distinguish each and treat accordingly. Assessment focuses on the present and past medical and pain history, along with the physical exam.

General History

- History of present illness—May have had recent fall or injury
- Current medications—Medications may result in myalgias.

- Medication allergies—Acute allergic reaction to particular medications or comorbidity that would be a contraindication to analgesics
- Past medical history—May have a chronic component to acute pain episode

Pain History

- Location—Where, radiation, sudden or gradual
- Quality—Sharp, dull, stabbing, pulsating, burning, and so on
- Modifying factors—What makes it better or worse?
- Impact on function—Affects sleep, appetite, activities, and mood
- Effect of treatments—Medications or therapy that work
- Severity or intensity—Measurement of pain can be challenging. Poor memory, depression, and sensory impairment can limit the ability to accurately report pain in the elderly. There are a variety of tools available such as the Visual Analog Scales (VAS) that measure the intensity or magnitude of sensations by marking on a continuum. Descriptors are placed at each end that are easily understood and identify the intensity from low to high. The numeric rating scale (NRS) is another tool utilizing 0 to 5 or 0 to 10 with the high number representing highest severity. When quantifying pain cannot be measured numerically the Verbal Descriptor Scale (VDS) with simple categories such as mild, moderate, severe, or extreme pain may be useful. Most important is to use a consistent tool that is accepted within each institution and understood by the patient.

Physical Exam

- Focused physical examination with emphasis on body or region in pain
- Vital signs with special attention to pulse, blood pressure, and respiratory rate. Subtle

changes may be the only manifestation in patients who are noncommunicative or confused.

- Mental status, neurological assessment with emphasis on sensory dysfunction and musculoskeletal status is important in determining specific areas of pain, possible etiology, and facilitating treatment choices.
- Functional assessment—Change in functional status or alteration
- Cognitively impaired—Emphasize nonverbal symptoms (Table 22-2)

Essential Diagnostic and Laboratory Tests

Diagnostic tests are based on specific findings identified from the history or physical exam. The facilities' resources and capabilities must be taken into consideration when ordering studies. Extensive diagnostic workup may not be in the patient's best interest if time and the patient's condition are in question.

Common laboratory tests include the following:

- Hemoglobin and hematocrit (if anemia is suspected)
- Blood urea nitrogen and creatinine (to assess renal function—especially if analgesics are prescribed)
- Liver profile (if liver disease is suspected; also important when using analgesics)
- Urinalyis (if infection, urolithiasis, or other genitourinary disease is suspected)
- Uric acid (if gout is suspected)

Common radiological studies include the following:

- Routine X-ray of skeletal system (if considering possible fracture or bony disease)
- Spine X-rays (if recurrent compression fractures are being considered)
- CT or MRI scan (if spinal stenosis is suspected)

TABLE 22-2   Nonspecific Signs and Symptoms Suggesting Presence of Pain in Cognitively Impaired
• Frowning, grimacing, fearful facial expressions, grinding teeth
• Bracing, guarding, rubbing
• Fidgeting, increased restlessness
• Striking out, increasing or recurring agitation
• Poor sleeping or eating habits
• Sighing, groaning, crying, breathing heavily
• Change in gait or behavior
• Loss of function

Source: Adapted from American Medical Directors Association, 2003.

See Table 22-3. Differential Diagnosis

TABLE 22-3 Differential Diagnosis of Pain			
CLASSIFICATION OF PAIN	**SOMATIC PAIN**	**VISCERAL PAIN**	**NEUROPATHIC PAIN**
Physiologic Structures	Cutaneous: skin and subcutaneous tissues	Generalized	Radiating or specific
Patient Description or Characteristics of Pain	Pin prick, stabbing, or sharp Localization of cutaneous pain: well localized Localization of deep somatic pain: less well defined	Ache, pressure, or sharp	Burning, prickling, tingling, electric shocklike, or lancinating
Mechanism of Pain	Activation of nociceptors. Located in the periphery	Activation of nociceptors	Dermatomal—(peripheral), or nondermatomal (central) Injury to nervous system structures, nonnociceptive
Clinical Examples	Superficial lacerations Superficial burns Intramuscular injections Venous access Otitis media Stomatitis Extensive abrasion	Periosteum, joints Muscles Colic and muscle spasm pain Sickle cell Appendicitis Kidney stone	Trigeminal Avulsion neuralgia Post-traumatic neuralgia Peripheral neuropathy (diabetes, human immunodeficiency virus) Limb amputation Herpetic neuralgia
Sources of Acute Pain	Postoperative pain— incisional Pain at insertion site—tubes Bone or hip fractures Skeletal muscles	Chest and abdominal tubes and drains Bladder distention or spasms Intestinal distention Pericarditis Constipation	Phantom limb pain Postmastectomy pain Nerve compression
Sources of Chronic Pain	Degenerative or osteoarthritis Rheumatoid arthritis Compression fractures for osteoporosis Back pain Peripheral vascular disease Chronic stasis ulcers Bony metastases	Chronic hepatitis Organ metastases Spastic bowel Hiatal hernia	Diabetic neuropathy Herpes zoster-related Cancer pain Chronic phantom limb pain Trigeminal neuralgia Central poststroke pain Postmastectomy syndrome
Most Responsive Treatments	Cold packs Tactile stimulation Acetaminophen Nonsteroidal anti-inflammatory drugs (NSAIDs) Opioids Local anesthetic (either topically or by infiltration)	NSAIDs Opioid via any route Interspinal local anesthetic agents	Anticonvulsants Tricyclic antidepressants Neural blockade

Source: Adapted from Institute for Clinical Systems Improvement, 2004; Polomano, 2002.

Management Plan

Treating pain in long-term care uses both pharmacologic and nonpharmacologic methods. The most common is the use of pharmacotherapy. Medications are not without risk, and knowledge of the medications and side effects are essential. Principles of pain management are similar for both acute and chronic pain and require the following to be taken into consideration (Adult Pain, 2001):

- The underlying diagnoses or conditions that are causing or contributing to pain
- The severity, location, nature, and causes of pain
- Degree of physical debilitation
- Confounding psychological variables (depression and anxiety)
- Cognitive or mental status
- The patient's preferences or wishes expressed or as identified in the advance directive
- Cost-effectiveness (for instance, costly treatment that is likely to result in a minimal increase in patient comfort may not be justified).
- Use of over-the-counter medications or herbal preparations that may interfere or result in interactions

Pharmacologic

For a systematic approach to pain management the World Health Organization (WHO) developed a three-step process to treat both acute and chronic pain (Figure 22-1) (Curriculum Emanuel L.L, 1999).

Step 1 Analgesics For mild pain, utilizing nonopioids (Table 22-4) and adjuvants (Table 22-5). Nonopioids include acetaminophen, nonsteroidal anti-inflammatory drugs (NSAIDs) and cyclo-oxygenase-2 (COX-2) drugs. These are effective for either chronic or acute pain

with antipyretic or analgesic properties. Physical dependence is not a concern for this group; however, there is a maximum ceiling effect for their analgesic potential. Given the many side effects of these medications the American Geriatrics Society advocates the use of opioids for persistent pain (American Geriatrics Society (AGS) Panel on Persistent Pain in Older Persons, 2002; Henkel, 2002). NSAIDs are used with caution given their side effects. Common risks of gastrointestinal bleeding may be decreased with proton-pump inhibitors; however, nothing substantially reduces the risks of renal impairment or the interactions with other medications. COX-2 selective drugs were recommended when NSAIDs were not indicated for long-term management of chronic pain from inflammation such as osteoarthritis. However recent studies have shown questionable risks versus benefit related to cardiovascular side effects in certain populations (Juni, et al., 2004). The Federal Drug Administration (FDA) now requires a "black box" warning be added to product labeling (National Pharmaceutical Council & Joint Commission on Accreditation of Healthcare Organizations, 2005) thus affirming the need for caution before prescribing these medications in the elderly population.

Adjuvant therapy (Table 22-5) utilizes drugs developed for purposes outside of pain relief that have been found to alter, ease, or modify pain perception. These drugs can be used alone or in combination with other analgesics to treat many different persistent pain conditions, especially neuropathic. They include: corticosteroids, anticonvulsants, tricyclic antidepressants, and local anesthetics. Each classification requires titrating to desired effects along with ongoing reassessment of analgesia and adverse reactions.

Step 2 and 3 of the Ladder Approach to Managing Moderate to Severe Pain Opioids are

---

FIGURE 22-1   Step Approach to Pain Management

Step 3, Severe Pain

↑ Morphine
Hydromorphone
Methadone
Levorphanol
Fentanyl
Oxycodone
± *Nonopioid analgesics*
± *Adjuvants*

Step 2, Moderate Pain

↑ Acet or ASA +
Codeine
Hydrocodone
Oxycodone
Dihydrocodeine
Tramadol (not available with ASA or Acet)
± *Adjuvants*

Step 1, Mild Pain

Aspirin (ASA)
Acetaminophen (Acet)
Nonsteroidal anti-inflammatory drugs (NSAIDs)
± *Adjuvants*

"Adjuvants" refers either to medications that are coadministered to manage an adverse effect of an opioid, or to so-called adjuvant analgesics that are added to enhance analgesia.

---

added to the treatment plan providing a combined approach to pain management, reducing the opioid requirement and side effects. To assist the nurse practitioner in prescribing and monitoring patients safely and effectively, Table 22-6 lists a set of guidelines.

Opioid Analgesics The use of opioids in long-term care is appropriate for moderate to severe pain that is not relieved by other categories of analgesics (Hanks & Cherry, 1998).

Several are available as immediate-release (short-acting) preparations or in combination with aspirin or acetaminophen. The immediate release preparations may be beneficial for breakthrough pain or before painful procedures. Opioids have been found to be safe and effective in relieving a variety of pain syndromes including both nociceptive and neuropathic pain. All opioids react basically in the same way, reaching their peak plasma level approximately 60–90 minutes after oral or rectal route and 30 minutes after subcutaneous or intramuscular dosing. The metabolites are excreted by the kidneys making it important for the nurse practitioner to assess renal function when considering dosing. Unfortunately, the use of opioids in long-term care carries many misconceptions and fears by both providers and patients regarding addiction, tolerance, and physical dependence, thus limiting their use. It is important for the nurse practitioner to acknowledge these concerns and educate all members of the team including staff, patient, and family about their use. See Table 22-7.

Managing the Side Effects of Opioids An integral part in prescribing and managing opioids is to understand the most common side effects. Monitoring for side effects includes observing for neurologic, gastrointestinal, and cognitive changes. Most common are constipation, sedation or impaired cognition, and nausea. Other effects such as myoclonus, impaired consciousness, hypoxia, or life-threatening respiratory depression are rare, especially when doses are started low and escalated slowly (American Geriatrics Society, 2002). Overall tolerance to most of the opioid side effects, except constipation, develops over time (AHCPR, 1994).

TABLE 22-4   Nonopioids for Pain Management in Long-Term Care

DRUG	STARTING DOSE (MAXIMUM DOSE)	TITRATION	POSSIBLE ADVERSE EFFECTS	COMMENTS
Acetaminophen	325–500 mg every 4–6 hrs (3000 mg/ 24 hrs)	After 4–6 doses	Toxic to liver if maximum dose exceeded	Reduce maximum dose 50–75% if liver disease or alcohol use Check liver function periodically in chronic use
NSAIDs (nonsteroidal anti-inflammatory drugs)			Bleeding, sodium retention Renal impairment GI bleed, platelets < 50,000	Avoid use with anticoagulants, corticosteroids, chemotherapy Dehydrated patients increased risk for renal failure
Ibuprofen	1600 mg/day every 6–8 hrs dosing (3200 mg/day)	After 4–6 doses	Dose dependent: gastric bleeding, renal impairment Abnormal platelet function Constipation, confusion, and headaches may be more common in elders	Avoid high doses for extended periods May be associated with chronic heart failure exacerbations Use with caution in patients with chronic renal failure
Naproxen	500 mg/day every 8–12 hrs dosing (1000 mg/day)	After 4–6 doses	Similar to ibuprofen	Avoid high doses for prolonged periods
Choline magnesium trisalicylate	500–750 mg every 8–12 hrs dosing (3000 mg/24 hrs)	After 4–6 doses	Prolonged half-life (8–12 hrs) Similar toxicity to ibuprofen	Periodic testing for salicylate level May allow daily or twice daily dosing after steady state is reached

Source: Adapted and revised from American Geriatrics Society, 2002.

TABLE 22-5   Adjunct Therapy for Pain Management in Long-Term Care

DRUG	STARTING DOSE (MAXIMUM DOSE)	TITRATION	POSSIBLE ADVERSE EFFECTS	COMMENTS
Corticosteroids (prednisone)	5 mg daily (variable)	After 2–3 doses	Increased risk of hyperglycemia	Avoid high doses in long-term osteopenia, and Cushings
Decadron	6–8 mg 2–4 times daily (8–20 mg)	Slow taper 7–10 days	Swelling, hyperglycemia	Immune suppressant seen in long-term use and proximal muscle wasting
Tricyclics (nortriptyline, doxepin amitriptyline, imipramine)	10 mg at bedtime (variable)	After 3–7 days	Anticholinergic effects Highly sedating	Not used if cardiac conduction abnormalities Nortriptyline least problematic Reduce dose or change if significant side effects
Anticonvulsants Carbamazepine (Tegretol)	100 mg at bedtime	After 3–5 days	Many drug interactions; thrombocytopenia, SIADH	Monitor LFTs, CBC, BUN/CR
Clonazepam (Klonopin)	0.25–0.5 mg at bedtime (20 mg)	After 3–5 days	May cause sedation, memory problems, depression	Useful for anxiety and opioid myoclonus Monitor CBC
Gabapentin (Neurontin)	100 mg at bedtime	After 1–2 days	Sedation, ataxia, edema	First line for neuropathic pain
Mexiletine	150 mg	After 3–5 days titrate to 2–4 times daily dosing	Bradyarrhythmia, tremor, dizziness, unsteadiness, paraesthesias	Useful for neuropathic pain Avoid in conduction problems Initial EKG and follow-up
Baclofen (Lioresal)	5 mg	After 3–5 days	Muscle weakness, irritability, rebound spasticity	For neuropathic pain and muscle spasms Monitor urinary function Abrupt discontinuation affects CNS
Clonidine	0.1 mg every 8–12 hrs (variable)	After 2–3 days	Hypotension, sedation	Useful for post-herpetic pain Diabetic neuropathy
Calcitonin	100 units Sq/IM Usual dose 50 units	Given 1–3 days	Nausea, vomiting, local irritation	Used for bone pain in cancer Allergy as with salmon

Local Anesthetics

Lidocaine 5% patch   Topical relief of postherpetic neuropathy, and other pain syndromes

• Placed on intact skin

• Use up to three patches

• Can be used over painful area and left in place up to 12 hours, then remove for 12 hours

• May be cut to size

Topical Analgesics

Counterirritants   E.g., menthol, methylsalicylate, trolamin salicylate

• Supplied as liniments, creams, ointments, sprays, gels, or lotions

• May be effective for arthritic pain, but effectiveness is limited when pain affects multiple joints

• Can cause skin injury, especially when used with heat or with an occlusive dressing

---

TABLE 22-5   (*Continued*)

Capsaicin cream 0.025% and 0.075%

- Derived from red peppers
- Desensitizes nerve fibers associated with pain
- May cause skin irritation and need for frequent application
- Use routinely for effectiveness. Begin with low dose and advance if necessary. Used for 6 weeks before termed treatment failure.

Abbreviations: IM, intramuscular; Sq, subcutaneous.
Source: Adapted and revised from American Geriatrics Society, 1998.

TABLE 22-6   Guidelines for Opioid Therapy in Long-Term Care

- "Start low and go slow"; begin with lower doses of less-potent, short-acting opioids.
- Be aware of peak effects and duration. Trial of short-acting opioids at half starting dose may be considered for frail elderly.
- Initial prescribing should allow for longer dosing intervals to assess response.
- When starting always start with immediate release preparation. Once daily dose established, convert to sustained-release preparation that is given every 8–12 hours for persistent pain.
- Breakthrough or rescue dosing is based on 10–15% of the daily dose every 1–10 hours as needed. If breakthrough medication is required more than 4 times per day the routine dose is increased accordingly.
- Avoid use of multiple opioids when possible
- Combined opioid preparations (e.g., Tylenol #3) for mild to moderate pain can be used short term.
- Consider lower doses of short-acting opioid without combination products such as Dilaudid for severe pain since it can be titrated for pain relief without concern of added toxicity as is the case with the combination products.
- Transdermal fentanyl (Duragesic) appropriate only for continuous pain control. Not used for episodic management or as initial therapy. Not used in opioid-naïve. Patients must be able to tolerate a daily dose of 30–40 mg of oxycodone or hydrocodone.
- Use conversion table when converting or adjusting opioids.
- When adding adjunct agents for pain control, allow ample time (at least 1–2 days) before giving new agents with potential psychoactive effects.
- Manage opioid-related side effects.
- Monitor and reassess for response to therapy.

Source: Adapted and revised from American Medical Directors Association, 2003; American Geriatrics Society, 2002.

TABLE 22-7   Opioids in Long-Term Care

DRUG	STARTING DOSE (MAXIMUM DOSE)	TITRATION	COMMENTS OR CONSIDERATIONS
Codeine	15 mg every 4–6 hrs (360 mg/24 hrs)	After 3–4 doses	Constipation common side effect. Frequently used with Tylenol or other agents for cough suppression.
Hydrocodone (Vicodin, Lorcet, Lortab)	5 mg every 4–6 hrs (see comments)	After 3–4 doses	Useful for acute, recurrent episodic, or breakthrough pain. Daily dose limited by fixed-dose combinations with Tylenol.
Oxycodone, immediate release (Percocet, Tylox)	5 mg every 4–6 hrs (see comments)	After 3–4 doses	Useful for acute, recurrent episodic or breakthrough pain. Daily dose limited by fixed-dose combinations with Tylenol.
Oxycodone, sustained release (OxyContin)	10 mg every 12 hrs (variable)	After 3–4 doses	Usually started after initial dose determined by effects of immediate-release opioid. Do not crush sustained-release tablets given rapid absorption leading to possible overdose.
Morphine, immediate release (Roxinal)	2.5–10 mg every 4 hrs (variable)	After 1–2 doses	Oral liquid concentrate recommended for breakthrough pain.
Morphine, sustained release (MSContin, Kadian)	15 mg every 12 hrs (variable)	After 3–5 days	Usually started after initial dose determined by effects of immediate-release opioid; metabolites may limit use or dose adjustment in renal insufficiency or at end of life.
Hydromorphone (Dilaudid, Hydrostat)	2 mg every 3–4 hrs (variable)	After 3–4 doses	For breakthrough pain or for routine dosing
Transdermal fentanyl (Duragesic)	25 µg/hr patch every 72 hr	After 2–3 patch changes	Usually started after initial dose determined by effects of immediate-release opioid; lowest dose recommended if patient receiving 60 mg per 24 hrs morphine equivalent. Peak effect first dose 18–24 hrs. Duration effect 72 hrs may range from 48 to 96 hrs. Not used in acute pain.
Methadone	2.5–5 mg every 3–4 hrs	After 7 days	Long half-life making it difficult in conversion and dosing. May result in QT prolongation predisposing to arrhythmia.
Atypical Opioids Tramadol (Ultram)	25 mg every 4–6 hrs (300 mg/24 hrs)	After 4–6 doses	Mixed opioid and central neurotransmitter action; monitor for opioid side effects including drowsiness and nausea.

Medications to Be Avoided

Demerol, an opioid, not recommended in long-term use or in elderly. Metabolized in liver to normeperidine which is excreted through kidneys. Elderly with poor renal function can develop toxicity resulting in myoclonus, seizures, and hyperreflexia.

Propoxyphene is a weak opioid agonist; when administered at typical doses it has similar effects to aspirin or Tylenol. Not indicated in elderly given excitotoxic metabolite norpropoxyphene, which can accumulate in individuals with renal insufficiency resulting in central nervous system toxicity.

Source: Adapted and revised from American Geriatrics Society, 1998; Hanks-Bell, Halvey, & Paice, 2004.

Constipation, the most common side effect, requires the initiation of a prophylactic bowel program when opioids are prescribed:

- Assessment of bowel function initially and on follow-up visits while on analgesics
- Mild laxatives such as Milk of Magnesia, senna products, or lactulose should be started routinely along with stool softeners.
- Bulking agents are to be avoided if immobile or where adequate hydration is a question.
- Encourage adequate fluid intake.
- Routine exercise, ambulation, and regular toileting habits are to be encouraged.
- If fecal impaction occurs, relieve with enema or manual removal.

Sedation or impaired cognition is anticipated when opioids are initiated or escalated. Care to prevent falls and accidents is mandatory. Profound sedation, unconsciousness or respiratory depression (respiratory rate less than 8/min or oxygen saturation less than 90%) should be treated with naloxone titrated slowly to avoid abrupt, complete opioid antagonism (American Geriatric Society, 1998). Prolonged sedation affecting quality of life may require switching to an alternate opioid.

Severe or persistent nausea may require the use of antiemetic drugs for relief:

- Generally mild nausea occurring with initiation of opioids clears spontaneously in a few days.
- Trial of alternative opioid if nausea persists
- Choice of antiemetic is directed by the least side effects occurring in the elderly.

Nonpharmacologic

Pharmacological approaches have been the basis of pain management for many years. However as public interest has guided medical care to alternative treatments for pain it is important to consider the use of complementary therapy at all levels of pain. The use of different physical and behavioral treatments alone or in combination with appropriate drug therapy often improves overall pain management (Hanks-Bell, Halvey, & Paice, 2004). Most therapies are effective when combined with analgesic medication used as adjuvant pain treatment (Griffie et al., 2002). In the long-term care setting many of the therapies may be requested by family or patients. It is important to recognize that although many of the therapies may not have a research base, few have side effects. Fostering an environment that promotes family and patient participation may also be instrumental in pain management. Recognizing that pain is a multidimensional experience based on spiritual, cultural, psychological, and social beliefs, acknowledges that not all pain can be relieved by medication. The pain of loss and loneliness, for instance, is not effectively treated with drug therapy. Understanding all aspects to the patient's pain allows for proper intervention and appropriate referrals as necessary. See Table 22-8.

ACUTE PAIN

Pain as previously described is from an identifiable cause signaling tissue injury. It may follow trauma, infection, inflammation, ischemia, or surgery and generally diminishes as healing occurs. Despite the etiology of pain, age-related physiologic changes and comorbidities (e.g., chronic obstructive pulmonary disease, coronary artery disease, and diabetes) place the elderly at increased risk for adverse effects of untreated acute pain (Egbert, 1996).

Proposed Etiology or Source of Pain and Symptoms

Pain can be somatic, visceral, or neuropathic depending on location and etiology (refer to Table 22-3 for specifics).

TABLE 22-8   Complementary Therapies

Complementary (Nonpharmacologic) Therapies for which Evidence of Effectiveness Exists

- Education
- Cognitive/behavioral therapy
- Exercise

Other Complementary Therapies

Although no scientific evidence supports the effectiveness of these therapies in elderly patients in the long-term care setting, they may be beneficial to some individuals.

Physical Therapies

- Physical and occupational therapy
- Positioning (e.g., braces, splints, wedges)
- Cutaneous stimulation (e.g., superficial heat or cold, massage therapy, pressure, vibration)
- Neurostimulation (e.g., acupuncture, transcutaneous electrical nerve stimulation)
- Chiropractic
- Magnet therapy

Nonphysical Therapies

- Psychological counseling
- Spiritual counseling
- Peer support groups
- Alternative medicine (e.g., herbal therapy, naturopathic, and homeopathic remedies)
- Aromatherapy
- Music, art, drama therapy
- Biofeedback
- Meditation and other relaxation techniques
- Hypnosis

Source: Adapted and revised from American Medical Directors Association, 2003.

Common Presenting Signs and Symptoms

Physiologic and autonomic responses—Tachycardia, hypertension, tachypnea, diaphoresis, and dilated pupils.

Pain is generally well localized and may be accompanied by restlessness, apprehension, and anxiety.

Essential Diagnostic and Laboratory Tests

Lab studies, X-rays, or other diagnostic test may be needed depending on results of history and physical exam.

Management Plan

- Depending on acuity of problem, patient may require transfer to acute setting.
- Pharmacological agents based on WHO step ladder approach (Figure 22-1)
- Specialty consults such as general surgery or orthopedic may be necessary.
- Complementary therapy (see Table 22-8)

Patient, Family, and Staff Education

- Identify educational needs of patient, family, and/or staff regarding pain, treatment, side effects, and prevention.
- Provide ongoing information to staff regarding assessment and nonpharmacologic and pharmacologic interventions.

▉▉ CHRONIC PAIN

Persisting beyond the expected time of healing, pain becomes a disease process not just a symptom. Transition to chronic pain marks changes in both physiological and psychological responses with a focus on adaptation.

Etiology or Source of Pain and Symptoms

Chronic pain, like acute pain, can be nociceptive (somatic and visceral) and neuropathic depending on location and etiology (refer to Table 22-3). However chronic nociceptive pain:

- Commonly occurs from arthritis and myofascial pain
- Cumulative effects often result in decline in function.

- May affect psychological functioning resulting in depression, anxiety, frustration, and anger, or it may present with sleep disorders or irritability.

Essential Diagnostic and Laboratory Tests

- Lab studies are rare unless used to determine renal, liver, or electrolyte functions prior to initiating pharmacologic therapies.
- Radiological studies may be necessary to rule out progression of disease or to assess condition prior to initiating specific therapy.

Management Plan

Follow the management plan as outlined in the section on acute pain with the addition of possible referral to physical therapy and/or pain clinic for maintenance of function and enhanced quality of life along with social worker or psychologist for coping strategies.

Patient, Family, and Staff Education

- Inform the patient and family regarding chronic nature of pain and different therapies with emphasis on maintenance of function and pain control.
- Educate the staff, patient, and or family regarding pain to dispel myths.
- Inform the staff regarding importance of adjuvant therapy along with nonpharmacologic interventions for pain control.

▰▰▰ CANCER PAIN

Eighty percent of the elderly with cancer experience significant pain as the cancer advances or from cancer-related treatment and procedures (McCaffery, 1999). Flexibility is the key to therapy, based on the stage of disease, response to interventions, and patient's beliefs or goals of care. Pain can be

both acute and chronic requiring multiple modalities in treatment.

Etiology or Source of Pain and Symptoms

- Bone pain
  - Primary malignancy or metastasis common in multiple myeloma, lung, breast or prostate cancer
  - Common sites include spine, pelvis, ribs, and proximal long bones
- Tests and procedures
  - Biopsies
  - Catheter insertions for drug administration
  - Scans and studies depending on positioning and comfort and as tolerated
- Flare response to medications such as hormonal therapy with prostate cancer
  - Chronic gynecomastia and breast tenderness most common with diethylstilbestrol
  - Chronic painful peripheral neuropathy secondary to chemotherapy (e.g., vincristine)
- Spinal cord compression
  - Result of metastasis to epidural space or by tumor extension
  - Weakness, sensory loss, autonomic dysfunction (e.g., urinary retention), reflex abnormalities
- Postradiation pain syndrome
  - Brachial and lumbosacral plexopathies—Weakness and sensory changes C5, C6, lymphedema, skin irritation; pain is usually progressive.
  - Chronic radiation myelopathy is most common after radiation of nasopharyngeal cancer or cervical spine with pain preceding development of motor dysfunction.

- Chronic radiation enteritis/proctitis
  - Delayed complication of abdominal or pelvic radiation
  - Involves rectum and rectosigmoid most often
  - Symptoms of bloody diarrhea, or cramping, pain from stricture or proctitis
  - Colicky abdominal pain may be associated with nausea or malabsorption indicating small-bowel damage.
- Chemotherapy-related neuropathies
  - Avascular necrosis of femoral or humeral head secondary to corticosteroids
  - Pain of hip, thigh, knee, shoulder, upper arm, or elbow
  - Oral mucositis
  - Peripheral neuropathy

Essential Diagnostic and Laboratory Tests

Assessment is crucial. Sudden severe pain in patients with cancer is recognized as a medical emergency. Lab studies, X-rays or other diagnostic tests based on history, physical exam, patient preferences, and goals of care. Primary focus is to rule out infection, anemia, or progression of disease.

Management Plan

Pharmacologic
- Treatment is individualized based on WHO step ladder approach (Figure 22-1)
- Biophosphates should be considered in addition to conventional analgesic techniques for all patients with multiple myeloma and for breast cancer who have pain due to metastatic bone disease.
- Transdermal fentanyl is an effective alternative to oral morphine but is best reserved for patients with stable opioid requirements.
- Neuropathic pain should have a trial of a tricyclic antidepressant and/or an anticonvulsant

- A trial of steroids should be considered for increased intracranial pressure, severe bone pain, nerve infiltration or compression, pressure due to soft tissue swelling/infiltration, or cord compression.
- When using antitumor therapy, effective analgesics are required.

Nonpharmacologic
- Complementary therapy (Table 22-8)
- Specialty consults such as psychology for behavioral techniques and coping strategies, radiation oncologist, chaplain for spiritual support

Patient, Family, and Staff Education
- Identify educational needs of patient, family, and/or staff regarding pain, pharmacologic and nonpharmacologic treatment, and side effects.
- Provide ongoing information to staff regarding importance of continual assessment along with specific treatments for pain.

■ PAIN AT END OF LIFE

Pain occurring at end of life can be from various sources and requires careful assessment and management. Recognizing pain in patients who have decreased consciousness makes assessment complicated. Behavioral cues such as a furrowed brow, change in respiratory rate, or stiffened body posturing all may be pain responses requiring treatment.

Etiology or Source of Pain and Symptoms

Assessment
- Observe for change of behavior
- Rule out potential cause of distress (constipation, bladder distention, delirium, positioning)
- Monitor for possible myoclonus, hallucinations or hyperirritable state. May be result of drug metabolites.

Management Plan

- Remove pain or irritating stimulus if identified.
- Administer short-acting dose of opioid that can be titrated up as necessary. Dose may be decreased during final hours given decreased renal function and perfusion.
- Use short-acting benzodiazepines or neuroleptics such as haldol if necessary for hyperactivity or myoclonus.
- Provide a quiet relaxing environment.
- Provide comfort to staff and family.
- Referral to specialty services as indicated (e.g., chaplain, psychology, social work)

Patient, Family, and Staff Education

- Use of medications at end of life to manage pain is appropriate therapy.
- "The principle of double effect" as an important concept for staff and family to understand.
- Importance of continued frequent monitoring and reassessment of symptoms.

■ SUMMARY

Pain management in long-term care involves establishing a treatment plan that is reasonable not only for the patient but also the family, facility, and staff. Limited resources and staff turnover in many facilities can make providing care to the elderly most challenging. Simplifying medication regimens by using sustained-release preparations can provide longer durations of comfort and better utilization of staff. Educating staff on pain management, different nonpharmacological treatments, and the importance of the interdisciplinary approach to care can result in more effective pain relief. Pain is a common experience in long-term care and nurse practitioners have a responsibility to evaluate and treat pain appropriately.

■ WEB SITES

- American Pain Society—www.ampainsoc.org
- American Medical Association: Pain Management: The Series—www.ama-cmeonline.com
- American Pain Foundation (APF)—www.painfoundation.org
- American Association of Colleges of Nursing (AACN), End-of-Life/Palliative Care Education Resource Center—www.aacn.nche.edu/elnec
- American Cancer Society—www.cancer.org
- End-of-Life/Palliative Care Education Resource Center, Fast Facts: Pain—www.eperc.mcw.edu/ff_index.htm
- Education in Palliative and End-of-Life Care—www.epec.net
- Hartford Center of Geriatric Nursing Excellence—www.nursing.upenn.edu/centers/hcgne/palliativecare.htm
- Promoting Excellence in End-of-Life Care (University of Montana)—www.promotingexcellence.org
- University of Michigan. Pain Management—www.med.umich.edu/pain

■ REFERENCES

Adult Pain Management and Staff Education. (2001). Retrieved February 22, 2005, from http://www.med.umich.edu/pain/apainmgt.htm#class

American Geriatric Society. (1998). The management of chronic pain in older persons. *Journal of American Geriatrics Society, 46,* 635–651.

American Geriatrics Society. (2002). The management of persistent pain in older persons. *Journal of American Geriatrics Society, 50*(Suppl. 6), S205–S224.

American Medical Directors Association. (AMDA). (2003). *Pain Management in Long-Term Settings: Clinical practice guidelines (Pain in Long-Term Care).* Columbia, MD: Author.

Egbert, A. M. (1996). Postoperative pain management in the frail elderly. *Clinical Geriatric Medicine, 12*(3), 583–599.

Eisenber, E., Borsook, D., & LeBell, A. A. (1996). Pain in the terminally ill. In D. Borsook (Ed.), *The Massachusetts General Hospital handbook of pain management* (pp. 310–326). Boston, MA: Little Brown & Co.

Galer, B. S., & Dworkin, R. H. (2002). *A clinical guide to neuropathic pain.* Minneapolis, MN: McGraw-Hill.

Griffie, J., Mckinnon, P., Berry, H., & Heidrich, E. (2002). Pain. In *End of life care: Clinical practice guidelines* (pp. 345–382). Philadelphia, PA: Sanders.

Hanks, G., & Cherry, N. (1998). Opioid analgesic therapy. In *Oxford Textbook of Palliative Medicine* (2nd ed., pp. 331–355). Oxford, England: Oxford University Press.

Hanks-Bell, M., Halvey, K., & Paice, J. A. (2004). Pain assessment and management in aging. *Online Journal of Issues in Nursing.* Retrieved March 20, 2005, from www.nursingworld.org/topic21/tpc21_6.htm

Helm, R. D., & Gibson, S. J. (1999). Pain in older people. In I. K. Crombie, P. R. Croft, S. J. Linton, M. Von Korff, & L. LeResche (Eds.), *Epidemiology of pain* (pp. 103–112). Seattle, WA: IASP.

Henkel, G. (July, 2002). Opioids can safely ease chronic non-malignant pain. *Caring for the Aged.* Retrieved February 6, 2005, from http://www.amda.com/publications/caring/july2002/opioids.cfm

Institute for Clinical Systems Improvement (ICSI). (2004). *Assessment and management of acute pain* (National Guideline Clearinghouse). Bloomington, MN: U.S. Government Printing Office. Retrieved May 15, 2005, from http://www.icsi.org/knowledge/detail.asp?catID=29&itemID=152

Jacox, A. K., Carr, D. B., Payne, R., Berde, C. B., Breitbart, W., Cain, J. M., et al. (Eds.). (1994). *Management of cancer pain: Clinical guideline* (AHCPR Pub. No. 94–0592). Rockville, MD: Public Health Service, Agency for Health Care Policy and Research.

Joint Commission of Accreditation of Healthcare Organization (JCAHO), & National Pharmaceutical Council (NPC). (2001). Pain: Current understanding of assessment, management and treatment. *National Pharmaceutical Council, 1.* Retrieved May 15, 2005, from http://www.npcnow.org/resources/alphabetical.asp#P

Juni, P., Nartey, L., Reichenbach, S., Sterchi, R., Dieppe, P. A., & Egger, M. (2004). Risk of cardiovascular events and rofecoxib: Cumulative meta-analysis. *Lancet, 364*, 2021–2029.

McCaffery, M. (1999). Pain in the elderly. In *Pain clinical manual* (2nd ed., pp. 674–710). St. Louis, MO: Mosby.

National Pharmaceutical Council & Joint Commission on Accreditation of Healthcare Organizations. (2005). *Pain: Current understanding of assessment, management, and treatments* (Addendum to clinical advances in pain management). Washington, DC: Author.

Parmelee, P. A., Katz, I. R., & Lawton, M. P. (1991). The relation of pain to depression among institutionalized aged. *Journal of Gerontology, 64*, 143–152.

Polomano, R. (2002). Pain. In V. T. Cotter, & N. E. Strumpf (Eds.), *Advanced practice nursing with older adults* (pp. 333–360). New York: McGraw-Hill.

BIBLIOGRAPHY

Adult Pain Management Staff Education. (2005). Retrieved May 15, 2005, from http://www. med. umich.edu/pain/apainmgt.htm.

EPEC. (1999). Pain management [Electronic version]. In *Education for Physicians on End-of-Life* (pp. 1–15). Princeton, NJ: Author.

Portenoy, R. K. (1998). Adjuvant analgesics in pain management. In *Textbook of palliative medicine* (pp. 361–390). Oxford, England: Oxford University Press.

CHAPTER 23

End-of-Life Care

Pegi Black

Nursing homes are increasingly viewed as the site for end-of-life care for our aging population. Statistics from 2001 reveal approximately 22% of all deaths occurred in nursing homes (National Center for Health Statistics, 2001). Estimates suggest the number of deaths will climb to 40% by 2020 (Brock & Foley, 1998). Nursing home residents are more medically complex, suffering from at least one chronic condition where cure is not an option and death is inevitable (Carter & Chichin, 2003). As the number of deaths increase in nursing homes care at end-of-life (EOL) must not be overlooked. Quality of life and death can be improved when EOL issues are addressed. Byock (1997) speaks of the prospect for growth at the end of life. Dying can be a time of love, reconciliation, and a time of transcendence of suffering.

The role of the nurse practitioner continues to evolve in response to the healthcare needs of society. There is a trend in health care to utilize nurse practitioners in long-term care as primary care providers who are important in guiding and managing patients with advanced chronic illness and providing care through the end of life. According to the International Council of Nurses (1997), nurses have a unique and primary responsibility for ensuring that individuals at end of life experience a peaceful death.

Recognizing the important role that nurses serve in providing care at EOL, the American Association of Colleges of Nursing (AACN), developed a position statement on a peaceful death with recommendations for competencies and curricular guidelines. The common belief is that individuals live until the moment of death and care is to be coordinated, with sensitivity to diversity, physical, psychological, social, and spiritual concerns of both the patient and family (American Association of Colleges of Nursing, 1997).

Contemporary end-of-life care in the United States started in the 1970s with the hospice philosophy of caring for the sick and dying (Egan & Labyak, 2001). This was based on the work of Dame Cicely Saunders (nurse, social worker, and physician) who developed the concept shortly after World War II. Care was to focus on comfort, dignity, and personal growth at life's end, a "biopsychosocial" model rather than a "disease" model of care (Fine & MacLow, 2004). It is the goal of this chapter to provide guidelines for the nurse practitioner in long-term care regarding the end of life. Much of the material is taken from the Education for Physicians on End-of-Life Care (EPEC) and the End-of-Life Nursing Education Consortium (ELNEC). Both programs were sponsored by a grant from the Robert Wood Johnson Foundation to improve end-of-life care through education and collaboration with medical and nursing colleagues.

THE EVOLUTION OF HOSPICE AND PALLIATIVE CARE IN THE UNITED STATES

Initially, hospice was primarily a home-based care model. However, in the late 1960s as society became more aware of the famous work and study on death and dying by Dr. Elizabeth Kubler Ross, the long-ignored problems of care for the dying became apparent. The growth of hospice programs prompted Medicare coverage in 1982 and was the impetus for shifting the care to nursing homes (Fine & MacLow, 2004). In 1995 the publication of the *Study to Understand Prognosis and Preferences for Outcomes and Risks of Treatments* (SUPPORT) revealed that Americans were dying in pain and often without dignity (Kuebler & Berry, 2002). Results of the study prompted a review of our healthcare system for those with life-limiting illness. This generated the palliative care philosophy and an initiation of a comprehensive approach earlier in the treatment plan for those with advanced chronic disease.

The goal of palliative care is to prevent and relieve suffering while promoting the best quality of life for both the patient and family with a life-limiting disease (Quaglietti, Blum, & Ellis, 2004). It is both a philosophy of care and a structured delivery system that expands the traditional disease-model approach and can be provided along with life-prolonging care as the main focus (National Consensus Project for Quality Palliative Care, 2004). This is done through early recognition of appropriate patients, careful assessment and treatment of pain and other distressing symptoms, along with integration or physical, spiritual, social, cultural, and psychological aspects to care (Quaglietti, Blum, & Ellis, 2004). As palliative care is initiated earlier in the course of disease

a more comprehensive approach to care is provided while focusing on both patients and families values along with goals of care. Given the relatively new field of palliative care, many confuse it with hospice and view it only for the terminally ill (Quaglietti, Blum, & Ellis, 2004). This limits care to patients with chronic illness who can many times benefit from the multidimensional approach of palliative care. For ease in understanding the two different yet similar approaches to care, consider palliative care as a model for all patients with debilitating and life-threatening illnesses that when initiated early can provide a seamless transition to appropriate end-of-life care.

BARRIERS AND BENEFITS TO APPROPRIATE END-OF-LIFE CARE

Historically there were barriers to initiating hospice in long-term care. Problems included clinical staff's views on life-sustaining treatments, prognostication in noncancer diagnoses, reimbursement issues, and advance care planning (Carter & Chichin, 2003). However as laws and regulations have changed, the benefits of the hospice philosophy in long-term care have become apparent to the patient, family, clinical staff, and facility. The interdisciplinary team approach to planning care, with a primary focus on pain and symptom management along with grief and bereavement for patient, family, and staff, is found to enhance quality of life and decrease the suffering of patients with advanced chronic illness (Knight, 1998).

The Medicare/Medicaid Issue

Most patients in long-term care are covered by Medicare or Medicaid. The Medicare Hospice Benefit (MHB) initiated in 1982 was prompted by the growth of hospice programs and has been the impetus for shifting the care to nursing homes (Kuebler & Berry, 2002). Currently the MHB covers a full range of palliative medical and support services and is covered under Medicare Part A (hospital insurance). The criteria for coverage had always been a prognosis of 6 months or less, if the terminal illness were to run its normal course, and is based on the provider's best clinical judgment. The focus of treatment is comfort as opposed to cure. Despite what many believe, to utilize the MHB does not require a "do not resuscitate" order or limits of care (decision against artificial nutrition and hydration, palliative radiation, or chemotherapy) to qualify for hospice. However, individual hospice providers may have more limiting policies.

Recent developments in hospice and palliative care, through the Medicare Prescription Drug, Improvement, and Modernization Act of 2003, encourage the use of the MHB implying the importance of hospice care. As of January 1, 2004, MHB allows coverage for a Medicare beneficiary, if terminally ill, to receive a hospice consult in an effort to explore issues of end-of-life care. Further advancements effective October 1, 2004, changed the definition of *attending physician* to include nurse practitioners, though it excludes nurse practitioners from certifying a patient's terminal illness. The bill does however allow the nurse practitioner to manage patients in long-term care and continue to bill for services when caring for those who may elect hospice. This provides an opportunity to encourage the continuity of care between the patient and their primary professional healthcare provider if they elect hospice (Fine & MacLow, 2004).

What Patients Are Appropriate?

In the past, hospice was geared towards patients with a cancer diagnosis, although that is now changing. Most nursing home residents have more than one chronic illness with advanced disease. This makes the curative approach to treatment unrealistic and of little benefit. For example, for a patient with chronic heart failure, or chronic obstructive pulmonary disease, cure is not a viable option. Undergoing

diagnostic procedures that will unlikely change the course of events or relieve suffering may not be an appropriate form of care. Shifting the goals to care as opposed to a curative approach relieves suffering in advanced disease (Emanuel & von Gunten, 1999).

The nurse practitioner frequently inherits patients from prior healthcare systems or providers where a life limiting diagnosis may have been given; however, the discussions regarding disease, prognosis, values, goals, and limits have many times never been addressed. The nurse practitioner has an important challenge to establish an appropriate plan of care for each patient based on the prognosis of the disease, the patient's goals, and values. It is difficult to establish rapport with the patient and family on an initial meeting and address all the needs for a chronically ill patient. Being able to clearly identify residents at risk with objective data helps to provide a prognosis when approaching both the patient and family to discuss goals of care.

Given the difficulty in determining prognosis, the National Hospice Organization published guidelines to help determine appropriateness of chronically ill patients for hospice care (refer to Table 23-1) (Standards & Accreditation Committee, Medical Guidelines Task Force, 1996). These guidelines generally combine disease-specific information with functional and nutritional measures. The focus of the guidelines has been on noncancer diagnoses that would raise suspicion for limited life expectancy (Keay & Schonwetter, 1998). However cancer, as the number one cause of death in people aged 65–74, and the second after age 74, has become the disease of the elderly, and must not be forgotten (Extermann, 2002).

In the elderly, one of the most sensitive but nonspecific indicators of limited life expectancy is an unexplained 10% weight loss over a period of 6 months, or a body mass index (BMI) < 22 kg/m^2 that require hospitalization regardless of diagnosis. These individuals are seen to have the highest mortality in the 6 months after

TABLE 23-1	Medical Guidelines for Determining Prognosis of 6 Months or Less	
CONDITION	**PRIMARY CRITERIA**	**SECONDARY CRITERIA/NOTES**
Heart disease	1. Has a poor response to (or chooses not to pursue) optimal treatment with diuretics, vasodilators, and/or ACE inhibitors 2. Has angina pectoris, at rest, that is resistant to standard nitrate therapy 3. Is not a candidate for or declines invasive procedures 4. Significant symptoms of recurrent CHF at rest and/or refractory angina 5. Is classified as NYHA IV	1. Treatment-resistant symptomatic supraventricular or ventricular arrhythmias 2. History of cardiac arrest or resuscitation and unexplained syncope 3. Brain embolism of cardiac origin 4. Ejection fraction of 20% or less 5. Concomitant HIV disease

HIV/AIDS	1. CD4+ count < 25 cells/mcL or persistent viral load > 100,000 copies/mL
	2. Karnofsky < 50%
	3. One of the following:
	  a. CNS lymphoma
	  b. Loss of 33% lean body mass
	  c. Mycobacterium avium complex bacteremia, untreated, unresponsive to treatment, or treatment refused
	  d. Progressive multifocal leukoencephalopathy
	  e. Systemic lymphoma, with advanced HIV disease and partial response to chemotherapy
	  f. Visceral Kaposi's sarcoma unresponsive to therapy
	  g. Renal failure in the absence of dialysis
	  h. Cryptosporidium infection
	  i. Toxoplasmosis, unresponsive to therapy
	  j. Advanced dementia
		1. Chronic persistent diarrhea for one year
		2. Persistent serum albumin < 2.5
		3. Concomitant, active substance abuse
		4. Age > 50 years
		5. Foregoing antiretroviral, chemotherapeutic, and prophylactic drug therapy related specifically to HIV disease
		6. CHF, NYHA Class IV
		Note: A Karnofsky performance score of < 50% denotes considerable assistance and frequent medical care.

Pulmonary disease	1. Severe chronic lung disease as documented by both a and b:
	  a. Disabling dyspnea at rest, unresponsive to bronchodilators, with decreased functional capacity
	  b. Progression of end-stage pulmonary disease, evidence including prior increasing visits to the emergency department or prior hospitalizations for pulmonary infections and/or respiratory failure
	2. Hypoxemia at rest on room air; evidence: $pO_2 \leq 55$ mm Hg or oxygen saturation $\leq 88\%$, or hypercapnia: evidence $pCO_2 \leq 50$ mm Hg.
		1. Cor pulmonale and right heart failure secondary to pulmonary disease (e.g., not secondary to left heart disease or valvulopathy)
		2. Unintentional progressive weight loss of greater than 10% of body weight over the preceding 6 months
		3. Resting tachycardia > 100/minute
		4. FEV1 after bronchodilator < 30% of predicted for normal patients
		5. Decreased FEV1 on serial testing > 40 mL per year

Renal disease	For chronic renal failure: 1. The patient is not seeking dialysis or renal transplant 2. Creatinine clearance < 10 cc/minute (< 15 cc/minute for diabetes) 3. Serum creatinine > 8.0 mg/dL (> 6.0 mg/dL for diabetes)	1. Mechanical ventilation 2. Malignancy—other organ system 3. Chronic lung disease 4. Advanced cardiac or liver disease 5. Sepsis

TABLE 23-1	*(Continued)*	
CONDITION	PRIMARY CRITERIA	SECONDARY CRITERIA/NOTES
	Signs and symptoms of renal failure: 1. Uremia 2. Oliguria (< 400 cc/day) 3. Intractable hyperkalemia (> 7.0) not responsive to treatment 4. Uremic pericarditis 5. Hepatorenal syndrome 6. Intractable fluid overload, not responsive to treatment	1. Immunosuppression/HIV disease 2. Cachexia or albumin < 3.5 gm/dL 3. Age > 75 years 4. Platelets < 25,000 5. Gastrointestinal bleed 6. Disseminated intravascular coagulation

ALS	Patients are considered to be in the terminal stage of ALS if one of the following three situations occurs within the 12 months preceding initial hospice certification:
	1. Critically impaired breathing capacity as demonstrated by all of the following characteristics 12 months before initial hospice certification:
	  ○ Vital capacity less than 30% of normal
	  ○ Significant dyspnea at rest
	  ○ Requiring supplemental oxygen at rest
	  ○ Patient declines artificial ventilation
	2. Rapid progression of ALS and critical nutritional impairment demonstrated by all of the following characteristics:
	  a. Rapid progression:
	    ■ Progression from independent ambulation to wheelchair or bedbound status
	    ■ Progression from normal to barely intelligible or unintelligible speech
	    ■ Progression from normal to pureed diet
	    ■ Progression from independence in most or all ADLs to major assistance by caretaker in all ADLs
	  b. Critical nutritional impairment:
	    ■ Oral intake of nutrients and fluids insufficient to sustain life
	    ■ Continuing weight loss
	    ■ Dehydration or hypovolemia
	    ■ Absence of artificial feeding methods
	3. Both rapid progression of ALS and life-threatening complications:
	  a. Rapid progression of ALS, see 2.a. above; and
	  b. Life-threatening complications:
	    ■ Recurrent aspiration pneumonia (with or without tube feedings)
	    ■ Upper urinary tract infection (e.g., pyelonephritis)
	    ■ Sepsis
	    ■ Recurrent fever after antibiotic therapy
		Some general considerations:
		1. ALS tends to progress in a linear fashion over time; the overall rate of decline in each patient is fairly constant and predictable.
		2. Multiple clinical parameters are required to judge the progression of ALS.
		3. Although ALS usually presents in a localized anatomic area, the location of initial presentation does not correlate with survival time.
		4. Progression of disease differs markedly from patient to patient.
		5. In end-stage ALS, two factors are critical in determining prognosis: ability to breathe and, to a lesser extent, ability to swallow.

(Continued)

TABLE 23-1	Medical Guidelines for Determining Prognosis of 6 Months or Less (*Continued*)	
CONDITION	PRIMARY CRITERIA	SECONDARY CRITERIA/NOTES

Stroke	The following are important indicators of functional and nutritional status, respectively, and support a terminal prognosis if met:
	1. A Palliative Performance Scale score of ≤ 40.
	   a. Degree of ambulation: mainly in bed
	   b. Activity/extent of disease: unable to do work; extensive disease
	   c. Ability to do self-care: mainly assistance
	   d. Food/fluid intake: normal to reduced
	   e. State of consciousness: either fully conscious or drowsy/confused
	2. Inability to maintain hydration and caloric intake with one of the following:
	   a. Weight loss > 10% during previous 6 months
	   b. Weight loss > 7.5% in previous 3 months
	   c. Serum albumin < 2.5 g/dL
	   d. Current history of pulmonary aspiration without effective response to speech language pathology interventions
	   e. Calorie counts documenting inadequate caloric/fluid intake
		If the patient does not meet both of the primary criteria, there should be documentation that describes a relevant comorbidity and/or rapid decline.

Alzheimer's disease and related disorders	Identification of specific structural/functional impairments, together with any relevant activity limitations, should serve as the basis for palliative interventions and care planning. In addition, any comorbid and/or secondary conditions such as delirium or pressure ulcers.	The FAST Scale has been used for many years to describe Medicare beneficiaries with Alzheimer's disease and a prognosis of 6 months or less.

NYHA, New York Heart Association Classification.

Source: Adapted and revised from Standards and Accreditation Committee, Medical Guidelines Task Force (1996).

discharge. Along with weight loss, progressive decline in activities of daily living are also an important predictor of 6-month mortality. These factors are very important to recognize, document, and consider when caring for patients in an effort to establish appropriate plans of care (Fine & MacLow, 2004). Tools utilized in long-term care such as the minimum data set (MDS) are utilized to assess a resident's function and health and may also be a way of determining patients at risk for decline and who are appropriate for referral to hospice or palliative care (Carter & Chichin, 2003). The current thought is that, ideally, palliative care is initiated at the time of initial diagnosis; unfortunately, that is rarely possible in long-term care.

ESTABLISHING GOALS OF CARE

Nurse practitioners in long-term care frequently acquire patients with preestablished diagnoses that may or may not have clearly defined goals of care. This is extremely important given the frailty of nursing home patients with high risks for acute events. Initiating discussions during a crisis event can result in decisions that may negatively affect quality of life. Issues raised early in the course of the illness with both patients and families allows for a more meaningful discussion rather than a technical approach to care (Fine & MacLow, 2004).

Many believe having a living will or durable power for health care is sufficient. Little time is spent on discussing the more important issues of cardiopulmonary resuscitation, acute hospitalization, artificial hydration and nutrition, and the use of antibiotics. Clarifying resident's goals of care is one of the most important jobs of the nurse practitioner in long-term care. Nurse practitioners must document all discussions that have taken place with the patient and/or family and any decisions made regarding end-of-life care.

Cardiopulmonary Resuscitation

Cardiopulmonary resuscitation (CPR) is often the first question to be raised after a nursing home admission, along with the decision of healthcare proxy. In an effort to ensure an informed decision is made it is important to have a clear discussion about the risks and benefits with emphasis on the probable outcomes. Multiple studies report poor outcomes from CPR in nursing home patients; however, many residents and loved ones are never informed of these outcomes (Kane & Burns, 1997). An explanation of the resident's primary disease and functional status is important to include in the discussion as both can affect the likelihood of a meaningful recovery. Such an explanation is essential to clarify any misconceptions or unrealistic expectations (Carter & Chichin, 2003).

Acute Care Transfers

Transferring to the acute care setting is a difficult topic for a resident, family, or even staff to understand. There are many variables in the decision to transfer. Certainly this is one decision that may change as the course of illness shifts. The key is to identify what the primary goal of a transfer is, along with its benefits and burdens. A baseline discussion with the resident, family, or decision maker helps to eliminate crisis decisions. It is important to reassure both resident and family that "do not hospitalize" does not mean "do not care or treat" (Hallenbeck, 2003a).

Artificial Nutrition and Hydration

Artificial nutrition and hydration raise some of the most challenging issues in long-term care for patients, families, and staff. Fears of starvation, dehydration, and suffering are the most common concerns. The meaning of food and fluids is many times based on an individual's psychosocial and cultural beliefs. In an effort to establish the plan of care it is important to investigate the patient's and their family's values. Are the procedures intended to prolong life or to enhance one's quality of life? Prolonging life does not always equate with quality of life. Certainly if the goal is for comfort and enhancing the quality of one's life, then life preserving is no longer relevant (Hallenbeck, 2003a). The role of the nurse practitioner in long-term care is to provide the patients and family with appropriate information so that decisions can be made to meet their goals.

Hydration has both risks and benefits. The beneficial aspects of hydration are believed by many to relieve dehydration, thirst, and dry mouth, all common problems at end of life. Ellershaw and Sutcliff (1995) in a study of dying patients found no difference between the symptoms of thirst or dry mouth in hydrated versus dehydrated patients. However, hydration has been found to be of benefit in individuals who may be experiencing delirium at end of life (Lawlor, 2000). Each situation needs to be addressed with clear goals of care with an emphasis on enhancing or prolonging life.

Nutrition is even more emotionally charged given each individual's beliefs and customs surrounding food. Eating is seen as a means of pleasure, comfort, nurturing, socialization, and nourishment. For many not eating or providing nutrition is seen as starvation. The role of artificial nutrition at end of life requires a purpose, and Hallenbeck's (2003a) question puts it into perspective. Is it "life prolonging" or "life enhancing"?

The nurse practitioner is obligated to be knowledgeable about current research and literature to facilitate the discussion of artificial nutrition. Frequently clinicians offer artificial nutrition without reviewing the true goals of therapy and understanding if it will be of benefit or burden. Many believe using tube feedings will prevent the risk of aspiration pneumonia, prolong life, or even enhance one's life. In an effort to facilitate discussions and decision making with families and patients regarding this most difficult topic guidelines were developed by the Education for Physicians on End of Life Care Project (EPEC). These guidelines review data on the value of nonoral feeding in dying and seriously ill patients (Table 23-2).

TABLE 23-2   Tube Feedings or Not?

Tube feeding is frequently used in chronically ill and dying patients. The bullets below summarize some of what is known and not known about tube feeding for specific indications.

TUBE FEEDING AS A MEANS TO PREVENT ASPIRATION PNEUMONIA

- No study has demonstrated a reduction in the incidence of pneumonia through tube feeding.
- No randomized control studies have been published. Three retrospective cohort studies that compare patients with and without tube feeding demonstrated no advantage to tube feeding for this purpose.
- Swallowing studies, such as videofluoroscopy, lack both sensitivity and specificity in predicting who will develop aspiration pneumonia. Croghan's (1994) study of 22 patients undergoing videofluoroscopy demonstrated a sensitivity of 65% and specificity of 67% in predicting who would develop aspiration pneumonia within one year. No reduction in the incidence of pneumonia was demonstrated in those tube fed.
- Swallowing studies may be helpful in providing guidance regarding swallowing techniques for populations who are amenable to instruction.
- Numerous observational studies have been published, demonstrating a high incidence of aspiration pneumonia in those who have been tube fed.

TUBE FEEDING TO PROLONG LIFE VIA CALORIC SUPPORT

- Data is strongest for patients with reversible illness in a catabolic state (such as acute sepsis).
- Data is weakest in advanced cancer. No improvement in survival has been found (few exceptions noted).
- Nonrandomized, retrospective studies have found no survival advantage in patients with dementia.
- Tube feeding may be life prolonging in the following select circumstances:
  1. Patients with proximal GI obstruction and a high functional status
  2. Patients receiving chemotherapy/radiation therapy involving the proximal GI tract
  3. Certain patients with AIDS and wasting syndromes

TUBE FEEDING TO ENHANCE QUALITY OF LIFE AND REDUCE SUFFERING

- Where true hunger and thirst exist, quality of life may be enhanced (i.e., very proximal GI obstruction).
- Most actively dying patients do *not* experience hunger or thirst (although dry mouth is common).
- Dry mouth is *not* improved by tube feeding (or IV hydration).
- A recent literature review using palliative care and enteral nutrition as search terms found no studies demonstrating improved quality of life through tube feeding (limited to a few observational studies).
- Tube feeding may adversely affect quality of life by increased need for physical restraints, infections, pain, indignity, cost, and the denial of the pleasure of eating.

Source: Weissman, 2000.

More times than not the issues of artificial nutrition are based on one's psychosocial and cultural beliefs as opposed to a scientific base. Therefore identifying the patient's and the family's true goals of care and values will help to maintain a focus when the issues of nutritional support arise or need to be addressed.

Antibiotics

The role of antibiotics in patients suffering from debilitating and rapidly deteriorating illness is an important topic for all involved (Hallenbeck, 2003a). Treating a bacterial infection is standard practice and would be considered neglect if not instituted. However in long-term care the declining resident who frequently experiences illness, febrile or not, antibiotics need to be addressed based on the goal of treatment. The question again is whether antibiotics are being used to prolong the individual's life or enhance their quality of life? Certainly antibiotics may affect both quantity and quality of life in complex ways (Freer & Bentley, 1995). Relieving the symptoms of fevers, dyspnea, cough, and delirium by treating pneumonia certainly enhances the quality of one's life. However the many negative effects of antibiotic administration in long- term care include: difficulty with access, utilizing intramuscular injections, multiple drug resistances, along with the significant side effect of developing *Clostridium difficile* diarrhea resulting from bacterial overgrowth secondary to destruction of normal gut flora. All of which can have a negative impact on the quality of one's life. The issue of prolonging life through the use of antibiotics is also of question. Studies indicate that the use of antibiotics in patients with advanced dementia does not alter survival (Fabiszewski, 1990). It has become a principle in end of life and palliative care that the closer to death a patient is, the less difference antibiotics will make in prolonging life. Certainly there are specific conditions such as pain of sinusitis, dental abscess, cellulitis, and parotitis that are best treated with antibiotics as opposed to morphine. The benefit or burden to the use of antibiotics in prolonging or enhancing one's life in long-term care is truly an individual's decision. More times than not antibiotics are requested based on a psychosocial and cultural need of the family showing that hope continues to exist and quality care is still being given (Hallenbeck, 2003a).

PAIN AND SYMPTOM MANAGEMENT

Pain and symptom management are important aspects to the care of the chronically ill with advanced disease in long-term care. Pain is discussed in a separate chapter and will not be addressed here. Common symptoms encountered in nursing home residents will be addressed in other chapters; however, some of the more common and troubling symptoms at end of life such as dyspnea, nausea, vomiting, anorexia, constipation, and depression are addressed here.

Before addressing the specific symptoms it is essential to mention the importance of ongoing staff education in the assessment and management of symptoms that occur at end of life. Nursing staff in the long-term care facilities are the mainstay of care for patients at end of life. Their understanding and commitment is the mainstay of quality care at end of life, not just the treatment plan established by the nurse practitioner. To provide effective care the staff has to be committed to the plan. For instance, "prn" or breakthrough morphine may not be given if the staff is uncomfortable or fearful of depressing respirations or causing death. These are common fears among many and need to be addressed if quality care is to be rendered.

A comprehensive approach to care includes both pharmacological and nonpharmacological treatment for symptom management. Many of the nonpharmacological strategies can be perceived as difficult or time consuming by staff and will not be carried out. Therefore it is imperative that staff becomes a partner in the plan of care.

Dyspnea

Dyspnea, tachypnea, and "breathlessness" all are viewed as one of the most common symptoms in advanced disease (Carter & Chichin, 2003). The etiology of the symptoms can be multidimensional and the nurse practitioner in long-term care needs to be aware of the many different approaches to treatment. As is in all symptoms the underlying cause should be treated whenever possible or feasible. Medications most commonly used are steroids, opioids, bronchodilators, and anxiolytics to correct or control the symptoms (Table 23-3).

Anorexia and Dysphagia

Additional problems frequently encountered in the nursing home setting are anorexia (lack of appetite) and dysphagia (difficulty in swallowing). Both are prevalent in advanced cancer and in many advanced and chronic illnesses such as degenerative dementias, cerebrovascular disease, end-stage heart/lung/kidney disease, and many other progressive illnesses that put the nursing home resident at risk for poor oral intake (Carter & Chichin, 2003). The "withering" away viewed by loved ones and staff causes great difficulty when discussing or deciding on treatment options. Clarifying the resident's goals helps to determine the course of treatment and provide information on the natural progression of the disease. Additional information

TABLE 23-3   Dyspnea Management

NONPHARMACOLOGIC	PHARMACOLOGIC
Breathing retraining Deep breaths slowly through nose and exhaling through pursed lips, with the exhalation twice as long as the inhalation.	Oxygen: • Benefit with hypoxia • Use with caution in COPD • Use with exertional activities
Positioning: sitting upright, leaning forward Plan care and activities to decrease exertional dyspnea.	Morphine sulfate, 5 mg or 10–15 mg orally or sublingually every 3 hours or as needed Reduces inappropriate tachypnea and overventilation of the large airways, making breathing more efficient and without CO_2 retention. For the opioid naïve, begin with 2.5 mg–5 mg.
Provide calming effect by reassurance	Bronchodilators—Beta agonists and anticholinergics. Care given side effects of nausea, tremors, vomiting, cardiac arrhythmias, blurred vision, dry mouth, and dizziness.
Encourage relaxation by gentle voice, touch, and guiding slow breaths.	May use antibiotics if acute bacterial infection present
Keep room cool and control humidity. Complementary therapy (massage, visualization, acupuncture and hypnosis)	Steroids—reduce to lowest effective dose. Monitor for hypertension, diabetes, mental changes, purpura
Move air in room by fan or open window.	Anxiolytics for the anxiety element

Source: Grenon, 2001.

that is frequently viewed as comforting to families and staff is that hunger and thirst are not commonly experienced in the terminally ill. However, for many with anorexia an appetite stimulant is requested. The most common pharmacological agents used include progestational agents, corticosteroids, prokinetic agents, and cannabinoids. Although research in this area continues, current studies have not been supportive in demonstrating that an increase in appetite improves the quality of one's life (Kuebler & McKinnon, 2002). Treatment options, including the use of IV hydration and artificial nutrition as previously mentioned, frequently need to be addressed regarding the patients goals along with burdens versus benefits to therapy.

Nausea and Vomiting

Gastrointestinal symptoms of nausea and vomiting are common in the nursing home population. The symptoms can affect the quality of one's life and cause serious suffering. Frequently the cause is multifactoral and can be the result of advanced cancer, balance disturbances, gastrointestinal infections, medication side effects, constipation/obstruction, or poor absorption of enteral feedings (Hallenbeck, 2003b). Treatment of choice is generally antiemetics in an effort to manage the symptom. However, frequently they prove to be ineffective due to an incomplete or incorrect diagnosis and or inadequate dosage (Griffie & McKinnon, 2002). The treatment focus is based on the cause of the symptom, and it is important to remember this especially in the frail and terminally ill. Many medications to treat nausea and vomiting can have secondary side effects that may lead to further suffering (Carter & Chichin, 2003). For instance, the use of anticholinergics can create further bowel slowing compounding the problem of constipation or obstruction. Treating nausea and vomiting can be extremely challenging in the nursing home setting where many patients are unable to communicate their needs.

Depression

Depression is a common symptom experienced in advanced chronic disease and requires aggressive treatment. It is important for the nurse practitioner to recognize that many of the somatic complaints of advanced disease (weight loss, sleeping alterations, agitation, and easy fatigue) can also be related to depression. Psychological symptoms of depressed mood, lack of interest in activities, inability to concentrate, and recurrent death wishes are potential signs of depression (Kuebler, 2002). However, it is important to note that in patients who do not communicate verbally, recognizing the symptoms become more challenging. The nurse practitioner also needs to be alert to withdrawal that may be the result of one's disconnecting in preparation for death, and differentiating it from depression. For the treatment strategies of depression refer to the specific chapter on depression. Overall depression affects many in long-term care, and must not be forgotten in managing the patient at end of life.

THE DYING PROCESS WHEN TIME IS NEAR

The goals of care change as death approaches. Medications are adjusted as the patient's condition declines. Antihypertensives, replacement hormones, supplements, iron, antiarrhythmics, and diuretics need to be discontinued unless essential to patient comfort (Griffie, Heidrich, & Berry, 2002). Oral medications may need to be administered by alternative routes. According to the *Palliative Care Clinical Guidelines* developed by the National Hospice and Specialist Palliative Care Services, the only medications necessary in the final days of life are analgesics, anticonvulsants, antiemetics, antipyretics, anticholinergics, and sedatives (Griffie, Heidrich, & Berry, 2002). The issue of corticosteroids in intracranial malignancy requires special consideration given their purpose to control seizures and intracranial swelling that can result in pain and suffering.

The change the body goes through as it approaches death is important for the nurse practitioner to recognize. This helps to alert the family in planning for the death. Has everyone who wanted to say goodbye had an opportunity? Do they have any regrets? Do they want to be present at the time of death; do they have special music, family rituals, or customs that need to be addressed? Byock (1997) suggests that patients and families be given an opportunity to share these thoughts: "Forgive me, I forgive you, thank you, I love you, and goodbye." Obviously it is impossible to know the exact time when death will occur; however, it is important to allow the families an opportunity to share their feelings if in the event they are unable to be present at the time of death. It is just as important to inform the families that

saying goodbye and letting the patient know that those left behind will be all right, is a way of giving the patient permission to die.

Physiologic changes that occur near death can be very distressing to loved ones. Educating families in advance regarding the normal physiologic changes in dying helps to alleviate fears and allows for a more peaceful transition for all (Table 23-4) (Berry, 2002).

GRIEF AND BEREAVEMENT

Grief and bereavement are an important part of end-of-life care in the long-term care setting. Grief is a normal response to loss, occurring every day in the nursing home (Carter & Chichin, 2003). Residents lose their independence, their belongings, and over time many

TABLE 23-4 Physiologic Changes with Dying and Interventions

NORMAL PROGRESSION OF DYING	SUGGESTED INTERVENTION
Sensation and Perception Impairment in ability to grasp ideas and reason. Episodes of alertness along with disorientation and restless.	Provide reassurance that changes are normal. Visualizations such as seeing people who have died before may be comforting. Explain this is a time for family to share memories and engage in conversation when patient is lucid.
Loss of visual acuity, increased sensitivity to bright light Enhanced auditory sensation	Keep sensory stimulation to minimum. Remind families to be mindful of what is said since hearing remains acute. Speak slowly, soft, and clearly.
Unconsciousness, eyes open, absent blink response	May enjoy music or reading of favorite books or poems
Cardiorespiratory Increased pulse and respirations Agonal respirations or sounds of gasping without discomfort Episodes of apnea or Cheyne-Stokes	Normalize by explanation of normal dying process Reassurance of comfort, assess and treat respiratory distress as appropriate. Reposition to left side lying in effort to pool secretions into one lung field and decrease rattling.
May use anticholinergic drugs (transdermal scopolamine, hyoscyamine) as appropriate Skin becomes cool to touch, may be moist Coloring becomes mottled, pulses weak	Suctioning rarely needed given stimulation for more secretions. May use gentle oral suction. Explanation as body is shutting down. Families may want to keep mouth moistened and skin dry.
Renal/Urinary Decreased urinary output—incontinence or retention. May exhibit precipitous drop in urinary output.	Foley or condom catheter Close monitoring for retention; may present as restlessness
Musculoskeletal Gradual weakness with progressive muscle loss, generally starting in legs to arms.	Explanation to families regarding the need initially to reposition for pressure relief; however, as body begins to shut down, minimize turning and repositioning.

may lose their function and health. It is important to acknowledge that the nursing home resident with advanced disease is especially prone to grief related to loss (Carter & Chichin, 2003).

Managing patients at end of life includes facilitating healthy grieving and observing for signs of complicated grief. Complicated or pathologic grief is commonly defined as intensified grief that is overwhelming and results in maladaptive behavior (Worden, 1991). Such patients cannot move through the mourning process and may exhibit self-destructive behaviors or severe depression. If a complicated grief reaction is suspected, then a referral to a professional who deals with grief is warranted. Responding to loss by grieving is a natural reaction. The initial shock of impending or actual loss establishes a new relationship with the person or object. This occurs over time as in waves, with each wave getting less intense. There is no set time table, and each person grieves differently (Hallenbeck & Weissman, 2000).

Anticipatory grief refers to the process of mourning an impending loss. It involves reviewing one's life, and for families it may mean reviewing what their life will be without the loved one (Roberts & Berry, 2002). Some interventions to assist in mourning include allowing a resident or family to talk openly without judgment about the loss and be honest when talking about impending loss or diagnosis.

Bereavement is grief following the death or loss (Carter & Chichin, 2003). Grief tends to be experienced as sadness; however, it can be expressed with anger, guilt, anxiety, loneliness, helplessness, relief, and numbness (Roberts & Berry, 2002). Loss is also experienced by the staff in long-term care, and they may also experience grief and bereavement as the residents decline and die (Carter & Chichin, 2003). Many staff in nursing homes are like extended family to the residents. They have developed close relationships and need to be remembered when providing support and guidance. Nurse practitioners in long-term care are frequently viewed as an added support to staff in bereavement and grieving after the loss of patients. This may affect the retention of quality caregivers by recognizing and acknowledging the staff's sense of loss may positively affect the retention of caregivers.

ETHICAL ISSUES

As health needs change in the frail elderly, frequent questions surrounding the end of life are raised. Historically, decisions regarding care for the elderly at the end of life were resolved by the physician, patient, and family. Today with the advances in medical technology, people are living much longer resulting in greater confusion surrounding treatment at the end of life. In an effort to answer the multifaceted questions surrounding such issues, the courts have been employed to provide answers. Many of these landmark bioethical cases have become the foundation of our current practice (Emanuel & von Gunten, 1999). It is important for nurse practitioners to be aware of legal and ethical issues that can affect their practice surrounding end-of-life care.

The principle of double effect is a moral challenge that occurs frequently when managing residents at end of life. The nurse practitioner is faced with prescribing treatment where benefit is not possible without potentially causing harm (Schwarz, 2001). The most recognized example is the terminally ill patient with pulmonary disease who is suffering in pain with a low respiratory rate. Treatment of choice is morphine, which would take care of the pain, but which has the likelihood of depressing the respirations. Morally, the nurse practitioner is obligated to remove the pain, but such an action conflicts with preservation of life. The American Nurses Association (1996) position statement on promotion of comfort and relief of pain in dying patients acknowledges the obligation of nurses to relieve pain and other symptoms in dying patients. Nurses should not hesitate to use full and effective doses of pain medication for the proper management of pain for the dying patient (Scanlon, 2001).

COMPETENCY

The question of competency is also raised frequently when caring for the elderly in nursing homes. This becomes of particular interest when considering the ability to make decisions for care. Competency is actually a legal term referring to a decision made by a court (Schwarz, 2001).

Decision-making capacity refers to a physician's determination that a patient can make medical decisions for him or herself. This is generally documented based on two physicians' determination in the following categories:

- Ability to comprehend the information including the impact of the disease, consequences of treatment, and the consequences of foregoing treatment

- Ability to make a decision that is consistent over time and to compare risks and benefits of each treatment option

- Ability to communicate choices (Emanuel & von Gunten, 1999).

Lack of decision-making capacity can occur any time there is a disruption in the ability to understand, reason, and evaluate or communicate a decision. When a patient lacks decisional capacity to make informed choices a surrogate is identified. That can be anyone the patient chooses; however, in the event that has not occurred, each state law dictates a list of eligible individuals. Most often this list includes spouse, family members, or others. In the event no available person is identified, a conservator may be appointed by the courts. Advance practice nurses have an important role in connecting with the surrogate decision maker to make sure the issues surrounding end of life have been addressed and thoroughly understood by all. Despite patient's wishes, decisions become difficult for grieving families, when issues of withholding or withdrawing treatment arise.

WITHHOLDING OR WITHDRAWING TREATMENT

Goals of care shift as the patient's condition changes. Controversies such as withdrawing or withholding treatment are frequently based on legal and ethical beliefs. All states in the United States have laws covering issues related to withholding or withdrawing life-sustaining treatments (Emanuel & von Gunten, 1999c). Nurse practitioners working in EOL care must become familiar with the specific laws of the state of practice. These situations require working collaboratively with physicians to address the legal and ethical base of treatment. However it is important to note that withholding or withdrawing life-sustaining medical treatment is considered neither homicide nor suicide. Courts have drawn a distinction between intentionally causing death versus allowing a person to die resulting from removal of life-sustaining treatment. Also there is a legal consensus that both withdrawing and withholding treatment, if not wanted by the patient or ineffective, can be justifiable (Emanuel & von Gunten, 1999).

ASSISTED SUICIDE

Lastly, assisted suicide remains a very passionate issue that fosters much controversy. Nurse practitioners need to know it is not uncommon for ill or dying patients to look forward to death or have thoughts of suicide (Schwarz, 2001). Recognition of a request to assist with death is a cry for help and needs to be investigated. Most often the issues are related to the need for better symptom management or spiritual and psychosocial support. Once symptoms are better controlled, the dying process can become more tolerable. The American Nurses Association position statement on assisted suicide (1994) opposes nurse involvement in both active euthanasia (the deliberate and intentional act of causing death) and assisted suicide (an act of providing a means to end life). It is viewed as a breach of the Code for Nurses and the ethical traditions of the profession.

Death is a part of life that calls for quality end-of-life care. As primary care providers, nurse practitioners in long-term care have a responsibility to patients, family, staff, and themselves to make the end-of-life transition a smooth and comfortable process. Remembering the words of Dame Cicely Saunders, "How people die remains in the memories of those who live on" and helps to guide us in providing that care (Kuebler & Berry, 2002).

WEB SITES

- Education in Palliative and End-of-Life Care—www.epec.net
- National Hospice and Palliative Care Organization—www.nhpco.org
- American Academy of Hospice and Palliative Medicine—www.aahpm.org
- American Board of Hospice and Palliative Medicine—www.abhpm.org
- Center to Advance Palliative Care—www.capc.org
- American Association of Colleges of Nursing (AACN), End-of-Life/Palliative Care Education Resource Center—www.aacn.nche.edu/elnec
- Hartford Center of Geriatric Nursing Excellence—www.nursing.upenn.edu/centers/hcgne/palliativecare.htm
- Promoting Excellence in End-of-Life (University of Montana)—www.promotingexcellence.org
- End-of-Life/Palliative Care Education Resource Center—www.eperc.mcw.edu

REFERENCES

American Association of Colleges of Nursing (AACN). (1997). *Peaceful Death: Recommended competencies and curricular guidelines for end-of-life nursing care*. Washington, DC: Author.

American Nurses Association. (1994). *Ethics and human rights position statements: Assisted suicide* (position statement). Silver Spring, MD: American Nurses Association.

Brock, D. B., & Foley, D. J. (1998). Demography and epidemiology of dying in the U.S. with emphasis on the deaths of older persons. *Hospice Journal, 13*(1–2), 49–60.

Byock, I. (1997). *Dying well: The prospect for growth at the end-of-life*. New York: Riverhead Trade.

Carter, J. M., & Chichin, E. (2003). Palliative care in the nursing home. In R. S. Morrison & D. E. Meir (Eds.), *Geriatric palliative care* (pp. 357–374). New York: Oxford University Press.

Egan, K. A., & Labyak, M. J. (2001). Hospice care: A model for quality end-of-life care. In B. Ferrell & N. Coyle (Eds.), *Textbook of palliative nursing* (pp. 7–27). New York: Oxford University Press.

Ellershaw, J., & Sutcliff, J. (1995). Dehydration and the dying patient. *Journal of Pain and Symptom Management, 10*, 192–197.

Emanuel, L. L., von Gunten, C. F., & Ferris, F. F. (1999). Goals of Care [Electronic version]. In *Education for Physicians on End-of-life Care Participant's Handbook* (No. Module 7, pp. M7–1–13). Chicago: EPEC. Retrieved January 15, 2005, from http://www.endoflife.northwestern.edu/eolc_goals_of_care.cfm

Emanuel, L. L., & von Gunten, C. F. (1999). Legal Issues [Electronic version]. In *The education in palliative and end-of-life care participant's handbook* (Plenary 2 (pp. P2–1–13). Chicago: EPEC. Retrieved January 15, 2005, from http://www.eperc.mew.edu

Extermann, M. (2002). Cancer in the older patient: A geriatric approach. *Annals of Long-Term Care, 10*(1). Retrieved February 14, 2005, from http://www.annalsoflongtermcare.com/article/155

Fabiszewski, K. J. (1990). Effect of antibiotic treatment on outcome of fevers in institutionalized Alzheimer patients. *Journal of American Medical Association, 263*, 3168–3172.

Fine, P., & MacLow, C. (2004). *Hospice referral and care: Practice guidance for clinicians*. Retrieved February 18, 2005, from http://www.medscape.com/viewprogram/3345.

Freer, J. A., & Bentley, D. (1995). The role of antibiotics in comfort care. In E. Olson, E. R. Chichin, &
L. S. Libow (Eds.), *Controversies in ethics in long-
term care* (pp. 91–107). New York: Springer Press.

Grenon, N. N. (2001). Pulmonary disease [Mono-
graph]. *Hospice and Palliative Nurses Association
Treatment of End-Stage Non-cancer Diagnoses, IV,*
21–30.

Griffie, J., & Mckinnon, S. (2002). Nausea and Vomiting. In K. K. Kuebler, P. H. Berry, & D. E. Heidrich
(Eds.), *End-of-life care: Clinical practice guidelines*
(pp. 333–345). Philadelphia: Saunders.

Griffie, J., Heidrich, D. E., & Berry, P. H. (2002).
Dying process. In K. K. Kuebler, P. H. Berry, &
D. E. Heidrich (Eds.), *End-of-life care: Clinical
practice guidelines* (pp. 39–51). Philadelphia:
Saunders.

Hallenbeck, J. L. (2003a). Hydration, nutrition, and
antibiotics in end-of-life care. In *Palliative care
perspectives* (pp. 117–127). New York: Oxford
University Press.

Hallenbeck, J. L. (2003b). Non-pain symptom management. In *Palliative care perspectives* (pp. 75–117).
New York: Oxford Press.

Hallenbeck, J., & Weissman, D. (Series Eds.), & End of
Life Palliative Education Resource Center. (2000).
Fast fact and concept #10: Tube feed or not tube feed?
Retrieved January 18, 2005, from http://www.
eperc.mcw.edu/FastFactPDF/Concept%20010.pdf

International Council of Nurses. (1997). *Basic principles of nursing care.* Washington, DC: American
Nurses Publishing.

Kane, R. S., & Burns, E. A. (1997). Cardiopulmonary
resuscitation policies in long-term care facilities.
Journal of American Geriatrics Society, 45, 154–157.

Keay, T. J., & Schonwetter, R. S. (1998). *Hospice care
in the nursing home* (3rd ed., Vol. 57). Retrieved
January 10, 2005, from http://www.aafp.org/
afp/980201ap/keay.html

Knight, A. L. (1998). The integration of hospice programs in nursing homes. *American Family Physician, 57*(3), 1–2.

Kuebler, K. K. (2002). Depression. In K. K. Kuebler,
P. H. Berry, & D. E. Heidrich (Eds.), *End-of-life
care: Clinical practice guidelines* (pp. 269–281).
Philadelphia: Saunders.

Kuebler, K. K., & McKinnon, S. (2002). Cachexia
and anorexia. In K. K. Kuebler, P. H. Berry, &

D. E. Heidrich (Eds.), *End-of-life care: Clinical
practice guidelines* (pp. 213–234). Philadelphia:
Saunders.

Kuebler, P. H., & Berry, P. H. (2002). End-of-life care.
In K. K. Kuebler, P. H. Berry, & D. E. Heidrich
(Eds.), *End-of-life care: Clinical practice guidelines*
(pp. 23–39). Philadelphia: Saunders.

Lawlor, P. G. (2000). Delirium at the end-of-life.
Journal of American Medical Association, 284(19),
2427–2479.

National Center for Health Statistics. (2001).
Deaths by place, age, race and sex: US (Mortality).
Washington, DC: U.S. Government Printing Office. Retrieved February 16, 2005, from http://
www.cde.gov/nchs/data/statb/mortfinal2001_
work309.pdf

National Consensus Project for Quality Palliative
Care. (2004). *Clinical guidelines for quality palliative
care.* Brooklyn, NY: National Consensus Project.

Quaglietti, S., Blum, L., & Ellis, V. (2004). The role
of the adult nurse practitioner in palliative care.
Journal of Hospice and Palliative Nursing, 6(4),
209–214.

Roberts, K. F., & Berry, P. H. (2002). Grief and bereavement. In K. K. Kuebler, P. H. Berry, & D. E.
Heidrich (Eds.), *End-of-life care: Clinical practice
guidelines* (pp. 53–65). Philadelphia: Saunders.

Scanlon, C. (2001). Public policy and end-of-life. In
B. Ferrell & N. Coyle (Eds.), *Textbook of palliative
nursing* (pp. 682–689). New York: Oxford Press.

Schwarz, J. K. (2001). Ethical aspects of palliative
care. In M. Matzo & S. Sherman (Eds.), *Palliative
care nursing quality care to the end-of-life* (pp.
140–180). New York: Springer.

Standards & Accreditation Committee, Medical
Guidelines Task Force. (1996). *Medical guidelines
for determining prognosis in selected non-cancer
diseases* (National Hospice Organization). Arlington, VA: Standards and Accreditation Committee.

Worden, J. W. (1991). *Grief counseling and grief therapy: A handbook for the mental health practitioner*
(2nd ed.). New York: Guilliford Press.

▓▓▓ BIBLIOGRAPHY

Ahronheim, J. C. (1996). Nutrition and hydration in
the terminal patient. *Clinic in Geriatrics, 12*(2),
379–391.

Emanuel, L. L., & von Gunten, C. F. (1999). Depression, anxiety, delirium [Electronic version]. In *Education for physicians on end-of-life care participant's handbook* (Module 6, pp. M6–1–13). Chicago: EPEC.

Finucane, T. E. (1996). Use of tube feeding to prevent aspiration pneumonia. *Lancet, 348,* 1421–1424.

Finucane, T. E., Christmas, C., & Travis, K. (1999). Tube feeding in patients with advanced dementia. *Journal of American Medical Association, 282,* 1365–1369.

Warm, E. (Series Ed.), & End of Life Palliative Education Resource Center. (2001). *Fast fact and concept #32: Grief and bereavement (Part 1).* Retrieved January 15, 2005, from http:// www. eperc.mcw. edu/FastFactPDF/Concept% 20032. pdf

INDEX

FIM™ Instrument

L E V E L S	7 Complete Independence (timely, safely) 6 Modified Independence (device)	NO HELPER
	Modified Dependence 5 Supervision (subject = 100%) 4 Minimal Assistance (subject = 75%+) 3 Moderate Assistance (subject = 50%+) **Complete Dependence** 2 Maximal Assistance (subject =25%+) 1 Total Assistance (subject = less than 25%)	HELPER

	ADMISSION	DISCHARGE	FOLLOW-UP
Self-Care A. Eating B. Grooming C. Bathing D. Dressing - Upper Body E. Dressing - Lower Body F. Toileting			
Sphincter Control G. Bladder Management H. Bowel Management			
Transfers I. Bed, Chair, Wheelchair J. Toilet K. Tub, Shower			
Locomotion L. Walk/Wheelchair M. Stairs	W Walk C Wheelchair B Both	W Walk C Wheelchair B Both	W Walk C Wheelchair B Both
Motor Subtotal Score			
Communication N. Comprehension O. Expression	A Auditory V Visual B Both A Auditory V Visual B Both	A Auditory V Visual B Both A Auditory V Visual B Both	A Auditory V Visual B Both A Auditory V Visual B Both
Social Cognition P. Social Interaction Q. Problem Solving R. Memory			
Cognitive Subtotal Score			
TOTAL FIM™ SCORE			

NOTE: Leave no blanks. Enter 1 if patient is not testable due to risk.

APPENDIX

THE	Patient Name:	_____
BARTHEL	Rater Name:	_____
INDEX	Date:	_____

Activity   Score

FEEDING
  0 = unable
  5 = needs help cutting, spreading butter, etc., or requires modified diet
  10 = independent   _____

BATHING
  0 = dependent
  5 = independent (or in shower)   _____

GROOMING
  0 = needs to help with personal care
  5 = independent face/hair/teeth/shaving (implements provided)   _____

DRESSING
  0 = dependent
  5 = needs help but can do about half unaided
  10 = independent (including buttons, zips, laces, etc.)   _____

BOWELS
  0 = incontinent (or needs to be given enemas)
  5 = occasional accident
  10 = continent   _____

BLADDER
  0 = incontinent, or catheterized and unable to manage alone
  5 = occasional accident
  10 = continent   _____

TOILET USE
  0 = dependent
  5 = needs some help, but can do something alone
  10 = independent (on and off, dressing, wiping)   _____

TRANSFERS (BED TO CHAIR AND BACK)
  0 = unable, no sitting balance
  5 = major help (one or two people, physical), can sit
  10 = minor help (verbal or physical)
  15 = independent   _____

MOBILITY (ON LEVEL SURFACES)
  0 = immobile or < 50 yards
  5 = wheelchair independent, including corners, > 50 yards
  10 = walks with help of one person (verbal or physical) > 50 yards
  15 = independent (but may use any aid; for example, stick) > 50 yards   _____

STAIRS
  0 = unable
  5 = needs help (verbal, physical, carrying aid)
  10 = independent   _____

TOTAL (0–100): _____